Withdrawn from University of Oregon Library

ADVANCES IN PROSTAGLANDIN, THROMBOXANE,
AND LEUKOTRIENE RESEARCH
VOLUME 21A

Prostaglandins and Related Compounds
Seventh International Conference, Florence, Italy

Advances in Prostaglandin, Thromboxane, and Leukotriene Research

Series Editors: Bengt Samuelsson and Rodolfo Paoletti
(Formerly *Advances in Prostaglandin and Thromboxane Research* Series)

Vols. 21A and 21B: Prostaglandins and Related Compounds, *edited by B. Samuelsson, P.W. Ramwell, R. Paoletti, G. Folco, and E. Granström*, 1012 pp., 1991.

Vol. 20: Trends in Eicosanoid Biology, *edited by B. Samuelsson, S.-E. Dahlén, J. Fritsch, and P. Hedqvist*, 264 pp., 1990.

Vol. 19: Taipei Conference on Prostaglandin and Leukotriene Research, *edited by B. Samuelsson, P. Y.-K. Wong, and F. F. Sun*, 723 pp., 1989.

Vol. 18: Mass Spectra of Prostaglandins and Related Products, *by Cecil Robert Pace-Asciak*, 565 pp., 1989.

Vols. 17A and 17B: Prostaglandins and Related Compounds, *edited by B. Samuelsson, R. Paoletti, and P. W. Ramwell,* 1216 pp., 1987.

Vol. 16: Leukotrienes and Prostaglandins in Health and Disease, *edited by U. Zor, Z. Naor, and F. Kohen*, 405 pp., 1986.

Vol. 15: Advances in Prostaglandin, Thromboxane, and Leukotriene Research, *edited by O. Hayaishi and S. Yamamoto,* 776 pp., 1985.

Vol. 14: Chemistry of the Prostaglandins and Leukotrienes, *edited by J. E. Pike and D. R. Morton, Jr.,* 458 pp., 1985.

Vol. 13: Platelets, Prostaglandins, and the Cardiovascular System, *edited by G. V. R. Born, J. C. McGiff, G. G. Neri Serneri, and R. Paoletti*, 424 pp., 1985.

*Vol. 12: Advances in Prostaglandin, Thromboxane, and Leukotriene Research, *edited by B. Samuelsson, R. Paoletti, and P. W. Ramwell,* 544 pp., 1983.

*Vol. 11: Advances in Prostaglandin, Thromboxane, and Leukotriene Research, *edited by B. Samuelsson, R. Paoletti, and P. W. Ramwell,* 576 pp., 1983.

Vol. 10: Prostaglandins and the Cardiovascular System, *edited by John A. Oates,* 400 pp., 1982.

Vol. 9: Leukotrienes and Other Lipoxygenase Products, *edited by Samuelsson and R. Paoletti,* 382 pp., 1982.

Vol. 8: Advances in Prostaglandin and Thromboxane Research, *edited by B. Samuelsson, P. W. Ramwell, and R. Paoletti,* 609 pp., 1980.

Vol. 7: Advances in Prostaglandin and Thromboxane Research, *edited by B. Samuelsson, P. W. Ramwell, and R. Paoletti,* 606 pp., 1980.

Vol. 6: Advances in Prostaglandin and Thromboxane Research, *edited by B. Samuelsson, P. W. Ramwell, and R. Paoletti,* 600 pp., 1980.

*Vol. 5: Methods in Prostaglandin Research, *edited by J. C. Frölich,* 256 pp., 1978.

Vol. 4: Prostaglandins and Perinatal Medicine, *edited by F. Coceani and P. M. Olley,* 432 pp., 1978.

Vol. 3: Prostaglandins and Phospholipases, *edited by C. Galli, G. Galli, and G. Porcellati,* 224 pp., 1978.

Vol. 2: Advances in Prostaglandin and Thromboxane Research, *edited by B. Samuelsson and R. Paoletti,* 1028 pp., 1976.

Vol. 1: Advances in Prostaglandin and Thromboxane Research, *edited by B. Samuelsson and R. Paoletti* 506 pp., 1976.

INTERNATIONAL ADVISORY BOARD

Sune Bergström, *Stockholm*
E. J. Corey, *Cambridge (U.S.)*
Pierre Crabbe, *Grenoble*
Kenneth E. Eakins, *New York*
Josef Fried, *Chicago*

Richard Gryglewski, *Krakow*
Osamu Hayaishi, *Kyoto*
William E. M. Lands, *Ann Arbor*
John E. Pike, *Kalamazoo*

Peter W. Ramwell, *Washington, D.C.*
John R. Vane, *London*
Gerald Weissmann, *New York*
D. A. Willoughby, *London*

*Out of print

Advances in Prostaglandin, Thromboxane,
and Leukotriene Research
Volume 21A

Prostaglandins and Related Compounds
Seventh International Conference, Florence, Italy

Editors

Bengt Samuelsson, M.D.
*Department of Physiological
 Chemistry
Karolinska Institutet
Stockholm, Sweden*

Peter W. Ramwell, Ph.D.
*Department of Physiology and
 Biophysics
Georgetown University Medical
 Center
Washington, D.C.*

Rodolfo Paoletti, M.D.
*Istituto di Scienze Farmacologiche
Università di Milano
Milan, Italy*

Giancarlo Folco, Ph.D.
*Istituto di Scienze Farmacologiche
Università di Milano
Milan, Italy*

Elisabeth Granström, M.D.
*Department of Reproductive Endocrinology
Karolinska Hospital
Stockholm, Sweden*

Raven Press ● New York

Raven Press, 1185 Avenue of the Americas, New York, New York 10036

© 1991 by Raven Press, Ltd. All rights reserved. This book is protected by copyright. No part of it may be reproduced, stored in a retrieval system, or transmitted, in any form or by any means, electronic, mechanical, photocopying, or recording, or otherwise, without the prior written permission of the publisher.

Made in the United States of America

International Standard Book Number 0-88167-742-6
Library of Congress Catalog Card Number 83-645438

Papers or parts thereof have been used as camera-ready copy as submitted by the authors whenever possible; when retyped, they have been edited by the editorial staff only to the extent considered necessary for the assistance of an international readership. The views expressed and the general style adopted remain, however, the responsibility of the named author. Great care has been taken to maintain the accuracy of the information contained in the volume. However, neither Raven Press nor the editors can be held responsible for errors or for any consequences arising from the use of information contained herein.

The use in this book of particular designations of countries or territories does not imply any judgment by the publisher or editors as to the legal status of such countries or territories, of their authorities or institutions, or of the delimitation of their boundaries.

Some of the names of products referred to in this book may be registered trademarks or proprietary names, although specific reference to this fact may not be made; however, the use of a name without designation is not to be construed as a representation by the publisher or editors that it is in the public domain. In addition, the mention of specific companies or of their products or proprietary names does not imply any endorsement or recommendation on the part of the publisher or editors.

The authors were responsible for obtaining the necessary permission to reproduce copyright material from other sources. With respect to the publisher's copyright, material appearing in this book prepared by individuals as part of their official duties as government employees is only covered by this copyright to the extent permitted by the appropriate national regulations.

9 8 7 6 5 4 3 2 1

Preface

Volumes 21A and 21B of *Advances in Prostaglandin, Thromboxane, and Leukotriene Research* contain the papers presented at the Seventh International Conference on Prostaglandins and Related Compounds held in Florence, Italy, on May 28–June 1, 1990. The conference showed the vitality of this broad area of research and its impact on both basic research and clinical medicine.

Arachidonic acid is metabolized by oxygenation and further transformations after release from cell membranes. The derivatives include prostaglandins, thromboxanes, leukotrienes, lipoxins, and other oxygenated compounds. The release and transformation of arachidonic acid serves to transform various signals to the cells into biological responses. These processes are of importance not only in the normal physiology of cells, but also in many pathophysiological mechanisms. Therefore, there is a growing interest in developing drugs related to the formation and action of prostaglandins and related compounds.

Considerable progress was reported in the area of leukotriene antagonists during the conference. The respiratory, cardiovascular, renal, nervous, and endocrine systems were given extensive coverage, as were the topics of biosynthesis and metabolism of eicosanoids and the molecular biology of prostaglandins. Other sections dealt with cytochrome P-450 and arachidonic acid metabolism, platelet-activating factor and its antagonists, eicosanoids and their role in inflammation, immunology and allergy, dietary and tissue precursors, and the contol of precursor release. Blood cells, cytoprotection, and cell differentiation and proliferation were also discussed.

In addition to a section devoted entirely to cancer, a round table was held on eicosanoids in cancer cell metastasis. Round tables were also held on cytokines and lipid mediators, as well as on the new frontiers in prostaglandin therapeutics.

We hope that this volume on prostaglandins and related compounds will serve as reference work for medical researchers and clinicians involved in the areas described above.

The Editors

Acknowledgments

We would like to express our gratitude to all the staff of the Fondazione Giovanni Lorenzini for their important work in connection with the conference. We are also grateful to Drs. F. Berti and S. Nicosia, the organizing and advisory committees, and the international program committee for their valuable contributions. It is also a pleasure to acknowledge the generous financial support from a number of pharmaceutical companies.

We hope that the rapid publication of this volume, which was made possible by the prompt submission of the papers by the authors, will further stimulate the development of this exciting area of research.

The Editors

Contents

Volume 21A

Molecular Biology

1 Characterization of the Promoter of the Human 5-Lipoxygenase Gene
B. Samuelsson, S. Hoshiko, and O. Rådmark

9 Regulation of the Production and Action of Leukotrienes by MK-571 and MK-886
A. W. Ford-Hutchinson

17 5-Lipoxygenase mRNA is Expressed in Rat Pancreatic Islets
M. H. Nathan and S. B. Pek

21 Immunohistochemical Study on Arachidonate 5-Lipoxygenase of Porcine Leukocytes
N. Ueda, K. Natsui, S. Yamamoto, N. Komatsu, and K. Watanabe

25 Expression of Cloned Human 15-Lipoxygenase in Eukaryotic and Prokaryotic Systems
D. L. Sloane, R. A. F. Dixon, C. S. Craik, and E. Sigal

29 Cloning and Expression of Arachidonate 12-Lipoxygenase cDNA from Porcine Leukocytes
T. Yoshimoto, H. Suzuki, S. Yamamoto, T. Takai, C. Yokoyama, and T. Tanabe

33 Polymerase Chain Reaction Cloning and Expression of Eicosanoid Metabolizing Enzymes from Blood Cells
C. D. Funk, L. Furci, and G. A. FitzGerald

37 Biochemical and Immunohistochemical Evidence for Selective Expression of Novel Epithelial Lipoxygenases
V. R. Shannon, J. R. Hansbrough, Y. Takahashi, N. Ueda, S. Yamamoto, and M. J. Holtzman

41 Leukotriene A_4-Hydrolase in Two Human Cell Lines
O. Rådmark, J. F. Medina, L. Macchia, C. Barrios, C.D. Funk, O. Larsson and J. Haeggström

45 The Biochemical and Pharmacological Manipulation of Cellular Cyclooxygenase (COX) Activity
K. Seibert, J. L. Masferrer, F. Jiyi, A. Honda, A. Raz, and P. Needleman

53 Induction of Fatty Acid Cyclooxygenase in Mouse Osteoblastic Cells (MC3T3-El)
S. Yamamoto, T. Oshima, M. Kusaka, T. Yoshimoto, C. Yokoyama, T. Takai, T. Tanabe, and M. Kumegawa

61 Cloning and Characterization of Human Cyclooxygenase Gene and Primary Structure of the Enzyme
C. Yokoyama, H. Toh, A. Miyata, and T. Tanabe

65 Serum Induction and Superinduction of PGG/H Synthase mRNA Levels in 3T3 Fibroblasts
D. L. DeWitt, S. A. Kraemer, and E. A. Meade

69 Regulation of Prostaglandin Synthesis by Differential Expression of the Gene Encoding Prostaglandin Endoperoxide Synthase
M. S. Simonson, J. A. Wolfe, and M. J. Dunn

73 Elevated Prostaglandin H Synthase Gene Expression in *Ras*-transformed Cells
R. R. Gorman, M. J. Bienkowski, and A. H. Lin

77 The Aspirin and Heme Binding Sites of PGG/H Synthase
W. L. Smith, D. L. DeWitt, and T. Shimokawa

81 Properties of Trypsin-Cleaved PGH Synthase
R. Odenwaller, C. Young O'Gara, and L. J. Marnett

85 The Structure and Function of Prostaglandin F Synthase
K. Watanabe, Y. Fujii, H. Hayashi, Y. Urade, and O. Hayaishi

Eicosanoid Biosynthesis and Metabolism

89 Conversion of Leukotriene A_4 to Lipoxins by Human Nasal Polyps and Bronchial Tissue
J. Å. Lindgren, C. Edenius, M. Kumlin, B. Dahlén, and A. Änggård

93 Lipoxin and Leukotriene Production During Receptor-Activated Interactions Between Human Platelets and Cytokine-Primed Neutrophils
S. Fiore, M. Romano, and C. N. Serhan

97 Lipoxin Formation in Human Platelets
C. Edenius, I. Forsberg, L. Stenke, and J. Å. Lindgren

101 Purification of 15-Lipoxygenase from Human Leukocytes, Evidence for the Presence of Isozymes
T. Izumi, O. Rådmark, and B. Samuelsson

105 Selective Incorporation of 15-HETE in Phosphatidylinositol: Agonist-Induced Deacylation and Transformation of Stored HETEs by Human Neutrophils
C. N. Serhan and M. E. Brezinski

109 Inhibition of 5-Lipoxygenase: Development of Hydroxamic Acids and Hydroxyureas as Potential Therapeutic Agents
J. A. Salmon, W. P. Jackson, and L. G. Garland

113 Inhibition of Leukotriene C_4 Output from Rat Isolated Heart and Lung by the Sulphasalazine Derivative Ph CL28A
Y. S. Bakhle, M. Nakamura, and J. J. Pankhania

117 Transformations of α-Linolenic Acid in Leaves of Corn (ZEA MAYS L.)
M. Hamberg

125 Formation of Unique Biologically Active Prostaglandins In Vivo by a Non-Cyclooxygenase Free Radical Catalyzed Mechanism
J. D. Morrow, K. E. Hill, R. F. Burk, T. M. Nammour, K. F. Badr, and L. Jackson Roberts, II

129 A Novel Prostaglandin Metabolic Pathway from a Marine Mollusc: Prostaglandin-1,15-Lactones
V. Di Marzo, G. Cimino, G. Sodano, A. Spinella, and G. Villani

133 Leukotriene A_4 Hydrolase in the B-Lymphocytic Cell Line *Raji*
B. Odlander, J. Haeggström, T. Bergman, O. Rådmark, A. Wetterholm, and H-E. Claesson

137 PGH Synthase: Interaction with Hydroperoxides and Indomethacin
R. J. Kulmacz, Y. Ren, A-L. Tsai, and G. Palmer

141 Evidence for Two Pools of Prostaglandin H Synthase in Human Endothelial Cells
A-L. Tsai, R. Sanduja, and K. K. Wu

145 Prostacyclin Secretion and Specific Intracellular Protein Phosphorylation
J. H. Grose, L. Caron, M. Lebel, and J. Landry

149 Inhibition of De Novo Synthesis and Message Expression of Prostaglandin H Synthase by Salicylates
R. Sanduja, D. Loose-Mitchell, and K. K. Wu

153 Effects of Non-Steroidal Anti-Inflammatory Drugs on the In Vivo Synthesis of Thromboxane and Prostacyclin in Humans
V. Drvota, O. Vesterqvist, and K. Gréen

157 Rebound Elevation in Urinary Thromboxane B_2 and 6-Keto-$PGF_{1\alpha}$ Excretion After Aspirin Withdrawal
J. H. Vial, L. J. McLeod, and M. S. Roberts

161 Mechanism-Based Inactivation of Thromboxane A_2 Synthase
F. A. Fitzpatrick, D. Jones, S. Winitz, and H. T. Fish

165 Selective Thromboxane Synthase Inhibition Does Not Increase In Vivo Synthesis of Prostacyclin in Healthy Humans
O. Vesterqvist, K. Gréen, P. Henriksson, G. Rasmanis, and O. Edhag

169 Eicosanoid Synthesis in Murine Macrophages Can Be Shifted from Prostaglandins to Leukotrienes But Not *Vice Versa* by Specific Inhibitors of Cyclooxygenase or 5'-Lipoxygenase Activity
V. Kaever and K. Resch

173 Synthesis and Biological Evaluation of 2,3,5-Trimethyl-6-(3-Pyridylmethyl)-1,4-Benzoquinone (CV-6504), a Dual Inhibitor of TXA_2 Synthase and 5-Lipoxygenase with Scavenging Activity of Active Oxygen Species (AOS)
S. Terao, S. Ohkawa, Z. Terashita, Y. Shibouta, and K. Nishikawa

177 Metabolism of Radioisotopic Variants of LTE_4 in Human Subjects and Excretion of Urinary Metabolites
A. Sala, N. Voelkel, J. Maclouf, and R. C. Murphy

181 Biosynthesis and Metabolism of Leukotriene B_4 by Rat Polymorphonuclear Leukocytes
W. S. Powell and F. Gravelle

Cytochrome P-450 and Arachidonic Acid Metabolism

185 The Cytochrome P450 Metabolic Pathway of Arachidonic Acid in the Cornea
M. L. Schwartzman, K. L. Davis, M. Nishimura, N. G. Abraham, and R. C. Murphy

193 Biosynthesis of P450 Products of Arachidonic Acid in Humans: Increased Formation in Cardiovascular Disease
F. Catella, J. Lawson, G. Braden, D. J. Fitzgerald, E. Shipp, and G. A. FitzGerald

197 A Novel Arachidonic Acid 18($\underline{R}$)-Hydroxylase and Eicosapentaenoic Acid w3-Epoxygenase of Seminal Vesicles
E. H. Oliw

201 Brain Synthesis and Cerebrovascular Action of Cytochrome P-450/Monooxygenase Metabolites of Arachidonic Acid
E. F. Ellis, S. C. Amruthesh, R. J. Police, and L. M. Yancey

205 An Epoxygenase Metabolite of Arachidonic Acid 5,6 Epoxy-Eicosatrienoic Acid Mediates Angiotensin-Induced Natriuresis in Proximal Tubular Epithelium
M. F. Romero, Z. T. Madhun, U. Hopfer, and J. G. Douglas

209 Ion Transport Inhibition in the Medullary Thick Ascending Limb of Henle's Loop by Cytochrome P450-Arachidonic Acid Metabolites
B. Escalante, D. Erlij, J. R. Falck, and J. C. McGiff

213 Synthesis and Biological Activity of Epoxyeicosatrienoic Acids (EETS) by Cultured Bovine Coronary Artery Endothelial Cells
M. Rosolowsky, J. R. Falck, and W. B. Campbell

Dietary and Tissue Precursors

217 Modification of the Eicosanoid System and Cell Signalling by Precursor Fatty Acids
P. C. Weber and A. Sellmayer

225 Dietary Fish and Prostanoid Formation in Man
G. Hornstra, A. C. van Houwelingen, G. A. A. Kivits, S. Fischer, and W. Uedelhoven

229 The Effect of Fish Oil on Plasma Lipids, Platelet and Neutrophil Function in Patients with Vascular Disease
T. A. Mori, R. Vandongen, F. Mahanian, and A. Douglas

233 Effects of EPA and DHA Ethylesters on Plasma Fatty Acids and on Platelets, PMN and Monocytes in Healthy Volunteers
E. Tremoli, C. Mosconi, P. Maderna, S. Colli, E. Stragliotto, C. R. Sirtori, and C. Galli

237 Eicosanoid Production and Membrane Related Properties of Endothelial Cells After Fatty Acid Modification In Vitro
R. C. R. M. Vossen, M. C. E. van Dam-Mieras, G. Hornstra, and R. F. A. Zwaal

241 Effect of Ingestion of Eicosapentaenoic Acid Ethyl-Ester on the Scavenger Activity for Acetylated LDL and the Production of Platelet-Derived Growth Factor in Rat Peritoneal Macrophages
H. Saito, I. Saito, K-J. Chang, Y. Tamura, and S. Yoshida

245 Effect of Oral N-3 Fatty Acid Supplementation on the Immune Response of Young and Older Women
S. N. Meydani, S. Endres, M. M. Woods, B. R. Goldin, C. Soo, A. Morrill-Labrode, C. A. Dinarello, and S. L. Gorbach

Control of Precursor Release

249 PAF Receptor Mediated PGE$_2$ Production in LPS Primed P388D$_1$ Macrophage-Like Cells
K. B. Glaser, R. Asmis, and E. A. Dennis

257 Arachidonic Acid Release in Rat Peritoneal Macrophages: Role of Calcium Ions
S. Nicosia and O. Letari

261 Modulation of Mast Cell Eicosanoid Synthesis by Attachment
B. A. Jakschik and L. Xu

265 A Novel Mechanism of Glucocorticosteroid (GC) Action in Suppression of Phospholipase A$_2$ (PLA$_2$) Activity Stimulated by Ca^{2+} Ionophor A23187: Induction of Protein Phosphates
U. Zor, E. Her, P. Braquet, E. Ferber, and N. Reiss

273 Purification of a Multimeric Phospholipase A$_2$ from Rabbit Renal Cortex
A. R. Morrison and C. Irwin

277 Activation of Group II Phospholipase A$_2$ Gene Via Two Distinct Mechanisms in Rat Vascular Smooth Muscle Cells
N. Arita, T. Nakano, O. Ohara, and H. Teraoka

281 The Eicosanoid Lipid Precursors Diacyl-Glycerol and Phosphatidic Acid are Formed by Phospholipase D in Neutrophils
M. M. Billah, S. Eckel, T. J. Mullmann, J-K. Pai, M. I. Siegel, and R. W. Egan

287 Phospholipase D in the Pancreatic Islet: Evidence Suggesting the Involvement of Phosphatidic Acid in Signal Transduction
S. Metz and M. Dunlop

291 Effect of Dexamethasone and Phorbol Myristate Acetate on Lipocortin 1, 2 and 5 mRNA and Protein Synthesis
E. Solito, G. Raugei, M. Melli, and L. Parente

Analytical Methods

295 A Critical Approach to Eicosanoid Assay
E. Granström and H. Kindahl

303 Development of Scintillation Proximity Assays for Prostaglandins and Related Compounds
P. M. Baxendale, R. C. Martin, K. T. Hughes, D. Y. Lee, and N. M. Waters

307 Immunoquantitation of Thromboxane Synthase in Human Tissues
R. Nüsing and V. Ullrich

311 Reverse Phase HPLC Profiling of Arachidonic Acid Metabolites in Blood Stimulated Ex Vivo
A. Odeimat, P. E. Poubelle, and P. Borgeat

315 A Stable Isotope Dilution Mass Spectrometric Assay for the Major Urinary Metabolite of PGD$_2$
J. D. Morrow, C. Prakash, T. A. Duckworth, W. E. Zackert, I. A. Blair, J. A. Oates, and L. J. Roberts II

319 Measurement of Leukotrienes by Enzyme Immunoassays Using Acetylcholinesterase as Label
C. Antoine, J. Maclouf, and P. Pradelles

323 A Novel Method for the Analysis of PAF and Alkyl-Ether Phospholipids by Mass Spectrometry
M. Balazy, J. Cluzel, and N. G. Bazan

327 Determination of Platelet-Activating Factor in Biological Samples by High Resolution Mass Spectrometry
F. Magni, F. Berti, L. De Angelis, G. Rossoni, and G. Galli

Receptors and Antagonists

331 Characterization of Thromboxane A$_2$/Prostaglandin H$_2$ Receptors of Various Tissues Using a New Radioiodinated Thromboxane A$_2$/Prostaglandin H$_2$ Mimetic, I-BOP
T. A. Morinelli, M. Naka, A. Masuda, J. E. Oatis, Jr., A. K. Okwu, D. E. Mais, D. L. Saussy, Jr., and P. V. Halushka

339 Purification and Characterization of the Human Platelet TXA$_2$/PGH$_2$ Receptor
S. Narumiya, F. Ushikubi, M. Nakajima, M. Hirata, and M. Okuma

347 Binding of a Radioiodinated Agonist to Thromboxane A$_2$/Prostaglandin H$_2$ (TXA$_2$/PGH$_2$) Receptors in Guinea Pig Lung Membranes
D. E. Mais, D. L. Saussy, Jr., D. E. Magee, and C. M. Williams

351 On the Mechanism of the Prolonged Action in Man of GR32191, a Thromboxane Receptor Antagonist
J. M. Ritter, H. S. Doktor, N. Benjamin, S. E. Barrow, and P. Stewart-Long

355 Effect of BAY U 3405, a New Thromboxane Antagonist, on Arachidonic Acid Induced Thromboembolism
F. Seuter, E. Perzborn, and V. B. Fiedler

359 Rational Design of Thromboxane A_2 Antagonists
N. Hamanaka, T. Seko, T. Miyazaki, and A. Kawasaki

363 Phorbol Ester-Induced Expression of the Common, Low-Affinity Binding Site for Primary Prostanoids in Vascular Smooth Muscle Cells
K. Hanasaki, M. Kishi, and H. Arita

367 Ca^{2+} Transients Evoked by Prostanoids in Swiss 3T3 Cells Suggest an FP-receptor Mediated Response
D. F. Woodward, C. E. Fairbairn, D. D. Goodrum, A. H-P. Krauss, T. L. Ralston, and L. S. Williams

371 Signal Transduction Coupled to Prostaglandin D_2
S. Ito, M. Negishi, K. Sugama, E. Okuda-Ashitaka, and O. Hayaishi

375 Characterisation of PGE_2 Receptors Mediating Increased Vascular Permeability in Inflammation
R. A. Armstrong, J. S. Matthews, R. L. Jones, and N. H. Wilson

379 GR63799X - A Novel Prostanoid With Selectivity for EP_3 Receptors
K. T. Bunce, N. M. Clayton, R. A. Coleman, E. W. Collington, H. Finch, J. M. Humphray, P. P. A. Humphrey, J. J. Reeves, R. L. G. Sheldrick, and R. Stables

383 Modulation of Platelet Activation by Prostaglandin E_2 Mimics
K-H. Thierauch and G. Prior

387 Biosynthesis and Function of Leukotriene B_4. Immunochemical Study of Leukotriene A_4 Hydrolase and Identification of Putative Leukotriene B_4 Receptor
T. Shimizu, N. Ohishi, I. Miki, M. Nakamura, and Y. Seyama

395 Photoaffinity Labeling of Leukotriene Binding Sites in Hepatocytes and Hepatoma Cells
M. Müller, E. Falk, R. Sandbrink, U. Berger, I. Leier, G. Jedlitschky, M. Huber, G. Kurz, and D. Keppler

399 Mechanisms of Leukotriene B_4-Specific Chemotactic Deactivation of Human Polymorphonuclear Leukocytes
J. M. Boggs and E. J. Goetzl

403 Desensitization of the Leukotriene B_4 Receptor by Partial Agonists
D. Kiel, R. E. Zipkin, and S. J. Feinmark

407 ONO-LB-457: A Novel and Orally Active Leukotriene B₄ Receptor Antagonist
K. Kishikawa, N. Matsunaga, T. Maruyama, R. Seo, M. Toda, T. Miyamoto, and A. Kawasaki

411 Synthesis and Structure-Activity Relationships of a Series of Substituted-Phenylpropionic Acids as a Novel Class of Leukotriene B₄ Antagonists
M. Konno, S. Sakuyama, T. Nakae, N. Hamanaka, T. Miyamoto, and A. Kawasaki

Respiratory System

415 Sulphidopeptide Leukotrienes in Asthma
T. H. Lee, S. P. O'Hickey, C. Jacques, R. J. Hawksworth, J. P. Arm, P. Christie, B.W. Spur, and A. E. G. Crea

421 Role of Arachidonic Acid Metabolites in the Pathogenesis of Actute Lung Injury
A. J. Lonigro, A. H. Stephenson, and R. S. Sprague

429 Further Evidence that Leukotrienes are the Major Mediators of Allergic Constriction in Human Bronchi
T. Björck, Y. Harada, B. Dahlén, O. Zetterström, G. Johansson, L. Rodriguez, P. Hedqvist, and S-E. Dahlén

433 Formation of PGD₂ After Allergen Inhalation in Atopic Asthmatics
K. Sladek, J. R. Sheller, G. A. FitzGerald, J. D. Morrow, and L. J. Roberts II

437 Metabolism of Arachidonic Acid by Foà-Kurloff Cells
P. Sirois, K. Maghni, C. Robidoux, A. Hallée, J. Laporte, S. Cloutier, and P. Borgeat

441 15(S)-Hydroxyeicosatetraenoic Acid (15-HETE) is the Major Arachidonic Acid Metabolite in Human Bronchi
M. Kumlin, E. Ohlson, T. Björck, M. Hamberg, E. Granström, B. Dahlén, O. Zetterström, and S-E. Dahlén

445 Metabolism of Arachidonic Acid in Human Alveolar Macrophages from Patients with Sarcoidosis
V. De Rose, M. T. Crivellari, T. Viganò, G. C. Folco, L. Trentin, M. Masciarelli, G. Semenzato, E. Pozzi, and G. Gialdroni Grassi

449 The Comparative Nasal Effects of Prostaglandin D₂ in Normal and Rhinitic Subjects
P. Howarth, S. Walsh, and C. Robinson

453 Inhibition of Endothelin-Induced Bronchoconstriction by OKY-046, a Selective Thromboxane A_2 Synthetase Inhibitor, in Guinea Pigs
F. Nambu, N. Yube, N. Omawari, M. Sawada, T. Okegawa, A. Kawasaki, and S. Ikeda

457 The Effects of a 5-Lipoxygenase Inhibitor on Antigen-Induced Mediator Release, Late-Phase Bronchoconstriction and Cellular Infiltrates in Primates
R. H. Gundel, C. A. Torcellini, C. C. Clarke, S. Desai, E. S. Lazer, and C. D. Wegner

461 Inhibition of Allergic Bronchoconstriction in Asthmatics by the Leukotriene-Antagonist ICI-204,219
S-E. Dahlén, B. Dahlén, E. Eliasson, H. Johansson, T. Björck, M. Kumlin, K. Boo, J. Whitney, S. Binks, B. King, R. Stark, and O. Zetterström

465 Effect of Leukotriene Antagonist on Experimental and Clinical Bronchial Asthma
T. Nakagawa, Y. Mizushima, A. Ishii, F. Nambu, M. Motoishi, Y. Yui, T. Shida, T. Miyamoto

469 The Pharmacological Profile of SK&F 104353-Z_2, a Potent, Selective Inhaled Antagonist of Cysteinyl Leukotrienes, in Normal Man
J. M. Evans, P. J. Piper, and J. F. Costello

473 Prostanoid Contractions in Human Isolated Pulmonary Muscle Preparations: Inhibition by BAY u3405
X. Norel, C. Labat, P. Gardiner, and C. Brink

477 WY-50,295 Tromethamine: A Novel Inhibitor of Leukotriene-Mediated Reactions
B. M. Weichman, J. W. Berkenkopf, D. Grimes, R. J. Heaslip, R. J. Sturm, and J. Y. Chang

*480a Leukotrienes in Cerebrospinal Fluid of the Conscious Cat: Effect of Platelet-Activating Factor and Pyrogens
F. Coceani, I. Bishai, J. Lees, and N. Hynes

Subject Index follows page 480d

Volume 21B

Immunology and Allergy

481 Eosinophil Phenotypes and LTC_4 Generation In Vitro and in Hypereosinophilic States
D. M. Sheff, W. F. Owen, Jr., K. F. Austen

---

*chapter added at press time

489 Murine Thymocyte Lysis by Inhibitors of Archidonic Acid Metabolism
A. M. Harford, G. M. Shopp, J. S. Goodwin, M. A. Ebbesen, L. Gibel, A. Y. Smith, and W. A. Sterling

493 Endogenous Leukotriene Production Elicited by Antigen Challenge of Sensitized Livers
W. Hagmann, I. Kaiser, and B. A. Jakschik

497 Prostaglandin E$_2$ Controls Antibody Affinity in Genetically Selected Mice
C. Phillips

501 Release of Peptide Leukotrienes into Nasal Secretions After Local Instillation of Aspirin in Aspirin-Sensitive Asthmatics
C. Picado, I. Ramis, J. Rosellò, O. Bulbena, V. Plaza, and E. Gelpí

503 CGP 45715 A: A Leukotriene D$_4$ Analogue with Potent Peptido-LT Antagonist Activity
M. A. Bray, W. H. Anderson, N. Subramanian, U. Niederhauser, M. Kuhn, M. Erard, and A. von Sprecher

509 Formation of Cyclooxygenase-Derived Eicosanoids by a Parasitic Intravascular Nematode
L. X. Liu, C. N. Serhan, and P. F. Weller

513 The Effect of Prostaglandin E$_2$ and Non-Steroidal Anti-Inflammatory Drugs on Cell-Associated Interleukin One
A. K. Bahl, J. C. Foreman, and M. M. Dale

517 5-Lipoxygenase Activation May Facilitate an Interleukin-1 Transduction Signal
K. G. Mugridge, M. Perretti, and L. Parente

521 Prostaglandin E$_2$ Down-Regulates the Expression of Tumor Necrosis Alpha Gene by Human Blood Monocytes
M. Spatafora, G. Chiappara, D. D'Amico, D. Volpes, M. Melis, E. Pace, and A. M. Merendino

525 High Urinary Leukotriene E$_4$ (LTE$_4$) and Thromboxane 2 (TXB$_2$) Levels are Associated with Capillary Leak Syndrome in Bone Marrow Transplant Patients
R. A. Cahill, Y. Zhao, R. Murphy, A. Sala, M. Foegh, T. Spitzer, and H. J. Deeg

529 Increased Formation of Thromboxane in the Antiphospholipid Syndrome
L. Årfors, O. Vesterqvist, and K. Greén

533 Definition of Platelet-Derived Histamine Releasing Factor (PDHRF) and Histaminergic Receptors Modulating Platelet Aggregation
E. Masini, A. Pistelli, F. Gambassi, M. G. Di Bello, and P. F. Mannaioni

Inflammation

537 Eicosanoids as Mediators and Modulators of Inflammation
P. Hedqvist, J. Raud, U. Palmertz, M. Kumlin, and S-E. Dahlén

545 Protein I of *N. Gonorrhoeae* Shows That Phosphatidate from Phosphatidylcholine *Via* Phospholipase C is an Intracellular Messenger in Neutrophil Activation by Chemoattractants
K. A. Haines and G. Weissmann

553 Lipoxins Trigger the Release But Not the Oxygenation of Arachidonic Acid in Human Neutrophils: Dissociation Between Lipid Remodeling and Adhesion
S. Fiore, S. Nigam, and C. N. Serhan

557 Generation and Biological Activities of Lipoxins in the Rainbow Trout - An Overview
A. F. Rowley, T. R. Pettitt, C. J. Secombes, G. J. E. Sharp, S. E. Barrow, and A. I. Mallet

561 Leukotriene B$_4$ Induced Neutrophil Functions in Chronic Granulomatous Disease (CGD)
B. Ringertz and J. Palmblad

565 The Role of Leukotriene B$_4$ as an Inflammatory Mediator in Skin and the Functional Characterisation of LTB$_4$ Receptor Antagonists
R. Ekerdt, B. Buchmann, W. Fröhlich, C. Giesen, J. Heindl, and W. Skuballa

569 Leukotoxin, 9,10-Epoxy-12-Octadecenoate, as a Burn Toxin Causing Adult Respiratory Distress Syndrome
T. Ozawa, M. Hayakawa, K. Kosaka, S. Sugiyama, T. Ogawa, K. Yokoo, H. Aoyama, and Y. Izawa

573 Altered Levels of Phospholipase A$_2$, Lipoperoxidation and Arachidonate Metabolism in Rat Pancreas Transplantation
G. Hotter, O. S. León, J. Roselloó-Catafau, J. Sánchez, P. Puig Parellada, M. A. López-Boado, A. Sáenz, R. D. Henriques, L. Fernández-Cruz, and E. Gelpí

Cardiovascular System

577 Mechanisms of Eicosanoid Action
G. A. FitzGerald, R. Murray, N. Moran, C. Funk, W. Charman, R. Clarke, L. Furci, and J. Fitzgerald

583 Iloprost, a Stable Analogue of PGI_2: Clinical Results and Pathophysiological Considerations
G. Stock, B. Müller, T. Krais, E. Schillinger

591 Cardio- and Hemodynamic Profile of Selective PGD_2 - Analogues
B. G. Schulz, R. Beckmann, B. Müller, G. Schröder, B. Maass, K-H. Thierauch, B. Buchmann, P. F. J. Verhallen, W. Fröhlich

595 A New Role for Prostaglandins in the Regulation of Peripheral Resistance
A. Koller and G. Kaley

599 Anti-Thrombotic Effect of ONO-8809, a Novel TxA_2/PG Endoperoxide Receptor antagonist
K. Wakitani, R. Matsumoto, H. Imawaka, Y. Kamanaka, M. Naka, N. Hamanaka, T. Okegawa, and A. Kawasaki

603 Maximal Blockade of TxA_2 Without Compromised PGI_2 Formation: A Superior Profile of the TxA_2 Receptor Blocking Drug GR32191 Over Aspirin
P. Lumley, R. J. Keery, K. A. Wharton, B. P. White, and I. S. Watts

607 Activation of Thromboxane and Prostacyclin Biosynthesis in Humans
K. Gréen, and O. Vesterqvist

611 Selective Inhibition of Platelet-Derived Thromboxane A_2 in Patients with Lupus Anticoagulant Using Low Doses Aspirin as Assessed by Enzyme Immunoassay
F. Lellouche, C. Falcon, L. Carreras, J. Maclouf

615 Relation Between Tobacco Consumption and Urinary Excretion of Thromboxane A_2 and Prostacyclin Metabolites in 756 Randomly Sampled Young Men
Å. Wennmalm, G. Benthin, E. F. Granström, L. Persson, A. S. Petersson, and S. Winell

619 Thromboxane-Dependent Platelet Activation as a Transducer of Enhanced Risk of Coronary and Cerebral Thrombosis
C. Patrono, G. Ciabattoni, and G. Davì

623 Involvement of Eicosanoids in Angiogenesis
S-I. Murota, T. Kanayasu, J. Nakano-Hayashi, and I. Morita

Blood Cells and Vascular Wall

627 Mediators from the Endothelial Cell
J. R. Vane and R. Botting

637 Guanidino Compounds and Endothelium Dependent Relaxation
G. Thomas, M. Y. Farhat, K. F. Heim, and P. W. Ramwell

645 Increased Formation of Thromboxane A_2 and Prostacyclin in Anaphylactoid Purpura
B. Tönshoff, R. Momper, H. Schweer, K. Schärer, and H. W. Seyberth

649 Thromboxane and Leukotriene Generation by Mononuclearcytes from Cardiac Transplant Patients
Y. Zhao, N. Katz, E. Lefrak, J. Macoviak, M. Foegh

655 Interaction Between Prostacyclin and Molsidomine in Blood Cells and Plasma
R. J. Gryglewski, K. Bieroń, A. Dembińska-Kieć, E. Kostka-Trabka, and A. Zembowicz

659 Cooperation of Adipocytes and Endothelial Cells is Necessary for Catecholamine-Stimulated PGI_2 Production by Rat Adipose Tissue
J. Parker, J. Lane, and L. Axelrod

663 Studies of Leukotriene A_4-Hydrolase and Leukotriene C_4-Synthase in Human Endothelial Cells: Enzymes Involved in the Metabolism of Monocyte Released Leukotriene A_4
H-E. Claesson, H. Ax:son-Johnson, O. Rådmark, and P-J. Jakobsson

667 13-HODE Synthesis in Internal Mammary Arteries and Saphenous Veins: Implications in Cardiovascular Surgery
S. J. Brister, T. A. Haas, M. C. Bertomeu, J. Austin, and M. R. Buchanan

671 Nitric Oxide But Not Prostacyclin Has An Autocrine Function in Porcine Aortic Endothelial Cells
H. Schröder, C. Machunsky, H. Strobach, and K. Schrör

Renal System

675 Cytrochrome P450-Dependent Arachidonate Metabolites, Renal Function and Blood Pressure Regulation
J. C. McGiff and M. A. Carroll

683 Functional Significance of Lipoxygenase Metabolites of Arachidonic Acid in the Glomerular Microcirculation
K. Takahashi and K. F. Badr

689 Increased Renal Production of Cytochrome P450-Dependent Metabolites of Arachidonic Acid in Cyclosporine-Induced Nephrotoxicity
D. Sacerdoti, M. Borsato, P. Rigotti, P. Amodio, P. Angeli, M. Ferraresso, M. Plebani, and A. Gatta

693 Mechanism of Renal Vasoconstriction with Thromboxane Mimetic: Engagement of Tubuloglomerular Feedback
W. J. Welch, C. S. Wilcox, and W. H. Folger

697 Synthesis and Metabolism of Cysteinyl Leukotrienes by the Isolated Pig Kidney
K. P. Moore, J. Wood, C. Gove, K. C. Tan, J. Eason, G. W. Taylor, and R. Williams

701 Regulation of Lipoxins (LX) and Leukotriene B_4 (LTB_4) Production in Rat Mesangial Cells (MC)
R. Garrick, A. Goodman, S. T. Shen, S. Ogunc, and P. Y-K. Wong

707 Inhibition by FCE 22178 of Platelet and Glomerular Thromboxane Synthase in Animal and Human Kidney Disease
P. Alessandrini, P. Salvati, F. Pugliese, G. Ciabattoni, C. Patrono

711 Defibrotide, a Prostacyclin Releasing Agent, Protects the Rabbit Kidney from Acute Failure
G. Bianchi, P. Alberico, R. Tettamanti, M. Mantovani, G. Prino, G. Rossoni, and F. Berti

Nervous System

715 Identification of Neuromodulators Produced by the 12-Lipoxygenase in Aplysia
S. J. Feinmark, M. Abe, E. Shapiro, V. Brezina, and J. H. Schwartz

723 Sleep-Wake Regulation by PGD2 and E2
O. Hayaishi, H. Matsumura, H. Onoe, Y. Koyama, and Y. Watanabe

727 Direct Opening of S-Type K^+ Channels of Aplysia Sensory Neurons by 12-Lipoxygenase Metabolites
A. Volterra, N. Buttner, and S. A. Siegelbaum

731 Formation of a Glutathionyl-Conjugate of Hepoxilin A_3 and its Action in Rat Brain
C. R. Pace-Asciak, O. Laneuville, N. Gurevich, P. Wu, P. L. Carlen, and E. J. Corey

735 PGE$_2$ Synthesis in Chick Spinal Cord and High Affinity PGE$_2$ Receptors on Motoneurons
  M-F. Vesin, E. Pralong, and B. Droz

739 Eicosanoid Synthesis by Spinal Cord Astrocytes is Evoked by Substance P; Possible Implications for Nociception and Pain
  D. Marriott, G. P. Wilkin, P.R. Coote, and J. N. Wood

743 Arachidonic Acid Cyclo and Lipoxygenase Pathways in Astroglial Cells
  A. Petroni, M. Blasevich, F. Visioli, and C. Galli

749 Studies on Eicosanoid Metabolism in the Fetal Rat Brain After Global Ischemia
  E. Yavin, B. Kuniewski, and S. Harel

Cytoprotection

753 Lipoxygenase Products in Gastric Damage and Protection
  B. M. Peskar

761 Vascular Interactions Between Endogenous Prostanoids and Vasoactive Peptide Mediators in Gastric Damage
  B. J. R. Whittle and J. V. Esplugues

767 Role of Prostaglandins in Mucus Synthesis in Rat Gastric Mucosa
  E. Quadros and D. E. Wilson

771 An Important Role of Leukotriene C$_4$ in Microcirculation During Ethanol-Induced Gastric Mucosal Injury in Rat
  M. Katori, K. Nishiyama, A. Ueno, and T. Ohno

777 Effect of Smoking on Prostaglandin, Thromboxane and Leukotriene Synthesis by Human Gastric Mucosa
  N. Hudson, T. K. Daneshmend, S. Hurst, N. K. Bhaskar, N. S. Brown, and C. J. Hawkey

781 Effect of Acute Alcohol Administration on Prostaglandin E2 (PGE2) and F2α (PGF2α) Synthesis and Histological Damage in Human Gastric Mucosa
  M. C. Parodi, P. Cognein, M. Marugo, G. Iaquinto, and L. Cuccurullo

785 Effects of Protective and Damaging Substances on Human Gastric Mucosal Eicosanoids
  I. A. Tavares, R. K. Goel, and A. Bennett

789 A Double Blind Randomized Placebo-Controlled Study Demonstrates the Protective Efficacy of Rosaprostol on Aspirin-Induced Gastrointestinal Bleeding in Man
G. Calcamuggi, G. Babini, C. Arduino, M. Lanzio, G. Anfossi, D. Ciani, G. Emanuelli

793 Nocloprost, a Unique PGE2 Analog, with Local Gastroprotective and Ulcer Healing Activity
S. J. Konturek, T. Brzozowski, D. Drozdowicz, E. Krzyzek, J. Garlicki, J. Majka, and I. Amon

Endocrine System and Reproductive Biology

799 The Role of Prostaglandins and Ovarian Hormones in the Regulation of Human Uterine Contractility
M. Bygdeman, K. Gemzell, M. L. Swahn

807 Altered Platelet Responses to P.A.F. in Pregnancy-Induced Hypertension
M. H. F. Sullivan, P. R. Tranter, Y. Ahmed, and M. G. Elder

811 Disappearance of Human Myometrial Adenylate Cyclase Activation by Prostaglandins at the End of Pregnancy. Comparison with β-adrenergic Response
M. Breuiller, F. Doualla-Bell, M. H. Litime, M. J. Leroy, and F. Ferré

815 The Steroidal Regulation of Arachidonic Acid Uptake by Human Endometrial Stromal Cells in Culture
J. S. Beesley, S. Franks, and R. C. Bonney

819 Prostaglandin (PG) Release from Human and Rabbit Endometrial Glandular Epithelial and Stromal Cell Cultures In Vitro
M. J. K. Harper, A. A. Alecozay, and M. Kasamo

823 Progesterone and Human Interferon α-2 Have a Different Effect on the Release of Prostaglandin F 2α from Human Endometrium
S. N. Mitchell and S. K. Smith

827 Role of Epoxygenase Metabolites of Arachidonic Acid in Intracellular Signal Transduction
A. Hirai, S. Yoshida, M. Nishimura, K. Seki, Y. Tamura, and S. Yoshida

Cell Differentiation and Proliferation

831 Phospholipase A_2 Activation is an Early Event in Erythropoietin Stimulated Murine Fetal Liver Cell Proliferation/Differentiation
B. S. Beckman, J-S. Tou, and M. Mason-Garcia

835 Child Syndrome: Fibroblasts from Involved Skin Fail to Proliferate in Response to Interleukin 1a Due to Induction of Excessive Prostaglandin E_2 Synthesis
M. E. Goldyne, L. Rea, and S. Z. Goldyne

839 Induction of Cyclooxygenase in Osteoblasts and Bone Metabolism
I. Morita, Y. Suzuki, K. Toriyama, and S-I. Murota

843 Transduction of the Epidermal Growth Factor Mitogenic Signal in BALB/c 3T3 Fibroblasts Involves Linoleic Acid Metabolism
T. E. Eling and W. C. Glasgow

847 Prostaglandin D_2 Stimulates Calcification by Human Osteoblastic Cells
Y. Koshihara, T. Amano, and R. Takamori

851 Effect of Di-M-PGE2 on T Cell Differentiation. Flow Cytometry Study at Thymus Level
A. Mastino, S. Grelli, C. Favalli, and E. Garaci

855 Endothelial or Cancer Cells Growth Regulation by PGE1 Analog Misoprostol
M. T. Foultier, T. Patrice, J. Harb, L. Robillard, G. Houillon, J. P. Galmiche, and L. Le Bodic

859 Effect of Cyclopentenone Prostaglandins on Glutathione Biosynthesis
M. Hirata and K. Ohno

863 LTB_4 Induces Formation of a Novel Polyphosphoinositide in Human Keratinocytes
V. A. Ziboh and W. Tang

Cancer

867 Induction of Heat Shock Protein Synthesis by Prostaglandins with Antineoplastic and Antiviral Activity
M. G. Santoro, E. Garaci, and C. Amici

875 Human Cancer Prostaglandins and Patient Survival
A. Bennett, I. F. Stamford, and D. Cooper

879 Involvement of Prostaglandins and Cytokines in Antitumor Cytostatic Activity of Human Peritoneal Macrophages
I. L. Bonta, S. Ben-Efraim, C. Tak, M. W. J. A. Fieren, and G. J. C. M. van den Bemd

883 Lipoxygenase Products in Myeloproliferative Disorders: Increased Leukotriene C_4 and Decreased Lipoxin Formation in Chronic Myeloid Leukemia
L. Stenke, B. Näsman-Glaser, C. Edenius, J. Samuelsson, J. Palmblad, and J. Å. Lindgren

887 Modulation of the Antiproliferative Activity of 9-Deoxy-Δ^9,Δ^{12} (E)-PGD$_2$ by Conjugation with Intracellular Glutathione
J. Atsmon, M. L. Freeman, M. J. Meredith, B. J. Sweetman, and L. J. Roberts II

891 Induction of 31,000 Protein by PGD$_2$-Treated Vascular Endothelial Cells
K. Koizumi, R. Yamauchi, A. Irie, T. Miyamoto, M. Negishi, and A. Ichikawa

Round Table on Eicosanoids in Cancer Cell Metastasis

895 Arachidonic Acid Metabolism of Cytosolic Fractions of Lewis Lung Carcinoma Cells
L. J. Marnett, M. T. Leithauser, K. M. Richards, I. Blair, K. V. Honn, S. Yamamoto, and T. Yoshimoto

901 Effects of Prostacyclin Analogues in In Vivo Tumor Models
M. R. Schneider, E. Schillinger, M. Schirner, W. Skuballa, S. Stürzebecher, and W. Witt

909 Endothelial Cell 13-HODE Synthesis and Tumor Cell Endothelial Cell Adhesion
M. R. Buchanan, M. C. Bertomeu, T. A. Haas, S. Gallo, and L. Eltringham-Smith

913 Antimetastatic Action of Stable Prostacyclin Analogs in Mice
T. Giraldi, V. Rapozzi, L. Perissin, and S. Zorzet

917 Mechanisms of the Antimetastatic Activity of Stable Prostacyclin Analogues: Modulation of Host Immunocompetence
V. Costantini, A. Giampietri, M. Allegrucci, G. Agnelli, G. G. Nenci, M. C. Fioretti

921 Antiproliferative Effects of Lipoxygenase Inhibitors on Human Leukemia Cells
D. S. Snyder

925 Tumour Cell Proliferation by Thromboxane A$_2$: A Receptor-Mediated Event
S. Nigam and A. Zakrzewicz

PAF and PAF Antagonists

929 From Ginkgolides to N-Substituted Piperidino-Thieno Diazepines, a New Series of Highly Potent Dual Antagonists
P. Braquet, J. P. Laurent, A. Rolland, C. Martin, J. Pommier, D. Hosford, and A. Esanu

939 Opposite Effects of PGI$_2$ and PAF Generated During Acute Myocardial Ischemia in the Perfused Rabbit Heart
F. Berti, F. Magni, G. Rossoni, L. De Angelis, and G. Galli

943 Platelet Activating Factor (PAF) Antagonists: Development of a Highly Potent PAF Antagonist, TCV-309
M. Takatani, N. Maezaki, Y. Imura, Z-I. Terashita, K. Nishikawa, and S. Tsushima

Round Table on New Frontiers in Prostaglandin Therapeutics

947 Role of Prostaglandins E in Inflammation and Immune Responses
R. B. Zurier

955 The Interactions of Cytokines, NSAIDs and Prostaglandins in Cartilage Destruction and Repair
J. T. Dingle and M. J. Shield

967 Role of Prostaglandins in NSAID-Induced Renal Dysfunction
R. D. Toto

Round Table on Cytokines and Lipid Mediators in the Regulation of CD 23/FcεRII Expression and IgE-Dependent Responses

975 Fc Epsilon Receptor II Expression in Parasitic Diseases: Effects of Cytokines on IgE-Dependent Activation of Eosinophils
M. Capron, R. L. Coffman, J. P. Papin, F. Ajana, and A. Capron

983 Role of CD23 in IgE Regulation... and Beyond
J. Gordon, L. Flores-Romo, J. A. Cairns, A. Veronesi, D. R. Stanworth, and A. A. Ghaderi

989 Role of PAF and Cytokines in the Modulation of FcεRII/CD23 Expression on Human Eosinophils
T. Kawabe, Y. Maeda, N. Maekawa, M. Tanaka, M. Mayumi, H. Mikawa, and J. Yodoi

977 Signalling Pathway Through the CD23 Molecule in Human B Cells
J. P. Kolb, B. Dugas, D. Renard, E. Génot, J. Poggioli, and G. Delespesse

1005 Biosynthesis and Biological Effects of Leukotriene B_4 in B Lymphocytes
P-J. Jakobsson, B. Odlander, K. A. Yamaoka, A. Rosén, and H-E. Claesson

Subject Index follows page 1012

Contributors

A
Abe, M., 715
Abraham, Nader G., 185
Åfors, L., 529
Agnelli, G., 917
Ahmed, Y., 807
Ajana, F., 975
Alberico, P., 711
Alecozay, A. A., 819
Alessandrini, P., 707
Allegrucci, M., 917
Amano, Toshikazu, 847
Amici, C., 867
Amodio, P., 689
Amon, I., 793
Amruthesh, S. C., 201
Anderson, W. H., 503
Anfossi, G., 789
Angeli, P., 689
Änggård, Anders, 89
Antoine, Catherine, 319
Aoyama, H., 569
Arduino, C., 789
Arita, H., 277,363
Arm, Jonathan P., 415
Armstrong, R. A., 375
Asmis, Reto, 249
Atsmon, J., 887
Austen, K. Frank, 481
Austin, J., 667
Axelrod, L., 659
Ax:son Johnson, Hélène, 663

B
Babini, G., 789
Badr, Kamal F., 125,683
Bahl, A. K., 513
Bakhle, Y. S., 113
Balazy, Michael, 323
Barrios, C., 41
Barrow, S. E., 351,557
Baxendale, P. M., 303
Bazan, Nicolas G., 323
Beckman, Barbara S., 831
Beckmann, R., 591
Beesley, J. S., 815
Ben-Efraim, S., 879
Benjamin, N., 351
Bennett, A., 785,875
Benthin, G., 615
Berger, U., 395
Bergman, Tomas, 133
Berkenkopf, Joseph W., 477
Berti, F., 327,711,939
Bertomeu, M. C., 667,909
Bhaskar, N. K., 777
Bianchi, G., 711
Bienkowski, Michael J., 73
Bieroń, K., 655
Billah, M. Motasim, 281
Binks, Sue, 461
Björck, Thure, 429,441,461
Blair, Ian A., 315,895
Blasevich, M., 743
Boggs, J. M., 399
Bonney, R. C., 815
Bonta, I. L., 879
Boo, Karin, 461
Borgeat, P., 311,437
Borsato, M., 689
Botting, Regina, 627
Braden, Greg, 193
Braquet, P., 265,929
Bray, M. A., 503
Breuiller, M., 811
Brezina, V., 715
Brezinski, Mark E., 105
Brink, C., 473
Brister, S. J., 667

Brown, N. S., 777
Brzozowski, T., 793
Buchanan, M. R., 667,909
Buchmann, B., 565,591
Bulbena, O., 501
Bunce, K. T., 379
Burk, Raymond F., 125
Buttner, N., 727
Bygdeman, M., 799

C

Cahill, R. A., 525
Cairns, Jennifer A., 983
Calcamuggi, G., 789
Campbell, W. B., 213
Capron, A., 975
Capron, M., 975
Carlen, P. L., 731
Caron, L., 145
Carreras, Luis, 611
Carroll, M. A., 675
Catella, Francesca, 193
Chang, Joseph Y., 477
Chang, Ke-Jian, 241
Charman, William, 577
Chiappara, G., 521
Christie, Pandora, 415
Ciabattoni, G., 619,707
Ciani, D., 789
Cimino, Guido, 129
Claesson, Hans-Erik, 133,663,1005
Clarke, Cosmos C., 457
Clarke, Robert, 577
Clayton, N. M., 379
Cloutier, S., 437
Cluzel, Jacques, 323
Coffman, R. L., 975
Cognein, P., 781
Coleman, R. A., 379
Colli, S., 233
Collington, E. W., 379
Cooper, D., 875
Coote, P. R., 739
Corey, E. J., 731

Costantini, V., 917
Costello, J. F., 469
Craik, Charles S., 25
Crea, Attilio E. G., 415
Crivellari, M. T., 445
Cuccurullo, L., 781

D

Dahlén, Barbro, 89,429,441,461
Dahlén, Sven-Erik, 429,441,461,537
Dale, M. M., 513
D'Amico, D., 521
Daneshmend, T. K., 777
Davì, G., 619
Davis, Karen L., 185
De Angelis, L., 327,939
Deeg, H. J., 525
Delespesse, G., 997
Dembińska-Kieć, A., 655
Dennis, Edward A., 249
De Rose, V., 445
Desai, Sudha, 457
DeWitt, David L., 65,77
Di Bello, M. G., 533
Di Marzo, Vincenzo, 129
Dinarello, Charles A., 245
Dingle, John T., 955
Dixon, Richard A. F., 25
Doktor, H. S., 351
Doualla-Bell, F., 811
Douglas, Andrea, 229
Douglas, Janice G., 205
Droz, Bernard, 735
Drozdowicz, D., 793
Drvota, Viktor, 153
Duckworth, Tanya A., 315
Dugas, B., 997
Dunlop, M., 287
Dunn, Michael J., 69

E

Eason, J., 697
Ebbesen, M. A., 489
Eckel, Stephen, 281

Edenius, Charlotte, 89,97,883
Edhag, Olof, 165
Egan, Robert W., 281
Ekerdt, R., 565
Elder, M. G., 807
Eliasson, Eva, 461
Eling, Thomas E., 843
Ellis, E. F., 201
Eltringham-Smith, L., 909
Emanuelli, G., 789
Endres, Stefan, 245
Erard, M., 503
Erlij, D., 209
Esanu, A., 929
Escalante, B., 209
Esplugues, J. V., 761
Evans, J. M., 469

F
Fairbairn, C. E., 367
Falck, J. R., 209,213
Falcon, Cristina, 611
Falk, E., 395
Farhat, Michel Y., 637
Favalli, C., 851
Feinmark, S. J., 403,715
Ferber, E., 265
Fernández-Cruz, L., 573
Ferraresso, M., 689
Ferré, F., 811
Fiedler, V. B., 355
Fieren, M. W. J. A., 879
Finch, H., 379
Fiore, Stefano, 93,553
Fioretti, M. C., 917
Fischer, S., 225
Fish, H. T., 161
Fitzgerald, Desmond J., 193,577
FitzGerald, Garret A., 33,193,433, 577
Fitzpatrick, F. A., 161
Flores-Romo, Leopoldo, 983
Foegh, M., 525,649
Folco, G. C., 445

Folger, Walter H., 693
Ford-Hutchinson, A. W., 9
Foreman, J. C., 513
Forsberg, Inger, 97
Foultier, M. T., 855
Franks, S., 815
Freeman, M. L., 887
Fröhlich, W., 565,591
Fujii, Yutaka, 85
Funk, Colin D., 33,41,577
Furci, Lucinda, 33,577

G
Galli, C., 233,743
Galli, G., 327,939
Gallo, S., 909
Galmiche, J. P., 855
Gambassi, F., 533
Garaci, E., 851,867
Gardiner, P., 473
Garland, Lawrence G., 109
Garlicki, J., 793
Garrick, R., 701
Gatta, A., 689
Gelpí, E., 501,573
Gemzell, K., 799
Génot, E., 997
Ghaderi, Abbas A., 983
Gialdroni Grassi, G., 445
Giampietri, A., 917
Gibel, L., 489
Giesen, C., 565
Giraldi, T., 913
Glaser, Keith B., 249
Glasgow, Wayne C., 843
Goel, R. K., 785
Goetzl, E. J., 399
Goldin, Barry R., 245
Goldyne, M. E., 835
Goldyne, S. Z., 835
Goodman, A., 701
Goodrum, D. D., 367
Goodwin, J. S., 489
Gorbach, Sherwood L., 245

Gordon, John, 983
Gorman, Robert R., 73
Gove, C., 697
Granström, Elisabeth F., 295,441, 615
Gravelle, Francine, 181
Gréen, Krister, 153,165,529,607
Grelli, S., 851
Grimes, David, 477
Grose, J. H., 145
Gryglewski, R. J., 655
Gundel, Robert H., 457
Gurevich, N., 731

H

Haas, T. A., 667,909
Haeggström, Jesper, 41,133
Hagmann, W., 493
Haines, Kathleen A., 545
Hallée, A., 437
Halushka, Perry V., 331
Hamanaka, N., 359,411,599
Hamberg, Mats, 117,441
Hanasaki, K., 363
Hansbrough, J. R., 37
Harada, Yoshiteru, 429
Harb, J., 855
Harel, S., 749
Harford, A. M., 489
Harper, M. J. K., 819
Hawkey, C. J., 777
Hawksworth, Richard J., 415
Hayaishi, Osamu, 85,371,723
Hayakawa, M., 569
Hayashi, Hideya, 85
Heaslip, Richard J., 477
Hedqvist, Per, 429,537
Heim, Kurt F., 637
Heindl, J., 565
Henriksson, Peter, 165
Henriques, R. D., 573
Her, E., 265
Hill, Kristina E., 125
Hirai, Aizan, 827
Hirata, Masaharu, 339,859

Holtzman, M. J., 37
Honda, Atsushi, 45
Honn, Kenneth V., 895
Hopfer, Ulrich, 205
Hornstra, G., 225,237
Hosford, D., 929
Hoshiko, Shigeru, 1
Hotter, G., 573
Houillon, G., 855
Howarth, P., 449
Huber, M., 395
Hudson, N., 777
Hughes, K. T., 303
Humphray, J. M., 379
Humphrey, P. P. A., 379
Hurst, S., 777

I

Iaquinto, G., 781
Ichikawa, A., 891
Ikeda, S., 453
Imawaka, H., 599
Imura, Yoshimi, 943
Irie, A., 891
Irwin, Carl, 273
Ishii, A., 465
Ito, Seiji, 371
Izawa, Y., 569
Izumi, T., 101

J

Jackson, William P., 109
Jacques, Crawford, 415
Jakobsson, Per-Johan, 663,1005
Jakschik, B. A., 261,493
Jedlitschky, G., 395
Jiyi, Fu, 45
Johansson, Gunnar, 429
Johansson, Helene, 461
Jones, D., 161
Jones, R. L., 375

K

Kaever, Volkhard, 169
Kaiser, I., 493
Kaley, Gabor, 595

Kamamaka, Y., 599
Kanayasu, Toshie, 623
Kasamo, M., 819
Katori, M., 771
Katz, N., 649
Kawabe, T., 989
Kawasaki, A., 359,407,411,453,599
Keery, R. J., 603
Keppler, D., 395
Kiel, D., 403
Kindahl, Hans, 295
King, Barbara, 461
Kishi, M., 363
Kishikawa, K., 407
Kivits, G. A. A., 225
Koizumi, K., 891
Kolb, J. P., 997
Koller, Akos, 595
Komatsu, N., 21
Konno, M., 411
Konturek, S. J., 793
Kosaka, K., 569
Koshihara, Yasuko, 847
Kostka-Trabka, E., 655
Koyama, Y., 723
Kraemer, Stacey A., 65
Krais, T., 583
Krauss, A. H-P., 367
Krzyzek, E., 793
Kuhn, M., 503
Kulmacz, Richard J., 137
Kumegawa, M., 53
Kumlin, Maria, 89,441,461,537
Kuniewski, B., 749
Kurz, G., 395
Kusaka, M., 53

L
Labat, C., 473
Landry, J., 145
Lane, J., 659
Laneuville, O., 731
Lanzio, M., 789
Laporte, J., 437

Larsson, O., 41
Laurent, J. P., 929
Lawson, John, 193
Lazer, Edward S., 457
Lebel, M., 145
Le Bodic, L., 855
Lee, D. Y., 303
Lee, Tak H., 415
Lefrak, E., 649
Leier, I., 395
Leithauser, Marie T., 895
Lellouche, Franck, 611
León, O. S., 573
Leroy, M. J., 811
Letari, O., 257
Lin, Alice H., 73
Lindgren, Jan Åke, 89,97,883
Litime, M. H., 811
Liu, Leo X., 509
Lonigro, Andrew J., 421
Loose-Mitchell, D., 149
López-Boado, M. A., 573
Lumley, P., 603

M
Maass, B., 591
Macchia, L., 41
Machunsky, Christine, 671
Maclouf, Jacques, 177,319,611
Macoviak, J., 649
Maderna, P., 233
Madhun, Zuhayr T., 205
Maeda, Y., 989
Maekawa, N., 989
Maezaki, Naoyoshi, 943
Magee, David E., 347
Maghni, K., 437
Magni, F., 327,939
Mahanian, Fariba, 229
Mais, Dale E., 331,347
Majka, J., 793
Mallet, A. I., 557
Mannaioni, P. F., 533
Mantovani, M., 711
Marnett, Lawrence J., 81,895

Marriott, D., 739
Martin, C., 929
Martin, R. C., 303
Marugo, M., 781
Maruyama, T., 407
Masciarelli, M., 445
Masferrer, Jaime L., 45
Masini, E., 533
Mason-Garcia, Meredith, 831
Mastino, A., 851
Masuda, Atsushi, 331
Matsumoto, R., 599
Matsumura, H., 723
Matsunaga, N., 407
Matthews, J. S., 375
Mayumi, M., 989
McGiff, J. C., 209, 675
McLeod, L. J., 157
Meade, Elizabeth A., 65
Medina, J. F., 41
Melis, M., 521
Melli, M., 291
Meredith, M. J., 887
Merendino, A. M., 521
Metz, S., 287
Meydani, Simin Nikbin, 245
Mikawa, H., 989
Miki, Ichiro, 387
Mitchell, S. N., 823
Miyamoto, T., 407, 411, 465, 891
Miyata, Atsuro, 61
Miyazaki, T., 359
Mizushima, Y., 465
Momper, Rita, 645
Moore, K. P., 697
Moran, Niamh, 577
Mori, Trevor A., 229
Morinelli, Thomas A., 331
Morita, Ikuo, 623, 839
Morrill-Labrode, Ann, 245
Morrison, Aubrey R., 273
Morrow, Jason D., 125, 315, 433
Mosconi, C., 233
Motoishi, M., 465

Mugridge, K. G., 517
Müller, M., 395
Müller, B., 583, 591
Mullmann, Theodore J., 281
Murota, Sei-itsu, 623, 839
Murphy, R. C., 177, 185, 525
Murray, Rosemary, 577

N
Naka, Masao, 331, 599
Nakae, T., 411
Nakagawa, T., 465
Nakajima, Masakazu, 339
Nakamura, Motonao, 113, 387
Nakano, T., 277
Nakano-Hayashi, Junko, 623
Nambu, F., 453, 465
Nammour, Tarek M., 125
Narumiya, Shuh, 339
Näsman-Glaser, Barbro, 883
Nathan, M. H., 17
Natsui, K., 21
Needleman, Philip, 45
Negishi, Manabu, 371, 891
Nenci, G. G., 917
Nicosia, S., 257
Niederhauser, U., 503
Nigam, Santosh, 553, 925
Nishikawa, Kohei, 173, 943
Nishimura, Motonobu, 185, 827
Nishiyama, K., 771
Norel, X., 473
Nüsing, R., 307

O
Oates, John A., 315
Oatis, John E. Jr., 331
Odeimat, A., 311
Odenwaller, Rebecca, 81
Odlander, Björn, 133, 1005
Ogawa, T., 569
Ogunc, S., 701
Ohara, O., 277

O'Hickey, Stephen P., 415
Ohishi, Nobuya, 387
Ohkawa, Sigenori, 173
Ohlson, E., 441
Ohno, Kouji, 859
Ohno, T., 771
Okegawa, T., 453, 599
Okuda-Ashitaka, Emiko, 371
Okuma, Minoru, 339
Okwu, Anselm K., 331
Oliw, Ernst H., 197
Omawari, N., 453
Onoe, H., 723
Oshima, T., 53
Owen, William F. Jr., 481
Ozawa, T., 569

P

Pace, E., 521
Pace-Asciak, C. R., 731
Pai, Jin-Keon, 281
Palmblad, Jan, 561,883
Palmer, Graham, 137
Palmertz, Ulla, 537
Pankhania, J. J., 113
Papin, J. P., 975
Parente, L., 291,517
Parker, J., 659
Parodi, M. C., 781
Patrice, T., 855
Patrono, C., 619,707
Pek, S. B., 17
Perissin, L., 913
Perretti, M., 517
Persson, L., 615
Perzborn, E., 355
Peskar, B. M., 753
Petersson, A. S., 615
Petroni, A., 743
Pettitt, T. R., 557
Phillips, Catherine, 497
Picado, C., 501
Piper, P. J., 469
Pistelli, A., 533

Plaza, V., 501
Plebani, M., 689
Poggioli, J., 997
Police, R. J., 201
Pommier, J., 929
Poubelle, P. E., 311
Powell, William S., 181
Pozzi, E., 445
Pradelles, Philippe, 319
Prakash, Chandra, 315
Pralong, Etienne, 735
Prino, G., 711
Prior, G., 383
Pugliese, F., 707
Puig Parellada, P., 573

Q

Quadros, E., 767

R

Rådmark, Olof, 1,41,101,133,663
Ralston, T. L., 367
Ramis, I., 501
Ramwell, Peter W., 637
Rapozzi, V., 913
Rasmanis, Gundars, 165
Raud, Johan, 537
Raugei, G., 291
Raz, Amiram, 45
Rea, L., 835
Reeves, J. J., 379
Reiss, N., 265
Ren, Yong, 137
Renard, D., 997
Resch, Klaus, 169
Richards, Karen M., 895
Rigotti, P., 689
Ringertz, Bo, 561
Ringotti, P., 689
Ritter, J. M., 351
Roberts, L. Jackson II, 125,315,433, 887
Roberts, M. S., 157
Robidoux, C., 437

Robillard, L., 855
Robinson, C., 449
Rodriguez, Louis, 429
Rolland, A., 929
Romano, Mario, 93
Romero, Michael F., 205
Rosellò, J., 501,573
Rosén, Anders, 1005
Rosolowsky, M., 213
Rossoni, G., 327,711,939
Rowley, A. F., 557

S

Sacerdoti, D., 689
Sáenz, A., 573
Saito, Hiroyuki, 241
Saito, Ichiro, 241
Sakuyama, S., 411
Sala, A., 177,525
Salmon, John A., 109
Salvati, P., 707
Samuelsson, Bengt, 1,101
Samuelsson, Jan, 883
Sánchez, J., 573
Sandbrink, R., 395
Sanduja, R., 141,149
Santoro, M. G., 867
Saussy, David L. Jr., 331,347
Sawada, M., 453
Schärer, Karl, 645
Schillinger, E., 583,901
Schirner, M., 901
Schneider, M. R., 901
Schröder, G., 591
Schröder, Henning, 671
Schrör, Karsten, 671
Schulz, B. G., 591
Schwartz, J. H., 715
Schwartzman, Michal Laniado, 185
Schweer, Horst, 645
Secombes, C. J., 557
Seibert, K., 45
Seki, Koichi, 827
Seko, T., 359

Sellmayer, Alois, 217
Semenzato, G., 445
Seo, R., 407
Serhan, Charles N., 93,105,509,553
Seuter, F., 355
Seyama, Yousuke, 387
Seyberth, Hannsjörg W., 645
Shannon, V. R., 37
Shapiro, E., 715
Sharp, G. J. E., 557
Sheff, Daniel M., 481
Sheldrick, R. L. G., 379
Sheller, J. R., 433
Shen, S. T., 701
Shibouta, Yumiko, 173
Shida, T., 465
Shield, Michael J., 955
Shimizu, Takao, 387
Shimokawa, T., 77
Shipp, Elizabeth, 193
Shopp, G. M., 489
Siegel, Marvin I., 281
Siegelbaum, S. A., 727
Sigal, Elliot, 25
Simonson, Michael S., 69
Sirois, P., 437
Sirtori, C. R., 233
Skuballa, W., 565,901
Sladek, K., 433
Sloane, David L., 25
Smith, A. Y., 489
Smith, S. K., 823
Smith, W. L., 77
Snyder, D. S., 921
Sodano, Guido, 129
Solito, E., 291
Soo, Cynthia, 245
Spatafora, M., 521
Spinella, Aldo, 129
Spitzer, T., 525
Sprague, Randy S., 421
Spur, Bernd W., 415
Stables, R., 379
Stamford, I. F., 875

Stanworth, Dennis R., 983
Stark, Ron, 461
Stenke, Leif, 97,883
Stephenson, Alan H., 421
Sterling, W. A., 489
Stewart-Long, P., 351
Stock, G., 583
Stragliotto, E., 233
Strobach, Hans, 671
Sturm, Robert J., 477
Stürzebecher, S., 901
Subramanian, N., 503
Sugama, Kazushige, 371
Sugiyama, S., 569
Sullivan, M. H. F., 807
Suzuki, H., 29
Suzuki, Yoshiharu, 839
Swahn, M. L., 799
Sweetman, B. J., 887

T

Tak, C., 879
Takahashi, Kihito, 683
Takahashi, Y., 37
Takai, T., 29,53
Takamori, Riko, 847
Takatani, Muneo, 943
Tamura, Yasushi, 241,827
Tan, K. C., 697
Tanabe, Tadashi, 29,53,61
Tanaka, M., 989
Tang, Wilson, 863
Tavares, I. A., 785
Taylor, G. W., 697
Terao, Shinji, 173
Teraoka, H., 277
Terashita, Yumiko, 173
Terashita, Zen-ichi, 173,943
Tettamanti, R., 711
Thierauch, K-H., 383,591
Thomas, George, 637
Toda, M., 407
Toh, Hiroyuki, 61
Tönshoff, Burkhard, 645

Torcellini, Carol A., 457
Toriyama, Kazuhiro, 839
Toto, Robert D., 967
Tou, Jen-sie, 831
Tranter, P. R., 807
Tremoli, E., 233
Trentin, L., 445
Tsai, Ah-Lim, 137,141
Tsushima, Susumu, 943

U

Ueda, N., 21,37
Uedelhoven, W., 225
Ueno, A., 771
Ullrich, V., 307
Urade, Yoshihiro, 85
Ushikubi, Fumitaka, 339

V

van Dam-Mieras, M. C. E., 237
van den Bemd, G. J. C. M., 879
Vandogen, Robert, 229
Vane, John R., 627
van Houwelingen, A. C., 225
Verhallen, P. F. J., 591
Veronesi, Arianna, 983
Vesin, Marie-Francoise, 735
Vesterqvist, Ole, 153,165,529,607
Vial, J. H., 157
Viganò, T., 445
Villani, Guido, 129
Visioli, F., 743
Voelkel, N., 177
Volpes, D., 521
Volterra, A., 727
von Sprecher, A., 503
Vossen, R. C. R. M., 237

W

Wakitani, K., 599
Walsh, S., 449
Watanabe, Kikuko, 21,85
Watanabe, Y., 723
Waters, N. M., 303

Watts, I. S., 603
Weber, P. C., 217
Wegner, Craig D., 457
Weichman, Barry M., 477
Weissmann, Gerald, 545
Welch, William J., 693
Weller, Peter F., 509
Wennmalm, Å., 615
Wetterholm, Anders, 133
Wharton, K. A., 603
White, B. P., 603
Whitney, Jeff, 461
Whittle, B. J. R., 761
Wilcox, Christopher S., 693
Wilkin, G. P., 739
Williams, Carl M., 347
Williams, L. S., 367
Williams, R., 697
Wilson, D. E., 767
Wilson, N. H., 375
Winell, S., 615
Winitz, S., 161
Witt, W., 901
Wolfe, Julie A., 69
Wong, P. Y-K., 701
Wood, J. N., 697,739
Woods, Margo M., 245
Woodward, D. F., 367
Wu, Kenneth K., 141,149
Wu, P., 731

X
Xu, L., 261

Y
Yamamoto, S., 21,29,37,53,895
Yamaoka, Kunio A., 1005
Yamauchi, R., 891
Yancey, L. M., 201
Yavin, E., 749
Yodoi, J., 989
Yokoo, K., 569
Yokoyama, Chieko, 29,53,61
Yoshida, Setsuko, 827
Yoshida, Sho, 241,827
Yoshimoto, T., 29,53,895
Young O'Gara, Coleen, 81
Yube, N., 453
Yui, Y., 465

Z
Zackert, William E., 315
Zakrzewicz, Andreas, 925
Zembowicz, A., 655
Zetterström, Olle, 429,441,461
Zhao, Y., 525,649
Ziboh, Vincent A., 863
Zipkin, R. E., 403
Zor, U., 265
Zorzet, S., 913
Zurier, Robert B., 947
Zwaal, R. F. A., 237

*Bishai, I., 480a
*Coceani, F., 480a
*Hynes, N., 480a
*Lees, J., 480a

---

*added at press time

CHARACTERIZATION OF THE PROMOTER OF THE HUMAN 5-LIPOXYGENASE GENE

Bengt Samuelsson, Shigeru Hoshiko*, and Olof Rådmark

*Department of Physiological Chemistry
Karolinska Institutet
S-104 01 Stockholm, Sweden*

* Permanent address: Pharmaceutical Laboratories, Meiji Seika Kaisha Ltd., Kohoku-ku, Yokohama 222 (Japan)

ABBREVIATIONS

base pair(s) (bp); kilobase pairs (kb); chloramphenicool acetyltransferase (CAT); 12-O-tetradecanoylphorbol 13-acetate (TPA); dimethyl sulfoxide (DMSO); 5-lipoxygenase (5-LO).

The enzyme 5-lipoxygenase (arachidonate:oxygen 5-oxidoreductase, EC 1.13.11.34) catalyzes formation of 5(S)-hydroperoxy-6-trans-6,11,14-cis-eicosatetraenoic acid (5HPETE) from arachidonic acid, as well as the following step in leukotriene biosynthesis, viz. the conversion of 5-HPETE to leukotriene A_4 (LTA$_4$, 5(S),6-oxido-7,9,11-trans-14-cis-eicosatetraenoic acid). The enzyme was purified from several sources, and clones corresponding to 5-lipoxygenase have been isolated from cDNA libraries derived from human placenta, differentiated HL60 cells, and rat basophilic leukemia cells (reviewed in ref 13). Also the human 5-lipoxygenase gene has been isolated and characterized (4). Several features of the putative promoter region were characteristic for so called house keeping genes (3) (no TATAA nor CCAAT, GC-rich, multiple GGGCGG sequences). Here, we report on further studies regarding the 5-LO gene promoter. A sequence containing five GGGCGG repeats was required for efficient transcription of CAT gene constructs and gel shift assays showed that the transcriptional factor Sp1 could bind to DNA containing this GC-rich region. For methodology, it is referred to the original paper (6).

RESULTS

<u>Identification of the promoter region</u>. Chimaeric genes between various parts of the 5-LO gene promoter and the CAT reporter gene were constructed. Thus, the region (-5900 to +20) was excised from the genomic clone 1x 12A (4), and

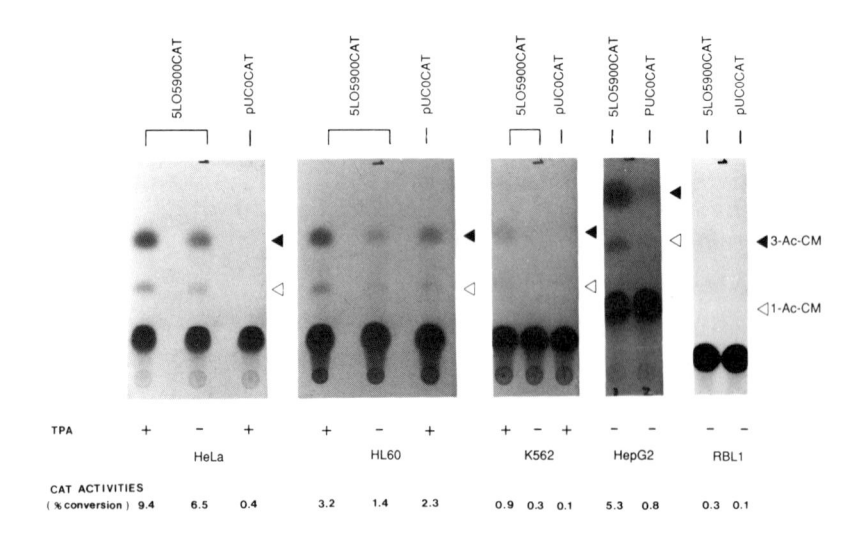

Fig. 1 Human 5-lipoxygenase promoter-driven expression of chloramphenicol acetyltransferase. The autoradiograms show the conversion of [^{14}C] chloramphenicol to monoacetylated derivatives by extracts from HeLa, HL60, K562, HepG2 and RBL1 which were transfected with 20 μg of 5LO5900CAT and pUC0CAT (negative control plasmid lacking promoter) respectively. Extracts (250 to 1000 μg of proteins, equivalent amounts for each set of experiments) were used. Transfected cells were treated with (+) or without (-) TPA (30 ng/ml) from 24 hr to 48 hr after transfection. The amounts of acetylated [^{14}C] chloramphenicol was determined on thin layer chromatography plates. Following autoradiography the acetylated products were excised and counted in a liquid scintilation counter. Positions of chloramphenicol (CM), 1-acetyl chloramphenicol (1-AcCM) and 3-acetylchloramphenicol (3-AcCM) are indicated by the arrows. Also, the percentage conversions of [^{14}C] chloramphenicol to acetylated forms are shown.

inserted to a plasmid already containing the CAT reporter gene (+1 is A in ATG start codon). The resulting plasmid (5LO5900CAT) was transiently introduced to HeLa and HepG2 cells, as well as to the myeloid cell lines HL60, K562 and RBL1. It was clear that the 5900 bp DNA fragment had promoter activity in all cell tested (Fig. 1). Before further analysis of the 5-LO gene promoter, it was also confirmed that CAT expression observed after transfection with 5LOCAT derivatives, was truly under control of the 5-LO gene promoter. For this purpose poly(A)+ RNA was prepared from HeLa cells transfected with three different 5LOCAT-constructs, and the transcriptional initiation sites for the chimaeric RNA species were determined by S1 nuclease protection assay. RNA-DNA hybrids originating between nucleotides -65 and -62 were found. This is practically identical to the initiation of 5-LO gene transcription in human leukocytes, showing that observed CAT activities were really controlled by the 5-LO gene promoter.

Deletion analysis of the promoter region. A set of plasmids with different deletions in the 5-LO gene promoter was constructed. HeLa cells were transfected with the various constructs. The resulting CAT activities, reflecting the activities of the corresponding promoters, are shown in Fig. 2. First, evidence for the essential role for a -179 to -56 DNA stretch (containing the transcriptional initiation sites and most of the GC-boxes) were obtained. When this DNA segment was absent, the promoter activity decreased considerably (in both HeLa and HL-60 cells). Also, succesive deletion mutants (in the downstream direction from the KpnI site at -5900) revealed two positive regulatory elements (-5900 to -3700 and -931 to -854) and two negative regulatory elements (-3400 and -1557, and -727 and -292).

Specific interaction of the 5-LO gene promoter region with nuclear proteins from HeLa and HL60 cells. A NarI-BglII fragment containing the DNA (-212 to -88) essential for promoter activity, was excised from the plasmid 5LO292-88CAT. After radiolabelling with [α-^{32}P] dideoxy ATP and terminal deoxynucleotidyl transferase, binding of proteins from nuclear extracts to the probe was examined by gel retardation assay. First, nuclear extracts from HeLaS3 cells were examined. The nonadherant HeLaS3 cells were used in this case, for convenient preparation of nuclear proteins. When gel retardation assay was performed with HeLa proteins, in presence of the nonspecific competitor poly(dI-dC), a number of shifted bands appeared in the electrophoresis, the two major

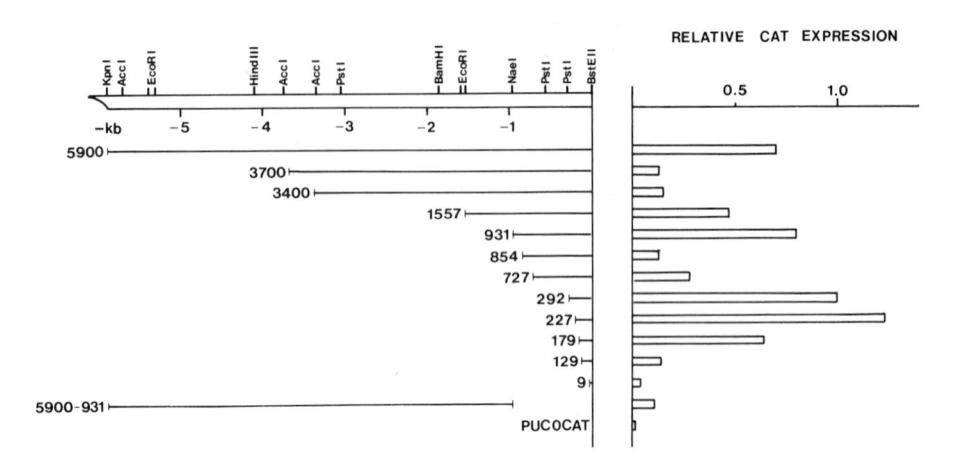

Fig. 2 Structure and activity of 5LOCAT chimaeric genes. HeLa cells (1 to 2 x 10⁶ cells) were transfected with 20 μg of the recombinant plasmids, carrying various parts of the 5-LO gene promoter. Also, 1 or 2 μg of a plasmid carrying the luciferase gene (pSV2ALΔ5') was included in all transfections, allowing for normalization of differing transfection efficiencies. CAT assays were performed using 250 to 500 μg of cellular protein, incubation times were 2 to 6 hr (at 37°C). The DNA fragment derived from the 5-lipoxygenase genomic clone lx12A (4), is shown on top as a wide bar. Representative restriction enzyme cleavage sites are shown above the bar. Nucelotide positions of the 5' flanking sequence are numbered in negative from the translation start codon. The normalized CAT activities of transfected HeLa cells are expressed in relation to the values obtained with 5LO292CAT.

are marked with arrows in Fig. 3A. Next, the assay was performed in presence of monomers of the Sp1 competitor oligonucleotide (d(GGGGCGGGGCTCGA)), the shifted bands were still formed. However in presence of concatemers of the Sp1 competitor, (d(GGGGCGGGGCTCGA)n) formation of the shifted bands was inhibited. The results indicate that the transcription factor Sp1 was present in the HeLa cell nuclear extracts, and that it can bind to the stretch of promoter region (-212 to -88). In line with this finding, the -212 to -88 stretch contains six (out of total ten) GC-boxes (the putative Sp1 binding motifs).

Nuclear extracts were also prepared from HL60 cells, either nondifferentiated or after treatment with TPA (24 hr) or DMSO (120 hr). When gel retardation assays were carried out with the three different HL60 extracts, shifted bands appeared in all three preparations (see arrows in Fig. 3B; no difference between nondifferentiated and differentiated cells). However,

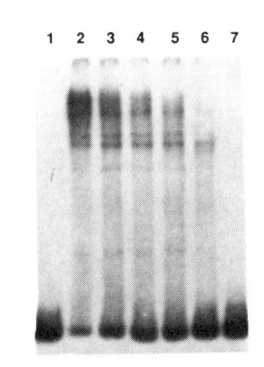

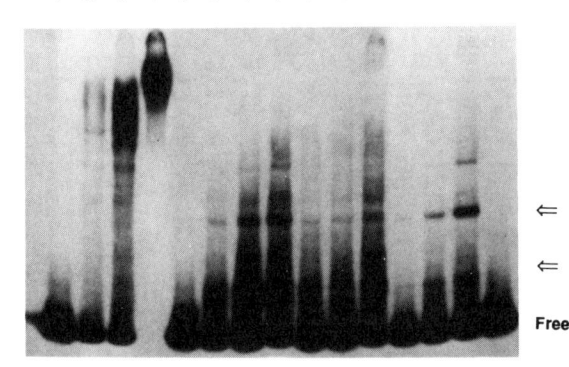

Fig. 3 Gel retardation analysis of nuclear protein extracts from HeLa and HL60 cells. **A.** Binding reactions were conducted using the radiolabeled NarI-BglII fragment (2×10^5 cpm, 90 fmol, 3.5 ng), poly(dI-dC) (200 µg/ml) and nuclear extracts from HeLa cells (2 µg of protein). Lanes 1 and 7 : No extract, probe alone; Lane 2: Probe with extract; Lane 3: Probe plus 50 molar excess of monomer Sp1 competitor, with extract; Lane 4: Probe plus 250 molar excess of monomer competitor, with extract; Lane 5: Probe plus 50 molar excess of concatemer form of Sp1 competitor, with extract; Lane 6: Probe plus 250 molar excess of concatemer competitor, with extract. Bands whose appearance were blocked by the concatemer form of the Sp1 competitor are indicated by arrows, as well as the position of the free DNA. **B.** Comparison of gel retardation patterns obtained with HeLa and HL60 nuclear extracts. Binding reactions were performed as in A. Lane 1,5 and 15: No extract, probe alone; Lane 2-4: Probe plus extract of HeLa cells (1.0, 3.0 and 9.0 µg of protein respectively) ; Lane 6-8: Probe plus extract of nontreated HL60 cells (1.0, 3.0 and 9.0 µg of protein, respectively) ; Lane 9-11: Probe plus extract of TPA treated HL60 cells (1.0, 3.0 and 9.0 µg of protein, respectively); Lane 12-14 : Probe plus extract of DMSO treated HL60 cells (1.0, 3.0 and 9.0 µg of protein, respectively). Distinct bands which are observed with HL60 nuclear extracts are indicated by the arrows.

these novel bands were not present in assays with nuclear proteins from HeLa cells. On the other hand the major bands obtained with HeLa nuclear protein were poorly formed with HL60 nuclear protein. This indicates that different factors binding to the 5-LO promoter region are present in HeLa and HL60 cells respectively.

DISCUSSION

Expression of the human 5-LO gene appears to be regulated in a cell specific manner. Substantial production of 5-LO metabolites is well documented for cells of myeloid lineage such as granulocytes, basophils and macrophages. Differentiation of immature cells to granulocytes or macrophage lineage is associated with enhanced 5-LO activity, exemplified by studies using HL60 cells (8) and chicken myelomonocytic cells (5). Our observations regarding transacting factors binding to the 5-LO gene promoter, apparently specific for HL-60 cells, may reflect the cell specific expression of 5-LO.

Endogenous 5-LO mRNA was present in HL60 cells (particularly after induction of differentiation by DMSO), but it was not at all detectable in HeLa cells. The probable reason for the observed expression of the chimaeric genes in HeLa cells, in spite of this cell being nonpermissive for expression of endogenous 5-LO, is that additional negative regulatory region(s) and/or positive regulatory region(s) specific for particular cells such as DMSO-differentiated HL60 cells, are located outside the analyzed part of the promoter. For the 5-LO gene, this implies that such regulatory elements should be present upstream of the -5900 KpnI site or in intron sequences. Similar findings have been presented in several other reports, i.e., that chimaeric gene with a certain promoter was active in cells that were nonpermissive for the gene of origin. For HeLa cells in particular, previous examples of this phenomenon are ε-globin (1) and retinol binding protein (2).

In order to identify regulatory DNA elements of the 5'-portion, a 1844 nucleotides stretch of the 5-LO gene promoter was sequenced. Several motifs were recognized as possible cis-acting sequences, binding to characterized transcriptional factors (10). The ten Spl to binding core motifs have already been mentioned. Five of these were located in a cluster. Deletion of promoter DNA involving the five clustered Sp1 binding motifs, caused drastic losses of CAT activity of transfected cells.

The transcriptional factor AP-2 mediates many effects of TPA on gene expression (9). Sequences similar to the AP-2 binding motif were identified in the 5-LO gene promoter, at -135 and -302. Thus the apparent TPA-stimulation of CAT activities in cells transfected with 5-LO gene promoter chimaeras (Fig. 1) may reflect regulation of 5-LO gene expression possibly related to TPA-primed cell differentiation. However, it might be premature to propose a mechanism for 5-LO gene regulation involving TPA, since it is unclear if TPA actually stimulates expression of endogeneous 5-LO.

Finally, a DNA sequence was found, which matched the binding motif for the myb protooncogene product previously described for the mim-1 gene promoter (7). A study using chicken myelomonocytic cells and myb containing oncovirus indicated a downregulatory effect of the myb protein on 5-LO gene expression with concomitant inhibition of macrophage lineage differentiation (5). Another observation in line with this reasoning, is that c-myb protooncogene expression was found to decline in HL60 cells during maturation (11).

The rabbit erythroid cell specific 15-lipoxygenase gene was recently cloned and sequenced (12). Comparison with the human 5-LO gene revealed similarities as well as differencies. Most striking was the identical exon/intron organizations of the 5-LO and 15-LO genes. This provides a strong argument for the development of the lipoxygenase family from a common ancestral gene. Regarding the promoter, also the 15-LO gene was GC-rich and one putative Sp1 binding GC-box was identified in the promoter region, showing similarity to house keeping gene promoters. The similar gene organizations of the human 5-LO and the rabbit 15-LO genes suggest conserved expression mechanisms. However the different cell specificities of expression of the various lipoxygenases indicates that different regulatory DNA elements should have been added to the genes in this family, after gene divergence.

ACKNOWLEDGEMENTS

We thank Suresh Subramani, George Khoury and Cornelia M. Gorman for providing various plasmids required for these studies. We also thank Tsutomu Nakamura for discussions. This study was supported by fellowships from Meiji Seika Kaisha Ltd. (to S.H.) and by grants from the Swedish Medical Council (03X-217, 03X-7467).

REFERENCES

1. Cao, S.X., Gutman, P.D., Dave, H.P.D., and Schechter, A. (1989) : *Proc. Natl. Acad. Sci. USA.* **86**: 5306-5309.
2. Colantuoni, V., Pirozzi, A., Blance, C. , and Cortese, R. (1987): *EMBO. J.* **6**: 631-636.
3. Dynan, W.S. (1986): *Trends Genet.* **2**: 196-197.
4. Funk, C.D., Hoshiko, S., Matsumoto, T., Rådmark, O., and Samuelsson, B. (1989): *Proc. Natl. Acad. Sci. USA.* **86**: 2587- 2591.
5. Habenicht, A.J.R., Goerig, M., Rotche, D.E.R., Specht, E., Ziegler, R., Glomset, J.A. and Graf, T. (1989): *Proc. Natl. Acad. Sci. USA.* **86**: 921-924.
6. Hoshiko, S., Rådmark, O., and Samuelsson, B. (1990): *Proc. Natl. Acad. Sci. USA,* in press.
7. Imagawa, M., Chiu, R., and Karin, M. (1987): *Cell* **51**: 251-260.
8. Kargman, S., Rouzer, C.A. (1989): *J. Biol. Chem.* **264**: 13313-13320.
9. Lenardo, M., and Baltimore, D. (1989): *Cell* **8**: 227-229.
10. Mitchell, P.J., and Tjian, R. (1989): *Science* **245**: 371-378.
11. Ness, S.A., Marknell, Å., and Graf, T. (1989): *Cell* **59**: 1115-1125.
12. O'Prey, J., Chester, J., Thiele, B.J., Janetzki, S., Prehn, S., Fleming, J., and Harrison, P.R. (1989): Gene **84**: 493-499
13. Samuelsson, B., and Funk, C.D. (1989): *J. Biol. Chem.* **264**: 19469-19472.

REGULATION OF THE PRODUCTION AND ACTION OF LEUKOTRIENES BY MK-571 AND MK-886

A. W. Ford-Hutchinson

Merck Frosst Centre for Therapeutic Research
P. O. Box 1005
Pointe-Claire-Dorval
Quebec H9R 4P8
Canada

INTRODUCTION

Leukotrienes have been proposed as key mediators of various human diseases including bronchial asthma. Because of this, therapeutic approaches to either inhibit the production or antagonize the action of these mediators have been developed. One approach has been to develop highly selective, potent leukotriene D_4 receptor antagonists and an example of such a compound, MK-571 (7), is described below together with an outline of some of the clinical data obtained to date in normal individuals and asthmatic patients. An alternative approach is to inhibit the production of all leukotrienes by blocking the action of the enzyme 5-lipoxygenase. This will prevent not only the synthesis of the peptidolipid leukotrienes, which appear to be important mediators of human asthma, but also of leukotriene B_4 which may be an important mediator of inflammatory conditions, such as inflammatory bowel disease. Up until recently the majority of 5-lipoxygenase inhibitors described can be classified as "redox" compounds. Such compounds include phenols, quinones, flavones and hydroxamic acids which all have the potential to reduce the enzyme (presumably by reducing the iron at the active site), and in doing so may generate radical intermediates through a pseudoperoxidase cycle. It also seems likely that the more potent the inhibitor the more likely it is that the radical species generated by the enzyme may be highly reactive and may form covalent adducts with macromolecules. Redox inhibitors may also react with other redox-based biological systems, a common problem being the formation of methemoglobin in dogs. Such inhibitors have other problems including insolubility, poor bioavailability, rapid metabolism and problems in showing biochemical efficacy *in vivo*. An alternative approach is through the use of leukotriene biosynthesis inhibitors, such as MK-886 (5), and the elucidation of the novel mechanism of action of this compound is described below.

MK-571

MK-571 (structure as shown in Figure 1) is a racemate, the two enantiomers both being potent, selective, orally active leukotriene D_4 receptor antagonists (7). During the development process one of the individual entantiomers, MK-679, has shown some advantages and is currently under development. However, all the published data so far relates to MK-571 and this will be described below. MK-571 has a high affinity for leukotriene D_4 receptor sides on both guinea-pig and human lung parenchymal membranes (IC_{50} values ~ 1 and 8 nM respectively). The compound is a potent competitive inhibitor or leukotriene D_4 responses on multiple smooth muscle preparations from both man and the guinea-pig and is highly selective in that it does not affect contractions induced by a variety of other spasmogens. In addition, MK-571 has shown potent activity in a number of antigen challenge animal models providing pre-clinical evidence that leukotrienes may have an important role in antigen-induced bronchoconstriction in man.

Early clinical trials with MK-571 have been carried out using intravenous infusions which have allowed for an accurate correlation of clinical efficacy with therapeutic blood levels. Studies in normal volunteers are summarized in Table 1.

CLINICAL EXPERIENCE WITH MK-571 STUDIES IN NORMAL VOLUNTEERS

Human kinetics and tolerability of intravenous MK-571	The drug was well tolerated at doses up to 1500mg with maximum blood levels of 300 µg/ml	Van Hecken et al. Europ.J.Pharmacol. in press (4)
Antagonism of LTD_4-induced bronchoconstriction in man	Complete antagonism of LTD_4-induced responses at doses achieving plasma concentrations of 110,6 & 1 µg/ml. No effect on baseline airway function	Kips et al. Am.Rev.Respir.Dis. in press (8)

These studies have shown that the compound is extremely well tolerated by the intravenous route at doses up to 1500 mg which achieved mean maximal plasma concentrations of approximately 300 µg/ml. In these normal individuals no effect of the drug on baseline airway function was observed and in a second study the compound proved to be a potent antagonist of leukotriene D_4-induced bronchoconstriction. Subsequent studies have been carried out in asthmatic patients and are summarized in Table 2.

CLINICAL EXPERIENCE WITH MK-571 STUDIES IN ASTHMATIC PATIENTS

Antagonism of LTD_4-induced bronchoconstriction in asthmatic men	Increase in baseline airway calibre following infusion of MK-571. Induction of shifts in the LTD_4 dose response curve of ≥80- & ≥40-fold at plasma concentrations of 20 & 2 µg/ml	Kips et al. Europ.Resp.J.2, supplement 8(1989) (9)
Effects in mild to moderate asthma. Interactions with albuterol	Bronchodilatation with MK-571, no interference with the effects of albuterol. The effects of MK-571 and albuterol appear to be additive	Gaddy et al. J.Allergy Clin. Immunol.85,197A (1990) (4)
Attenuation of dual responses to inhaled antigen	Attenuation of early and late responses indicates that LTD_4 is an important mediator of antigen-induced responses	Hendeles et al. J.Allergy Clin. Immunol.85,197A (1990) (6)

Following LTD_4 challenge of asthmatic patients, MK-571, at doses which achieved plasma concentrations of approximately 20 and 2 µg/ml, produced shifts in the LTD dose response curves of ≥ 80- and ≥ 40-fold respectively. Unlike the studies in normal individuals the intravenous administration of MK-571 to asthmatic patients increased baseline airway calibre as measured by specific airway conductance. This suggests that leukotriene D_4 may contribute to basal airway tone in asthmatics and was confirmed in a subsequent study in twelve patients with mild to moderate asthma studied in a double blind placebo controlled, randomized, crossover study. In this trial MK-571 caused significant improvements in FEV_1 within twenty minutes of administration compared to placebo control. In addition the compound did not interfere with the bronchodilator effect of albuterol and interestingly the effects of albuterol and MK-571 appeared to be additive. Finally a study with MK-571 has shown that leukotriene D_4 is an important mediator of antigen-induced bronchoconstriction. In a randomized crossover study, highly significant attenuation of both the early and late phase bronchoconstrictor responses to inhaled antigen were observed. These results indicate that leukotriene D_4 may be an important mediator of human bronchial asthma and that leukotriene antagonists such as MK-571 or MK-679 may have therapeutic actions with minimal side effects. Chronic asthma studies with such compounds will be required to confirm such suggestions.

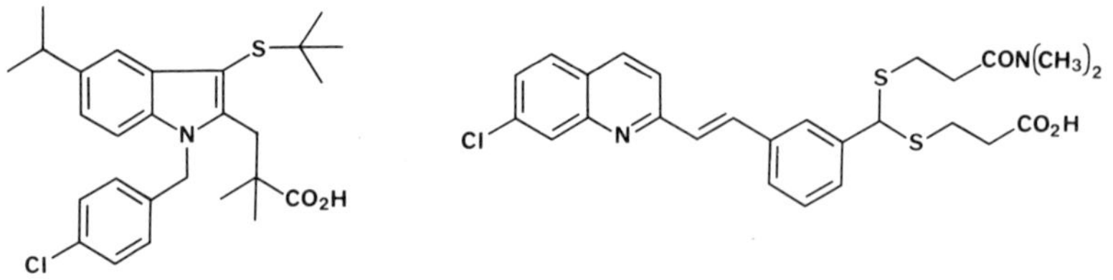

Figure 1. Structures of MK-571 and MK-886

MK-886

MK-886 is a potent inhibitor of the production of leukotrienes in a variety of intact cell types (neutrophils, eosinophils, mast cells and monocytes) exposed *in vitro* to a variety of stimuli. The compound is also a potent inhibitor of leukotriene production *in vivo* which is reflected in functional inhibition of antigen-induced bronchoconstriction in animal models. Although MK-886 inhibits leukotriene production in all intact cells examined to date and exposed to physiological stimuli, the compound has no effect on either the 5-lipoxygenase enzyme itself or on the availability of the substrate, arachidonic acid. A number of observations have suggested that 5-lipoxygenase might require an activation step before leukotriene synthesis could occur. In particular Rouzer and Kargman have demonstrated that following neutrophil activation, 5-lipoxygenase translocated from the cytosol to the cell membrane where it could be detected by western blot analysis as dead enzyme, presumably having undergone suicide inactivation (12). A clue to the mechanism of action of MK-886 came from similar studies in intact human polymorphonuclear leukocytes where MK-886 was shown to prevent, in a concentration dependent fashion, the translocation of 5-lipoxygenase to the membrane. In addition this inhibition of translocation could be correlated with inhibition of leukotriene biosynthesis for a range of structural analogs of MK-886 (13). These results suggested that translocation to the membrane was a key activation step for 5-lipoxygenase.

As MK-886 shows activity at nM concentrations this suggests that it binds to a molecular target with high affinity. In order to search for a putative binding protein two series of chemical tools were synthesized. The first were radioactive photoaffinity probes based on the structure of MK-886 and the second a series of affinity chromotography columns to which MK-886 or structural analogs were coupled with a variety of chemical linkages (11). Incubation of the photoaffinity probe (^{125}I-L-669,083 containing a photoactivatible azido group) with neutrophils, followed by irradiation with ultraviolet light resulted in the labelling of a number of proteins. However the labelling of only a single protein was specifically inhibited by MK-886, this protein having a molecular weight of 18kD. The 18kD protein was only present in the membrane (100,000 X g pellet) of leukocytes and was not present in a variety of other cell lines known not to have 5-lipoxygenase (11). Purification of the protein was achieved from CHAPS solubilized extracts of rat leukocyte membranes using affinity columns, elution with MK-886 and subsequent purification through Superose 12 and TSK-3000 columns (11). Sequence information on the rat protein was obtained from the native protein and cynogen bromide and tryptic cleavage products. Immunoprecipation experiments using a polyclonal rabbit antibody to the internal sequence of the rat protein demonstrated that the protein identified by the photoaffinity probe was the same as that purified by the affinity column. Using the partial amino acid sequence of the purified rat protein, cDNA clones were isolated from both rat RBL1 and human HL60 cell line cDNA libraries (3). Both cDNA clones encoded proteins of 161 amino acids which were 92% identical and contained all the peptide sequence derived from the originally purified rat protein. The proteins are very hydrophobic as indicated by hydropathy plots and which is consistent with their membrane localization. Using hydrophobic moment analysis three hydrophobic transmembrane spanning regions were predicted and thus the proposed structure of the protein consists of three transmembrane domains connected by two hydrophilic loops with the N and C termini on opposite sides of the membrane. This protein has been termed 5-lipoxygenase activating protein (FLAP). Comparison of sequence of FLAP with those of other proteins revealed that FLAP is not identical to any other known protein but does show some similarities to several integral membrane proteins. These similarities are with hydrophobic residues in the proposed transmembrane regions rather than significant primary sequence homologies.

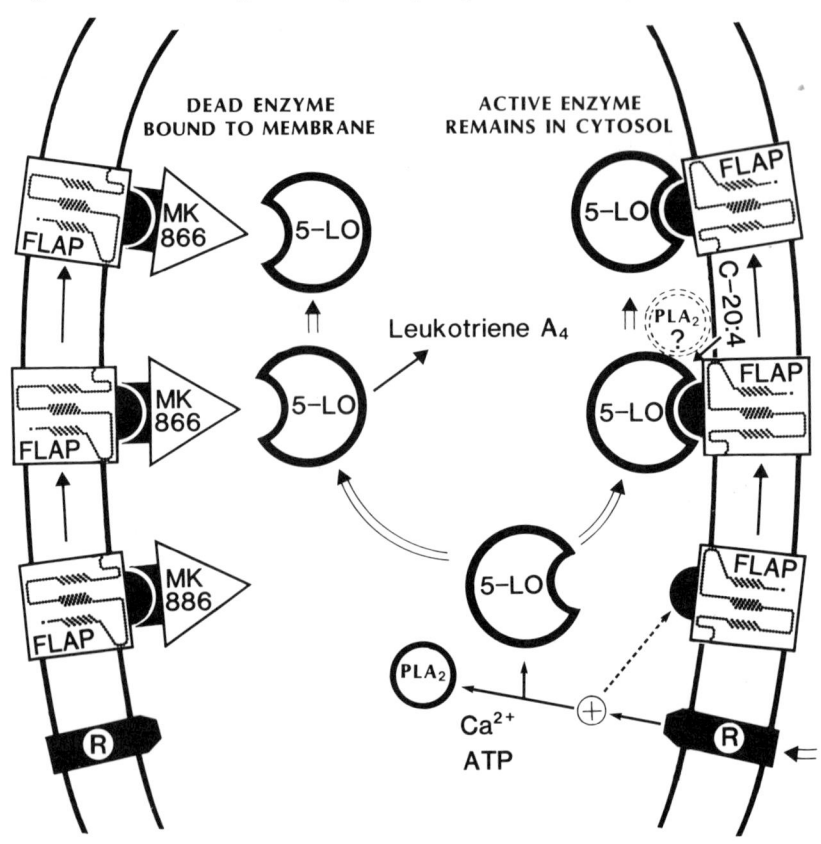

Figure 2. Involvement of FLAP and 5-lipoxygenase in leukotriene synthesis: inhibition by MK-886.

The next step was to demonstrate that the presence of FLAP was necessary for cellular leukotriene synthesis. This was achieved in a series of transfection experiments in osteosarcoma cells (3). These demonstrated that expression of FLAP together with 5-lipoxygenase was essential for cellular leukotriene biosynthesis. Thus the binding of MK-886 to FLAP can explain the mechanism of inhibition of leukotriene biosynthesis by this compound. The current hypothesis is shown in Figure 2. Following activation of 5-lipoxygenase through elevations in intracellular calcium after receptor activation, the enzyme translocates to the membrane and is attached to a "docking" protein, FLAP. In this proposed model, a stable complex will be required to form at the membrane between activated 5-lipoxygenase and FLAP as well as possibly other components of the leukotriene synthetic pathway (e.g. phospholipase A_2). The formation of this complex would regulate the interaction of the enzyme with its substrate, arachidonic acid, and the attachment of MK-886 to FLAP would prevent this association. This mechanism may be of more general interest as a number of other proteins, such as protein kinase C and phospholipase C may translocate to the membrane (2,10). If this represents a general process then other "docking" proteins could serve as novel therapeutic target. Clearly this mechanism represents a novel approach to inhibition of leukotriene synthesis which overcomes many of the problems of direct "redox" 5-lipoxygenase inhibitors. In this context MK-886 has undergone early clinical evaluation, shown inhibition of leukotriene B_4 production following *ex vivo* challenge with ionophore A23187 and has shown significant attenuation of the early phase of antigen-induced bronchoconstriction in asthmatic patients (1).

REFERENCES

1. Bel, E.H., Tanaka, W., Spector, R., Friedman, B., von de Veen, H., Dijkman, J.H., and Sterk, P.J. (1990): *Am. Rev. Respir. Dis.* 141: A31.
2. Creutz, C.E., Dowling, L.G., Kyger, E.M., and Franson, R.C. (1985): *J. Biol. Chem.* 260: 7171.
3. Dixon, R.A.F., Diehl, R.E., Opas, E., Rands, E., Vickers, P.J., Evans, J.F., Gillard, J.W., and Miller, D.K. (1990): *Nature* 343: 282-284.
4. Gaddy, J., Bush, R.K., Margolskee, D., Williams, V.C., and Busse, W. (1990): *J. Allergy Clin. Immunol.* 85: 197A.
5. Gillard, J., Ford-Hutchinson, A.W., Chan, C., Charleson, S., Denis, D., Foster, A., Fortin, R., Leger, S., McFarlane, C.S., Morton, H., Piechuta, H., Riendeau, D., Rouzer, C.A., Rokach, J., Young, R., MacIntyre, D.E., Peterson, L., Bach, T., Eiermann, G., Hopple, S., Humes, J., Hupe, L., Luell, S., Metzger, J., Meurer, R., Miller, D.K., Opas, E., and Pacholok, S. (1989): *Can. J. Physiol. Pharmacol.* 67:456-464.
6. Hendeles, L., Davison, D., Blake, K., Harman, E., Cooper, R., and Margolskee, D. (1990): *J. Allergy Clin. Immunol.* 85: 197A.
7. Jones, T.R., Zamboni, R., Belley, M., Champion, E., Charette, L., Ford-Hutchinson, A.W., Frenette, R., Gauthier, J-Y., Leger, S.,

Masson, P., McFarlane, C.S., Piechuta, H., Rokach, J., Williams, H., Young, R.N., DeHaven, R.N., and Pong, S.S. (1989): *Can. J. Physiol. Pharmacol.* 67: 17-28.
8. Kips, J.C., Joos, G., Margolskee, D., DeLepeleire, I., Rogers, J.D., Pauwels, R., and Van der Straeten, M. (1989): *Am. Rev. Respir. Dis.* 139: A63.
9. Kips, J., Joos, G., Margolskee, D., DeLepeleire, I., Pauwels, R., and Van der Straeten, M. (1989): *Eur. Respir. J.* 2: Suppl.8.
10. Melloni, E., Pontremoli, S., Michetti, M., Sacco, O., Sparatore, B., Salamino, F., and Horecker, B.L. (1985): *Proc. Natl. Acad. Sci. USA* 82: 6435-6439.
11. Miller, D.K., Gillard, J.W., Vickers, P.J., Sadowski, S., Léveillé, C., Mancini, J.A. Charleson, P., Dixon, R.A.F., Ford-Hutchinson, A.W., Fortin, R., Gauthier, J-Y., Rodkey, J., Rozen, R., Rouzer, C., Sigal, I.S., Strader, C.D., and Evans, J.F. (1990): *Nature* 343: 278-281.
12. Rouzer, C.A., and Kargman, S. (1988): *J. Biol. Chem.* 263: 10980-10988.
13. Rouzer, C.A., Ford-Hutchinson, A.W., Morton, H.E., and Gillard, J.W. (1990): *J. Biol. Chem.* 265: 1436-1442.
14. Van Hecken, A., De Schepper, P.J., Margolskee, D.J., Hsieh, J.Y.K., Robinette, R.S., Buntinx, A., and Rogers, J.D. (1989): *Europ. J. Clin. Pharmacol.* 36: Supplement.

5-LIPOXYGENASE mRNA IS EXPRESSED IN RAT PANCREATIC ISLETS

M. H. Nathan, and S. B. Pek

The University of Michigan, Ann Arbor, Michigan 48109-0678, USA

We have reported that exogenous leukotriene B_4 (LTB_4), LTC_4, LTD_4 and LTE_4 stimulate the release of insulin from isolated perfused rat pancreas, in the concentration range of 10^{-11} to 10^{-7} M, in the presence of 5.6 mM glucose (1). In the perfused pancreas, nordihydroguaiaretic acid (NDGA), an inhibitor of lipoxygenases, inhibited insulin release stimulated by glucose or arginine; we interpreted this finding as an indication that endogenous lipoxygenase pathway products of arachidonate metabolism play an amplifying role in insulin secretion (2,3). We observed in isolated pancreatic islets, that arachidonic acid is converted to compounds which behave like peptidyl LTs in high-performance liquid chromatography (HPLC) (4). The 5-lipoxygenase (5-LOX) enzyme catalyzes the conversion of arachidonic acid to LTs. Recently, the 5-LOX gene has been cloned from an human DNA library (5,6). In order to solidify the evidence that islet cells are capable of producing LTs, we explored the expression of 5-LOX mRNA in pancreatic islets; we found significant amounts of it in islet cells.

MATERIALS AND METHODS

The cDNA probes for human 5-LOX and rat proinsulin-I were kindly provided by Dr. R. A. Dixon of Burroughs-Wellcome Labs. (5), and by Drs. S. J. Chan and D. F. Steiner of the University of Chicago (7), respectively. Each probe was propagated further in *E. coli* (8).

Pancreatic islets of normal rats were isolated by a collagenase (type V, Sigma) digestion method (9). The islets were maintained overnight (37°C, 5% CO_2 in air) in RPMI-1640 growth medium (GIBCO) which contained 11 mM glucose. The next day, the islets were washed with Krebs-Ringers-Hepes (KRH) buffer, any cellular debris or extracellular RNA was eliminated. Aliquots of 200 islets were placed in fresh growth medium containing 11 mM glucose, in the absence or presence of 10 µM NDGA (Sigma), and incubated at 37°C for 90 minutes. Thereafter, the samples were chilled rapidly and centrifuged (2,000 rpm, 2 min). Insulin concentrations in the supernatants were measured by a rat insulin radioimmunoassay. After adding 500 µl guanidinium thiocyanate (GTC, Fluka), the pellets were stored at -70°C for subsequent extraction of RNA.

To serve as positive and negative controls, respectively, for the expression of 5-LOX mRNA, rat lung and liver tissues were frozen in liquid nitrogen immediately upon removal, enriched with GTC, and stored at -70°C.

Total RNA in each sample was extracted by a single-step technique, using phenol/chloroform/isoamyl alcohol and precipitated with isopropanol (10). The RNA pellet was dissolved in 50 µl water treated with diethyl pyrocarbonate (DEPC). Using 10-µl aliquots, the concentration of total RNA in each sample was determined spectrophotometrically at 260 nm.

Aliquots of 250, 500 and 1000 ng of total RNA was slot-blotted onto Nytran membranes and baked at 82°C for 1 h. The blotted RNA was prehybridized at 42°C for 4 h with excess salmon sperm DNA in Denhardt's solution, and then hybridized overnight at 42°C in a solution containing excess salmon sperm DNA, 50% formamide, and 5-LOX [^{32}P]cDNA which had been labelled using [^{32}P]dCTP. After hybridization, the membranes were washed serially with solutions of saline/sodium citrate and sodium dodecylsulfate, and submitted to autoradiography. The intensity of radioactivity in individual slots was quantified by computer-driven laser densitometry, and expressed as area/µg total RNA.

After quantifying 5-LOX mRNA, the Nytran membranes were stripped of any DNA by boiling for 1 h in saline/sodium citrate and sodium dodecylsulfate (8). The RNA samples of the membranes were hybridized with rat proinsulin-I [^{32}P]cDNA, following a protocol similar to that used for hybridization with 5-LOX cDNA (8).

RESULTS

Tissue immediately frozen for RNA extraction, demonstrated that the expression of 5-LOX mRNA was high in the lung, undetectable in the liver, and detectable but 37% of that in the lung in islets (Fig 1).

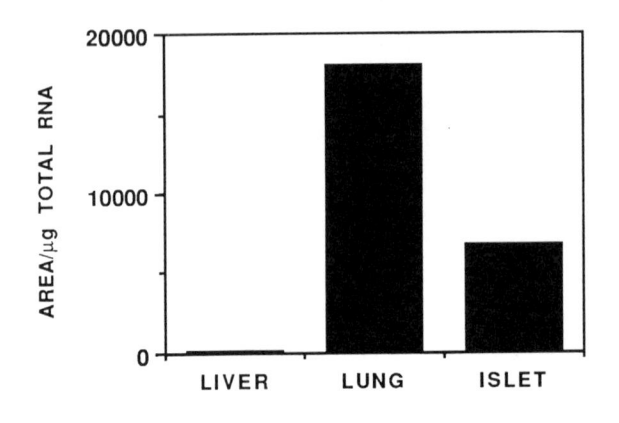

FIGURE 1: Relative amounts of 5-LOX mRNA in rat pancreatic islets, as compared to rat lung and liver tissues. Autoradiograms were quantified by laser densitometry.

In islets, exposure to 10 μM NDGA over 90 min in the presence of 11 mM glucose reduced the expression of 5-LOX mRNA by 80% (p <0.05), but had no effect on the expression of proinsulin mRNA (Fig 2).

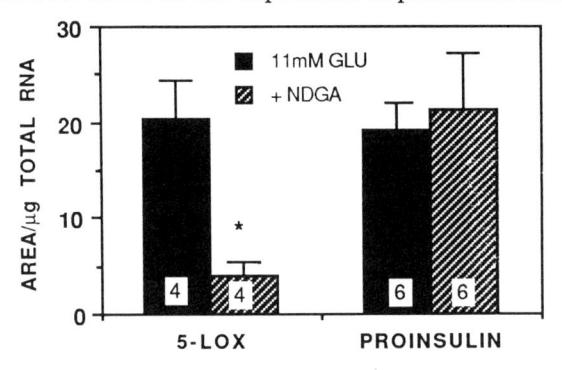

FIGURE 2: Effect of 90-min exposure to NDGA on the steady-state levels of 5-LOX mRNA and proinsulin mRNA in rat islets, as quantified by laser densitometry. [*] p <0.01 vs no NDGA.

In the presence of 11 mM glucose, NDGA inhibited the secretion of insulin from 0.66 to 0.37 μU per islet/min (p <0.05) (Fig 3).

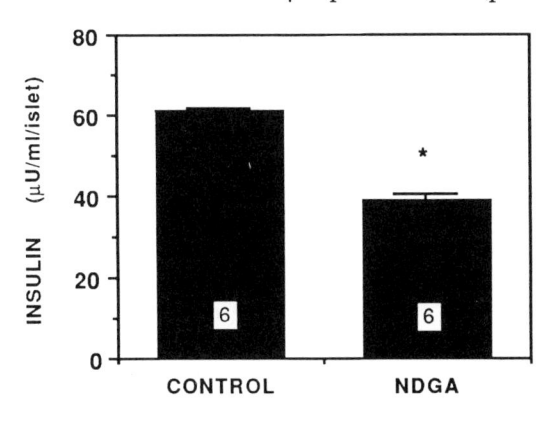

FIGURE 3: Effect of NDGA on insulin release from rat islets over 90 min, in the presence of 11 mM glucose. Mean±SE, N=6. [*] p <0.05 vs no NDGA.

DISCUSSION

Our observation that normal rat pancreatic islet cells express the 5-LOX mRNA confirms the presence of the enzyme essential for the biosynthesis of LTs, and extends the existing HPLC and radioimmunoassay evidence for the production and release of LTs in islets (4,11). The islet-cell types which have the capability to synthesize 5-LOX are yet to be identified. Regardless of whether the insulin-producing ß-cells themselves possess 5-LOX activity or not, LTs produced in any part of the islet would be capable of acting as paracrine regulators of insulin biosynthesis and secretion.

The attenuation of the expression of 5-LOX mRNA by NDGA in islets indicates that this compound reduces the availability of 5-LOX enzyme in tissues, in addition to inhibiting its activity.

The failure of NDGA to affect proinsulin mRNA, at a time it inhibited insulin secretion and 5-LOX mRNA expression, suggests that endogenous

LTs may be involved in the regulation of secretion rather than biosynthesis of insulin.

The experimental protocols which we employed are not suitable to determine whether the observed changes in the expression of 5-LOX mRNA in response to NDGA represent changes in transcription, translation or degradation. However, given the short (90 minutes) duration of exposure to NDGA, which did not affect proinsulin mRNA levels, NDGA is likely to have inhibited the transcription or translation of 5-LOX mRNA, rather than increasing its degradation.

We conclude the following: [1] Normal pancreatic islets contain 5-LOX mRNA and thus are capable of producing LTs. [2] The inhibitory effects of NDGA are due, at least in part, to reduced cellular levels of lipoxygenase. [3] Endogenous LTs are likely to contribute to the regulation of secretion rather than biosynthesis of insulin.

REFERENCES

1. Pek, S. B., and Walsh, M. F. (1984): *Proc. Natl. Acad. Sci. USA*, 81: 2199-2202.
2. Walsh, M. F., and Pek, S. B. (1984): *Life Sci.*, 34: 1699-1706.
3. Walsh, M. F., and Pek, S. B. (1984): *Diabetes*, 33: 929-936.
4. Pek, S. B., and Walsh, M. F. (1986): *Excerpta Medica Intl. Cong. Ser.*, 700: 198-202.
5. Dixon, R. A. F., Jones, R. E., Diehl. R. E., Bennett, C. D., Kargman, S., and Rouzer, C. A. (1988): *Proc. Natl. Acad. Sci. USA*, 85: 416-420.
6. Funk, C. D., Hoshiko, S., Matsumoto, T., Radmark, O., and Samuelsson, B. (1989): *Proc. Natl. Acad. Sci. USA,* 86: 2587-2591.
7. Chan, S. J., Keim, P., and Steiner, D. F. (1976): *Proc. Natl. Acad. Sci. USA,* 73: 1964-1968.
8. Sambrook, J., Fritsch, E. F., and Maniatis, T. (1989): In *Molecular Cloning, A Laboratory Manual.* (2nd Ed.), Cold Springs Harbor Laboratory Press, N.Y.
9. Gotoh, M., Maki, T., Kiyoizumi, T., Satomi, S., and Monaco, A.P. (1985): *Transplantation,* 40: 437-438.
10. Chomczynski, P., and Sacchi, N. (1987): *Anal. Biochem.*, 162: 156-159.
11. Morgan, R. O., and Laychock, S. B. (1988): *Prostaglandins,* 35: 609-623.

IMMUNOHISTOCHEMICAL STUDY ON ARACHIDONATE 5-LIPOXYGENASE OF PORCINE LEUKOCYTES

N. Ueda, K. Natsui, S. Yamamoto, *N. Komatsu, and *K. Watanabe

Department of Biochemistry, Tokushima University
School of Medicine, Tokushima 770, Japan,
and *Department of Pathology, Tokai University
School of Medicine, Isehara 259-11, Japan

The activity of arachidonate 5-lipoxygenase is found in various types of leukocyte such as neutrophil, eosinophil, monocyte, macrophage, and mast cell (3,7). Several lines of leukemia cell are utilized as rich sources of 5-lipoxygenase. Thus, 5-lipoxygenase has been recognized generally as a leukocyte enzyme, and the studies on the molecular and catalytic properties have been performed with the enzymes purified from leukocytes (8,10).

Previously we were successful in the purification of 5-lipoxygenase from porcine leukocytes by immunoaffinity chromatography using a monoclonal anti-5-lipoxygenase antibody (9). Recently, we raised an antiserum in a rabbit with the purified enzyme as an antigen. The polyclonal antibody was purified to an IgG fraction, and applied to immunohistochemical studies on the distribution of 5-lipoxygenase in porcine leukocytes and other tissues.

Western blotting analysis confirmed an immunospecificity of the polyclonal antibody against porcine leukocyte 5-lipoxygenase. The cytosol fraction of porcine leukocytes showed a major band associated with the 5-lipoxygenase protein purified from porcine leukocytes. The polyclonal antibody did not cross-react with 12-lipoxygenase, which was contained in porcine leukocytes in a much higher amount than 5-lipoxygenase (1).

Leukocytes were collected from porcine peripheral blood, and fixed with periodate-lysine-paraformaldehyde. Then, the frozen section was prepared, and stained with the anti-5-lipoxygenase antibody according to the indirect peroxidase-labeled antibody method of Nakane and Pierce (4). Peroxidase reaction was carried out with diaminobenzidine and hydrogen peroxide as substrates, and the sections were counterstained with methyl green.

As observed by light microscopy, positive cells were mainly polymorphonuclear cells, while negative cells were mononuclear cells. A control experiment using non-immunized rabbit IgG indicated that the positive staining was not attributed to an endogenous peroxidase, which was inactivated by the treatment with hydrogen peroxide in methanol.

An immunoelectron microscopic observation indicated that most of the positively stained leukocytes were neutrophils and eosinophils (FIG. 1A). The enzyme was localized exclusively in the cytoplasm of these cells, but not found in the plasma membrane, nucleus, and granules. This finding was in agreement with the results of differential centrifugation demonstrating that 5-lipoxygenase activity was predominantly in the cytosol (5). Unlike the human leukocyte enzyme (6), when porcine neutrophils were challenged with 10 μM of calcium ionophore A23187, immunoelectron microscopy did not show an obvious translocation of the enzyme from the cytosol to the membrane. Since the cytoplasmic granules of eosinophils showed a high electron density by conventional electron microscopy, the density of the granules seemed unrelated to 5-lipoxygenase. Basophils were also positively stained. In contrast, lymphocytes were not stained (FIG. 1A).

Previously we developed a peroxidase-linked immunoassay of sandwich-type for quantification of 5-lipoxygenase (1). Among various porcine tissues, peripheral leukocytes showed by far the highest content of 5-lipoxygenase. Moreover, ileum, lung, pancreas, and several other organs contained smaller but significant amounts of the enzyme (1). Therefore, we attempted to identify the 5-lipoxygenase-containing cells in these porcine organs.

When porcine ileum was observed by light microscopy, mucosal surface was totally unstained, and the immuno-stained cells were found in the lamina propria mucosae. No stained cells were found in a control experiment using non-immunized rabbit IgG. Electron microscopic observation demonstrated that the positive cells in the lamina propria mucosae were mostly eosinophils. Mast cells were also immuno-stained.

Porcine lung was treated with anti-5-lipoxygenase antiserum. Certain cells in bronchiolar epithelium were strongly stained concomitant with eosinophils and mast cells found in the interstitium. Alveolar macrophages were stained more weakly than eosinophils and mast cells. As shown in the electron micrograph of FIG. 1B, the positive cells in bronchiolar epithelium possessed microvilli and filaments. These cells were distinguishable from various types of leukocyte.

Previously, the 5-lipoxygenase metabolites were related to pancreatic exocrine and endocrine functions (2,11). Therefore, we noted the result of the enzyme immunoassay detecting a significant amount of 5-lipoxygenase in the pancreas. Upon light microscopy, acinar cells of porcine pancreas were positively stained with the anti-5-lipoxygenase antibody. However, Langer-

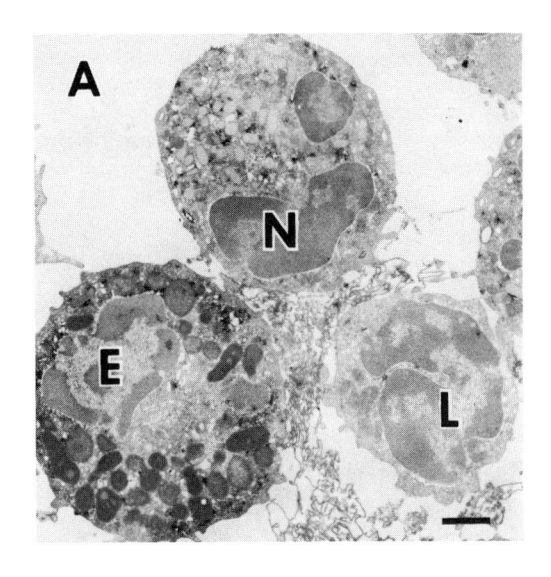

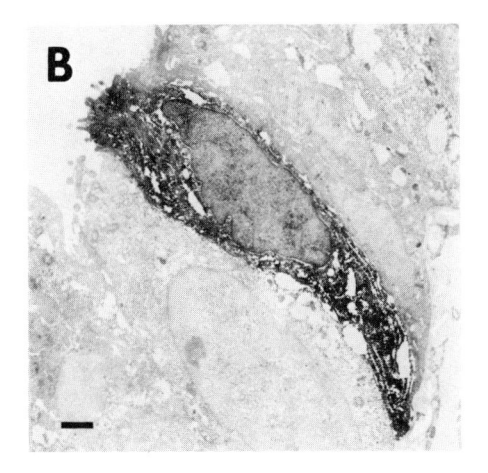

FIG. 1. Immunoelectron microscopic localization of 5-lipoxygenase in porcine peripheral leukocytes (A) and lung (B). N, neutrophil; E, eosinophil; L, lymphocyte. Original magnifications: A x 6,900, B x 5,000. Bar = 1 μm

hans islets and lymphatic nodules were not significantly stained. Positively stained granulocytes were hardly detected. By immunoelectron microscopy 5-lipoxygenase was detected around the nuclear membrane of the pancreatic acinar cells. Cytoplasm, plasma membrane, and subcellular organelles such as zymogen granules and endoplasmic reticulum were not stained. However, we could not rule out a possible artificial translocation of 5-lipoxygenase from the cytosol to the nuclear membrane during the immunostaining procedures.

REFERENCES

1. Kaneko, S., Ueda, N., Tonai, T., Maruyama, T., Yoshimoto, T., and Yamamoto, S. (1987): J. Biol. Chem., 262:6741-6745.

2. Konturek, S.J., Pawlik, W., Czarnobilski, K., Gustaw, P., Jaworek, J., Beck, G., and Jendralla, H. (1988): Am. J. Physiol., 254:G849-G855.

3. Lewis, R.A., and Austen, K.F. (1984): J. Clin. Invest., 73: 889-897.

4. Nakane, P.K., and Pierce, G.B., Jr. (1967): J. Cell. Biol., 33:307-318.

5. Ochi, K., Yoshimoto, T., Yamamoto, S., Taniguchi, K., and Miyamoto, T. (1983): J. Biol. Chem., 258:5754-5758.

6. Rouzer, C.A., and Kargman, S. (1988): J. Biol. Chem., 263: 10980-10988.

7. Samuelsson, B. (1983): Science, 220:568-575.

8. Samuelsson, B., and Funk, C.D. (1989): J. Biol. Chem., 264: 19469-19472.

9. Ueda, N., Kaneko, S., Yoshimoto, T., and Yamamoto, S. (1986): J. Biol. Chem., 261:7982-7988.

10. Yamamoto, S. (1989): Prostaglandins Leukotrienes and Essential Fatty Acids, 35:219-229.

11. Yamamoto, S., Ishii, M., Nakadate, T., Nakaki, T., and Kato, R. (1983): J. Biol. Chem., 258:12149-12152.

EXPRESSION OF CLONED HUMAN 15-LIPOXYGENASE IN EUKARYOTIC AND PROKARYOTIC SYSTEMS

David L. Sloane,[1] Richard A.F. Dixon,[4] Charles S. Craik[3] and Elliott Sigal[1,2]

[1]Cardiovascular Research Institute and Departments of [2]Medicine and [3]Pharmaceutical Chemistry, University of California, San Francisco, CA 94143 and [4]Department of Molecular Biology, Merck, Sharp and Dohme Research Laboratories, West Point, PA 19486

The enzyme 15-lipoxygenase (15-LO) catalyzes the insertion of molecular oxygen into arachidonic acid at carbon 15 and can also oxygenate a variety of polyenoic free fatty acids and phospholipids [1,2,3]. This ability to perform lipid peroxidation is manifested in multiple biological systems. For example, 15-LO appears to contribute to cellular differentiation in the reticulocyte [2] and to the generation of inflammatory mediators in leukocytes [1,4] and in human airway epithelial cells [5]. These potential biological actions for 15-LO have led to increasing interest in understanding the molecular mechanism of the enzyme. We recently isolated from a human reticulocyte library a cDNA encoding 15-LO [6] and showed that the encoded protein was immunologically related to the 15-LOs of airway cells, leukocytes, and reticulocytes [7]. In this paper we summarize our expression studies that have led to the verification of the catalytic function of the encoded enzyme, to the generation of antibodies to human 15-LO, and to the development of an expression system in bacteria designed for mechanistic studies using site-directed mutagenesis.

The plasmid pCMV15LOX was constructed by inserting the 15-LO cDNA, 15LOX [6], downstream of the CMV promoter in the mammalian expression vector pR135 which conveys hygromycin resistance [8]. Plasmids with and without the 15-LO cDNA were transfected into human osteosarcoma cells, and individual hygromycin-resistant clones were screened for 15-LO activity as described [7]. Enzyme activity was not detected in the nontransfected cells or in any of the colonies (n=5) transfected with the vector alone. In contrast, 6 out of 10 clones transfected with the cDNA for 15-LO exhibited enzyme activity. The most highly expressing clone, OS15LOX(+), was selected for further characterization, and clone OS15LOX(-), which contained the vector but no insert, was used to determine basal levels of lipoxygenase expression. Incubation of OS15LOX(+) cells with arachidonic acid resulted in the predominant generation of 15-HETE (2817 ± 200 pmol/10^6 cells, n=8) and 12-HETE (328 ± 20 pmol/10^6 cells, n=8), with lesser amounts of 15-keto-ETE, four isomers of 8,15-diHETE, and one isomer of 14,15-diHETE, as determined by HPLC, mass spectra, and ultraviolet spectra [7]. Incubation of cells with linoleic acid resulted in predominant generation of 13-HODE and lesser amounts of 13-keto-ODE. Cells transformed with the vector alone did not metabolize either linoleic or arachidonic acid. The formation of 15-HETE was inhibited by preincubation with the inhibitor ETYA in a dose-dependent manner, and there was no inhibition of enzyme activity seen with indomethacin (10^{-4} M).

A 21-amino-acid peptide sequence corresponding to the predicted amino acids 37-57 deduced from the cDNA 15LOX [6] was synthesized and used to generate rabbit antisera. Antisera to this peptide (1:100 dilution) hybridized to one major band (70 kDa) in an immunoblot analysis of enriched human leukocyte 15-LO. To obtain antibodies to multiple epitopes of the enzyme, the cDNA was subcloned into the bacterial expression vector pJC264 [9], which resulted in the production of 15-LO fused with the bacterial protein CheY. This insoluble fusion protein was readily purified by differential solubility, and the bacterial proteins from multiple transformants were analyzed by SDS-PAGE (fig. 1, A). This heterologously expressed protein and its partial translation products were immunoreactive to the peptide-derived antibody on immunoblots (fig. 1, B). The immunoreaction could be inhibited by preincubation with peptide, and the peptide-derived antibody did not hybridize to extracts from bacteria that did not contain the 15LOX expression plasmid (fig. 1, B). A polyclonal antibody raised to the CheY-15-LO fusion protein hybridized (1:3000 dilution) to the same band (70 kDa) of human leukocyte 15-LO as did the peptide-derived antibody (fig. 1,C, D). Furthermore, these antibodies hybridized to one major band (70 kDa) in the extract from the human osteosarcoma cell line, OS15LOX(+), the extract from the human tracheal epithelial cells, and purified rabbit reticulocyte 15-LO but not to the cell clone OS15LOX(-) which did not express lipoxygenase activity [7].

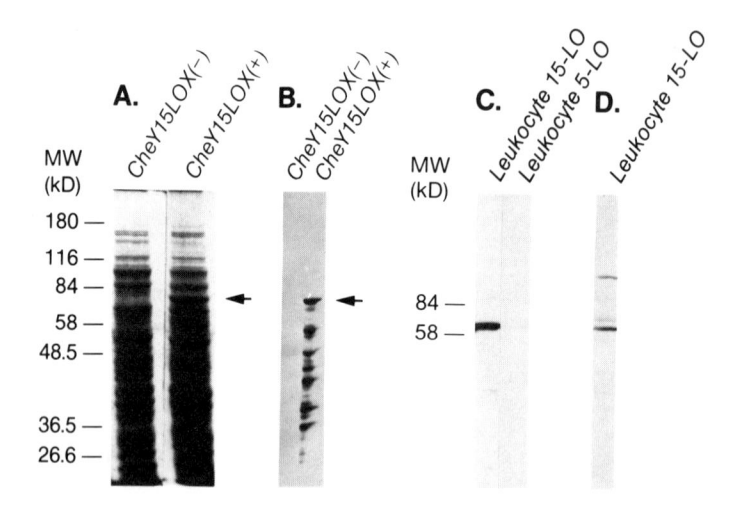

FIG. 1. **Expression of CheY-15-LO fusion protein in *E. coli*.** Bacterial proteins from colonies with and without 15LOX were separated by SDS-PAGE and were either stained with Coomassie blue or transferred to nitrocellulose. A) The fusion protein (arrow) was detected on Coomassie blue-stained gels of colonies containing 15LOX, CheY15LOX(+), but not of colonies without 15LOX, CheY15LOX(-). B) An immunoblot using the peptide-derived antisera (1:100) demonstrated immunoreactivity to the fusion protein and to multiple degradation products. C) Antibodies to the CheY-15-LO fusion (1:3000 dilution) recognized one major band in human leukocyte 15-LO and did not cross-react to human 5-LO. D) The peptide-derived antisera recognized the same band in leukocyte 15-LO as did the antibodies to the fusion protein. (Reproduced with permission from [7]).

To obtain expression of active 15-LO in bacteria, the plasmid pUCLOX was constructed as an in-frame fusion of 15LOX with the *lac Z* gene on the plasmid pUC12 [10]. The fusion gene codes for the first ten amino acids of β-galactosidase fused to the eight amino acids prior to the start codon of the 15LOX gene. The DH5α strain containing pUCLOX was tested for the production of the fusion protein. An immunoblot analysis of the whole cell extract of DH5α transformed with pUC12 and DH5α transformed with pUCLOX is shown in fig. 2. A specific immunoreactive band of approximately the same molecular weight as rabbit reticulocyte lipoxygenase is apparent in the lanes loaded with extracts of uninduced and induced cultures of DH5α carrying pUCLOX. In contrast, the lanes loaded with uninduced and induced cultures of DH5α carrying pUC12 do not show an immunoreactive 70 kDa band. Presumably, the induction with IPTG is not required because the copy number of the expression plasmid used in these studies is sufficiently high to exceed the levels of the endogenous repressor protein lacI.

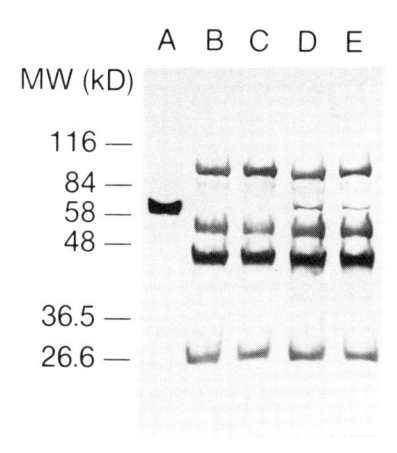

FIG. 2. **Immunoblot of active 15-LO expressed in *E. coli*.** Proteins were analyzed with the antibodies to the CheY-15-LO fusion protein. A) Rabbit reticulocyte lipoxygenase. Whole cell extracts of bacteria transformed without 15LOX cDNA and grown without (B) or with (C) IPTG. Whole cell extracts of bacteria transformed with 15LOX cDNA and grown without (D) or with (E) IPTG. (Reproduced with permission from [10]).

The soluble supernatants of cells with and without 15LOX were used to assay for lipoxygenase activity using either linoleic acid or arachidonic acid as substrate. Lysates of cells without 15LOX showed no HETE production whereas lysates of cells with 15LOX catalyzed the production of 59.3 pmol of 15-HETE and 6 pmol 12-HETE in 15 min at 37°C per μg protein. From this specific activity, we estimate that the lipoxygenase represents approximately 0.1% of the total cellular proteins. The enzyme also converted linoleic acid to 13-HODE, and the formation of both 15-HETE and 13-HODE was inhibited by ETYA.

To construct a vector for performing mutagenesis, an origin of single-stranded DNA replication from the bacteriophage f1 was inserted into pUCLOX. This construction was then used to generate single-stranded DNA. The *lacZ* sequence was deleted using loop-out mutagenesis so that the start codon of

15-LO was placed the same distance away from the ribosome binding site as the original *lacZ*. This resulted in the expression of non-fused, intact 15-LO at the same levels as the β-galactosidase-15-LO fusion. The resulting plasmid, pSS15LO, is being used to generate site-specific mutants of 15-LO.

In summary, cloned 15-LO has been expressed in active form in both eukaryotic and prokaryotic systems, establishing the authenticity of the previously isolated 15-LO cDNA. The expressed 15-LO possesses the ability to perform 12-lipoxygenation, suggesting that the enzyme is multifunctional. The predicted sequence from the cDNA together with the expressed 15-LO have led to the generation of new antibodies to human 15-LO. Immunoblots using these antibodies suggest that the 15-LOs of airway epithelial cells, leukocytes, and reticulocytes are antigenically related. Finally, the expression of active 15-LO in bacteria will facilitate more detailed mechanistic studies using site-directed mutagenesis. Having a convenient expression system is essential to any molecular genetic analysis, and questions concerning substrate specificity, the catalytic mechanism, and the iron-binding site of lipoxygenase can now be addressed more readily.

ACKNOWLEDGMENTS

We gratefully acknowledge the work of Coleman Gross, Ella Highland, Lawrence Costello, and Dorit Grunberger in these studies. Patty Snell assisted in the preparation of the manuscript. This work was supported in part by NIH Program Project Grant HL-24136, a Cystic Fibrosis Foundation RDP Center Grant, the Council for Tobacco Research Grant 2489 (E.S.), and NSF Grant GM8608086 (C.S.C.). E.S. is a recipient of NIH Clinical Investigator Award HL-02047 and an Arthritis Investigator Award from the Arthritis Foundation.

REFERENCES

1. Samuelsson, B., Dahlen, S. -E., Lindgren, J. A., Rouzer, C. A., and Serhan, C. N. (1987): *Science*, 237:1171-1176.
2. Rapoport, S. M., Schewe, T., Wiesner, R., Halangk, W., Ludwig, P., Janicke-Hohne, M., Tannert, C., Hiebsch, C., and Klatt, D. (1979): *Eur. J. Biochem.*, 96:545-561.
3. Murray, J. J., and Brash, A. R. (1988): *Arch. Biochem. Biophys.*, 263:514-523.
4. Turk, J., Mass, R. L., Brash, A. R., Roberts, L. J., II, and Oates, J. A. (1982): *J. Biol. Chem.*, 257:7068-7076.
5. Hunter, J. A., Finkbeiner, W. E., Nadel, J. A., Goetzl, E. J., and Holtzman, M. J. (1985): *Proc. Natl. Acad. Sci. USA*, 82:4633-4637.
6. Sigal, E., Craik, C. S., Highland, E., Grunberger, D., Costello, L. L., Dixon, R. A. F., and Nadel, J. A. (1988): *Biochem. Biophys. Res. Commun.*, 157:457-464.
7. Sigal, E., Grunberger, D., Highland, E., Gross, C., Dixon, R. A. F., and Craik, C. S. (1990): *J. Biol. Chem.*, 265:5113-5120.
8. Rouzer, C. A., Rands, E., Kargman, S., Jones, R. E., Register, R. B., and Dixon, R. A. F. (1988): *J. Biol. Chem.*, 263:10135-10140.
9. Gan, Z. -R., Condra, J. H., Gould, R. J., Zivin, R. A., Bennett, C. D., Jacobs, J. W., Friedman, P. A., and Polokoff, M. A. (1989): *Gene*, 7:159-166.
10. Sloane, D. L., Craik, C. S., and Sigal, E. (1990) *Biomed. Biochem. Acta*, (in press).

CLONING AND EXPRESSION OF ARACHIDONATE

12-LIPOXYGENASE cDNA FROM PORCINE LEUKOCYTES

T. Yoshimoto, H. Suzuki, S. Yamamoto,
*T. Takai, *C. Yokoyama, and *T. Tanabe

Department of Biochemistry, Tokushima University,
School of Medicine, Tokushima 770, Japan
*Department of Pharmacology, National Cardiovascular Center Research Institute,
Osaka 565, Japan

Arachidonate 12-lipoxygenase introduces a molecular oxygen into the C-12 of arachidonic acid to yield 12S-hydroperoxy-5, 8, 10, 14-eicosatetraenoic acid. Despite the fact that 12-lipoxygenase was first described in human platelets among mammalian lipoxygenases, the physiological significance of this enzyme has not yet been elucidated. Previously, we found a 12-lipoxygenase in porcine leukocytes, and immunoaffinity-purified the enzyme to near homogeneity using monoclonal antibody against the enzyme (8). As a molecular biological approach to the 12-lipoxygenase of porcine leukocytes, we isolated a cDNA clone of the enzyme (9).

RESULTS AND DISCUSSION

The purified 12-lipoxygenase of porcine leukocytes (0.25 mg) was digested by *Achromobacter* proteinase I (3 µg) which specifically cleaved on the carboxyl side of lysine residue. The peptide fragments were separated by reverse-phase HPLC. Amino acid sequences of these peptide fragments and the native enzyme were determined by a gas-phase sequencer and a PTH-amino acid analyzer (Applied Biosystems). Based upon these partial amino acid sequences, two oligonucleotide probes were synthesized: probe A, 5'-ATYTCCATNGTRTA-3' (Tyr-Thr-Met-Glu-Ile) and probe B, 5'-TGRTCRAADATNCC-3' (Gly-Ile-Phe-Asp-Gln), where R is A or G; Y is C or T; D is A, G or T; and N is A, G, T or C. These probes were labeled with ^{32}P, and used in the screening of a cDNA library constructed from poly (A)$^+$ RNA of porcine leukocytes. A clone which hybridized with both probes was obtained, and designated as pLOX-89. The clone had a DNA insert of 2.3 kb, but did not contain the N-terminal coding region of the 12-lipoxygenase gene. Therefore, we constructed another cDNA library with specific primers I and II as shown in FIG. 1. From this primer-extention library, the clones pLOX-96 and 134 were obtained. The sequence of these cDNA clones was determined by the dideoxy-nucleotide chain termination method. The cDNA for 12-lipoxygenase contained an open reading frame encoding 662 amino acids and 900 base-pairs of 3'-noncoding region.

The calculated molecular weight of 74,911 was close to that (72,000) of the purified 12-lipoxygenase as examined by SDS-polyacrylamide gel electrophoresis (8). Hydropathicity analysis indicated that the central portions of the enzyme (amino acid #293-298 and 374-383) are considerably hydrophobic, but the protein is overall hydrophilic. The result was in agreement with our previous finding that the enzyme was localized in the cytosol of porcine leukocytes as examined by both differential centrifugation and immunohistochemical study.

As shown in FIG. 2, a well-conserved histidine-containing sequence was proposed as a putative iron-binding domain of soybean lipoxygenases (6) and human reticulocyte 15-lipoxygenase (7). This sequence is found in our 12-lipoxygenase at amino acid #356-393. However, mutations of His-362 or His-372 of human 5-lipoxygenase to serine residues did not affect 5-lipoxygenase activity, suggesting these histidines were not essential for iron coordination (4). We noted a short cysteine-containing sequence Cys-X_3-Cys-X_3-His-X_3-His (amino acids #533-545) in our 12-lipoxygenase which matches the sequence Cys-X_{2-4}-Cys-X_{2-15}-Cys/His-X_{2-4}-Cys/His. This sequence is found in many metal-

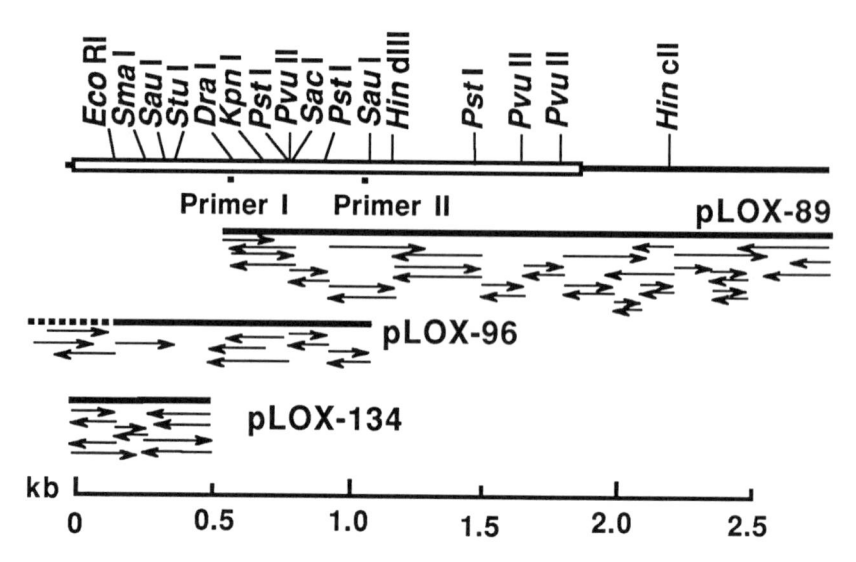

FIG. 1. Restriction endonuclease map of porcine 12-lipoxygenase cDNA.

```
              #356                                      #393 #533      #545
    Conserved:H----H-L--H---E----A--R-L---HP--KL---H  C---C---H---H
      Pig 12-LO:HELHSHLLRGHLMAEVIAVATMRCLPSIHPIFKLLIPH CIFTCTGQHSSNH
    Human 15-LO:HELQSHLLRGHLMAEVIVVATMRCLPSIHPIFKLIIPH CIFTCTGQHASVH
   Rabbit 15-LO:HELNSHLLRGHLMAEVFTVATMRCLPSIHPVFKLIVPH CIFTCTGQHSSIH
    Human 5-LO:HQTITHLLRTHLVSEVFGIAMYRQLPAVHPIFKLLVAH VIFTASAQHAAVN
      Rat 5-LO:HQTITHLLRTHLVSEVFGIAMYRQLPAVHPLFKLLVAH VIFTASAQHAAVN
   Soybean LO-1:HQLMSHWLNTHAAMEPFVIATHRHLSVLHPIYKLLTPH IIWIASALHAAVN
```

FIG. 2. Putative metal-binding domain of lipoxygenases (LO).

binding proteins such as cytochrome c and metallothionein (1). This sequence was also found in the 15-lipoxygenases of human (7) and rabbit (3), but not in 5-lipoxygenase (2,5) and soybean lipoxy-genase (6).

FIG. 3 shows the comparison of the predicted amino acid sequence of the 12-lipoxygenase to those of 15- and 5-lipoxygenases by Harr plots. The amino acid sequence of 12-lipoxygenase shows 86% and 41% identity with 15- and 5-lipoxygenases, respectively. This result, taken together with enzymological properties of lipoxygenases, indicates that 12-lipoxygenase is evolutionarily more related to 15-lipoxygenase than to 5-lipoxygenase.

As illustrated in FIG. 4, an expression vector was constructed from pKK-223 with *tac* promoter. The 12-lipoxygenase cDNA fragments were excised from the plasmids pLOX-89, 96 and 134, and were ligated to the expression vector. The enzyme expressed in *E. coli* system was incubated with arachidonic acid, and the borohydride-reduced products were analyzed by reverse-phase HPLC. The major reaction product was identified as 12-HETE. In addition, a small peak correspond-ing 15-HETE was detected in 5% amount of 12-HETE. Such a minor production of 15-HETE was also observed by the purified enzyme from porcine leukocytes. Furthermore, the expression of the 12-lipoxygenase was demonstrated by Western blotting analysis utilizing anti-12-lipoxygenase antibody. The enzyme protein was not detected in the extract of *E. coli* transformed with a control plasmid containing no 12-lipoxygenase cDNA. Site-directed mutagenesis experiment will clarify the structure of the active site controling the positional specificity of our 12-lipoxygenase.

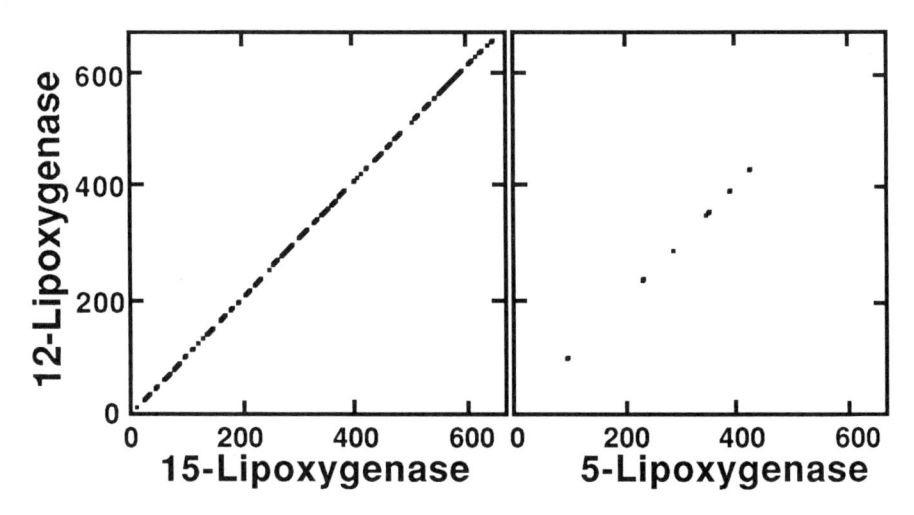

FIG. 3. Comparison of porcine 12-lipoxygenase to human 15- and 5-lipoxygenases by Harr plots.

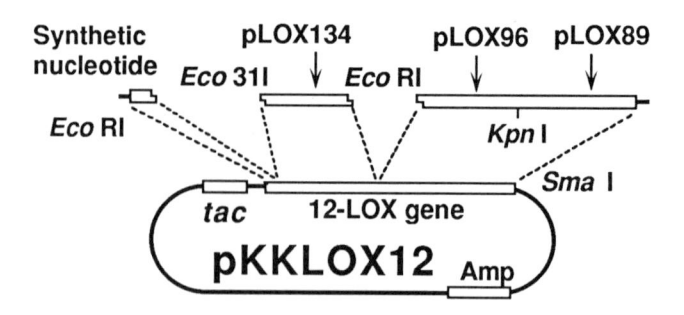

FIG. 4. Construction of an expression vector for porcine 12-lipoxygenase.

ACKNOWLEDGEMENTS

This work has been supported by grants-in-aid from the Ministry of Education, Science and Culture and the Ministry of Health and Welfare of Japan, and grants from the Japanese Foundation of Metabolism and Diseases, Takeda Science Foundation, Tokyo Biochemical Research Foundation, and Uehara Memorial Foundation.

REFERECES

1. Berg, J. M. (1986): *Science*. 232: 485-487.
2. Dixon, R. A. F., Jones, R.E., Diehl, R.E., Bennett, C.D., Kargman, S., and Rouzer, C.A. (1988): *Proc. Natl. Acad. Sci. USA*. 85: 416-420.
3. Fleming, J., Thiele, B.J., Chester, J., O'Prey, J., Janetzki, S., Aitken, A., Rapoport, S.M., and Harrison, P.R. (1989): *Gene*. 79: 181-188.
4. Funk, C. D., Gunne, H., Steiner, H., Izumi, T., and Samuelsson, B. (1989): *Proc. Natl. Acad. Sci. USA*. 86: 2592-2596.
5. Matsumoto, T., Funk, C., Rådmark, O., Höög, J.-O., Jörnvall, H., and Samuelsson, B. (1988): *Proc. Natl. Acad. Sci. USA*. 85: 26-30.
6. Shibata, D., Steczko, J., Dixon, J.E., Andrews, P.C., Hermodson, M., and Axelrod, B. (1988): *J. Biol. Chem*. 263: 6816-6821.
7. Sigal, E., Craik, C.S., Highland, E., Grunberger, D., Costello, L.L., Dixon, R.A.F., and Nadel, J.A. (1988): *Biochem. Biophys. Res. Commun*. 157: 457-464.
8. Yokoyama, C., Shinjo, F., Yoshimoto, T., Yamamoto, S., Oates, J.A., and Brash, A.R. (1986): *J. Biol. Chem*. 261: 16714-16721.
9. Yoshimoto, T., Suzuki, H., Yamamoto, S., Takai, T., Yokoyama, C., and Tanabe, T. (1990): *Proc. Natl. Acad. Sci. USA*. 87: 2142-2146.

POLYMERASE CHAIN REACTION CLONING AND EXPRESSION OF EICOSANOID METABOLIZING ENZYMES FROM BLOOD CELLS.

C.D. Funk, L. Furci, and G.A. FitzGerald

Vanderbilt University,
Division of Clinical Pharmacology,
Nashville, TN 37232

The polymerase chain reaction (PCR) has become an essential tool for the rapid and specific amplification of DNA molecules. Since certain blood cells, for example platelets, contain minute amounts of RNA, it is virtually impossible to construct cDNA libraries by conventional means. In these studies, we have successfully used PCR to isolate the cDNA encoding the platelet localized 12-lipoxygenase and the erythrocyte/reticulocyte 15-lipoxygenase. These lipoxygenases, as well as human leukocyte 5-lipoxygenase have been expressed in simian COS-M6 cells.

METHODS

RNA was isolated from washed human platelets and red blood cells by the method of Chomczynski and Sacchi (1). An aliquot was taken for first strand cDNA synthesis (final volume 25 μl) using avian myeloblastosis virus reverse transcriptase and the downstream oligonucleotide (~ 25-50 pmol) used as primer. The mixture was diluted to 100 μl and adjusted to PCR conditions (100 mM Tris HCl, pH 8.3, 50 mM KCl, 2 mM $MgCl_2$, 0.2 mM dNTP, 25-50 pmol each primer set and 2.5 U Thermus aquaticus DNA polymerase (Taq polymerase) and amplification of target DNA was performed for 30 cycles. PCR conditions were adjusted empirically for the different target DNAs in order to achieve maximal amplification. Typical conditions were as follows: denaturation, 94°C-1 min; annealing, 37-50°C-45 sec. to 1 min 45 sec; and extension, 72°C-1 to 3 min.

Amplified DNAs for the three lipoxygenases were subcloned into the mammalian cell expression vector pcDNA-1 (Invitrogen, San Diego, CA) and were introduced into simian COS-M6 cells by calcium phosphate mediated transfection. Cells were assayed for lipoxygenase activity basically as previously described (2).

RESULTS AND DISCUSSION

5-lipoxygenase and 15-lipoxygenase share certain highly homologous regions. We hypothesized that 12-lipoxygenase would also contain similar homologous segments. Therefore, we synthesized mixed oligonucleotide primers based on the amino acid sequences 347-355 and 427-434 of human 5-lipoxygenase (3) (amino acids 340-348 and 420-427 of human reticulocyte 15-lipoxygenase (4)).

Using these primers and platelet cDNA template, a 0.26 kb DNA species (PL12lx;Fig.1) was amplified by PCR. When sequenced, this DNA was found to contain a single open reading frame. The translated sequence was found to be 76% identical with human 15-lipoxygenase and 60% identical to human 5-lipoxygenase. Since platelets contain only 12-lipoxygenase, we had good reason to believe that we had isolated a short segment of the 12-lipoxygenase cDNA. In order to isolate the complete cDNA for 12-lipoxygenase, we chose to screen a cDNA library constructed from RNA isolated from phorbol-myristate acetate stimulated human erythroleukemia cells with the ^{32}P-labeled PL12lx clone. These cells carry many platelet/megakaryocytic markers (6). Three clones were isolated, purified and sequenced after screening two different cDNA libraries (Fig. 1). The clones covered the complete cDNA including 42 bp of 5' noncoding region, a 1989 bp open reading frame and a 0.31 kb 3' noncoding region. A consensus AATAAA polyadenylation signal was found 15 bp upstream of a poly (A)$^+$ tail. The open reading frame would encode a 663 amino acid protein with a molecular weight of 75,000. There are no predictions for membrane spanning domains which is consistent with the cytosolic localization of 12-lipoxygenase.

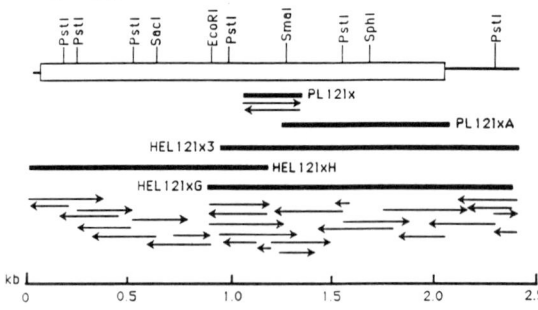

Fig. 1 Partial restriction map and sequencing strategy for cloned cDNAs encoding human platelet/erythroleukemia cell 12-lipoxygenase. Direction and extent of sequencing determinations are indicated by arrows. The open box indicates the protein coding region.

To confirm further the platelet origin of the 12-lipoxygenase clone PL12lx, we designed new oligonucleotide primers based on the sequence information obtained from clones HEL 12lx3, HEL 12lxG and HEL 12lxH.

An additional clone PL12lxA was obtained by PCR from platelet cDNA (Fig. 1) and did not arise from genomic DNA contamination. Combined sequence data from clones PL12lxA and PL12lx indicate that these clones are identical to the HEL cell-derived clones and are presumed to encode an identical 12-lipoxygenase. 12-lipoxygenase displays an overall similar hydrophobicity profile to other lipoxygenases and is 65% identical to both human reticulocyte 15-lipoxygenase and a recently described porcine leukocyte 12-lipoxygenase (7), and is 40% identical to human 5-lipoxygenase. In contrast, the reticulocyte 15-lipoxygenase and porcine leukocyte 12-lipoxygenase are 86% identical indicating that these proteins are much more closely related to each other then to the human platelet 12-lipoxygenase.

Human erythrocyte/reticulocyte 15-lipoxygenase cDNA was cloned by PCR in a two-step procedure using oligonucleotide primers based on the known sequence of Sigal et al. (4). The cDNAs for the three major mammalian lipoxygenase forms, 5-, 12- and 15-lipoxygenase were constructed into the pcDNA-1 expression vector.

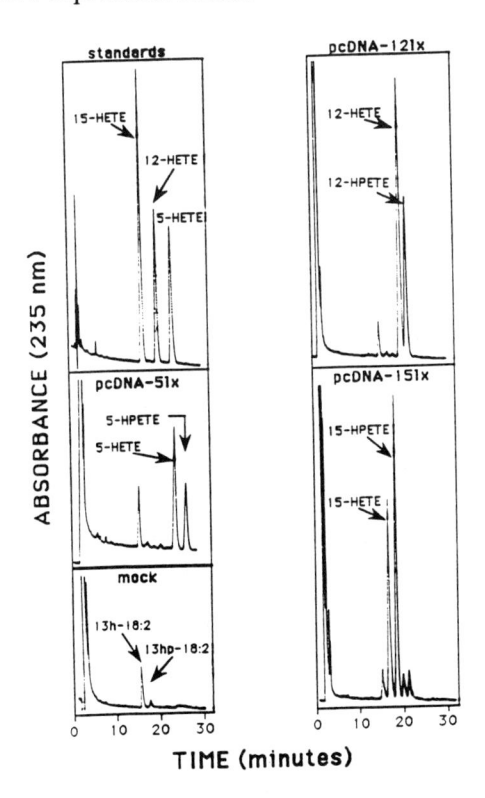

Fig. 2 Reverse phase-HPLC chromatograms of lipoxygenase products from transfected COS-M6 cells. 13-hydroperoxy-octadecadienoic acid (13hp-18:2) was added to incubations to enhance lipoxygenase activation. 13h-18:2 is its reduced metabolite.

These expression constructs, under the control of the cytomegalovirus promoter, were introduced into COS-M6 cells and the expression of lipoxygenase enzyme activity was monitored in the 10,000 x g supernatants 2-3 days post-transfection. Normal COS-M6 cells or mock-transfected cells produced no detectable lipoxygenase products (Fig. 2). However, incubations from each of the pcDNA-5lx, pcDNA-12lx and pcDNA-15lx transfected cells were able to produce their respective hydroperoxy- and hydroxy-eicosatetraenoic acid metabolites from added arachidonic acid (Fig. 2). pcDNA-15lx transfected cells also made small amounts of 12-HETE and 12-HPETE as recently demonstrated in transfected osteosarcoma cells (5).

CONCLUSIONS

We have cloned the cDNA for the human platelet/erythroleukemia cell 12-lipoxygenase and have successfully expressed all three major mammalian lipoxygenase forms in COS-M6 cells. The expression system described here will be ideally suited for studying the structure/function properties of these enzymes.

REFERENCES

1. Chomczynski, P. and Sacchi, N. (1987): Anal. Biochem., 132:6-13.
2. Funk, C.D., Gunne, H., Steiner, H., Izumi, T., and Samuelsson, B. (1989): Proc. Natl. Acad. Sci. USA, 86:2592-2596.
3. Matsumoto, T., Funk, C.D., Rådmark, O., Höög, J-O., Jörnvall, H., and Samuelsson, B. (1988): Proc. Natl. Acad. Sci. USA, 85:26-30, and correction (1988): Proc. Natl. Acad. Sci. 85:3406.
4. Sigal, E., Craik, C.S., Highland, E., Grunberger, D., Costello, L.L., Dixon, R.A.F., and Nadel, J.A. (1988): Biochem. Biophys. Res. Commun., 157:457-464.
5. Sigal, E., Grunberger, D., Highland, E., Gross, C., Dixon, R.A.F., and Craik, C.S. (1990): J. Biol. Chem., 265:5113-5120.
6. Tabilio, A., Rosa, J-P., Testa, U., Kieffer, N., Nurden, A.T., Del Canizo, M.C., Breton-Gorius, J., and Vainchenker, V. (1984): EMBO J., 3:453-459.
7. Yoshimoto, T., Suzuki, H., Yamamoto, S., Toshiyuki, T., Yokoyama, C., and Tanabe, T., (1990): Proc. Natl. Acad. Sci. USA, 87:2142-2146.

BIOCHEMICAL AND IMMUNOHISTOCHEMICAL EVIDENCE FOR SELECTIVE EXPRESSION OF NOVEL EPITHELIAL LIPOXYGENASES

V. R. Shannon, J. R. Hansbrough, Y. Takahashi*, N. Ueda*, S. Yamamoto*, and M. J. Holtzman

Department of Medicine, Washington University School of Medicine, St. Louis, Missouri 63110 and *Department of Biochemistry, Tokushima University School of Medicine, Tokushima 770, Japan

The epithelial cell surface serves as an active interface between environmental agents and the underlying cells. Several findings suggest that the epithelial cells carry out their sentinel role in part by releasing lipid mediators: (i) the cells contain abundant stores of fatty acid substrates for oxygenation, (ii) they have the capacity to release these substrates through the action of specific phospholipases, (iii) they express enzymatic pathways for selective oxygenation of fatty acids at a high level relative to other cell types, and (iv) the oxygenated metabolites have potent effects on endorgans such as smooth muscle, nerves, and glands and on epithelial cells themselves (reviewed in ref. 5). Studies of isolated epithelial cells from skin and lung demonstrate that all three of the enzymatic pathways capable of fatty acid oxygenation—cyclooxygenase, lipoxygenase, and monooxygenase are expressed selectively under different culture conditions (3-5). One of the most novel results to date is the identification of an arachidonate 15-lipoxygenase in human tracheal epithelial cells that is present at a high level relative to other cell types (3). Because the availability of human tissue is limited, further investigation of this epithelial lipoxygenase has been difficult. For that reason, we explored the possibility that other species might express a related lipoxygenase that in turn might be used to develop reagents to further characterize the human enzyme.

BIOCHEMICAL CHARACTERIZATION OF EPITHELIAL LIPOXYGENASES

Epithelial cells were isolated from bovine, canine, porcine, and ovine tracheal mucosa by enzymatic dissociation and tested for cellular capacity to lipoxygenate arachidonic acid. In each species, chromatographic and mass spectrometric analysis of oxygenation products showed that the cells convert arachidonate to 12-HETE with smaller amounts of 15-HETE as well as 8,15- and 14,15-diHETEs, and hydroxyepoxy-ETEs. This pattern of product formation is consistent with an arachidonate 12-lipoxygenase. The level of enzymatic activity is similar to the highest levels reported for other types of mammalian cells and to the level of 15-lipoxygenase activity in human tracheal epithelial cells (1).

Similarities between tracheal epithelial 12-lipoxygenase in animals and epithelial 15-lipoxygenase in humans are noteworthy. Both enzymes exhibit nearly identical concentration-response relationships during incubation with exogenous substrate, and both lead to evanescent detection for some of their lipoxygenation products (e.g., hydroperoxy acids). Both convert arachidonic acid predominantly to 15- and 12-HETE (although in differing proportions), and this dual capability enables both to generate an identical series of dihydroxylated conjugated triene derivatives (3). For other fatty acid substrates, the predominant product of the two lipoxygenases may even be identical. For example, both enzymes convert linoleic acid to its 13-hydroperoxy analogue. The preservation of a functional domain for fatty acid lipoxygenation may be specifically essential for tracheal epithelial function, but the basis for the variability between species is uncertain.

Further studies of bovine tracheal epithelial cells have examined the characteristics of the 12-lipoxygenase in relation to the enzyme expressed in leukocytes and platelets. Several similarities were found: epithelial cell lipoxygenase activity was localized to the soluble cytoplasmic fraction of disrupted cells; 12-HPETE formation accompanied 12-HETE synthesis; 12S stereospecificity of product formation was absolute; and analysis of cytosolic enzymatic activity for pH dependence (maximum activity at pH 7.4-8.0), divalent cation effects (no dependence on cations), and kinetic characteristics (lag phase elimination by addition of hydroperoxide) all exhibited similarity to leukocyte and platelet 12-lipoxygenases.

Immunological characterization of 12-lipoxygenase demonstrated a degree of similarity between epithelial cell and leukocyte forms of the enzyme. Immunoprecipitation experiments were carried out using a monoclonal antibody directed against porcine leukocyte 12-lipoxygenase (*lox-2*), which cross-reacted with bovine leukocyte 12-lipoxygenase, and one directed against the human platelet 12-lipoxygenase (*HPLO-3*), which cross-reacted with bovine platelet 12-lipoxygenase (7). The epithelial 12-lipoxygenase reacted with anti-leukocyte *lox-2* but not with anti-platelet *HPLO-3* (2). Assays of resuspended *lox-2* immune complexes reflected a corresponding recovery of activity, so the antibody does not inactivate the enzyme. Immunoaffinity chromatography of the epithelial cytosolic fraction using *lox-2* linked to Affi Prep 10 yielded a single predominant protein band (M_r = 72,000) by SDS-PAGE identical in apparent mass to the bovine leukocyte lipoxygenase. Immunoblotting of the purified enzyme using a rabbit polyclonal antibody to leukocyte 12-lipoxygenase (6) showed peroxidase staining of the same 72 kDa protein band.

The 12-lipoxygenases from platelets, leukocytes, and epithelial cells showed considerable heterogeneity in activity. Activity assays of the immunoaffinity-purified enzymes demonstrated that the platelet 12-lipoxygenase is relatively restricted to arachidonic acid as a substrate and is incapable of converting 18-carbon fatty acid substrates to the corresponding monohydroxylated conjugated diene; the leukocyte 12-lipoxygenase has slightly broader substrate acceptability; and the epithelial form of the enzyme is the most efficient user of alternative substrates (Fig. 1). Confirmation that the purified enzymes were representative of

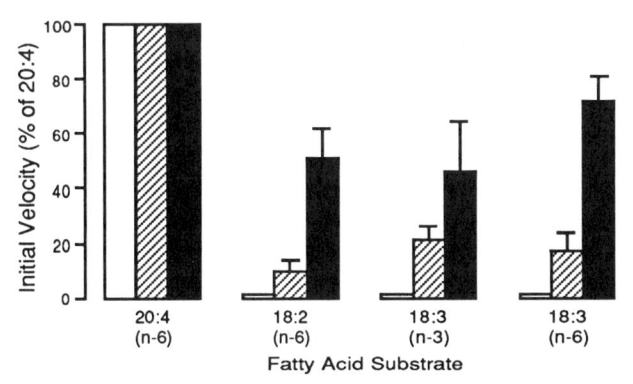

FIG. 1. Heterogeneity of 12-lipoxygenase activities from bovine platelets (open bars), leukocytes (striped bars), and epithelial cells (dark bars). Immunoaffinity-purified enzymes were incubated with 25 µM fatty acid substrate, and the initial reaction velocity was calculated from the rate of change in UV absorbance at 240 nm and compared to arachidonate (20:4, n-6).

the 12-lipoxygenase activities contained in epithelial cells and leukocytes was obtained when the cytosolic fraction prepared from epithelial cells also exhibited quantitatively higher activity for linoleic acid than did the fraction from leukocytes.

IMMUNOHISTOCHEMISTRY OF EPITHELIAL TISSUE

Lipoxygenase distribution in bovine trachea was examined by immunoperoxidase staining of formalin-fixed tissue using rabbit polyclonal anti-12-lipoxygenase antibody and a biotinylated secondary antibody linked to a streptavidin-horseradish peroxidase detection system. The 12-lipoxygenase antigen is present throughout the tracheal epithelium and is similar in staining intensity to keratin. Antigen was also present in submucosal glands and was easily detected in polymorphonuclear and mononuclear leukocytes in the submucosa. Antigen was not present in tracheal smooth muscle, a finding that correlates well with the absence of significant lipoxygenase activity in that tissue.

The same reagents were used to investigate the pattern of immunoperoxidase staining in human trachea. The distribution of the presumed 15-lipoxygenase antigen was similar in that epithelial cells and submucosal glands contained the antigen. In contrast to bovine trachea, submucosal leukocytes were not stained— an observation that fits with the absence of significant 12- or 15-lipoxygenase activity in this class of cells.

We also examined the distribution of the lipoxygenase antigen along the pulmonary airway in bovine and human lung. Distribution was assessed in each species by comparing staining of trachea to bronchus and to peripheral lung parenchyma. In both bovine and human tissue, the intensity of staining decreases markedly even by the level of the mainstem bronchus and staining is virtually absent in peripheral lung. The decrease in the level of lipoxygenase antigen does not appear to be due simply to a disappearance of specific epithelial cell types because virtually all the epithelial cells in the trachea stain positively, and these same cells do not stain at all in more distal airways. One notable difference between the pattern in human and bovine trachea was the positivity of smooth muscle staining in humans signifying potential lipoxygenase in that tissue.

SUMMARY

Human tracheal epithelial cells contain an arachidonate 15-lipoxygenase, while the same cells from animals (including bovine, ovine, canine, porcine) cells express a 12-lipoxygenase. The epithelial 12-lipoxygenase is antigenically related to the leukocyte 12-lipoxygenase but is biochemically distinct from platelet and leukocyte forms of the enzyme, in that it is more efficient at metabolizing a wider array of fatty acid substrates. We have suggested that this lipoxygenase heterogeneity may provide a basis for different functional roles for the enzyme in different cell types. In addition, animal epithelial 12-lipoxygenase and human epithelial 15-lipoxygenase are antigenically related and have similar but distinct distributions in the lung. Our findings might suggest that the species diversity for epithelial lipoxygenases represents molecular divergence within a family of closely related genes with perhaps closely related functions.

Acknowledgments—This work was supported in part by grants from the National Institutes of Health and from the Ministry of Health and Welfare of Japan and by the Schering Career Investigator Award from the American Lung Association.

REFERENCES

1. Hansbrough, J. R., Atlas, A. B., Turk, J., and Holtzman, M. J. (1989): *Am. J. Respir. Cell. Mol. Biol.* 1:237-244.
2. Hansbrough, J. R., Takahashi, Y., Ueda, N., Yamamoto, S., and Holtzman, M. J. (1990): *J. Biol. Chem.*, 265:1771-1776.
3. Holtzman, M. J., Hansbrough, J. R., Rosen, G. D., and Turk, J. (1988): *Biochim. Biophys. Acta,.* 963:401-413.
4. Holtzman, M. J., Turk, J., and Pentland, A. (1989): *J. Clin. Invest.* 84:1446-1453.
5. Holtzman, M. J. (1990): In: *The Airway Epithelium: Structure and Function in Health and Disease,* edited by S. G. Farmer and D. W. P. Hay, Marcel Dekker, New York.
6. Maruyama, T., Ueda, N., Yoshimoto, T., Yamamoto, S., Komatsu, N., and Watanabe, K. (1989): *J. Histochem. Cytochem.* 37:1125-1131.
7. Takahashi, Y., Ueda, N., and Yamamoto, S. (1988): *Arch. Biochem. Biophys.* 266:613-621.

Leukotriene A_4-hydrolase in two human cell lines.

Rådmark[1], O., Medina[1], J.F., Macchia[1], L., Barrios[2], C., Funk[1], C.D., Larsson[2], O. and Haeggström[1] J.

Departments of Physiological Chemistry[1] and Tumor Biology[2]
Karolinska Institutet
S-104 01 Stockholm, Sweden

Leukotriene A_4-hydrolase catalyzes the conversion of leukotriene A_4 (LTA_4) to the chemotactic dihydroxyacid leukotriene B (LTB_4). In studies of the tissue distribution of LTA_4-hydrolase, the enzyme was found to be widely spread. It could be demonstrated in almost all guinea pig, rat and human tissues examined (reviewed in ref 1). Phagocytes are probably the richest source of LTA_4-hydrolase, but in addition the human enzyme has been found in plasma, erythrocytes, umbilical vein derived endothelium, and in lymphocytes (reviewed in ref 1). Recent histochemical localization of LTA_4-hydrolase in guinea pig tissues demonstrated the enzyme in epithelial cells (airways, GI-tract), in vascular endothelium and in intestinal plexa (2). LTA_4-hydrolase activity was also found in human intestinal epithelium (Tornhamre et al, personal communication).

Here we demonstrate the presence of LTA_4-hydrolase in human fibroblast cell lines. Fibroblasts aswell as many of the cell types mentioned above are present in most tissues, thus providing an explanation for the wide tissue distribution of LTA_4-hydrolase. Also, the expression of LTA_4-hydrolase in HL-60 cells was studied. Of particular interest was the apparent inhibition by dexamethasone, of LTA_4-hydrolase activity in HL-60 cells, induced to differentiate[4] with dimethylsulfoxide.

Results and Discussion

LTA_4-hydrolase in fibroblast cell lines. Non-senescent human lung diploid fibroblasts (WI-38, passage 15-30) and SV-40 transformed human lung fibroblasts (WI-38 VA13) were obtained from Flow. Homogenates of these cells converted LTA_4 to LTB_4 as demonstrated by HPLC, UV-spectroscopy and GC-MS (see ref 3 for data aswell as methodology). Larger amounts of LTB_4 (threefold increase) were formed in homogenates of SV-40 transformed cells, indicating a higher LTA_4-hydrolase content in these cells. This was confirmed by Western blots of 10.000 x g supernatants from fibroblast homogenates (fig 1). The amount of enzyme in normal diploid cells was estimated to be about 0.5 mg/g soluble protein, approximately 20 % of the LTA_4-hydrolase content in human leukocytes. Also, LTA_4-hydrolase mRNA was detectable in Northern blots of fibroblast RNA, and there was a stronger signal from SV-40 transformed cells than from normal diploid cells (data not shown).

Thus, these fibroblast cell lines expressed LTA_4-hydrolase, but 5-lipoxygenase activity was undetectable. Assuming that this is the case also for fibroblasts in vivo, this is an argument for transcellular metabolism of LTA_4. The function of LTA_4-hydrolase in fibroblasts could be to augment the formation of LTB_4 around activated leukocytes, and thus the recruitment of leukocytes to inflammatory sites. Furthermore, LTB_4 is chemotactic also for fibroblasts (4), and transcellular metabolism of LTA_4 could augment migration of fibroblasts in inflammation and wound healing.

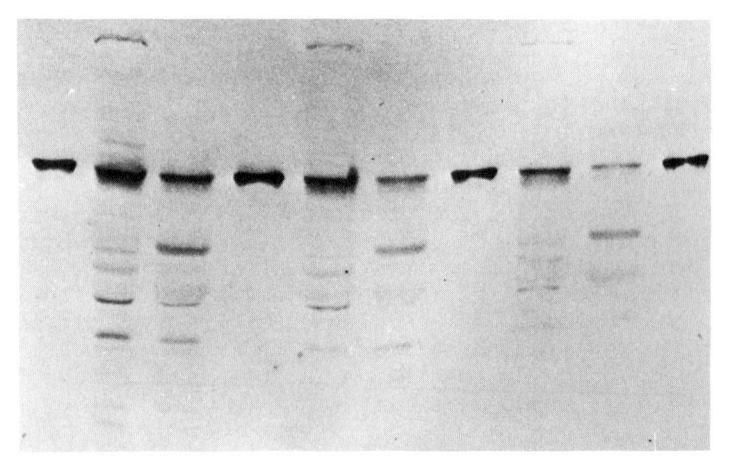

FIG 1. Western blot analysis of soluble proteins from fibroblast homogenates. After electrophoresis in a SDS-polyacrylamide gel and blotting to nitrocellulose, the membrane was incubated with a polyclonal LTA_4-hydrolase antiserum. Lanes 1, 4, 7 and 10 : standard LTA_4-hydrolase purified from human leukocytes (100 ng). Lanes 2, 5 and 8 : proteins from virus transformed cells, 45, 30 and 15 µg respectively. Lanes 3, 6 and 9 : proteins from normal diploid cells, 60, 40 and 20 µg respectively.

It is also possible that LTB_4 is involved in regulation of fibroblast cell growth. LTB_4 increases thymidine incorporation in fibroblasts stimulated by platelet derived growth factor (O.L. unpublished) and it may be speculated that the increased LTB_4 formation of the virus transformed cells bears some relation to their higher proliferative capacity.

LTA_4-hydrolase in HL-60 cells. The premyeloid human cell line HL-60 can be induced to differentiate to granulocytic or monocytic lineages. Treatment with DMSO leads to granulocytic differentiation, previously found to result in a higher capacity for leukotriene biosynthesis (5,6). In order to determine variations in LTA_4-hydrolase during DMSO induced differentiation, we incubated HL-60 cells with LTA_4. HL-60 cells were obtained from ATCC and cultured in RPMI 1640 or DMEM, with 10% foetal calf serum, penicillin and streptomycin. For differentiation, cells were seeded at 0.25×10^6 cells/ml, and dimethylsulfoxide (DMSO) and/or dexamethasone 21-phosphate was added as indicated. When the cells were harvested, after six days in culture, the viability was typically around 75% as judged by trypan blue exclusion.

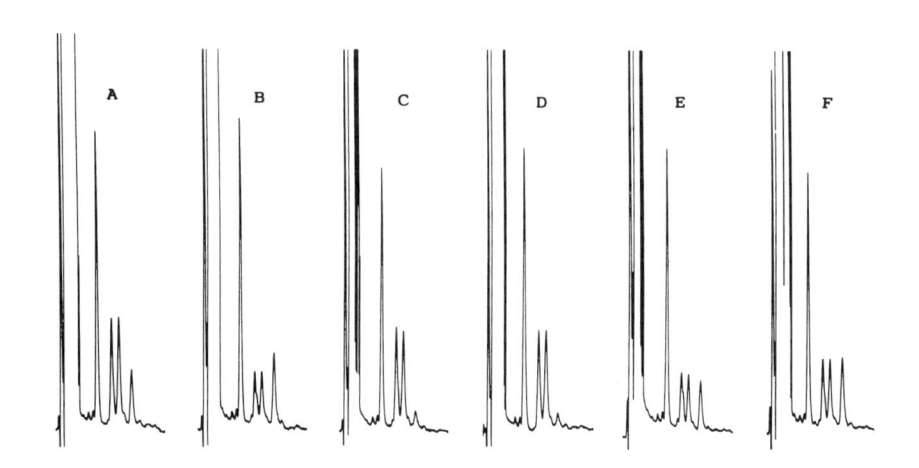

FIG 2. HPLC analysis of incubations of HL-60 cells with LTA_4. After six days in culture with different additions (see text), cells were harvested and resuspended in PBS with albumin (5 g/l). 30×10^6 cells (in 0.5 ml) were incubated with LTA_4 (5µM) for 15 min at $37°C$. The incubations were terminated by addition of methanol and internal standard prostaglandin B_1 (0.45 nmol). After solid phase extraction (C18) aliquots were analyzed by HPLC. A Nucleosil C18 column was eluted with methanol/ water/ TFA, 70/30/0.01 at 1 ml/min, with continous recording of the absorbance at 270 nm.

Representative HPLC tracings derived from incubations of equivalent numbers of intact cells (30×10^6) are shown in fig 2. Chromatogram A shows that nondifferentiated cells had a considerable basal LTA_4-hydrolase activity. After differentiation with DMSO (1.3%, v/v) for six days, the LTA_4-hydrolase activity (per cell) was increased (chromatogram B), and corresponded to 10-20% of the activity found in granulocytes prepared from peripheral blood. When the antiinflammatory steroid dexamethasone (1 or 10 µM) was added together with DMSO, this resulted in a decrease in the subsequent conversion of LTA_4 to LTB_4 (chromatograms C and D). However, when only dexamethasone (1 or 10 µM) was added to nondifferentiated cells, there was no apparent change in the subsequent conversion of LTA_4 (chromatograms E and F). This indicates that dexamethasone could attenuate the expression of LTA_4-hydrolase associated with differentiation, but not the basal expression in nondifferentiated cells. Total RNA was prepared from HL-60 cells, after culture for six days with different additions. When Northern blots were hybridized with the LTA_4-hydrolase probe, the signal corresponding to LTA_4-hydrolase mRNA was diminished after culture with both DMSO and dexamethasone, as compared to culture with DMSO only.

Whether these observations are of relevance for the supposed expression of LTA_4-hydrolase during maturation of granulocytes in vivo is a matter of speculation. However, the results are of interest in relation to the leukotactic role of LTB_4 in inflammation, and the observed effects of dexamethasone on leukocyte accumulation in vivo.

References

1. Rådmark, O. and Haeggström, J. (1990) In: Advances in Prostaglandin, Thromboxane and Leukotriene Research, edited by B. Samuelsson, S.E. Dahlén, J. Fritsch and P. Hedqvist. Raven Press, New York, vol. 20, in press.

2. Ohishi, N., Minami, M., Kobayashi, J., Seyama, Y., Hata, J., Yotsumoto, H., Takaku, F. and Shimizu, T. (1990) J. Biol. Chem., in press.

3. Medina, J.F., Barrios, C., Funk, C.D. Larsson, O., Haeggström, J. and Rådmark, O. (1990) Eur. J. Biochem., in press

4. Mensing, H. and Czarnetzki, B.M. (1984) J. Invest. Dermatol. 82, 9-12.

5. Anthes, J.C., Bryant, R.W., Musch, M.W., Kwokei, Ng and Siegel, M. I. (1986) Inflammation 10, 145-156.

6. Ziboh, V.A., Wong, T., Wu, M. and Yunis, A.A. (1986) J. Lab. Clin. Med., august issue, pp. 161-166.

THE BIOCHEMICAL AND PHARMACOLOGICAL MANIPULATION OF CELLULAR CYCLOOXYGENASE (COX) ACTIVITY.

Karen Seibert, Jaime L. Masferrer, Fu Jiyi, Atsushi Honda, Amiram Raz, and Philip Needleman*.

Washington University Medical School and the Monsanto Company*, St. Louis, Missouri USA.

INTRODUCTION

Inflammation is characterized morphologically by an influx of leukocytes into the interstitial space. Fibroblasts proliferate and fibrosis develops at the site. Tissue injury and inflammation are also commonly associated with enhanced eicosanoid release. Myocardial infarction (6), pulmonary fibrosis (4), renal ischemia (17) and hydronephrosis (18,22) are among the many examples of inflammatory pathologies characterized by exaggerated arachidonic acid release and metabolism. We hypothesize that the enhanced release of eicosanoids by infiltrating cells modulates the interactions among mononuclear cells, fibroblasts, platelets, and lymphocytes. These cell-cell interactions result in the release of inflammatory mediators coupled to arachidonate metabolism that collectively influence tissue injury.

Hydronephrosis can be induced by unilateral ureter obstruction in the rabbit and is characterized by a massive increase in arachidonic acid release and metabolism to PGE_2 and TxA_2 (20,24). Thromboxane synthetase activity, absent in the normal kidney, is markedly increased in the hydronephrotic kidney (HNK) (18,19). Angiotensin and bradykinin, endogenous inflammatory mediators, induce TxA_2 and PGE_2 production in the HNK compared to only modest changes in PGE_2 and no thromboxane production in a perfused normal kidney (22). Histologically, the post-obstructive kidney is characterized by a widening of the interstitial space and a marked influx of monocytes and macrophages to the nephrotic cortex followed by a massive proliferation of fibroblasts at the site (20,21,24). Interestingly, if the uretal obstruction is released, the macrophage population decreases accompanied by a decrease in arachidonate metabolism, while the fibrosis remains irreversible (24).

We assert that the invasion of macrophages into the HNK cortex and the proliferation of fibroblasts account for many of the metabolic changes observed in the nephrotic kidney, including the sustained increase in eicosanoid release. This hypothesis is supported by two observations: 1) perfusion of the HNK with endotoxin lipopolysaccharide (LPS), a macrophage agonist, results in a sustained and enhanced thromboxane response (23) and, 2) *in vivo* pretreatment with nitrogen mustard renders the rabbit leukopenic, blocking both the influx of macrophages to the nephrotic kidney cortex and the expected exaggerated thromboxane release (16). From these studies we conclude that monocytes and macrophages play a critical role in the tissue damage associated with hydronephrosis - not only as scavengers of necrotic tissue - but through the release of bioactive eicosanoids, proteolytic enzymes, and mononuclear cell factors (MNCF).

Our underlying hypothesis is that the release of eicosanoids and other bioactive compounds from monocytes, macrophages, fibroblasts, and lymphocytes contribute to the cellular basis of inflammation. We are now interested in understanding the temporal sequence of cell infiltration and how the biochemical regulation of the eicosanoids and other cellular mediators is involved in tissue injury and inflammation.

Anti-inflammatory glucocorticoids are widely employed for the treatment of acute and chronic inflammatory diseases. Glucocorticoids inhibit eicosanoid production, both *in vivo* and *in vitro*, in many cells and tissues including fibroblasts (27) and macrophages (9). The cellular mechanism of the glucocorticoids is unclear. It has been reported that dexamethasone (DEX) induces lipocortin I - a protein thought to inhibit phospholipase activity - resulting in a decrease in available arachidonate and eicosanoid production (7, 8, 11). However, recent reports indicate that lipocortin does not inhibit cellular phospholipase activity (13,28) nor do glucocorticoids induce the mRNA for lipocortin I in cells known to respond to DEX (3).

The following studies were designed to investigate the cellular mechanisms through which inflammatory mediators like the interleukins and LPS and the anti-inflammatory glucocorticoids modulate eicosanoid formation *in vitro* and *in vivo* in fibroblasts, monocytes, and macrophages.

Regulation of COX in Human Dermal Fibroblasts

Interleukin 1 (IL-1) is present in the synovial fluid of inflamed joints and is known to stimulate PGE_2 release in several cell types including dermal fibroblasts (10,14,26,29). We recently reported that fibroblasts respond to IL-1 in both a time and concentration dependent manner to stimulate the release of PGE_2 by increased COX activity (26); concentration of IL-1 as low as 0.1 U/ml significantly stimulate prostaglandin release into the cell culture medium with a maximum effect of IL-1 at 0.3 U/ml. Given that IL-1 increases COX activity, fibroblasts were labelled with [^{35}S]-methionine followed by immunoprecipitation with a specific rabbit anti-sheep polyclonal antibody for COX. We found that the increases in COX activity were coincident with IL-1 induced *de novo* synthesis of COX mass. Interestingly, the induction of COX in the fibroblasts could be separated into an early (actinomycin D sensitive) trancriptional phase and a later (cycloheximide but not actinomycin D sensitive) post-transcriptional phase. IL-1 exerted its effect on COX induction during the early transcriptional phase (Figure 1, lanes 3,4).

The anti-inflammatory agent, DEX, blocked the increase in COX activity seen following IL-1 stimulation (Figure 2, Panel A); a similar study reported that DEX inhibits the EGF-stimulated COX activity in aortic smooth muscle cells (25).

Immunoprecipitation of DEX-treated cells confirmed that the glucocorticoid inhibited induction of COX mass when added during the post-transcriptional "late" phase (Figure 1, lanes 1,3). Interestingly, the effect of DEX on COX could be blocked by the addition of actinomycin D (Figure 1, lane 2). Thus, the glucocorticoid effect on fibroblast COX appears to require new, dexamethasone-induced protein synthesis as it is both actinomycin D and cycloheximide sensitive. The effect of DEX on COX suggested a novel mechanism for the inhibition of PG release by glucocorticoid - quite different from an inhibition of phospholipase activity.

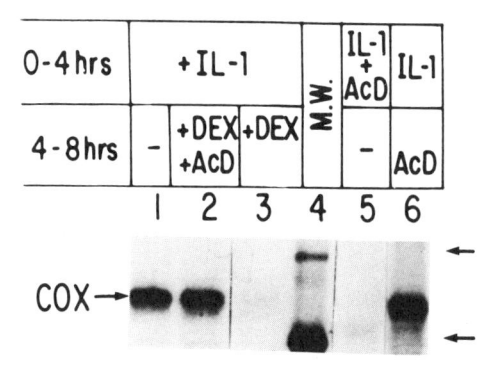

Figure 1. *De novo* synthesis of fibroblast COX. Fibroblasts were preincubated with IL-1 (0.3 U/ml) for 4 h and then further incubated for 4 h with or without dexamethasone (2 μM) or actinomycin D (1 μM). The cells were then incubated in methionine-poor DMEM plus [^{35}S]methionine for 6 h; solubilized cell preparations were processed for Staph A immunoprecipitation using a rabbit anti-sheep polyclonal antibody for COX and samples were analyzed by SDS-PAGE. Arrows indicate the position of molecular weight markers for phospholipase B (92 kDa) and BSA (68 kDa).

Endotoxin and Dexamethasone in Human Mononuclear Cells

Endotoxin lipopolysaccharide (LPS) is a monocyte/macrophage "agonist" that stimulates the release of arachidonic acid metabolites in mononuclear cells (1,15) as well as endothelial cells (2), neutrophils (2,5), and glomerular mesangial cells (30). We have recently found that LPS induces human blood monocytes in a time- and dose-dependent manner to release prodigious amounts of both prostaglandins and lipoxygenase products, with thromboxane the major metabolite formed (submitted for publication). Cells responded to as little as 1 ng/ml LPS to release PGE_2 and TxA_2 with maximal stimulation at 10 μg/ml (Figure 2, Panel B). DEX completely blocked the LPS-induced PG release with little effect on basal (i.e. unstimulated monocytes) COX activity. Immunoprecipitation of [^{35}S]methionine labelled cells confirmed that the effect of LPS and DEX on the monocyte could be a attributed to an increase or decrease, respectively, of COX mass.

The effect of LPS and DEX on phospholipase was examined following [^{3}H]arachidonic acid labelling of cells. Labelled cells, preincubated with LPS or DEX then stimulated with the ionophore A23187, demonstrated no difference in their ability to release [^{3}H]arachidonic acid which suggested that the effect of LPS on PG formation may be exclusive to the COX enzyme. In support of that observation, LPS and DEX exerted no apparent effect on lipoxygenase activity (measured by LTB_4 formation) or thromboxane synthetase activity (assessed as the conversion of exogenous PGH_2 to TxA_2) in the blood monocyte.

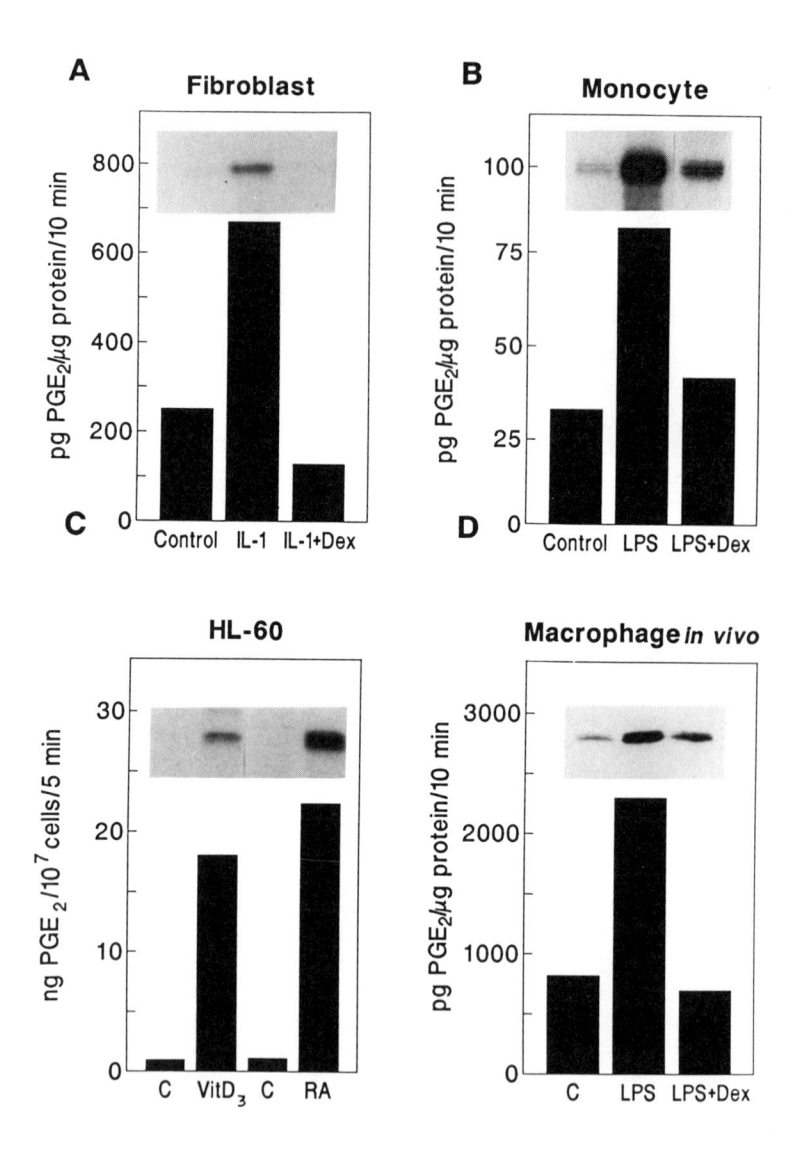

Figure 2. Modulation of COX by Dexamethasone. A. Fibroblasts were incubated in DMEM +/- IL-1 (0.3 U/ml) for 4 h, followed by DEX (2 μM) for 4 h. B. Monocytes were incubated +/- LPS (10 μg/ml) and DEX (2 μM) for 18 h. C. HL60 cells were incubated in RPMI + 10% FCS for 4 days + VitD$_3$ (26 nM) or 3 days + retinoic acid (1 μM). D. Mice were coinjected with LPS (50 μg/mouse, i.v.) and DEX (5 mg/kg, i.v.). After 12 h, macrophages were purified by adherence. COX activity and immunoprecipitations were as described (26).

It is interesting to note that two other mononuclear cell populations can respond to LPS and DEX *in vitro* similar to the human monocyte. The promyelocytic cell line, HL60, can be differentiated in culture to two different phenotypes: 1) with retinoic acid to a non-adherent granulocyte type that releases prodigious amounts of PGE_2 and 2) with $1\alpha,25$-dihydroxyvitamin D_3 to an adherent monocyte phenotype that produces PGE_2 as well as TxA_2 (12) (Figure 2, Panel C). In both cases the effect on prostaglandin release corresponds to an increase of *de novo* synthesized COX as measured by immunoprecipitation (submitted for publication). Preliminary observations suggest that vitamin D_3- differentiated HL60 cells respond to DEX similarly to human peripheral monocytes in culture.

Dexamethsone inhibits COX *In Vivo*

We have demonstrated that DEX inhibits *in vitro* COX activity by suppressing the *de novo* synthesis of COX in the dermal fibroblast, blood monocyte, human HL60 cell line, and the mouse peritoneal macarophage. Others have shown that steroids suppress COX mRNA levels and PG synthesis in cultured vascular cells (25). Glucocorticoids are therapeutically useful in the treatment of various systemic inflammatory disorders. We have recently found that *in vivo* administration of DEX will completely block the symptoms associated with endotoxemia following a single intravenous injection of LPS in mice (submitted for publication). LPS and/or DEX were coadministered and twelve hours later peritoneal macarophages were harvested and COX activity assessed. DEX completely blocked the increased COX activity produced by LPS; DEX also produced only a small decrease in basal (not LPS treated) macrophage COX activity (Figure 2, Panel D). The regulation observed in COX activity by LPS and DEX were mimicked by changes in COX mass as determined by immunoprecipitation. The effect on COX seemed localized to the peritoneal cells as there was no effect on COX by LPS or DEX in kidney microsomes. These studies bridge the gap between the *in vitro* observation made on COX and the potential theraeputic effect of DEX on COX activity and synthesis *in vivo*.

CONCLUSION

Inflammation involves many cell types - mononuclear cells, fibroblasts, lymphocytes - converging at the site of injury and interacting via eicosanoid and inflammatory mediator release. We have shown that the increase in PG release *in vitro* in fibroblasts, monocytes, and macrophages can, in all instances, be explained by an increase in COX activity via new protein synthesis. Furthermore, the anti-inflammatory glucocorticoid inhibits COX to block prostaglandin release not only *in vitro* but *in vivo* as well. It is interesting that the inhibition of basal (unstimulated) COX by DEX is minimal whereas DEX exhibits a much greater effect on a stimulated, or induced, COX. This suggests the possible existence of multiple COX pools - constitutive and stimulated - possibly under different regulatory controls.

The question of multiple COX pools remains to be answered; however COX does appear to be the critical regulatory enzyme in prostaglandin biosynthesis that is readily amenable to hormonal, cytokine, and pharmacologic manipulation.

ACKNOWLEDGEMENTS

This work was supported by National Institutes of Health Grants RO1-HL20787 and PO1-DK38111.

REFERENCES

1. Aderem, A.A., Cohen, D.S., Wright, S.D., and Cohn, Z. (1986) J. Exp. Med., 164:165-179.
2. Bottoms, G.D., Johnson, M.A., Lamar, C.H., Fessler, J.F., and Turek, J.J. (1985) Circ. Shock, 15:155-162.
3. Brönnegard, M., Anderson, O., Edwaull, D., Lund, J., Norstedt, G., and Carlstedt-Duke, J. (1988) Mol. Endocrinol., 2:732-739.
4. Clark, J.G., Kostal, K.M., and Marino, B.H. (1983) J. Clin. Invest., 72:2082-2091.
5. T. Doerfler, E.M., Danner, L.R., Shelhamer, H.J., and Parillo, E.J. (1989) J. Clin. Invest., 83:970-977.
6. Evers, A.S., Murphree, S., Saffitz, J.E., Jakschik, B.A., and Needleman, P. (1985) J. Clin. Invest., 75:992-999.
7. Flower, R.J. and Blackwell, G.L. (1979) Nature, 278:456-459.
8. Flower, R.J. (1989) Adv. Inflamm. Res., 8:1-34.
9. Fuller, W.R., Kelsey, R.C., Cole, J.P., Dollary, T.C., and MacDermot, J. (1984) Clin. Sci., 67:653-656.
10. Gerry, I. and Lepe-Zuniga, J.L. (1984) Lymphokines, 6:109-125.
11. Hirata, F., Schiffman, E., Venkatasubramanian, K., Solomon, D., and Axelrod, J. (1980) Proc. Natl. Acad. Sci. USA, 77:2533-2536.
12. Honda, A., Morita, I., Murota, S., and Mori, Y. (1986) Biophys. Biochem. Acta., 877:423-432.
13. Hullin, F., Raynal, P., Ragalo-Thomas, M.F.J., Fauvel, J. and Chap, H. (1989) J. Biol. Chem., 264:3506-3513.
14. Kampschmidt, R.F. (1984) J. Leukocyte Biol., 36:341-355.
15. Kurland, J.I. and Bockman, R. (1978) J. Exp. Med., 147:952-957.
16. Lefkowith, J.B., Okegawa, T., DeSchryver-Kecskemeti, K., and Needleman, P. (1984) Kid. Intl., 26:10-17.
17. McGiff, J.C., Crowshaw, K., Terragno, N.A., Lonigro, A.J., Strand, J.C., Williamson, M.A., Lee, J.B., and Ng, K.D.F. (1970) Circ. Res., 27:765-789.
18. Morrison, A.R., Nishikawa, K., and Needleman, P. (1977) Nature, 269:259-260.
19. Morrison, A.R., Nishikawa, K., and Needleman, P. (1978) J. Pharmacol. Exp. Ther., 205:1-8.
20. Nagle, R.B., Bulger, R.E., Cutler, R.E., Jervis, H.R., and Benditt, E.P. (1973) Lab. Invest., 28:456-467.
21. Nagle, R.B., Johnson, M.E., and Jervis, H.R. (1976) Lab. Invest., 35:18-22.
22. Nishikawa, K., Morrison, A.R., and Needleman, P. (1977) J. Clin. Invest., 59:1143-1150.
23. Okegawa, T., DeSchryver-Kecskemeti, K., and Needleman, P. (1983) J. Pharmacol. Exp. Ther., 225:213-218.
24. Okegawa, T., Jonas, P.E., DeSchryver, K., Kawasaki, A., and Needleman, P. (1983) J. Clin. Invest., 71:81-90.
25. Pash, M.J. and Bailey, M.J. (1988) Faseb J., 2:2613-2618.

26. Raz, A., Wyche, A., and Needleman, P. (1988) J. Biol. Chem., 263:3022-3028.
27. Raz, A., Wyche, A., and Needleman, P. (1989) Proc. Natl. Acad. Sci. USA, 86:1657-1661.
28. Russo-Marie, F. and Duval, D. (1982) Biochim. Biophys. Acta, 712:177-185.
29. Simon, P.L. and Willoughby, W.F. (1982) Lymphokines, 6:47-63.
30. Wang, J., Kester, M., and Dunn, J.M. (1988) Biochimica et Biophysica Acta, 963:429-435.

INDUCTION OF FATTY ACID CYCLOOXYGENASE
IN MOUSE OSTEOBLASTIC CELLS (MC3T3-E1)

S. Yamamoto[1], T. Oshima[1], M. Kusaka[1], T. Yoshimoto[1], C. Yokoyama[2], T. Takai[2], T. Tanabe[2], and M. Kumegawa[3]

[1] Department of Biochemistry, Tokushima University
School of Medicine, Tokushima 770
[2] National Cardiovascular Center Research Institute, Osaka 565
[3] Department of Oral Anatomy, Meikai University
School of Dentistry, Saitama 350-02, Japan

After the arachidonate release is triggered by phospholipase fatty acid cyclooxygenase is a rate-limiting enzyme. Therefore, studies on the regulatory property of the key enzyme are required for elucidation of the physiological and pathological roles of prostaglandins and thromboxanes. As an example, we will discuss the cyclooxygenase enzyme of mouse osteoblasts which produce PGE_2 as a bone-resorption factor. Arachidonic acid is transformed to PGH_2 via PGG_2 by the catalysis of PG endoperoxide synthase as a bifunctional enzyme with both cyclooxygenase and hydroperoxidase activities (4,6). The endoperoxide of PGH_2 is isomerized, and PGE_2 is produced (5). MC3T3-E1 cell, which we used in this work, was cloned from newborn mouse calvaria by Kodama et al. (1). The cell line differentiates into an osteoblast in the cell culture, and is characteristic of its calcification in vitro (8). Parameters of bone formation change in response to various hormones and growth factors (2).

Arachidonate metabolites were derivatized with 9-anthryl diazomethane, and the fluorescent derivatives were separated by HPLC. PGE_2 was found as an essentially sole arachidonate metabolite in this unique and useful cell line. The PGE_2 synthesis by MC3T3-E1 cells was markedly stimulated by the addition of epidermal growth factor(EGF) to the culture medium (10). A maximum stimulation was observed by the presence of about 1 ng of EGF in 1 ml of culture medium. After the addition of EGF, the PGE_2 production was initiated with a lag phase of about 1 h (FIG. 1). Transforming growth factor(TGF)-β also stimulated the PGE_2 release (9). The addition of 1 ng of TGF-β to 1 ml of culture medium gave a maximum stimulation. There was a lag phase of about 1 h before the start of PGE_2 release.

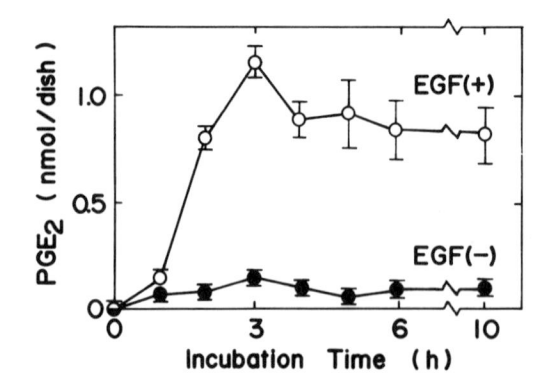

FIG. 1 PGE$_2$ relase by MC3T3-E1 cells stimulated by epidermal growth factor.

The biosynthesis of PGE$_2$ from endogenous arachidonic acid is considered to be triggered by phospholipase. We examined effect of these growth factors on the arachidonate release. The cells were prelabeled with ^{14}C-arachidonic acid, and then either TGF-β or EGF was added to the culture medium. As shown in FIG. 2, arachidonate release was fast, whereas PGE$_2$ synthesis started with a lag phase of more than 1 h. These observations indicate that the arachidonate liberation is triggered by EGF or TGF-β, but the cyclooxygenase reaction is a rate-limiting step after the arachidonate release. When aspirin was given to irreversibly inhibit cyclooxygenase, addition of EGF stimulated the PGE$_2$ release in the aspirin-treated cells as much as in the intact cells (10). The observation suggested a de novo synthesis of the enzyme protein rather than an activation of a constitutive enzyme.

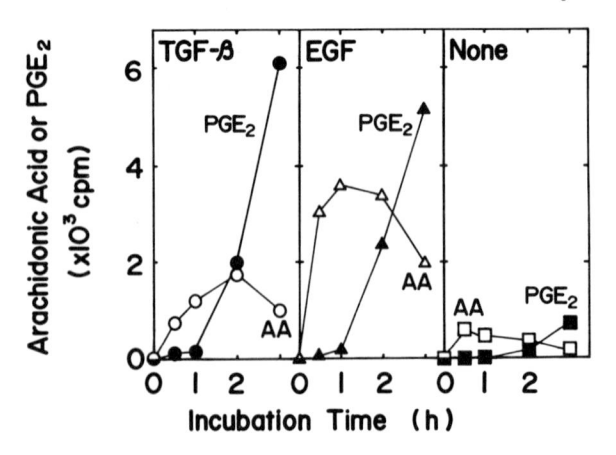

FIG. 2 Arachidonate relase and PGE$_2$ synthesis by MC3T3-E1 cells labeled with ^{14}C-arachidonic acid.

In addition to these peptidyl growth factors, we found that epinephrine was a stimulator of the PGE$_2$ synthesis (3). The PGE$_2$ release in the culture medium started about 1 h after addition of epinephrine, and reached a maximum after 3 h. FIG. 3 presents effect of epinephrine concentration on the PGE$_2$ synthesis. The PGE$_2$ release increased in a concentration-dependent manner, and about 0.1 μM epinephrine gave a maximal stimulation. In view of such a stimulatory effect of epinephrine on the PGE$_2$ synthesis we examined a possible involvement of adrenergic receptor (3). First, we tested various agonists and antagonists. Isoproterenol as a β-agonist was as active as epinephrine, while phenylephrine as an α-agonist was much less effective. Propranolol at 1 μM as a β-antagonist abolished the stimulatory effect of 1 μM epinephrine.

Since the results suggested the participation of a β-adrenergic receptor, we investigated whether cAMP was involved in the

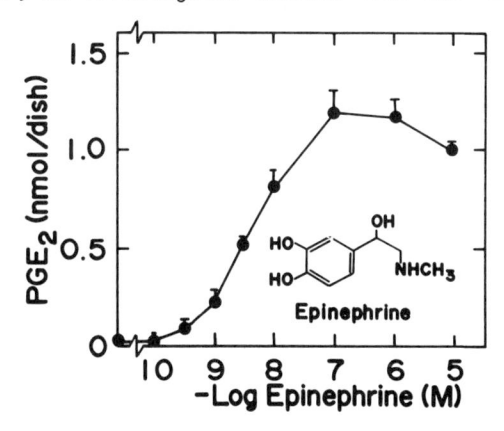

FIG. 3 PGE$_2$ release by MC3T3-E1 cells stimulated by epinephrine.

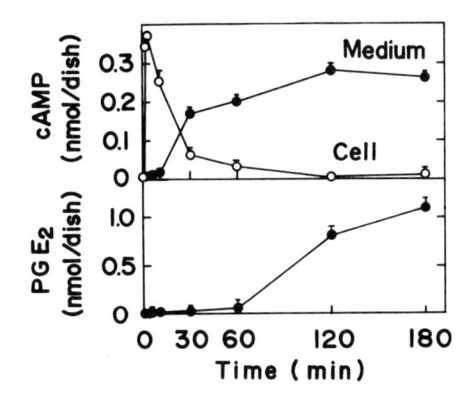

FIG. 4 Time courses of epinephrine-stimulated synthesis of cAMP and PGE$_2$ in MC3T3-E1 cells.

stimulation of PGE$_2$ production by MC3T3-E1 cells (3). As shown in FIG. 4, we found a rapid accumulation of cAMP within the cells depending on the epinephrine concentration. The time course of cAMP production was compared with that of the PGE$_2$ release. The intracellular cAMP level reached a maximum almost immediately when epinephrine was added to the cell culture. In contrast, no PGE$_2$ synthesis was observed for at least 1 h, and then the PGE$_2$ level increased reaching a maximum after 3 h. We applied other methods to increase the intracellular cAMP level (3). When cholera toxin was given to MC3T3-E1 cells, the intracellular cAMP level increased in a concentration-dependent manner. The release of PGE$_2$ also increased depending on the amount of cholera toxin. Forskolin, which also increased the intracellular cAMP, stimulated the PGE$_2$ synthesis. Both 8-bromo-cAMP and dibutyryl cAMP stimulated the PGE$_2$ production. All these data suggested that cAMP was involved in the stimulation of PGE$_2$ synthesis.

The enzymes for PGE$_2$ synthesis were localized in microsomes of bovine seminal vesicle (4). Therefore, the microsomes were prepared from the epinephrine-treated cells and the control cells (3). The conversion of arachidonic acid to PGH$_2$ occurred at a much higher rate with the microsomes from the epinephrine-treated cells. In contrast, the conversion of PGH$_2$ to PGE$_2$ was not significantly affected by the presence of epinephrine. Thus, the overall synthesis of PGE$_2$ was stimulated by epinephrine at the step of cyclooxygenase.

As shown in FIG. 5, the epinephrine-dependent stimulation of PGE$_2$ synthesis was inhibited by the presence of actinomycin D as a transcription inhibitor and cycloheximide as a translation inhibitor (3). These experimental results suggested that the cyclooxygenase protein was induced or synthesized de novo in the

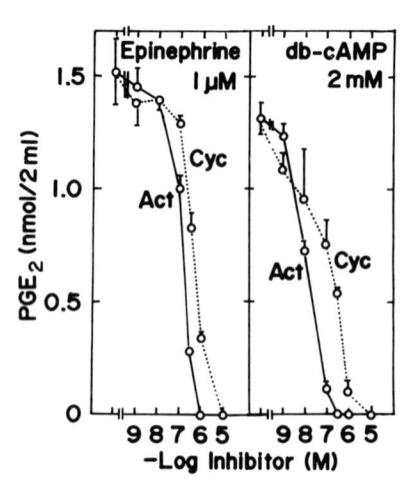

FIG. 5 Inhibition by actinomycin D and cycloheximide of PGE$_2$ synthesis stimulated by epinephrine and dibutyryl cAMP.

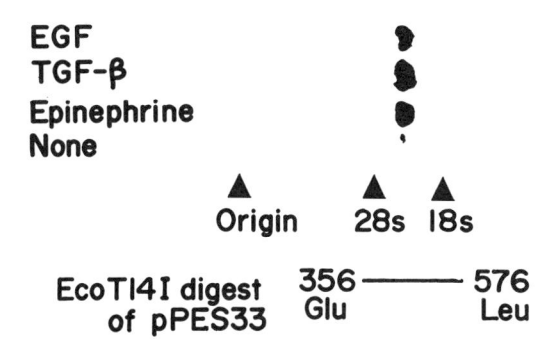

```
   EGF              •
   TGF-β            •
   Epinephrine      •
   None             ·

              ▲       ▲   ▲
            Origin   28s  18s

   EcoT14I digest   356 ——— 576
      of pPES33     Glu      Leu
```

FIG. 6 Northern blotting of cyclooxygenase mRNA in MC3T3-E1 cells.

presence of epinephrine. It should be noted that the PGE_2 synthesis stimulated by dibutyryl cAMP was also inhibited by actinomycin D and cycloheximide.

We carried out Western blotting to qualitatively demonstrate that the amount of the cyclooxygenase protein actually increased when the cells were treated with epinephrine. The cells were incubated with 1 μM epinephrine for various time intervals. Whole cells were treated with Tween 20. The cyclooxygenase in the high-speed supernatant was separated by SDS-polyacrylamide gel electrophoresis. The cyclooxygenase was immunostained with the aid of anti-cyclooxygenase antibody, which was raised against the enzyme of bovine seminal vesicle. The cyclooxygenase bands were denser depending on the iucubation time after the addition of epinephrine.

The next approach to clearly demonstrate the cyclooxygenase induction, was the determination of mRNA. A cDNA fragment, which encoded 220 C-terminal amino acids of the enzyme of ovine seminal vesicle, was isolated previously (11), and used in this work as a probe to specifically detect the cyclooxygenase mRNA (FIG. 6). Total RNA was isolated from the cells, and subjected to Northern blotting. A 3.4-kb mRNA was detected with ^{32}P-labeled probe. Autoradiograms of the Northern blots showed qualitatively higher levels of the cyclooxygenase mRNA from the cells which were treated with EGF, TGF-β and epinephrine, respectively. Each dark band was quantitated by the use of a laser densitometer. The cyclooxygenase mRNA increased depending on the epinephrine concentration. A maximum mRNA level was found with epinephrine at 0.1 μM. This concentration of epinephrine brought about a maximum enzyme activity. We examined effect of 8-bromo-cAMP and dibutyryl cAMP on the cyclooxygenase mRNA level. These compounds were as active as epinephrine. Similar results were obtained with forskolin and cholera toxin.

In order to find out whether the cyclooxygenase mRNA synthesis requires a continuous presence of epinephrine or only its transient presence is sufficient, we preincubated the cells with epinephrine for various time intervals, and then the culture medium was replaced by a fresh medium containing no epinephrine. Only 5-min preincubation was sufficient for the increase of both mRNA and activity of the cyclooxygenase. When the time course of the cyclooxygenase mRNA synthesis was followed after the addition of epinephrine, the mRNA level increased during the initial 1 h, and then slightly decreased for the following several hours. There was another rise of the mRNA level reaching a maximum 9 h after the epinephrine addition. The first rise in the mRNA was followed by increase of the enzyme activity which was determined by the overall synthesis of PGE_2 from exogenous arachidonic acid. The significance of the biphasic change in the mRNA level has not yet been fully understood. Recently we found a concomitant increase in the mRNA and activity of cyclooxygenase depending on the PGE_2 concentration. Therefore, the second rise of the mRNA may be attributable to the accumulating PGE_2.

cAMP is well known as an intracellular second messenger. It is produced in response to a transmembrane signal transduction, and activates protein kinase A which phosphorylates a variety of enzymes and proteins. Another cAMP function is a transcriptional role which was earlier found in bacterial cells. Recently the biosynthesis of various mammalian enzymes and bioactive proteins has been found to be controlled by cAMP at the gene level(7). As discussed in this paper, the PGE_2 synthesis in MC3T3-E1 cells is regulated by the cyclooxygenase induction, which is mediated by a certain transcriptional role of cAMP. Does cAMP activate protein kinase A, which may phosphorylate a still unkonwn transcriptional factor? Is there a cAMP-responsive element in the cyclooxygenase gene? Does cAMP stabilize preexisting mRNA for cyclooxygenase? These are questions to be answered by our further molecular biological investigations.

Acknowledgement This work has been supported by grants-in-aid from the Ministry of Education, Science and Culture and the Ministry of Health and Welfare of Japan

References

1. Kodama, H., Amagai, Y., Sudo, H., Kasai, S., and Yamamoto, S. (1981): Jpn. J. Oral Biol., 23:899-901.

2. Kumegawa, M., Hiramatsu, M., Hatakeyama, K., Yajima, T., Kodama, H., Usaki, T., and Kurisu, K. (1983): Calcif. Tissue Int., 35:542-548.

3. Kusaka, M., Oshima, T., Yokota, K., Yamamoto, S., and Kumegawa, M. (1988): Biochim. Biophys. Acta, 972:339-346.

4. Miyamoto, T., Ogino, N., Yamamoto, S., and Hayaishi, O. (1976): J. Biol. Chem., 251:2629-2636.

5. Ogino, N., Miyamoto, T., Yamamoto, S., and Hayaishi, O. (1977): J. Biol. Chem., 252:890-895.

6. Ohki, S., Ogino, N., Yamamoto, S., and Hayaishi, O. (1979): J. Biol. Chem., 254:829-836.

7. Roesler, W.J., Vandenbark, G.R., and Hanson, R.W. (1988): J. Biol. Chem., 263:9063-9066.

8. Sudo, H., Kodama, H., Amagai, Y., Yamamoto, S., and Kasai, S. (1983): J. Cell Biol., 96:191-198.

9. Sumitani, K., Kawata, T., Yoshimoto, T., Yamamoto, S., and Kumegawa, M. (1989): Arch. Biochem. Biophys., 270:588-595.

10. Yokota, K., Kusaka, M., Ohshima, T., Yamamoto, S., Kurihara, N., Yoshino, T., and Kumegawa, M. (1986): J. Biol. Chem., 261:15410-15415.

11. Yokoyama, C., Takai, T., and Tanabe, T. (1988): FEBS Lett., 231:347-351.

CLONING AND CHARACTERIZATION OF HUMAN CYCLOOXYGENASE GENE

AND PRIMARY STRUCTURE OF THE ENZYME

Chieko Yokoyama, Hiroyuki Toh[*], Atsuro Miyata
and Tadashi Tanabe

Department of Pharmacology, National Cardiovascular Center
Research Institute, Fujishiro-dai, Suita, Osaka 565, Japan
[*]Protein Engineering Research Institute,
Furuedai, Suita, Osaka 565, Japan

Cyclooxygenase (EC 1.14.99.1, Prostaglandin (PG) endoperoxide synthase, PGH synthase) is the enzyme catalyzing the first step of PG biosynthesis (1). Recently, cDNAs encoding sheep and mouse cyclooxygenase were isolated and their primary structures of the enzyme have been determined from the nucleotide sequences of the cDNA (2-5). Though cDNA for the human enzyme has been cloned (6), neither its nucleotide sequence nor the primary structure has been reported. Several groups have shown that hormones, growth factors, cAMP and interleukin-1 regulated messenger RNA levels of the enzyme in cultured mammalian cells. To study the gene expression of cyclooxygenase it is important to determine the gene structure of the enzyme. In this paper, we report isolation and partial characterization of human gene encoding cyclooxygenase, and the primary structure of the human enzyme, which has been deduced from nucleotide sequences of 11 exons (7).

We have previously reported the isolation of cDNA clones for sheep cyclooxygenase (2). The fragments of the sheep cDNA clones, (nucleotides -111-239, 116-701, 758-1442, 1002-1221, 1223-1310, 1311-1432, 1433-1922) were labeled with [α-^{32}P] dCTP and their mixture was used as a probe for screening of the human genomic library (Japanese peripheral blood) in EMBL3. Isolated four genomic DNA clones; λhPES 13, λ hPES 20, λ hPES 27 and λ hPES 29 covered approximately 40 kb of human gene.

The exons were determined by nucleotide sequencing. The translational initiation codon, ATG was assigned by comparing the sequence with those of sheep and human cDNAs. The nucleotide sequence surrounding the putative initiation codon agrees with the consensus sequence for eukaryotic initiation sites described by Kozak. The exon containing this initiation codon was tentatively named exon 1. Protein coding sequence appeared in 11 exons. A typical polyadenylation signal, AATAAA, appeared at 727-732 bp downstream from the first residue of the termination codon, TGA in the exon 11.

Human cyclooxygenase gene was analyzed by Southern blot hybridization. Ten μg each of the genomic DNA isolated from human leukocytes was digested with Eco RI, Hind III, a mixture of Eco RI and Hind III, Sma I, Bam HI, and Pvu II. After the agarose electrophoresis, genomic DNA fragments were transferred to a nylon membrane and hybridized with the Pst I-fragment(246 bp) of the isolated cyclooxygenase gene containing the exon 5 as a probe. Only one fragment was hybridized with the probe when the genomic DNA digested with each restriction enzyme (FIG. 1). The sizes of those fragments agreed with the estimated values from the restriction map determined from the isolated genomic clones. This result possibly implies that there may be one gene coding for human cyclooxygenase. More detailed study, however, will be necessary to determine the precise gene copy number.

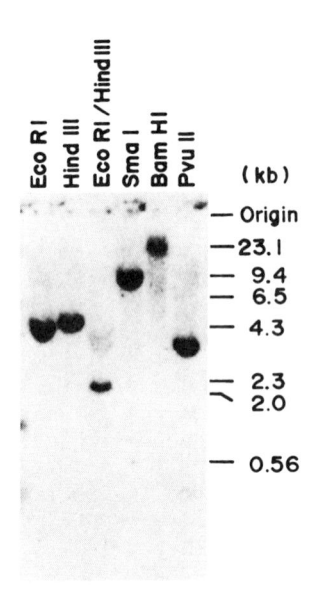

FIG. 1. Southern blot analysis of human cyclooxygenase gene.

RNA blot hybridization analysis was carried out using the RNA from human platelets and placenta. A cDNA fragment isolated from a cDNA library of human endothelial cells was used as a probe, which contains the sequences of the exon 11 and a part of the exon 10. As shown in FIG. 2, platelets cyclooxygenase mRNA appeared at the sizes of approximately 3 and 5.6 kilo nucleotides (5 μg of total RNA, lane 1). With use of 10 μg of total RNA from human placenta, mRNA of the enzyme was not detected (lane 2). However, a major band of 3 kilo-nucleotides and a minor band of a larger size were detectable when 15 µg of placenta poly(A)$^+$ RNA was analyzed (lane 3).

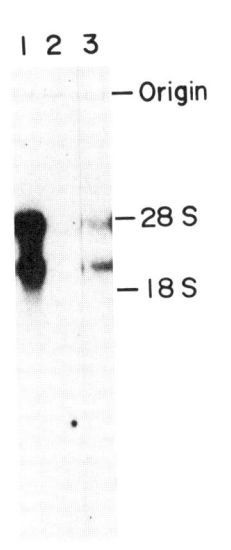

FIG. 2. RNA blot analysis of human cyclooxygenase mRNA. lane 1, 5 µg of human platelet total RNA; lane 2, 10 µg of human placenta total RNA; lane 3, 15 µg of human placenta poly(A)$^+$RNA.

The amino acid sequence of human cyclooxygenase deduced from the nucleotide sequence suggested that the precursor form of the human enzyme is composed of 599 amino acid residues with a molecular weight of 68,548. The primary structure of human cyclooxygenase exhibited approximately 90 % identity to those of the sheep (2) and mouse (5) enzymes and the nucleotide sequences of the open reading frames encoding the human and sheep enzymes showed a 88.5 % homology. The amino terminal 23-amino acid residues shows a characteristic sequence of the signal peptide as found in the sheep enzyme (2-4). Four potential asparagine-linked glycosylation sites and the aspirin acetylation site were found in the amino acid sequences of the animal enzymes (2-5, 7).

Various proteins have EGF-like sequences, though roles of the domains have not been known yet. The amino terminal part of the amino acid sequence of the sheep enzyme was shown to resemble that of EGF (8). Also the amino terminal parts of the amino acid sequences of the human and mouse enzymes resemble that of EGF and 6 cysteine residues and 3 glycine residues involved in construction of the protein structure of EGF are completely preserved. It is noteworthy that the EGF-like domain of the human enzyme (residues 33-71) encoded by the entire region of the exon 3 is highly identical with sequences of sheep and mouse enzyme. This fact may support the notion that the EGF-like domain of the enzyme has occured by exon-shuffling during the evolution of the enzyme (8).

Cyclooxygenase is homologous with the other peroxidases around the histidine-285 of the mature form which may bind heme (5). We searched the homology with various peroxidases more carefully; human, mouse and porcine thyroid peroxidase, human, rat and mouse myeroperoxidase, and human eosinophil peroxidase (9). The identical residues or residues showing conservative substitution appeared not only around the histidine-285 but in the wide region between residue 198 and C-terminus. A genealogical tree of the peroxidase domain was constructed based on the sequences of the homologous regions. The result suggested that cyclooxygenase was separated from other peroxidases in an early period of the evolution. Furthermore, the molecular evolutionary rate calculated among the human, sheep and mouse cyclooxygenase is very slow. This may support that cyclooxygenase plays a physiologically important role in animals.

ACKNOWLEDGEMENTS

This work has been supported in part by grants from the Ministry of Health, and Welfare and the Ministry of Education, Science and Culture of Japan, and by grants from ONO Medical Research Foundation, Yamanouchi Foundation of Research on Metabolic Disorders, Japan. Platelets was kindly donated by Osaka Red Cross Blood Center, Japan.

REFERENCES

1. Yamamoto, S. (1989): Prostag. Leukot. Essent. Fat. Acids, 35:219-229.
2. Yokoyama, C., Takai, T., and Tanabe, T. (1988): FEBS Lett., 231:347-351.
3. DeWitt, D.L., and Smith, W.L. (1988): Proc. Natl. Acad. Sci. USA, 85:1412-1416, and correction p.5056.
4. Merlie, J.P., Fagan, D., Mudd, J. and Needleman, P. (1988): J. Biol. Chem., 263:3550-3553.
5. DeWitt, D.L., El-Harith, E.A., Kraemer, S.A., Andrews, M.J., Yao, E.F., Armstrong, R.L. and Smith, W.L. (1990): J. Biol. Chem., 265:5192-5198.
6. Hla, T., Farrell, M., Kumar, A., and Bailey, J.M. (1986): Prostaglandins, 32:829-845.
7. Yokoyama, C. and Tanabe, T. (1989): Biochem. Biophys. Res. Commun., 165:888-894.
8. Toh, H.(1989): FEBS Lett., 258:317-319.
9. Toh, H., et al., submitted.

SERUM INDUCTION AND SUPERINDUCTION OF PGG/H SYNTHASE mRNA LEVELS IN 3T3 FIBROBLASTS

David L. DeWitt, Stacey A. Kraemer, and Elizabeth A. Meade

Department of Biochemistry, Michigan State University
East Lansing, Michigan, 48824 USA

Historically, prostaglandin synthesis has been assumed to be controlled solely by the activation of specific phospholipases that in turn liberate arachidonate from phospholipid stores. However, expression of prostaglandin endoperoxide (PGG/H) synthase, the enzyme which catalyzes the conversion of arachidonate to prostaglandin H_2, the precursor of $PGF_{2\alpha}$, PGE_2, PGD_2, prostacyclin, and thromboxane A_2, has also been shown to be regulated. Numerous animal and cell culture model systems have been described in which growth factors (4,5,13,14), cytokines (3,10,11), hormones (7,8), and tumor promoters (14), modulate PGG/H synthase protein levels, indicating that this may be a general mechanism for controlling prostaglandin synthesis. The goal of this research it to determine the molecular mechanisms regulating PGG/H synthase synthesis. To address this question we have used a recently cloned mouse PGG/H synthase cDNA (2) to examine PGG/H synthase gene expression in 3T3 fibroblasts, a cell system in which expression of PGG/H synthase appears to be under control of growth factors.

METHODS

3T3 cells were subcultured at a density of 2×10^5 cells per 100 mm dish in 10 ml of DME media containing 100 µg/ml penicillin, 100 µg/ml streptomycin, and 10% fetal calf serum and allowed to grow for seven days. Quiescence was confirmed by measuring ^{3}H-thymidine incorporation (data not shown). At time zero, spent medium was removed and 5 ml of fresh culture medium was added, with or without 10 µg/ml cycloheximide. Cells (1.5×10^7) were harvested by washing plates twice with 5 ml ice cold phosphate buffered saline (PBS), then by scraping the cells with a rubber policeman into 5 ml per plate of PBS. The cells were collected by centrifugation at 2000 rpm in a Beckman GLC centrifuge and cytoplasmic RNA was isolated (12). Poly(A+)RNA was separated from total cytoplasmic RNA by oligo-dt cellulose chromatography (12). This mRNA was fractionated by electrophoresis on a 1% formaldehyde agarose gel and transferred to nitrocellulose filters. These filters were then hybridized (12) for 18 hours simultaneously with [α-^{32}P]dCTP labeled probes for the mouse PGG/H synthase cDNA (3), the mouse

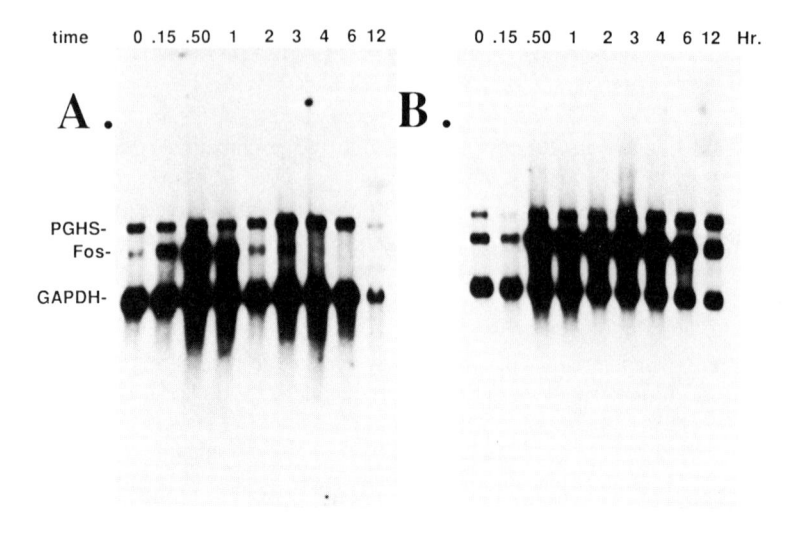

Figure 1- Autoradiogram of northern blots of poly(A+)RNA isolated from (A), serum; and (B), serum plus 10 µg/ml cycloheximide stimulated 3T3 fibroblasts. Blots were simultaneously hybridized with ^{32}P-labeled probe to the mouse c-fos gene, PGG/H synthase cDNA, and the GAPDH gene.

c-fos gene (ATCC-41041), and the glyceraldehyde-3-phosphate dehydrogenase gene (GAPDH) (1). After autoradiography, bands corresponding to the hybridized mRNA species were cut from the nitrocellulose and quantitated by scintillation counting. Values for the PGG/H synthase and c-fos were normalized to the values for the GAPDH to correct for variations in mRNA recovery and changes in total mRNA levels during mitogenesis.

RESULTS

Autoradiographs from northern blots of poly(A+)RNA isolated from serum stimulated 3T3 fibroblasts are presented in Figure 1. The values obtained for hybridization of the ^{32}P-labeled probes to both c-fos and PGG/H synthase mRNA normalized to the hybridization to GAPDH mRNA are presented in Figure 2. In serum stimulated cells (Fig. 1a, 2b) PGG/H synthase mRNA levels transiently increased to 1.5 fold zero time levels 3-4 hours after serum addition and returned to below 0 time levels at 12 hours. In cells stimulated in the presence of 10 µg/ml cycloheximide (Fig. 1b,2b), PGG/H synthase message levels increased for the duration of the experiment reaching 4-5 fold the 0 time levels by twelve hours. c-Fos message levels (Fig. 1,2a), which were monitored as an

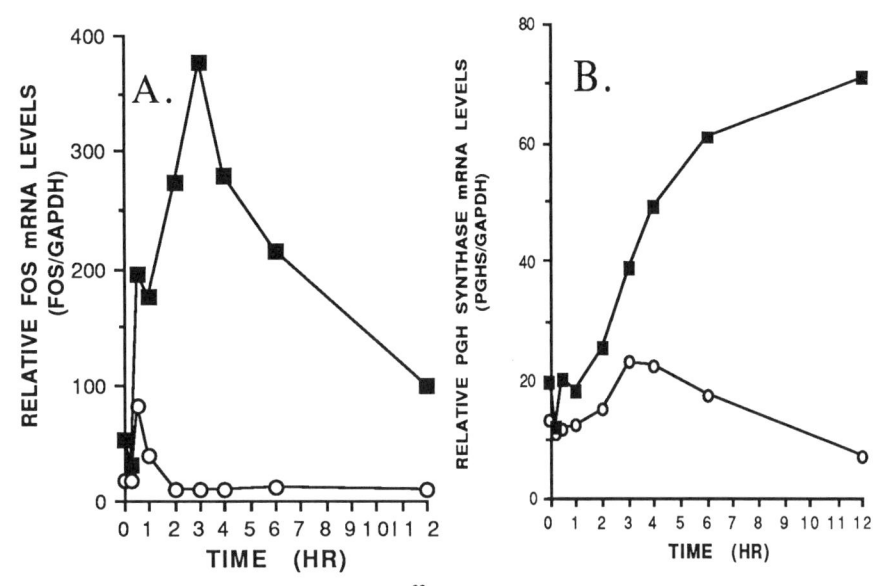

Figure 2. (A) Relative hybridization of ^{32}P-probes to c-fos mRNA as determined by scintillation counting of the corresponding nitrocellulose bands excised from the northern blots shown in figure 1. Values are normalized to the hybridization to GAPDH gene probe. (B) Relative hybridization to the PGG/H synthase mRNA. (Open circles, 10 % serum stimulated; solid squares, 10% serum plus 10 µg/ml cycloheximide stimulated.)

internal control, transiently increased in serum stimulated cells, and were both superinduced and stabilized in serum plus cycloheximide treated cells (6).

DISCUSSION

Both prostaglandin synthesis and PGG/H synthase activity have been reported to increase at from 3-4 hours after PDGF stimulation of Swiss 3T3 cells (4,5), suggesting that PDGF induces the de novo synthesis of the PGG/H synthase. Our experiment, using instead mitogenic stimulation with fetal calf serum, demonstrated a transient increase in PGG/H synthase mRNA levels 3-4 hours after serum addition which correlates well with the reported increase in PGG/H synthase expression. One possible mechanism for regulating PGG/H synthase expression in 3T3 cells thus, may be by regulating PGG/H synthase mRNA levels. In contrast with these results, Lin et al.(9), while observing similar PDGF stimulated increases in PGG/H synthase mRNA levels in NIH-3T3 cells, saw no increase in either PGG/H synthase protein expression, or prostaglandin synthesis in the 3-4 hour time frame. Additionally they see no superinduction of PGG/H synthase mRNA with cycloheximide. Differences in the cell lines used (NIH-3T3 vs. Swiss-3T3) or the culture conditions may explain these discrepancies. Lin et al. stimulated with PDGF in the near absence of serum (0.5%), while experiments that have demonstrated

PDGF stimulated increases in PGG/H synthase levels were conducted in the presence of 5% plasma derived serum (4,5). Serum may contain additional factors necessary for PGG/H synthase protein expression. In support of this explanation, experiments in MC3T3-E1 cells showed a dependence on serum for the increased expression of PGG/H synthase induced by either TGF-β or EGF (13,15).

That PGG/H synthase mRNA levels are superinducible in the presence of cycloheximide suggests several mechanisms for the regulation of PGG/H synthase message levels. Cycloheximide could inhibit the synthesis of a labile inhibitor of PGG/H synthase transcription and thus increase transcription of the gene. It might also inhibit the synthesis of a labile ribonuclease, and thus increase stability of the message. Alternatively, message stability may be linked to translation of the PGG/H synthase mRNA, and inhibition of translation by cycloheximide may increase PGG/H synthase mRNA stability. To differentiate between these possibilities it will be necessary to measure changes in the transcription of the PGG/H synthase gene and to measure changes in the stability of the PGG/H synthase mRNA.

REFERENCES

1. Bedard, P., Alcorta, D., Simmons, D.L., Luk, K., and Erikson, R.L. (1987) Proc. Natl. Acad. Sci. USA,84, 6715-6719.
2. DeWitt, D.L., El-Harith, E. A., Kraemer, S.A., Andrews, M.J., Yao, E.F, Armstrong, R.L., and Smith, W.L. (1990): J. Biol. Chem., 265 , 5192-5198.
3. Frasier-Scott, K, Hatzakis, H., Seong, D., Jones, C.M., and Wu, K.K., (1988): J. Clin. Invest., 82, 1877-1883.
4. Goerig, M., Habenicht, A.J.R., Zeh, W., Salbach, P., Burkhard, K., Rothe, D.E.R., Nastainczyk, W., and Glomset, J.A. (1988): J. Biol. Chem., 263, 19384-19391.
5. Habenicht, A. J. R., Goerig, M. Grulich, J., Rothe, D., Gronwald, R. Loth, U., Schettler, G., Kommerell, B., Ross, R. (1985): J. Clin. Invest., 75, 1381-1387
6. Greenberg, M.E., Hermanowski, A.L., and Ziff, E.B. (1986): Mol. Cell. Biol., 6, 1050-1057.
7. Huslig, R. L. Fogwell, R. L. , and Smith, W.L., (1979): Biol. Reprod., 21, 589-600.
8. Hedin, L. Gady-Kurten, D., Kurten, R., DeWitt, D.L., Smith, W.L. and Richards, J.S.(1987): Endocrinology, 121, 722-731.
9. Lin, A.H., Bienkowski, M.J., and Gorman, R.R. (1989): J. Biol. Chem., 29, 17379-17383.
10. Raz, A., Wych, A.L., Siegel, N., Needleman, P. (1988): J. Biol. Chem., 263, 3022-3028
11. Raz, A., Wyche, A.L., and Needleman, P. (1989): Proc. Natl. Acad. Sci. USA, 86, 1657-1661.
12. Sambrook, J., Fritsch, E.F., Maniatis, T. (1989): Molecular Cloning: A Laboratory Manual, Second Edition. Cold Spring Harbor Laboatory Press. New York.
13. Sumitani, K., Kawata, T., Yoshimoto, T., Yamamoto, S., and Kumegawa, M. (1989): Arch. Biochem. Biophys., 279, 588-595
14. Wu, K. W., Hatzakis, H., Lo, S. S., Seong, D. C., Sanduja, S. K., Tai, H. (1988):J. Biol. Chem., 263, 19043-19047.
15. Yokaota, K., Kusaka, M., Ohshima, T., Yomamoto, S., Kurihara, N., Hoshino, T., and Kumegawa, M. (1986): J. Biol. Chem., 15410-15415.

REGULATION OF PROSTAGLANDIN SYNTHESIS BY DIFFERENTIAL EXPRESSION OF THE GENE ENCODING PROSTAGLANDIN ENDOPEROXIDE SYNTHASE

Michael S. Simonson, Julie A. Wolfe, and Michael J. Dunn

Departments of Medicine and Physiology and Biophysics, Case Western Reserve University, Cleveland, Ohio 44106

Short-term activation of phospholipase A_2 by hormones, neurotransmitters, and other ligands has traditionally been considered the major mechanism regulating prostaglandin synthesis (see 1,2). Agonist/receptor-evoked phospholipase A_2 activity increases prostaglandin synthesis by elevating the concentration of free arachidonate substrate for prostaglandin endoperoxide synthase (PES, also cyclooxygenase) (2,3). While it may seem obvious that the availability of free arachidonate controls prostaglandin synthesis, recent evidence suggests that regulation also occurs at the level of PES gene expression (4,5). PES levels are increased by interleukin-1 (6), platelet-derived growth factor (7,8), phorbol esters (9), and epidermal growth factor (10), and these agents chronically elevate prostaglandin synthesis. Yet despite recent progress, little is known about the regulation of PES gene expression. Here we describe experiments to test whether the PES gene is inducible and whether induction of the gene results in increased prostaglandin synthesis.

RESULTS AND DISCUSSION

Induction of the PES gene was examined in serum-free (G_0) glomerular mesangial cells treated with heterologous serum, which induces many of the phenotypic alterations observed in glomerular inflammation (i.e., increased growth fraction, matrix accumulation, and elevated prostaglandin synthesis, see ref. 11). As shown in Fig. 1A, serum increased PGE_2 accumulation in control cells and in cells incubated with arginine vasopressin (AVP). To assess PES activity, serum-free and serum-treated cells were incubated with arachidonate under saturating conditions. These experiments showed that serum induced a ~4-fold increase in PES enzymatic activity (Fig. 1A). Concurrent experiments measuring [^{3}H]arachidonate release from equilibrium-labeled cells suggested that phospholipase A_2 activity was also induced by serum (data not shown). Consistent with increased PES expression by serum,

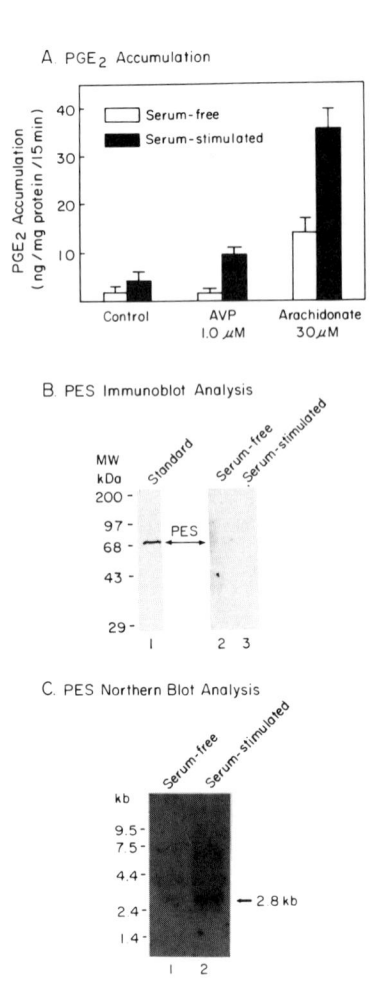

Fig. 1 Increased PES expression by serum in rat glomerular mesangial cells. **(A)** Serum-free (G_0) and serum-stimulated (24 h) mesangial cells were incubated for 15 min with medium alone (control), arginine vasopressin (AVP), or saturating concentrations of arachidonate and PGE_2 accumulation in the supernate was measured by radioimmunoassay. **(B)** Mesangial cell proteins (40 ug/lane) fractionated on 10% SDS-PAGE gels, electrophoretically transferred to nitrocellulose, and PES protein was detected by immunoblotting using a polyclonal antisera against PES and a peroxidase-labeled second antibody (6). **(C)** Total RNA (12 ug/lane) was fractionated on a 1.2% agarose gel, transferred to nitrocellulose, and probed with nick-translated [^{32}P]cDNA encoding murine PES (12). Final washing stringency was 0.1 x SSPE at 42°C.

immunoblot analysis demonstrated a large increase in a 70-kd immunoreactive PES protein after 24 h treatment with serum (Fig. 1B). Collectively, these data suggest that the PES gene is inducible and that serum increases PES expression.

To address the mechanisms by which serum induces PES expression we analyzed steady-state PES mRNA levels by Northern blotting. Identical concentrations of total RNA were electrophoretically fractionated, transferred to nitrocellulose, and the membranes were probed with nick-translated [^{32}P]cDNA encoding murine PES (12). Serum increased by 5-fold the steady-state level of a 2.8 kb PES mRNA transcript in mesangial cells (Fig. 1C). A larger, less abundant transcript was also present at 4.0 kb, but it was unclear whether this transcript arises via alternative mRNA splicing or represents unprocessed PES hnRNA (4,13). Increased expression of a 2.8 kb PES mRNA transcript is further evidence that serum induces expression of the PES gene in G_o mesangial cells.

In further experiments (data not shown), we asked whether induction of PES gene expression was necessary for increased PES activity in serum treated cells. Serum-induced PES activity was first apparent at 4 h and rose gradually to maximal levels at 24 h; the increase in PES activity was blocked by cycloheximide suggesting a requirement for *de novo* protein synthesis. An increase in PES mRNA was apparent at 3 h and increased gradually thereafter (data not shown), suggesting that the increase in PES activity by serum requires induction of the gene encoding PES.

CONCLUSIONS

The present data demonstrate that in rat mesangial cells (*i*) the PES gene is inducible, not constitutive, and that (*ii*) serum increases expression of the PES gene resulting in increased PGE$_2$ accumulation. Thus our data are consistent with the hypothesis that regulation of gene expression for enzymes of the arachidonic acid cascade controls, partially, prostaglandin synthesis. Increased expression of PES has been hypothesized (1,5,6) to account for the elevated levels of prostaglandin synthesis observed in chronic inflammatory diseases (14,15). It will be interesting to learn whether induction of glomerular levels of PES could contribute to the increased synthesis of prostaglandins commonly associated with glomerulonephritis (15).

ACKNOWLEDGEMENTS

We gratefully acknowledge Dr. David DeWitt (Dept. Biochemistry, Michigan State University) for providing the cDNA encoding murine PES and Drs. Philip Needleman and Ami Raz (Dept. of Pharmacology, Washington University) for providing the polyclonal antiserum to ram seminal vesicle PES. This work was supported by National Institutes of Health grant HL-22563.

REFERENCES

1. Smith, W. (1989): *Biochem. J.*, 259:315-324.
2. Dennis, E. (1987): *Bio/Technology*, 5:1294-1900.
3. Irvine, R. (1982): *Biochem. J.*, 204:3-16.
4. DeWitt, D., Meade, E., El-Harith, E., and Smith, W. (1989): In: *Platelets and Vascular Occlusions.* edited by C. Patrono, and G. Fitzgerald. pp. 109-118. Raven Press, New York.
5. Raz, A., Wyche, A., Fagan, D., and Needleman, P. (1989): In: *Renal Eicosanoids.* edited by M. Dunn, C. Patrono, and G. Cinotti. pp. 1-21. Plenum, New York.
6. Raz, A., Wyche, A., Siegel, N., and Needleman, P. (1988): *J. Biol. Chem.*, 263:3022-3028.
7. Habenicht, A., Goerig, M., Grulich, J., Rothe, D., Gronwald, R., Loth, U., Schletter, G., Kommerell, B., and Ross, R. (1985): *J. Clin. Invest.* 75:1381-1387.
8. Lin, A., Bienkowski, M., and Gorman, R. (1989): *J. Biol. Chem.* 264:17379-17383.
9. Wu, K., Hatzakis, H., Lo, S., Seong, D., Sanduja, S., and Tai, H-H. (1988): *J. Biol. Chem.* 263:19043-19047.
10. Bailey, J., Muza, B., Hla, T., and Salata, K. (1985): *J. Lipid Res.* 26:54-61.
11. Mene', P., Simonson, M., and Dunn, M. (1989): *Physiol. Rev.* 69:1347-1424.
12. DeWitt,D., El-Harith, E., Kraemer, S., Andrews, M., Yao, E., Armstrong, R., and Smith, W. (1990): *J. Biol. Chem.* 265:5192-5198.
13. Rosen, G., Birkenmeier, T., Raz, A., and Holtzman, M. (1989): *Biochem. Biophys. Res. Comm.* 164:1358-1365.
14. Dunn, M, and Weissmann, G., editors. (1987): *Drugs* 33(S1):1-66.
15. Scharschmidt, L., Simonson, M., and Dunn, M. (1986): *Am. J. Med.* 81(2B)30-42.

ELEVATED PROSTAGLANDIN H SYNTHASE GENE EXPRESSION IN *RAS*-TRANSFORMED CELLS

Robert R. Gorman, Michael J. Bienkowski and Alice H. Lin

Department of Cell Biology
The Upjohn Company
Kalamazoo, MI 49008 USA

INTRODUCTION

Once free arachidonate is mobilized from phospholipid stores, prostaglandin endoperoxide synthesis and all subsequent prostaglandin and thromboxane production are regulated by prostaglandin H synthase (PGHS) (1) (prostaglandin synthase, EC 1.14.99.1). Although this enzyme has been studied in considerable detail, little is known about factors which regulate cellular PGHS gene expression.

In this report we show that in wildtype NIH-3T3 cells recombinant platelet derived growth factor (rPDGF) induces PGHS mRNA levels, but that peak mRNA induction occurs after maximal PGE_2 synthesis is achieved. However, in cells transformed by the EJ-*ras* oncogene product p21, PGHS mRNA and enzyme levels are greatly elevated. In addition, this constitutive synthesis is not augmented by rPDGF.

RESULTS AND DISCUSSION

Control NIH-3T3 cells (transfected with only calf thymus DNA and pUCNeo DNA) grown for 24 hr in 1.25% PDS release significant amounts of PGE_2 as determined by RIA when exposed to rPDGF at 2 units/ml. The presence of PGE_2 in the culture medium is observed within minutes of PDGF addition, with maximal levels occurring 2 hr after exposure. In contrast, NIH-3T3 cells transfected with EJ-*ras* and pUC Neo DNA release only low levels of PGE_2 in response to rPDGF (Figure 1).

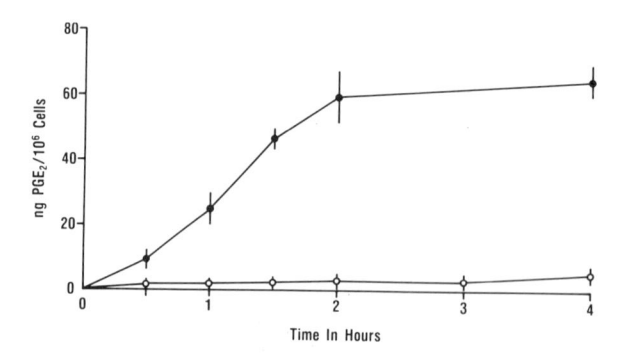

FIG 1. PDGF-stimulated PGE$_2$ release in control and EJ-*ras*-transformed cells. Data are reported as mean ± SEM of triplicate determinations. ● control + PDGF; ○ EJ-*ras*-transformed + PDGF.

Because of this difference, we were interested in measuring rPDGF-driven PGHS gene expression in both control and EJ-*ras* transformed cells. Figure 2 shows Northern blots of PGHS mRNA levels in control (upper panel) and EJ-*ras* transformed cells (lower panel) in response to rPDGF. PGHS mRNA levels peak at 3 hrs in control cells, but are not changed in *ras*-transformed cells. Note that PGHS mRNA levels are high in the *ras*-transformed cells when compared to control cells.

To assess the significance of the mRNA data, we also measured PGHS enzyme levels by immunoblot (Figure 3).

The immunoblots showed that neither control nor *ras*-transformed cells increase their total PGHS enzyme levels, but that the enzyme levels do mirror the mRNA measurements.

The *ras* transformed cells have significantly (approximately 4 fold) more PGHS enzyme than the control cells.

SUMMARY

1. rPDGF stimulates PGE$_2$ release in wild type, but not *ras* transformed NIH-3T3 cells.
2. *Ras* transformation blocks PGE$_2$ release by inhibiting phospholipase C activation, IP$_3$ synthesis, and Ca^{2+} mobilization.
3. rPDGF stimulation of wild type NIH-3T3 cells increases both prostaglandin H synthase (PGHS) mRNA levels and PGHS enzyme levels as measured by immunoblot. However, PGHS gene transcription is not required for PDGF-stimulated PGE$_2$ release.
4. *Ras* transformed NIH-3T3 cells display elevated basal PGE$_2$ synthesis, and very high levels of both PGHS mRNA and enzyme. rPDGF does not further stimulate PGHS gene transcription.
5. Exogenous PGE$_2$ attenuates rPDGF-stimulated cell proliferation in both wild type and *ras* transformed cells.

6. These data suggest that increased PGHS gene expression and enhanced basal PGE$_2$ synthesis may be in response to the unregulated growth of *ras* transformed cells.

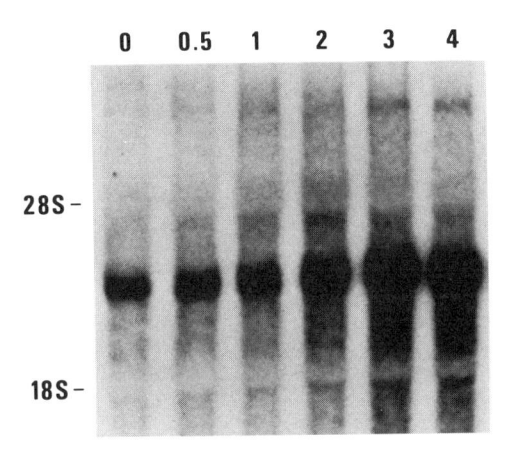

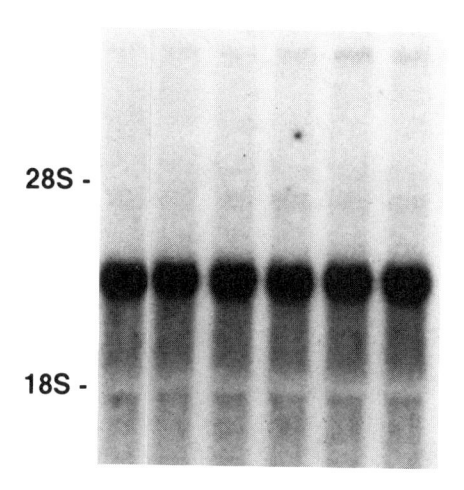

FIG. 2. Northern analysis of PGHS mRNA levels in rPDGF-stimulated cells. NIH-3T3 cells (5 x 10^6/dish) were cultured as described for Fig. 1 and stimulated with 20 ng/ml rPDGF. At zero time and 0.5, 1, 2, 3, and 4 h after the addition of rPDGF mRNA was quantitated. Upper panel control cells; lower panel EJ-*ras*-transformed cells.

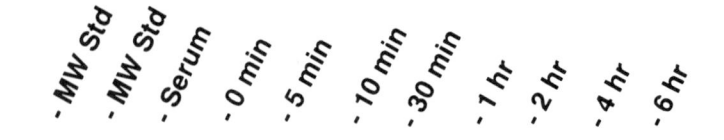

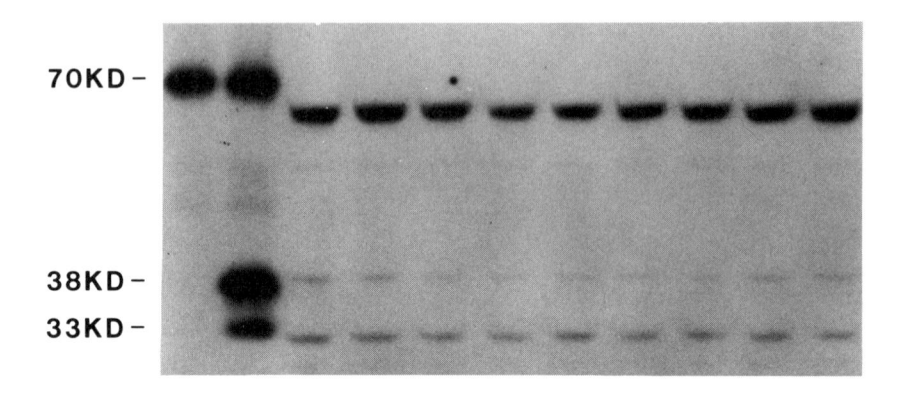

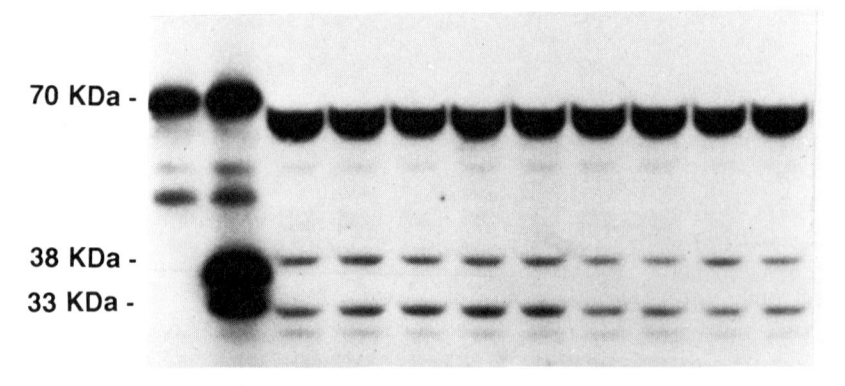

FIG 3. Immunoblot of PGHS enzyme levels in rPDGF-stimulated cells. NIH-3T3 cells (5 x 10^6/dish) were cultured either in 10% serum (designated "serum") or in 0.5% serum. At zero time, PGHS levels were quantitated in both the serum cells and the serum-deprived cells. Some of the deprived cells received 20 ng/ml rPDGF, and PGHS levels in these cells were determined by immunoblot at 5, 10, and 15 min and 1, 2, 4 and 6 h. Upper panel controls, lower panel *ras*-transformed.

REFERENCES

1. Lin, A.H.,, Bienkowski, J.M., and Gorman, R.R. (1989) *J. Biol. Chem.* 264:17379-17383.

THE ASPIRIN AND HEME BINDING SITES OF PGG/H SYNTHASE

W.L. Smith, D.L. DeWitt, and T. Shimokawa

Department of Biochemistry, Michigan State University,
East Lansing, Michigan, U.S.A., 48824

PGG/H synthase catalyzes the conversion of arachidonic acid to PGH_2. The enzyme has two activities: (a) a cyclooxygenase catalyzing a <u>bis</u>-oxygenation of arachidonate to yield PGG_2 and (b) a hydroperoxidase catalyzing a two electron reduction of PGH_2 to PGG_2. The goal of our present work is to determine which amino acids are essential for catalysis and substrate binding by PGG/H synthase. In the study reported here, we have investigated the role of the serine residue which, when acetylated by aspirin, leads to a selective loss of cyclooxygenase but not hydroperoxidase activity. In addition, we report preliminary studies to determine which histidine residues may be involved in the binding of heme to the active site of the enzyme.

LOCATION OF THE ACTIVE SITE SERINE RESIDUE

Shown in Fig. 1 are the deduced amino acid sequences of the sheep (2,8,11), mouse (1), and human (12) PGG/H synthases. The numbering system refers to the sheep enzyme and by convention begins with the methionine residue at the site of initiation of translation. Ser-530 was initially identified as the site of aspirin acetylation by comparing the amino acid sequence deduced from the cDNA sequence with the peptide sequence determined by Roth et al. (10) to contain the acetylated serine. It is of interest that the sequence in the region from residues 483-583 is very highly conserved. The last intron/exon junction in the coding region of the human protein is reported to occur at Glu-483 (12) so that residues 483-600 are from the same exon.

To determine if the hydroxyl group of Ser-530 is important in cyclooxygenase catalysis, we used site-directed mutagenesis to replace Ser-530 with an alanine. As shown in Table I, the Ala-530 mutant exhibited cyclooxygenase and hydroperoxidase activities similar in magnitude to the native Ser-530 PGG/H synthase. Moreover, the K_m values for arachidonate were the same for the native enzyme and the Ala-530 mutant. As expected, the Ala-530 mutant, which lacks a hydroxyl group at position 530, is insensitive to irreversible inactivation by

```
  1        10        20        30        40        50
MSRRSLSLWFPLLLLLLLPPTPSVLLADPGVPSPVNPCCYYPCQNQGVCVRFGLDNYQCD mse
: :^: : :::::^::::::: : :::: : :::::::::: ::::::::::::: :::
MSRQSISLRFP-LLLLLLSPSP-VFSADPGAPAPVNPCCYYPCQHQGICVRFGLDRYQCD shp
:::^^:::::: ::::::::::  ::::::: ::::::::::::::::::::::::::::
MSR-SLLLRF-LLLLLLLPPLP-VLLADPGAPTPVNPCCYYPCQHQGICVRFGLDRYQCD hmn

    60        70        80        90       100       110
CTRTGYSGPNCTIPEIWTWLRNSLRPSPSFTHFLLTHGYWLWEFVNATFIREVLMRLVLT mse
::::::::::::::::::::::.:::::::.::::::::.::.::::::::..:::::::
CTRTGYSGPNCTIPEIWTWLRTTLRPSPSFIHFLLTHGRWLWDFVNATFIRDTLMRLVLT shp
:::::::::::::.::::::::::::::::::::::::.::.:::::::::...:::::
CTRTGYSGPNCTIPGLWTWLRNSLRPSPSFTHFLLTHGRWFWEFVNATFIREMLLLVLT hmn

   120       130       140       150       160       170
VRSNLIPSPPTYNSAHDYISWESFSNVSYYTRILPSVPKDCPTPMGTKGKKQLPDVQLLA mse
::::::::::::.::::::::::::::::::::::::::::::::::::::::::...:
VRSNLIPSPPTYNIAHDYISWESFSNVSYYTRILPSVPRDCPTPMGTKGKKQLPDAEFLS shp
::::::::::::::::::::::::::::::::::::::::::::::::::::::::.:::
VRSNLIPSPPTYNSAHDYISWESFSNVSYYTRILPSVPKDCPTPMGTKGKKQLPDAQLLA hmn

   180       190       200       210       220       230
QQLLLRREFIPAPQGTNILFAFFAQHFTHQFFKTSGKMGPGFTKALGHGVDLGHIYGDNL mse
...:::::::.:::::::.::::::::::::::::::::::::::::::::::::::::
RRFLLRRKFIPDPQGTNLMFAFFAQHFTHQFFKTSGKMGPGFTKALGHGVDLGHIYGDNL shp
::::::::::::::::::::::::::::::::::::::::::::::::::::::::::::
RRFLLRRKFIPDPQGTNLMFAFFAQHFTHQFFKTSGKMGPGFTKALGHGVDLGHIYGDNL hmn

   240       250       260       270       280       290
ERQYHLRLFKDGKLKYQVLDGEVYPPSVEQASVLMRYPPGVPPERQMAVGQEVFGLLPGL mse
:::::::::::::::::::::::::::::::.::::::.:::::.::::::::::::::
ERQYQLRLFKDGKLKYQMLNGEVYPPSVEEAPVLMHYPRGIPPQSQMAVGQEVFGLLPGL shp
:::::::::::::::::::::.:::::::::::::::::::::::::::::::::::::
ERQYQLRLFKDGKLKYQVLDGEMYPPSVEEAPVLMHYPRGIPPQSQMAVGQEVFGLLPGL hmn

   300       310       320       330       340       350
MLFSTIWLREHNRVCDLLKEEHPTWDDEQLFQTTRLILIGETIKIVIEEYVQHLSGYFLQ mse
::.::::::::::::::::.::::::.:::::::::::::::::::::::::.::::::
MLYATIWLREHNRVCDLLKAEHPTWGDEQLFQTARLILIGETIKIVIEEYVQQLSGYFLQ shp
:::::::::::::::::::::::::::::::::::::::::::::::::::::::::::
MLYATLWLREHNRVCDLLKAEHPTWGDEQLFQTTRLILIGETIKIVIEEYVQQLSGYFLQ hmn

   360       370       380       390       400       410
LKFDPELLFRAQFQYRNRIAMEFNHLYHWHPLMPNSFQVGSQEYSYEQFLFNTSMLVDYG mse
::::::::..:::::::::::::::.::::::::::::::::::::::::::::::::::
LKFDPELLFGAQFQYRNRIAMEFNQLYHWHPLMPDSFRVGPQDYSYEQFLFNTSMLVDYG shp
:::::::::.::::::::::::::::::::::::::::::::::::::::::::::::::
LKFDPELLFGVQFQYRNRIATEFNHLYHWHPLMPDSFKVGSQEYSYEQFLFNTSMLVDYG hmn

   420       430       440       450       460       470
VEALVDAFSRQRAGRIGGGRNFDYHVLHVAVDVIKESREMRLQPFNEYRKRFGLKPYTSF mse
::::::::::.::::::::::: :::.::::::::::::..::::::::::..::::::
VEALVDAFSRQPAGRIGGGRNIDHHILHVAVDVIKESRVLRLQPFNEYRKRFGMKPYTSF shp
:::::::::::.:::::::::..::.::::::::::::::.::::::::::::::::::
VEALVDAFSRQIAGRIGGGRNMDHHILHVAVDVIRESREMRLQPFNEYRKRFGMKPYTSF hmn

   480       490       500       510       520       530
QELTGEKEMAAELEELYGDIDALEFYPGLLLEKCQPNSIFGESMIEMGAPFSLKGLLGNP mse
::::::::::::::::::::::::::::::::::.::::::::::::::::::::::::
QELTGEKEMAAELEELYGDIDALEFYPGLLLEKCHPNSIFGESMIEMGAPFSLKGLLGNP shp
:::.:::::::::::::::::::::::::::::::::::::::::.:.:::::::::::
QELVGEKEMAAELEELYGDIDALEFYPGLLLEKCHPNSIFGESMIEIGAPFSLKGLLGNP hmn

   540       550       560       570       580       590       600
ICSPEYWKPSTFGGDVGFNLVNTASLKKLVCLNTKTCPYVSFRVPDYPGDDGSVLVRRSTEL mse
:::::::::.::::.::::::.::.:::::::::::::::::.:::..::..:.:..:::
ICSPEYWKASTFGGEVGFNLVKTATLKKLVCLNTKTCPYVSFHVPDPRQEDRPGVERPPTEL shp
:::::::::::::::::::::::::::::::::::::::::::::::.:::.:..:::::
ICSPEYWKPSTFGGEVGFNIVKTATLKKLVCLNTKTCPYVSFRVPDASQDDGPAVERPSTEL hmn
```

FIG. 1. <u>Deduced amino acid sequences of PGG/H synthases.</u> Numbering is for the sheep sequence. Identical residues are marked with a colon (:); residues involving a one-letter change in the codon (i.e. conservative substitutions) are marked with a period (.); nonconservative changes involving two- or three-letter changes in the codon are unmarked. Alignments were performed using the FASTP sequence comparison program (6).

aspirin (1). The results obtained in comparing the properties of the Ala-530 mutant with those of the native enzyme suggest that the effect of acetylation may be to introduce a bulky acetyl substituent at Ser-530 which interferes with substrate binding. As an initial test of this hypothesis, we used site-directed mutagenesis to replace Ser-530 with Asn-530. As shown in Table II, the Asn-530 mutant lacked cyclooxygenase activity but retained hydroperoxidase activity; in fact, the hydroperoxidase activity of the Asn-530 appeared to be somewhat higher than that of the native enzyme. The finding that the Asn-530 mutant lacks cyclooxygenase activity is consistent with the concept that aspirin acetylation causes irreversible inhibition of cyclooxygenase activity by placing a bulky group at Ser-530 thereby interfering with the binding of arachidonate to the cyclooxygenase active site. It will be of interest to determine if substitution of Ser-530 with Thr-530 yields an enzyme with intermediate levels of cyclooxygenase activity and whether a Thr-530 containing enzyme can be irreversibly inactivated by aspirin.

TABLE 1. Effect of mutagenesis of Ser-530 on PGG/H synthase

Residue at Position 530	Cyclooxygenase (%)	Hydroperoxidase (%)
Ser (Native)	100	100
Acetylated Ser (aspirin)	0	100
Ala	89	102
Asn	0	141

HISTIDINE RESIDUES INVOLVED IN HEME BINDING

Comparison of the sequences for the sheep, mouse, and human PGG/H synthases (Fig. 1) indicates that there are thirteen histidine residues which are conserved among various species. These include His-90, His-95, His-134, His-204, His-207, His-226, His-232, His-309, His-320, His-386, His-388, His-443, and His-446. Interestingly, residues 303-312 which contain His-309 are quite similar to sequences found in both myeloperoxidase and thyroid peroxidase (3-5,9). We hypothesize, based on these sequence comparisons, that His-309 is the axial heme ligand of PGG/H synthase. The identity of the distal heme ligand is not obvious from sequence comparisons with other peroxidases although it is probably not His-274 (7) since His-274 is not a conserved histidine.

REFERENCES

1. DeWitt, D.L., El-Harith, E.A., Kraemer, S.A., Andrews, M.J., Yao, E., Armstrong, R.L., and Smith, W.L. (1990): *J. Biol. Chem.*, 265:5192-5198.

2. DeWitt, D.L., and Smith, W.L. (1988): *Proc. Natl. Acad. Sci. U. S. A.*, 85:1412-1416.

3. Johnson, K.R., Nauseef, W.M., Care, A., Weelock, J.J.C., and Rovera, G. (1987): *Nucleic Acids Res.*, 15:2013-2028.

4. Kimura, S., and Ikeda-Saito, M. (1988): *Proteins Struc. Func. Gene*, 3:113-120.

5. Kimura, S., Kotani, T., McBride, O.W., Umeki, K., Hirai, K., Nakayama, T., and Ohtaki, S. (1987): *Proc. Natl. Acad. Sci. U.S.A.*, 84:5555-5559.

6. Lipman, D., and Pearson, W.T. (1985): *Science*, 227:1435-1441.

7. Marnett, L.J., Chen, Y-N.P., Maddipati, K.R., Plé, P., and Labeque, R. (1989): *J. Biol. Chem.*, 263:16532-16535.

8. Merlie, J. P., Fagan, D., Mudd, J., and Needleman, P. (1988): *J. Biol. Chem.* 263:3550-3553.

9. Morishita, K., Kubota, N., Asano, S., Kaziro, Y., and Nagata, S. (1987): *J. Biol. Chem.*, 262:3844-3851.

10. Roth, G.J., Machuga, E.T., and Ozols, J. (1983): *Biochemistry*, 22:4672-4675.

11. Yokoyama, C., Taka, T., and Tanabe, T. (1988): *FEBS Lett.*, 231:347-351.

12. Yokoyama, C., and Tanabe, T. (1989): *Biochem. Biophys. Res. Commun.*, 165:888-894.

PROPERTIES OF TRYPSIN-CLEAVED PGH SYNTHASE

Rebecca Odenwaller, Coleen Young O'Gara,
and Lawrence J. Marnett

Department of Biochemistry
Center in Molecular Toxicology
Vanderbilt University School of Medicine
Nashville, TN 37232 USA

Figure 1 is a crude representation of the structural elements of the 70 kDa subunit of prostaglandin H (PGH) synthase purified from sheep seminal vesicles (2,12,14). Trypsin cleaves the native apoprotein at Arg[253] to produce fragments of 33 and 38 kDa (1). The 33 kDa fragment contains the N-terminus of the intact protein and three of the four carbohydrate binding sites (X). The 38 kDa fragment contains the C-terminus of the intact protein and the aspirin acetylation site (OH). A very hydrophobic sequence that may be a membrane-binding domain is located adjacent to the trypsin cleavage site (12). Binding of the heme prosthetic group or certain cyclooxygenase inhibitors to the protein reduces the susceptibility of Arg[253] to tryptic cleavage (1,5,9).

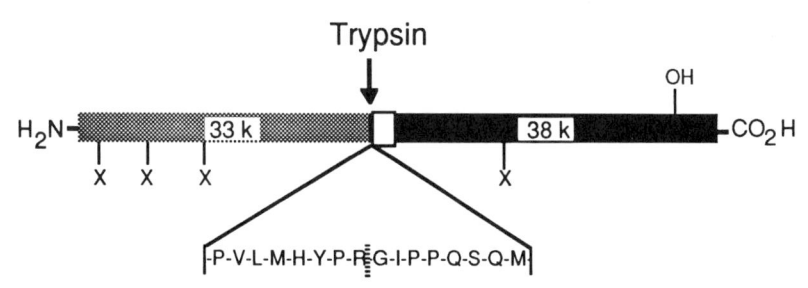

FIG. 1. Gross structural elements of ovine PGH synthase. X=Consensus carbohydrate attachment site; OH=Aspirin acetylation site; Broken line in expanded region shows trypsin cleavage site; The white annulus near the trypsin cleavage site indicates a highly hydrophobic sequence.

The 33 and 38 kDa fragments remain tightly associated under non-denaturing conditions (1). Titration of trypsin-cleaved PGH synthase (TPGH synthase) with heme demonstrates the loss of one high affinity heme-binding site (11). The EPR spectrum of heme-reconstituted TPGH synthase at 15°K exhibits maxima at g=6.3 and 7.3. The maxima exhibited by native enzyme at g=5.7 and 6.6 are absent in ^{T}PGH synthase. The EPR spectrum of ^{T}PGH synthase appears quite similar to the EPR spectrum of heat-denatured PGH synthase following heme reconstitution (3). This suggests the coordination site of the heme in ^{T}PGH synthase is different from that of native PGH synthase. Intact PGH synthase exhibits a trough in its circular dichroism spectrum at 410 nm that is absent in heme-reconstituted ^{T}PGH synthase (Figure 2). This is further evidence for significant differences in the heme-binding properties of ^{T}PGH synthase relative to native enzyme. In fact, the sum of the observations suggest most of the heme of ^{T}PGH synthase is non-specifically bound.

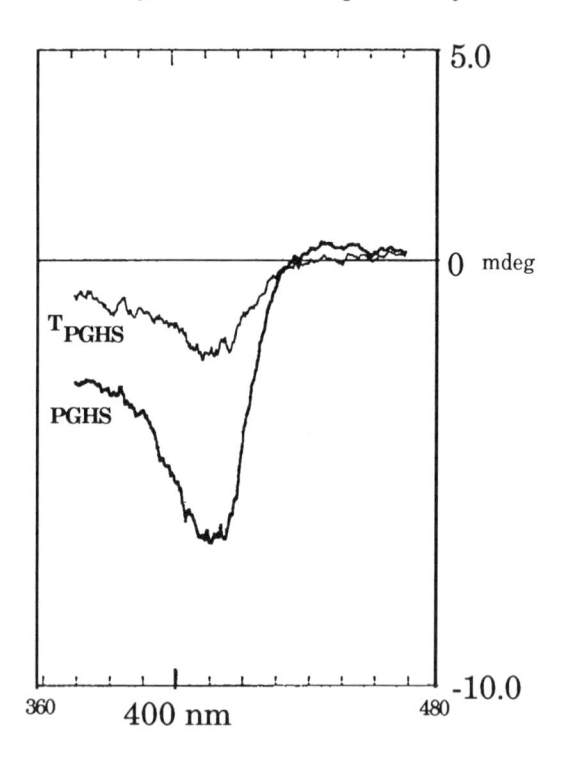

FIG. 2. Circular dichroism spectra of PGH synthase and ^{T}PGH synthase in the Soret region.

Controversy exists over the catalytic properties of ^{T}PGH synthase. Our laboratory reported that ^{T}PGH synthase retains 50-60% of the cyclooxygenase activity but only 10-20% of the peroxidase activity of native PGH synthase (11). The residual peroxidase activity corresponds to the amount of uncleaved protein remaining in the trypsin cleavage mixture. Kulmacz and associates (8-10) report ^{T}PGH synthase prepared in their laboratory retains neither cyclooxygenase nor peroxidase activity. In our hands, the differentiation of cyclooxygenase and peroxidase activities by tryptic cleavage is highly reproducible. Attempts to resolve the discrepancy between the two laboratories using different conditions of trypsin digestion or protein preparations of differing purity have been unsuccessful. ^{T}PGH synthase retains 50-60% of its cyclooxygenase activity but 10-20% of its peroxidase activity. The kinetic parameters of the cyclooxygenase activity of ^{T}PGH synthase are similar to those of native enzyme: K_m = 30 µM, k_{cat} = 1260 min^{-1} (TPGH synthase) vs K_m = 31 µM, k_{cat} = 1890 min^{-1} (PGH synthase).

^{T}PGH synthase may be an important tool in unraveling the complex mechanism of cyclooxygenase catalysis. Previous experiments have indicated a dependence of cyclooxygenase activity on a functioning peroxidase and a proposal has been made that the two activities are synergistically related (6,7). EPR spectra of PGH synthase reacted with organic hydroperoxides at 5°C reveal the presence of a tyrosyl radical formed by intramolecular electron transfer to an intermediate in peroxidase catalysis (4). The tyrosyl radical has been proposed to be the oxidizing agent that supports cyclooxygenase catalysis and the transducer of redox equivalents between the two separate but interdependent activities of PGH synthase (4). The fact that heme-reconstituted ^{T}PGH synthase exhibits cyclooxygenase activity but relatively low peroxidase activity is reminiscent of the properties of Mn^{3+}-protoporphyrin IX-reconstituted PGH synthase (13). The very low levels of peroxidase activity in these two proteins suggests they may be useful probes of the formation of the tyrosyl radical by higher oxidation states of the peroxidase and its relation to cyclooxygenase catalysis.

REFERENCES

1. Chen, Y.-N.P., Bienkowski, M.J., and Marnett, L.J. (1987): *J. Biol Chem.*, **252**:16892-16899.
2. DeWitt, D.L. and Smith, W.L. (1988): *Proc. Natl. Acad. Sci. USA*, **85**:1412-1416.
3. Karthein, R., Nastainczyk, W., and Ruf, H.H. (1987): *Eur. J. Biochem.*, **166**:173-180.
4. Karthein, R., Dietz, R., Nastainczyk, W., and Ruf, H.H. (1988): *Eur. J. Biochem.*, **171**:313-320.

5. Kulmacz, R.J., and Lands, W.E.M. (1982): *Biochem. Biophys. Res. Comm.*, **104**:758-764.
6. Kulmacz, R.J., and Lands, W.E.M. (1983): *Prostaglandins*, **25**:531-540.
7. Kulmacz, R.J., Miller, Jr., J.F., and Lands, W.E.M. (1985): *Biochem. Biophys. Res. Comm.*, **130**:918-923.
8. Kulmacz, R.J., and Wu, K.K. (1989): *Arch. Biochem. Biophys.*, **268**:502-515.
9. Kulmacz, R.J. (1989): *J. Biol. Chem.*, **264**:14136-14144.
10. Kulmacz, R.J. (1989): *Prostaglandins*, **38**:277-288.
11. Marnett, L.J., Chen, Y.-N.P., Maddipati, K.R., Ple, P., and Labeque, R. (1988): *J. Biol. Chem.*, **263**:16532-16535.
12. Merlie, J.P., Fagan, D., Mudd, J., and Needleman, P. (1988): *J. Biol. Chem.*, **263**:3550-3553.
13. Ogino, N., Ohki, S., Yamamoto, S., and Hayaishi, O. (1978): *J. Biol. Chem.*, **253**:5061-5068.
14. Yokoyama, C., Takai, T., and Tanabe, T. (1988): *FEBS Letts.*, **231**:347-351.

THE STRUCTURE AND FUNCTION OF PROSTAGLANDIN F SYNTHASE

Kikuko Watanabe[1], Yutaka Fujii[2], Hideya Hayashi[3], Yoshihiro Urade[4] and Osamu Hayaishi[1]

[1]Osaka Bioscience Institute, 6-2-4 Furuedai, Suita-shi, Osaka 565 Japan, [2]Department of Chemistry, Fukui Medical College, Fukui 910-11 Japan, [3]Bioscience Research Laboratories, Nippon Mining Co Ltd.,Saitama 335, Japan, [4]Bio-organic Research Department, International Research Laboratories,CIBA-GEIGY(Japan), Takarazuka 665 Japan.

Prostaglandin(PG) F synthase is a monomeric protein with a Mr of 36,666 and composed of 323-amino acid residues. It is a dual function enzyme catalyzing the reduction of PGH_2 to $PGF_{2\alpha}$ and PGD_2 to $9\alpha,11\beta\text{-}PGF_2$ at different active sites on the same molecule[1-3]. PGF synthase is distributed in the lung and spleen, judging from its immunoreactivity and from Northern blot analyses[4]. Moreover, in immunoperoxidase staining, this enzyme was localized in alveolar interstitial cells and nonciliated epithelial cells in lung, and in histiocytes and/or dendritic cells in spleen[4](Fig.1).

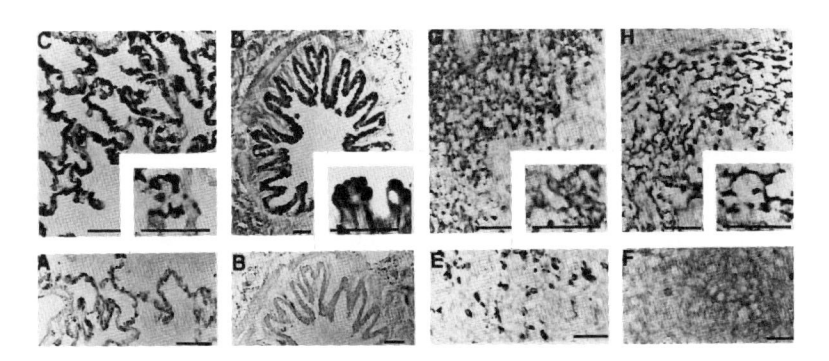

Fig 1. Immunohistochemical distribution of PGF synthase.
Cryosections of the alveoli(A,C) and bronchiole(B,D) of lung, and the red pulp(E,G) and white pulp(F,H) of spleen, were immunoperoxidase-stained with anti-(PGF synthase)IgG(C,D,G,H) or the antibody preabsorbed with an excess of the purified enzyme(A,B,E,F).

PGF synthase is a type of aldo-keto reductase (aldehyde reductase, aldose reductase and carbonyl reductase) in terms of Mr, substrate specificity, and cofactor requirement[1]. The amino acid sequence of PGF synthase shows about 65% similarity to those of human liver aldehyde reductase and rat lens aldose reductase, and shows 77% similarity to the partial amino acid sequence(225 residues) of the C-terminus of frog lens ρ-crystallin[3]. We purified ρ-crystallin to apparent homogeneity from the eye lens of the Japanese bullfrog(Rana catesbeiana) and determined the remaining portion of the N-terminal amino acid sequence(107 residues). The full amino acid sequence of ρ-crystallin also shows 77% similarity to that of PGF synthase[5]. These results suggest that they form a gene family. However, aldehyde reductase, aldose reductase, and ρ-crystallin do not cross react with antibody against PGF synthase and the antibody against ρ-crystallin does not cross react with other enzymes. Therefore, the antigenic determinants are different in these proteins.

To examine the role of these proteins in PG metabolism, the catalytic properties of these proteins were characterized with respect to the various PGs[5,6]. The human liver aldehyde reductase and the rat lens aldose reductase catalyze the reduction of PGH_2, but not that of PGD_2 and PGE_2 (Table 1).

Table 1 Substrate specificity of aldo-keto reductase

Substrate	PGF Synthetase Vmax	Km	Aldehyde Reductase Vmax	Km	Aldose Reductase Vmax	Km
	nmol/min.mg protein	μM	nmol/min.mg protein	μM	nmol/min.mg protein	μM
PGD_2	129	120	N.D.	-	<1	-
PGH_2	57	10	88	100	38	10
PGJ_2	42	230	190	500	-	-
Δ^{12}-PGJ_2	42	670	117	-	-	-
PGA_2	34	250	73	710	-	-
PGE_2	7		N.D.	-	<1	-

The reaction product from PGH_2 was identified as $PGF_{2\alpha}$ by reverse phase-HPLC and GC-MS analyses, and it was found that the reduction of PGH_2 to $PGF_{2\alpha}$ was not inhibited by other substrates, such as phenanthrenequinone and 4-nitrobenzaldehyde. These results suggest that the aldo-keto reductase has at least two active sites like PGF synthase.

On the other hand, PGH_2 reductase activity of ρ-crystallin was about 1.5% higher than that of PGF synthase, and PGD_2 reductase activity was lower than the detection limit of the method (0.1% of that of PGF synthase)(Table 2).

These results suggest that aldo-keto reductase is a dual function enzyme like PGF synthase, and that ρ-crystallin may have lost its active site(s) during differentiation.

PGF synthase utilizes NADPH as a cofactor. The binding number of NADPH to the enzyme is about 1 mol of the cofactor/mol of protein (Fig. 2), which is about the same as aldo-keto reductase and ρ-crystallin[5]

Table 2 Comparison of the molecular properties of PGF synthase and ρ-crystallin

	ρ-Crystallin	PGF Synthetase
Mr	36,801	36,517
Binding number of NADPH	1	1
PGD$_2$ 11-keto reductase activity	<0.1	100
PGH$_2$ reductase activity	1	44
Immunoreactivity		
anti-ρ-crystallin antibody	+++	-
anti-PGF synthetase antibody	-	+++

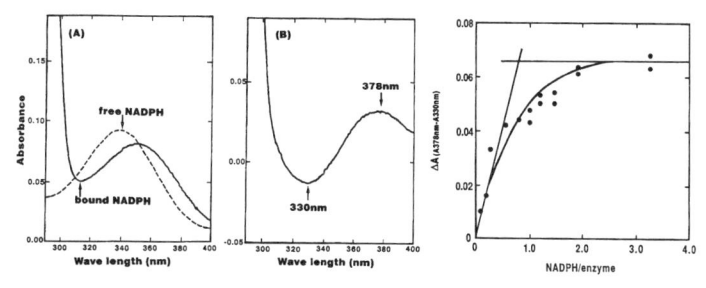

Fig 2. The binding number of NADPH and PGF synthase

The amino acid sequences of PGF synthase and ρ-crystallin are identical in a long stretch of the protein(residues 178-198) with only ^{195}Pro being different. ^{195}Pro was changed to Val of ρ-crystallin by site directed mutagenesis using cDNA of PGF synthase. PGD11-ketoreductase activity of the mutant decreased, but the PGH$_2$ reductase activity did not change. However, when ^{195}Pro was changed to Gly, both enzyme activites remained the same as that of the wild type(Table 3). This result suggests that ^{195}Pro may be related to the active site for PGD$_2$ of the enzyme.

Table 3. PGF synthase activity of wild type and mutants

	Mutant ^{195}Pro→Val	Mutant ^{195}Pro→Gly	Wild
	nmol/min.mg	nmol/min.mg	nmol/min.mg
PGD$_2$	14	78	56
PGH$_2$	28	8	10

PGF synthase, which is a dual function enzyme and catalyzes the reduction of PGH$_2$ and PGD$_2$ on a single protein, has one binding site for NADPH. The enzyme is constructed from at least two catalytic domains and ^{195}Pro is related to the active site for PGD$_2$ of PGF synthase.

ACKOWLEDGMENT

We thank Dr.Tsuji of Osaka Bioscience Institute for critical reading, and N.Eguchi, M.Miyata, and M.Ueta for techinical and assistance.

REFERENCE

1. Watanabe,K., Yoshida,R., Shimizu,T., an d Hayaishi,O.,(1985) *J.Biol.Chem.* **260**, 7035-7041
2. Watanabe,K.,Iguchi,Y.,Iguchi,S.,Arai,Y.,Hayaishi,O. and RobertsII, L.J., (1986) *Proc.Natl.Acad.Sci.U.S.A.* **83**, 1583-1587
3. Watanabe,K., Fujii,Y.,Nakayama,K.,OhkuboH.,Kuramitsu,S., Kagamiyama, H., Nakanishi,S., and Hayaishi,O. (1988) *Proc. Natl. Acad.Sci.U.S.A.* **85**, 11-15
4. Urade,Y.,Watanabe,K.,Eguchi,N.,Fujii,Y., and Hayaishi,O. (1990) *J.Biol.Chem.* in press
5. Fujii,Y.,Watanabe,K.,Hayashi,H.,Urade,Y.,and Hayaishi,O. (1990) *J.Biol.Chem.* in press
6. Hayashi,H.,Fujii,Y.,Watanabe,K.,Urade,Y.,and Hayaishi,O. (1989) *J.Biol.Chem.* **264**, 1036-1040
7. Watanabe,K., Fujii,Y., Nakayama,K., Ohkubo,H., Kuramitsu,S.,Hayashi,H., Kagamiyama,H.,Nakanishi,S., and Hayaishi,O. (1989) in Advances in Prostaglandin, Thromboxane, and Leukotriene Research, Vol19 pp.462-465 (B.Samuelsson, P.Y.-K.Wong, and F.F.Sun)

CONVERSION OF LEUKOTRIENE A4 TO LIPOXINS BY HUMAN NASAL POLYPS AND BRONCHIAL TISSUE

JAN ÅKE LINDGREN[1], CHARLOTTE EDENIUS[1], MARIA KUMLIN[1], BARBRO DAHLÉN[2] AND ANDERS ÄNGGÅRD[3]

Departments of Physiological Chemistry[1], Thoracic Medicine[2] and Oto-Rhino-Laryngology[3], Karolinska Institutet, S-104 01 Stockholm, SWEDEN.

The lipoxins were originally isolated and characterized after addition of exogenous 15-H(P)ETE to human leukocyte suspensions (11). In accordance, the importance of interaction between the 5-lipoxygenase (5-LO) and the 15-LO in lipoxin formation was postulated. However, the involvement of the latter enzyme in the formation of lipoxins from endogenous substrate has not been convincingly demonstrated. Recently, we described lipoxin production from endogenous sources of arachidonic acid via platelet-dependent lipoxygenation at C-15 of granulocyte-derived leukotriene (LT)A$_4$ (1). This 15-LO activity was probably exerted by the platelet 12-lipoxygenase (4,12).

Several reports indicate that human respiratory epithelium possess a highly active 15-LO. Thus, formation of 15-HETE as the major lipoxygenase product in nasal, tracheal and bronchial epithelium (5,6,10) as well as in bronchial tissue (7) has been described. Furthermore, 15-HETE has been isolated from nasal and bronchoalveolar lavage fluids (8,9). Therefore, it was of interest to investigate the capacity of tissue derived from the human upper and lower respiratory tract to synthesize lipoxins from authentic or granulocyte-derived LTA$_4$. The present paper demonstrates that human nasal polyps efficiently converted exogenous LTA$_4$ to lipoxin (LX)A$_4$ and isomers of lipoxins A$_4$ and B$_4$. In comparison, the capacity of human bronchial tissue to produce lipoxins from LTA$_4$ was much less pronounced as measured per gram tissue. Furthermore, transcellular formation of lipoxins A$_4$ and B$_4$ and their isomers in mixed suspensions of granulocytes and chopped nasal polyps is described.

METHODS

Surgical removal and preparation of chopped human nasal polyps and bronchial tissue, collection of human blood and preparation of polymorphonuclear granulocyte suspensions, as well as incubations of cells and tissues, lipoxygenase product purification and reversed-phase high-performance liquid chromatography (RP-HPLC) were performed as described (3).

RESULTS AND DISCUSSION

Incubation of chopped human nasal polyps (300 mg tissue/ml buffer) at 37°C for 30 min in the absence of exogenous stimulus, led to formation of 15-HETE (2.3 nmol/g tissue), while no 12- or 5-HETE was produced. Addition of arachidonic acid (75 µM) markedly increased the 15-HETE synthesis (23.3 nmol/g; wet weight) and induced a minor 12-HETE production, whereas no 5-HETE was formed. The conversion of arachidonic acid to 15- and 12-HETE was not significantly altered by the addition of ionophore A23187 (5 µM). No detectable amounts of 5-HETE or leukotrienes was observed after incubation with arachidonic acid and ionophore A23187, indicating the absence of significant amounts of contaminating leukocytes.

As judged by RP-HPLC analysis combined with on-line computerized UV-spectroscopy and co-elution with authentic standards, the nasal polyps transformed authentic LTA$_4$ (10 µM) to LXA$_4$, 6(S)-LXA$_4$, and the all-*trans*-isomers of LXA$_4$ and LXB$_4$. The major metabolite formed after 30 min incubation was LXA$_4$. In contrast, LXB$_4$ was not formed. Stimulation of the tissue with ionophore A23187 (1 µM) did not influence the lipoxin production from exogenous LTA$_4$. This indicates that contaminating platelets could not be responsible for the conversion of LTA$_4$ to lipoxins, since platelet dependent lipoxin formation is markedly stimulated by ionophore A23187 (2). No formation of lipoxins could be detected after incubation of nasal polyps with ionophore A23187 in the absence or presence of exogenous arachidonic acid.

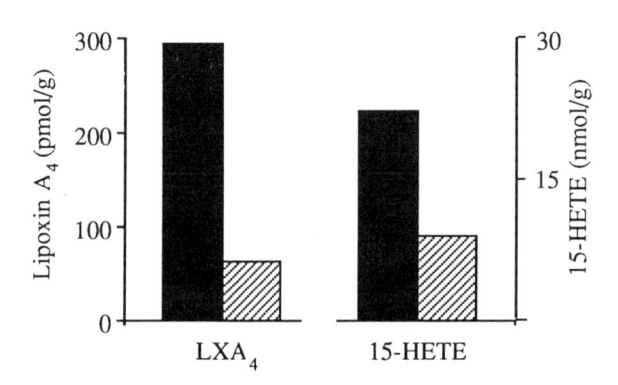

Fig 1. Comparison of lipoxin A$_4$ and 15-HETE formation in chopped human nasal polyps (n=3; filled bars) and bronchial tissue (n=3; hatched bars). The tissues were incubated with leukotriene A$_4$ (10 µM) or arachidonic acid (75 µM) for 30 min at 37°C.

Human bronchial tissue possessed less 15-LO activity than polyp tissue as judged by the conversion of exogenous arachidonic acid to 15-HETE (fig 1). Thus, 4.2-14.7 nmol 15-HETE/g (wet weight) of bronchial tissue was formed as compared to 8.3-43.4 nmol/g of polyp tissue. In parallel, bronchial tissue converted LTA$_4$ to lipoxins, but much less efficiently than nasal polyps (63 and 294 pmol LXA$_4$/g of bronchial or polyp tissue, respectively). The results are in agreement with a reported gradual decrease of immuno-reactive lipoxygenase along the human airways (13). However, it should be observed that the bronchial tissue may contain less epithelium per weight as compared to the nasal polyps.

Addition of granulocytes to chopped nasal polyps and stimulation of the mixture for 30 min with ionophore A23187 (1 µM) led to the formation of both LXA$_4$ and LXB$_4$. The synthesis of lipoxins increased about 3-fold in the presence of exogenous arachidonic acid (75 µM) (fig. 2).

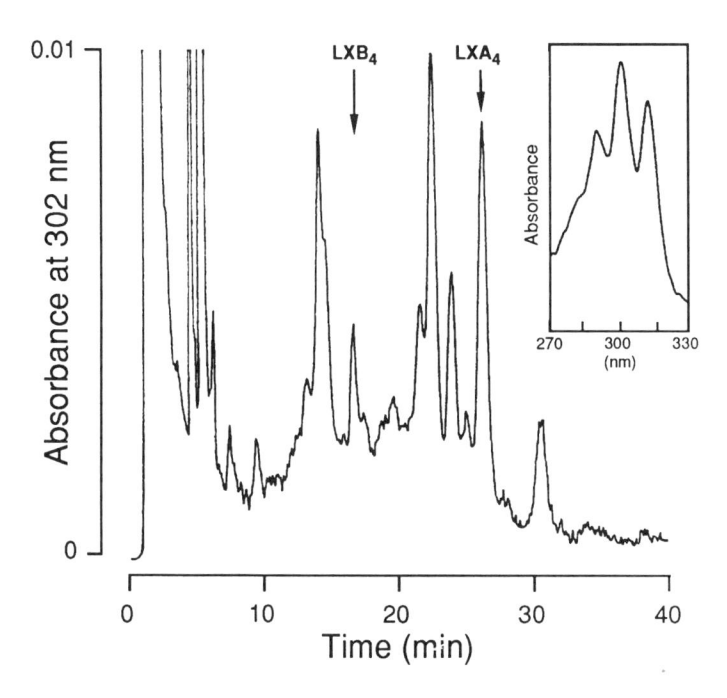

Fig 2. Reversed-phase HPLC-chromatogram of lipoxins formed in mixed suspensions of human granulocytes (15 x 10^6/ml) and chopped nasal polyps (150 mg/ml). Incubations were performed in the presence of ionophore A23187 (1 µM) and arachidonic acid (75 µM) for 30 min at 37°C. The retention times of synthetic lipoxin standards are indicated. Insert: on-line UV-spectrum of biosynthetic material eluting at the retention time of LXB$_4$.

The transcellular interactions between granulocytes and polyp tissue may lead to lipoxin formation via at least two pathways. First, leukotriene A$_4$, synthesized by the granulocyte 5-lipoxygenase, may be released and further converted to the tetraene intermediate 15-hydroxy-5(6)-epoxy-eicosatetraenoic acid by the 15-lipoxygenase in the polyp tissue. Subsequently, hydrolysis of this intermediate epoxide would lead to formation of the trihydroxylated lipoxins. This hypothesis is supported by the fact that nasal polyps transformed synthetic LTA$_4$ to lipoxins. Second, 15-H(P)ETE, synthesized by the polyp tissue, may be further converted to lipoxins by the granulocytes (11). The findings that nasal polyps released 15-HETE and that the production of this compound was markedly increased in the presence of exogenous arachidonic acid, which also stimulated the lipoxin formation in mixed granulocyte/nasal polyp incubations, support the second route of formation.

Interestingly, LXB$_4$ formation was observed exclusively in the presence of granulocytes, while pure nasal polyps only produced LXA$_4$ together with LXA$_4$- and LXB$_4$-isomers. These results are in agreement with the results obtained with mixed platelet-granulocyte suspensions (1,4). The findings indicate that the synthesis of LXB$_4$ is catalyzed by an epoxide hydrolase activity possessed by the granulocytes.

The present results indicate the importance of 15-LO for lipoxin formation in human respiratory mucosa. Transcellular formation of lipoxins may be of pathophysiological importance in nasal inflammatory disorders, since a number of pathological conditions include formation of an empyema with activated granulocytes in the sinusoidal cavities and/or an inflammatory reaction in the mucosa due to allergic or non-allergic rhinitis.

ACKNOWLEDGEMENTS

We thank Ms. Inger Forsberg and Ms. Barbro Näsman-Glaser for excellent technical assistance. This project was supported by the Swedish National Association against Heart and Lung Diseases and the Swedish Medical Research Council (proj no 03X-6805).

REFERENCES

1. Edenius, C., Haeggström, J. and Lindgren, J. Å. (1988): *Biochem. Biophys. Res. Commun.* 157: 801-807.
2. Edenius, C., Forsberg, I., Stenke, L. and Lindgren, J.Å. (1990): This volume.
3. Edenius, C., Kumlin, M., Dahlén, B., Änggård, A. and Lindgren, J.Å. (1990): To be published.
4. Edenius, C., Stenke, L. and Lindgren, J. Å. (1990): To be published.
5. Henke, D., Danilowicz, R. M., Curtis, J. F., Boucher, R. C. and Eling, T. E. (1988): *Arch. Biochem. Biophys.* 267: 426-436.
6. Hunter, J. A., Finkbeiner, W. E., Nadel, J. A., Goetzl, E. J.and Holtzman, M. J. (1985): *Proc. Natl. Acad. Sci. (USA)* 82: 4633-4637.
7. Kumlin, M., Ohlson, E., Björck, T., Hamberg, M., Granström, E., Dahlén, B., Zetterström, O. and Dahlén, S.-E. (1990): This volume.
8. Murray, J. J., Tonnel, A. B., Brash, A. R., Roberts, II, L. J., Gosset, P., Workman, R., Capron, A. and Oates, J. A. (1986): *N. Engl. J. Med.* 315: 800-804.
9. Ramis, I., Roselló-Catafau, J. and Bulbena, O. (1989): *J. Chromatog.* 496: 416-422.
10. Salari, H. and Chan-Yeung, M. (1989): *Am. J. Resp. Cell Mol. Biol.* 1: 245-250.
11. Samuelsson, B., Dahlén, S.-E., Lindgren, J. Å., Rouzer, C. A. and Serhan, C. N. (1987): *Science* 220: 568-575.
12. Serhan, C. N. and Sheppard, K.-A. (1990): *J. Clin. Invest.* 85: 772-780.
13. Shannon, V. R., Hansbrough, J.R., Takahashi, Y., Ueda, N., Yamamoto, S. and Holtzman, M. J. (1990): This volume.

LIPOXIN AND LEUKOTRIENE PRODUCTION DURING RECEPTOR-ACTIVATED INTERACTIONS BETWEEN HUMAN PLATELETS AND CYTOKINE-PRIMED NEUTROPHILS

Stefano Fiore, Mario Romano and Charles N. Serhan*

Hematology Division, Brigham and Women's Hospital and
Harvard Medical School, Boston, Massachusetts 02115

Cell-cell interactions can initiate transcellular routes for the biosynthesis of lipoxygenase (LO) derived eicosanoids (8). These transcellular routes may not only serve to amplify the levels of eicosanoids within a local milieu but may also lead to the generation of novel bioactive products. Studies on the interactions between human platelets and leukocytes have revealed several models for transcellular biosynthesis, which may also be operative within complex tissues (2,3,7,8,11). Platelets, for example, can utilize leukocyte-derived leukotriene A_4 to generate both peptido-leukotrienes (3,7) and lipoxins (2,11). Regulatory events between LOs which may be operative following receptor-mediated activation remain of interest. Along these lines, PMN primed by the cytokine GM-CSF can generate LTB_4 and its ω-oxidation products following stimulation by either the complement component C5a or the chemoattractant FMLP in quantities that are detectable by UV-RP-HPLC (1,9). Recent results indicated that coincubations of platelets and PMN stimulated with thrombin and FMLP leads to lipoxin production (11). Here, we have determined the relationship between leukotrienes and lipoxins generated by these receptor-mediated signals during coincubations of platelets with GM-CSF-primed PMN (in vitro).

MATERIALS AND METHODS

Human recombinant granulocyte-colony stimulating factor (GM-CSFrh) was purchased from Genzyme Co. (Boston, MA). Fresh peripheral blood was obtained from healthy donors who had not taken aspirin for at least 7 days. PMN were isolated by Ficoll-Hypaque gradient centrifugation and dextran sedimentation. These suspensions contained 98 ± 1% PMN as scored by light microscopy before incubation with GM-CSF (200 pM, 90 min, 37°C). Platelets were isolated using ACD (8) and enumerated using a Coulter Counter model ZM.

Incubations were terminated with methanol containing PGB_2 as internal standard and extracted (11). Following C18-Sep Pack (Waters Associates), materials within the methyl formate fractions (i.e. LTB_4, LXA_4) were chromatographed separately from those eluting within the methanol fractions (i.e. LTC_4). ω-oxidation products of LTB_4, LTB_4 and the lipoxins were resolved utilizing ED-UV detection with RP-HPLC (5,12). This system was equipped with a Lambda Max UV detector model 481 and an Electro Chemical detector (ED) model M 460 (Waters Associates). The column, a Beckman Ultrasphere-ODS (4.5 mm x 25

---

*For correspondence.

cm) was eluted with MeOH:H_2O (65:35, v/v), trifluoro acetic acid (1 mM). This system permits detection of lipoxins and LTB_4 in the picogram range (5). LTC_4, LTD_4 and LTE_4 were resolved using an RP-HPLC system equipped with an LC-75 UV detector (Perkin-Elmer, Norwalk, CT). LO products were routinely identified by comparison of their retention times with those obtained for standards in each HPLC system. Their quantities were determined by comparing peak heights obtained for calibrated standards in each system and the corresponding products from individual incubations following correction for the recovery of internal standard. Pentafluorobenzyl (PFB) ester derivatives were prepared as in (13). GC-MS (Hewlett-Packard model 5988A equipped with an HP 59970 workstation) was operated in the negative ion mode.

RESULTS AND DISCUSSION

<u>GM-CSF-primed PMN</u>. Primed PMN exposed to FMLP (10^{-7}M) generated both leukotrienes and lipoxins without the addition of exogenous substrates (Table 1). These results with LTB_4 and its ω-oxidation products are consistent with those reported (1,9). Peptido-LTs were not detected, while the levels of LXA_4, LXB_4 and their all-trans-isomers were obtained in amounts similar to those of LTB_4. The levels of lipoxins and their relationship to LTB_4 production with GM-CSF-primed PMN stimulated via a receptor-mediated agonist are drastically different from their relationship in ionophore-stimulated PMN. In the case of A_{23187}, PMN generate LTB_4 as a dominant product (12). Since both ED and UV detection with HPLC indicated that the lipoxins were formed in nanogram amounts (Table 1), it was necessary to utilize NICI-MS (13) to confirm the identity of the materials generated by GM-CSF-primed PMN stimulated with FMLP that coeluted with synthetic lipoxins on ED-UV-RP-HPLC. To this end, the materials were collected following HPLC, converted to PFB ester derivatives, treated with BSTFA, and analyzed by NICI-MS. The mass spectrum of the PFB ester, bis-TMS ether of the material which coeluted with LXA_4, showed an intense anion at m/e 567 which corresponded to [M-PFB]$^-$. Also present in its spectrum were ions at m/e 477 and m/e 387 corresponding to the loss of TMSOH and 2(TMSOH). These two ions were present in <5% of the spectrum and the ion at m/e 567 was the base peak. Together the physical characteristics of these products on ED-UV-RP-HPLC as well as ions present in their respective mass spectra recorded on GC-NICI-MS suggest that primed PMN stimulated with FMLP generate lipoxins.

<u>Coincubation of GM-CSFrh-primed PMN and platelets</u>. Simultaneous activation of PMN and platelets with thrombin and FMLP leads to the formation of both LXA_4 and LXB_4 (11). In addition, the platelet 12-LO can play a role in the formation of lipoxins from LTA_4 (2,11). Platelets can also utilize LTA_4 to generate LTC_4 (3,7); therefore, we evaluated the relationship between leukotrienes and lipoxins generated by GM-CSFrh-primed PMN coincubated with platelets (1:100 cell ratio). Following addition of FMLP (10^{-7}M), the peptido-LTs were generated (Table 1). Since human platelets do not possess either the 5-LO or the ω-oxidation system for LTB_4 (3,7,8), it is likely that the increased formation of ω-LTB_4 and the peptido-LTs observed with GM-CSF-primed PMN and platelets reflects, at least in part, the increased formation of LTA_4 by GM-CSF-primed PMN and the transfer of LTA_4 to platelets for LTC_4 production. The levels of LXB_4 and its trans-isomers were also increased in the presence of platelets, suggesting that multiple biosynthetic routes may contribute to the formation of lipoxins during the interactions of platelets with GM-CSF-primed PMN.

Addition of thrombin (0.1 U/ml) to coincubations led to an increase in LXA_4 and a decrease in the amounts of peptido-LTs. For purposes of comparison, the relationship between LXs and LTs was included for platelets coincubated with PMN stimulated with FMLP (10^{-7}M) and thrombin (0.1 U) in the absence of the cytokine. In this case, both lipoxins and leukotrienes were generated with LTC_4 (which can be derived from platelets; 3,7) and ω-oxidation products of LTB_4 (formed by PMN; 1,9) registered as the dominant products. GM-CSF-primed PMN coincubated with platelets also generated lipoxins and LTs when exposed to

Table 1. GM-CSFrh-primed Human PMN Coincubations with Platelets: Formation of Lipoxins and Leukotrienes

Incubation	t-LXB$_4$	LXB$_4$	t-LXA$_4$	LXA$_4$	LTC$_4$	LTD$_4$	LTE$_4$	ω_s-LTB$_4$	LTB$_4$
GM-CSF-primed PMN[a] + (FMLP 10^{-7}M)	11.4 ± 2.9	7.9 ± 2.8	14.2 ± 3.3	14.1 ± 5.9	c	c	c	51.7 ± 4.5	13.8 ± 3.5
PMN[b] and platelets (FMLP + thrombin)	21.0 ± 1.5	24.1 ± 1.7	17.5 ± 3.2	18.6 ± 4.5	52.3 ± 8.1	28.7 ± 8.7	15.7 ± 7.9	60.3 ± 7.3	6.2 ± 2.1
GM-CSF-primed PMN[a] and platelets (FMLP)	103.7 ± 58.4	54.0 ± 8.4	26.7 ± 3.1	22.9 ± 6.7	47.5 ± 7.2	54.7 ± 34.2	13.0 ± 5.3	77.7 ± 11.1	10.5 ± 4.4
GM-CSF-primed PMN[a] and platelets (FMLP + thrombin)	76.3 ± 30.9	35.5 ± 4.6	23.5 ± 4.8	29.6 ± 7.8	37.6 ± 8.0	21.6 ± 5.1	13.5 ± 5.7	75.6 ± 12.7	12.2 ± 3.0
GM-CSF-primed PMN[a] and platelets (A23187; 10^{-7}M)	134.1 ± 74.3	100.7 ± 26.3	45.2 ± 5.5	46.2 ± 12.4	88.3 ± 36.2	34.5 ± 9.6	21.5 ± 9.0	127.7 ± 35.6	21.3 ± 8.9

Isolated PMN (30 x 10^6/ml) were incubated for 90 min at 37°C in the [a]presence or [b]absence of GM-CSFrh (200 pM). Next, aliquots (0.5 ml) of each cell suspension were combined with 0.5 ml aliquots of isolated platelet suspensions (3 x 10^9/ml). Cell ratios were approximately 1:100 (PMN:platelet) in 1 ml. The suspensions were exposed to either A23187 (0.1 μM), FMLP (10^{-7}M), or FMLP (10^{-7}M) in combination with thrombin (0.1 U/ml). ω_s-LTB$_4$ denotes [20-OH-LTB$_4$ + 20-COOH-LTB$_4$] and t-LX denotes the two coeluting all-trans-isomers of LXA$_4$ and LXB$_4$, respectively (see ref. 12). The incubations (20 min at 37°C) were terminated and analyzed by RP-HPLC as described in Methods. Results are expressed in nanograms/incubation; mean ± SE of three separate experiments.

[c]Products not detected.

ionophore (A_{23187}, $10^{-7}M$). Since the ionophore does not interact with specific receptors, it may provide an index of the biosynthetic potential of these cells to generate individual LO products during the interaction of GM-CSF-primed PMN with platelets.

CONCLUSIONS

These results demonstrate the levels of both lipoxins and leukotrienes generated from endogenous sources by PMN primed with GM-CSFrh and in coincubations with platelets. Upon exposure to receptor-mediated stimuli (FMLP and thrombin), the levels of lipoxins generated were within the range of both LTB_4 and LTC_4. Additional experiments revealed that coincubation of [1-^{14}C]-arachidonate-labeled platelets with primed PMN followed by addition of thrombin and FMLP led to the formation of both 5- and 15-LO products which carried ^{14}C-label (4).

The profile of bioactions observed for LXA_4 (10) and its identification in human bronchoalveolar fluids (6) suggest that the generation of lipoxins may play a functional role in vivo. Thus, the generation of physiologically relevant levels of lipoxins by receptor-mediated activation of cytokine-primed PMN interacting with platelets (in vitro) by at least two separate biosynthetic routes, namely one which involves the donation of platelet-arachidonate to the 15-LO of PMN and the other PMN-derived LTA_4 transformation by platelets (bidirectional formation), may be important in both inflammation and in the interaction of these cells with the vessel wall.

Acknowledgments. The authors thank Kelly-Ann Sheppard for technical assistance and Mary Halm Small for skillful preparation of the manuscript. This work was supported in part by National Institutes of Health grants AI-26714 and GM-38765. Dr. Serhan is a Pew Scholar in the Biomedical Sciences. Dr. Fiore is the recipient of an American Heart Association, Massachusetts Affiliate Fellowship.

REFERENCES

1. Dahinden, C.A., Zingg, J., Maly, F.E., and de Weck, A.L. (1988): J. Exp. Med. 167:1281.
2. Edenius, C., Haeggström, J., and Lindgren, J.A. (1988): Biochem. Biophys. Res. Commun. 157:801-807.
3. Edenius, C., Heidvall, K., and Lindgren, J.A. (1988): Eur. J. Biochem. 178:81-86.
4. Fiore, S., and Serhan, C.N. (1990): (submitted).
5. Herrmann, T., Steinhilber, D., Knospe, J., and Roth, H.J. (1988): J. Chromatogr. 428:237.
6. Lee, T.H., Crea, A.E.G., Gant, V., Spur, B.W., Marron, B.E., Nicolaou, K.C., Reardon, E., Brezinski, M., and Serhan, C.N. (1990): Am. Rev. Respir. Dis. 141 (in press)
7. Maclouf, J.A., and Murphy, R.C. (1988): J. Biol. Chem. 263:174-181.
8. Marcus A.J., Broekman, M.J., Safier, L.B., Ullman, H.L., Islam, N., Serhan, C.N., Rutherford, L.E., Korchak, H.M., and Weissmann, G. (1982): Biochem. Biophys. Res. Commun. 109:130-137.
9. McColl, S.R., Krump, E., Naccache, P.H., and Borgeat, P. (1989): Agents and Actions 27:465-468.
10. Samuelsson, B., and Serhan, C.N. (1987): In Prostaglandins in Cancer Research, edited by E. Garaci, R. Paoletti, and M.G. Santoro, pp. 3-11. Springer-Verlag, Berlin, Heidelberg.
11. Serhan, C.N., and Sheppard, K.-A. (1990): J. Clin. Invest. 85:772-780.
12. Serhan, C.N. (1989): Biochim. Biophys. Acta 1004:158-168.
13. Strife, R.J., and Murphy, R.C. (1984): J. Chromatogr. 305:3.

LIPOXIN FORMATION IN HUMAN PLATELETS

CHARLOTTE EDENIUS, INGER FORSBERG, LEIF STENKE
AND JAN ÅKE LINDGREN

*Department of Physiological Chemistry, Karolinska Institutet,
Box 60 400, S-104 01 Stockholm, SWEDEN*

Several recent reports indicate that platelets may be important inflammatory cells interacting with various aspects of leukocyte function (11). Transcellular cooperation between platelets and granulocytes leads to formation of unique lipoxygenase products, such as 5(S),12(S)-dihydroxyeicosatetraenoic acid (DiHETE), which is formed via interaction of the platelet 12-lipoxygenase (12-LO) and the granulocyte 5-LO (7). Recently, we reported that human platelets possess a specific leukotriene (LT)C$_4$ synthase that utilize exogenous LTA$_4$, derived from e.g. granulocytes to produce LTC$_4$ (3). Furthermore, the platelets efficiently metabolize this compound to LTD$_4$ and LTE$_4$. In addition, lipoxin (LX) formation from endogenous substrate via platelet-dependent lipoxygenation of granulocyte-derived LTA$_4$ was demonstrated (2). The present report describes results derived from extended studies of platelet-dependent metabolism of LTA$_4$ to lipoxins (4,5).

METHODS

Preparation of platelet and granulocyte suspensions obtained from peripheral human blood, incubation of intact cells and subcellular fractions, platelet aggregation studies, sample purification and determination of lipoxygenase products using reversed-phase high-performance liquid chromatography (RP-HPLC), including on-line UV-spectroscopy were performed as described (2-5).

RESULTS AND DISCUSSION

Ionophore A23187 stimulation of mixed platelet/granulocyte suspensions led to a platelet-concentration dependent formation of LXA$_4$, LXB$_4$, 6(S)-LXA$_4$ and the all-*trans* isomers of LXA$_4$ and B$_4$ (2,4). In the absence of added platelets, no significant lipoxin formation could be observed. Furthermore, pure platelet suspensions converted exogenous LTA$_4$ to a similar profile of lipoxin isomers, although LXB$_4$ was not formed. The results suggest a platelet-dependent lipoxygenation of LTA$_4$ at C-15 leading to formation of the putative intermediate in lipoxin synthesis 5(6)-epoxy-15-HETE (12), which is further hydrolyzed to trihydroxy-lipoxins. The inability of pure platelets to convert LTA$_4$ to LXB$_4$ indicates that the formation of this lipoxin depends on an epoxide hydrolase activity expressed by the granulocytes.

Based on isolation of lipoxins from leukocyte suspension incubated with 15-H(P)ETE and ionophore A23187 it was postulated that lipoxins are formed via interaction between the 5- and the 15-lipoxygenase (11). Recent findings suggest this route of formation in human respiratory tissue (8). However, although human platelets possess minor 15-LO activity (2,18), only one principal lipoxygenase, the 12-LO has been described in these cells (6). The involvement of this enzyme in lipoxin formation was suggested by results obtained with 12-LO deficient platelets (5,17) derived from patients with chronic myelogenous leukemia (CML) (10). These platelets transformed exogenous arachidonic acid to the cyclo-oxygenase products 12-hydroxyheptadecatrienoic acid (HHT) and thromboxane B_2 but not to 12-HETE. In parallel, the cells lacked the capacity to convert exogenous LTA_4 to lipoxins. Granulocytes from these patients produced both 5-HETE and 15-HETE as well as leukotrienes C_4 and B_4 after incubation with exogenous arachidonic acid and ionophore A23187, indicating that the lipoxygenase deficiency was restricted to the platelet 12-LO.

A recent report by Serhan and Sheppard (14) confirms our findings of platelet-dependent lipoxin formation and suggests the 12-LO as the catalyzing enzyme. This hypothesis was based on parallel lipoxin formation and 12-LO activity in the 100 000 x g supernatant of human platelets. In the present study, the 12-lipoxygenase activity was recovered from both the soluble and particulate fractions with approximately 70 % of the total activity found in the cytosol (Table 1). The lipoxin formation showed a similar subcellular distribution with 54% of the total activity found in the cytosol and 46% in the particulate fraction. In addition, the specific activity of the 12-HETE and lipoxin formation was about 2-5 times higher in the particulate preparation, indicating an enrichment of the enzymatic activity in the membrane fraction (Table 1). In comparison, more than 95% of the human eosinophil 15-LO activity was found in the 100 000 x g supernatant, whereas the enzyme activity was negligible in the particulate fraction (16).

Table 1. Subcellular distribution of platelet 12-LO activity and lipoxin formation

	12-HETE formation			Lipoxin A_4 formation		
	Total activity (nmol)	%	Specific activity (nmol/mg prot)	Total activity (nmol)	%	Specific activity (nmol/mg prot)
Sonicate	83.6±20.4		29.7±5.1	2.01±1.1		0.70±0.24
Soluble	48.8±18.0	69.9	20.2±7.0	0.90±0.53	54.0	0.35±0.08
Particulate	20.6±1.80	31.1	42.8±11.6	0.70±0.21	46.0	1.41±0.35

The 100.000 x g supernatant (soluble fraction) and pellet (particulate fraction) were prepared from sonicated human platelet suspensions (400 x 10^6/ml). All three fractions were incubated with either arachidonic acid (20μM) or LTA_4 (20μM) prior to analysis of 12-HETE and LXA_4, respectively. 12-LO activity was assayed in the presence of indomethacin (1 μM). Mean of three experiments performed in duplicate ± S.D.

Taken together, the lack of lipoxin production in 12-LO deficient platelets and the similar subcellular distribution of 12-LO activity and lipoxin formation indicate the importance of this enzyme in platelet dependent lipoxin synthesis.

Activation of intact platelets by various concentrations of the Ca-ionophore A23187 led to a dose-dependent stimulation of the conversion of LTA$_4$ to lipoxins. Thus, increased lipoxin synthesis was observed already at 0.1 µM and maximal effect was obtained at 1 µM ionophore A23187 (Fig. 1, left panel). Concomitantly, a decrease in the formation of cysteinyl-containing leukotrienes was observed, probably due to substrate competition (Fig. 1, left panel).

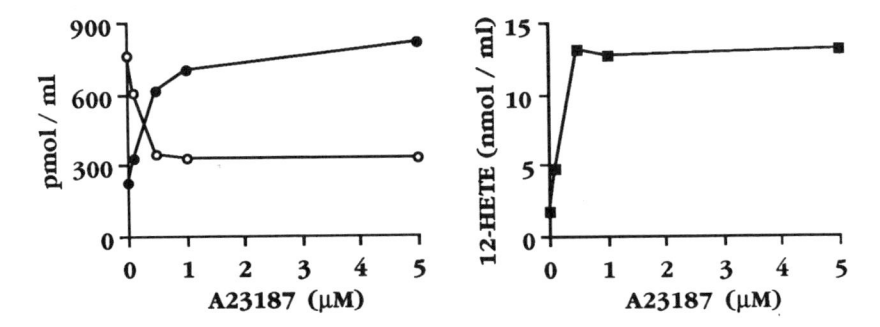

Fig. 1 Effect of ionophore A23187 on the conversion of LTA$_4$ (10 µM; left panel) to lipoxins (•) and cysteinyl-containing leukotrienes (o) and the transformation of arachidonic acid (10 µM; right panel) to 12-HETE (■) in human platelets.

In addition, 12-HETE production from exogenous arachidonic acid was stimulated in the presence of ionophore with a similar dose-response curve as demonstrated for lipoxin formation (Fig. 1, right panel). Furthermore, the conversion of LTA$_4$ to lipoxins was stimulated by receptor mediated activation of the platelets with thrombin. The results indicate a correlation between platelet activation and lipoxin formation. Preincubation with the anti-aggregatory prostaglandin E$_1$ led to a dose-dependent inhibition of ionophore A23187-induced aggregation, while the stimulatory effect of the ionophore on lipoxin synthesis was unaffected (Fig. 2).

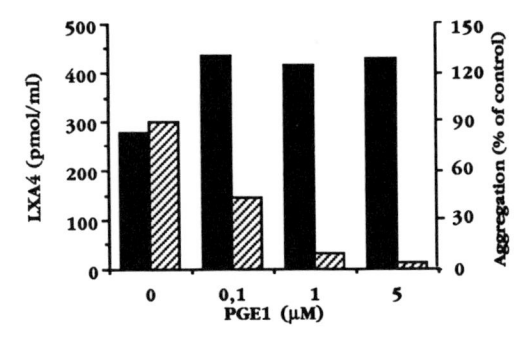

Fig. 2 Effect of PGE$_1$ on ionophore A23187-induced platelet aggregation and lipoxin formation. Platelet suspensions (400 x10^6 /ml) were preincubated with PGE$_1$ at 37°C for 2 min before addition of A23187 (0.2 µM) and LTA$_4$ (10 µM). Lipoxin production (filled bars) was analysed using RP-HPLC. Platelet aggregation (hatched bars) was studied as described (5).

This suggests that lipoxin formation is linked to an event in platelet activation but not directly to the aggregation. Calcium-dependent translocation of rat platelet 12-LO to the membrane leading to activation of the enzyme has been reported (1). Furthermore, prostacyclin has been demonstrated to inhibit ionophore A23187-induced platelet aggregation without affecting intracellular Ca-mobilisation induced by this compound (15). Therefore, mobilisation of calcium might be involved in the regulation of lipoxin synthesis in human platelets.

Transcellular interactions between granulocytes and platelets leads to an increased formation of cysteinyl-containing leukotrienes (3,9). The present observations demonstrate that this co-operation also results in the formation of lipoxins from endogenous substrate and that platelet activation leads to a more efficient conversion of LTA$_4$ to lipoxins. Thus, platelet dependent modulation of LTA$_4$ metabolism may be of importance in allergy and inflammation, since accumulation and activation of platelets have been reported under these conditions (11).

ACKNOWLEDGEMENTS

We thank Ms. Barbro Näsman-Glaser for skillful technical assistance. This project was supported by the Swedish National Association against Heart and Chest Disease, The Swedish Medical Research Council, The Swedish Cancer Society, King Gustaf V 80-years Fund, The Swedish Medical Society, Magnus Bergvalls Foundation and Karolinska Institutet´s Research Funds.

REFERENCES

1. Baba, A., Sakuma, S., Okamoto, H., Inoue, T. and Iwata, H. (1989) *J. Biol. Chem.* 264: 15790-15795.
2. Edenius, C., Haeggström, J. and Lindgren, J.Å. (1988) *Biochem. Biophys. Res. Commun.* 157: 801-807.
3. Edenius, C., Heidvall, K. and Lindgren, J.Å. (1988) *Eur. J. Biochem.* 178: 81-86.
4. Edenius, C., Stenke, L. and Lindgren, J.Å. (1990) Submitted.
5. Edenius, C. and Lindgren, J. Å. (1990) To be published
6. Hamberg, M. and Samuelsson, B. (1974) *Proc. Natl. Acad. Sci.* USA 71: 3400-3404.
7. Lindgren, J.Å., Hansson, G. and Samuelsson, B. (1981) *FEBS Lett.* 128: 329-335.
8. Lindgren, J. Å., Edenius, C., Kumlin, M., Dahlén, B. and Änggård, A. This volume.
9. Maclouf, J. and Murphy, R. C. (1988) *J. Biol. Chem.* 263: 174-181.
10. Okuma, M. and Uchino, H. (1979) *Blood* 54: 1258-1271.
11. Page, C.P. (1989) *Immunopharmacology* 17: 51-59.
12. Puustinen, T., Webber, S. E., Nicolaou, K. C., Haeggström, J., Serhan, C. N. and Samuelsson, B. (1986) *FEBS Lett* 207: 127-132.
13. Samuelsson, B., Dahlén, S.-E., Lindgren, J.Å., Rouzer, C.A. and Serhan, C. N. (1987) *Science* 220: 568-575.
14. Serhan, C. N. and Sheppard, K.-A. (1990) *J. Clin. Invest.* 85: 772-780.
15. Siess, W. and Lapetina, G. (1989) *Biochemical J.* 258: 57-65.
16. Sigal, E., Grunberger, D., Cashman, J. R., Craik, C. S.,Caughey, G. H. and Nadel, J. A. (1988) *Biochem. Biophys. Res. Commun.* 150: 376-383.
17. Stenke, L., Edenius, C. and Lindgren, J. Å. (1990) Submitted.
18. Wong, P.Y.-K., Westlund, P., Hamberg, M., Granström, E. Chao, P.H.-W. and Samuelsson, B. (1985) *J. Biol. Chem.* 260: 9162-9165.

PURIFICATION OF 15-LIPOXYGENASE FROM HUMAN LEUKOCYTES, EVIDENCE FOR THE PRESENCE OF ISOZYMES

T. Izumi, O. Rådmark, and B. Samuelsson

Department of Physiological Chemistry, Karolinska Institutet, Box 60 400, S-104 01, Stockholm, Sweden

Two different proteins with 15-lipoxygenase (15-LO) activity were purified to homogeneity from human leukocytes. The major 15-LO was clearly separated from the minor form on a Mono S column. The N-terminal amino acid sequence of the major 15-LO is similar, but not identical to the published sequence of reticulocyte 15-LO (6), while the minor 15-LO has the same N-ternimal sequence as reticulocyte enzyme. The minor protein was enriched in the leukocytes from a patient with eosinophilia, and Northern blot analysis revealed that an RNA-species of eosinophil-enriched leukocytes hybridized to a reticulocyte 15-LO cDNA but RNA of normal leukocytes did not. These results indicate that there are two isozymes of 15-LO in human leukocytes.

INTRODUCTION

The enzyme 15-LO catalyzes the insertion of molecular oxygen into arachidonic acid at carbon 15 to form 15-hydroperoxyeicosatetraenoic acid (15-HPETE). This enzyme is distributed in many mammalian cells (leukocytes, eosiophils, keratinocytes, and airway epithelial cells) and also in plants (soybean seed and pea seed). The mammalian 15-LOs were first purified to homogeneity from rabbit reticulocytes (4) and then from human eosinophil-enriched leukocytes (5). The cDNAs which encode these enzymes have been isolated (2, 6). It was reported that soybean contains at least four distinct isozymes and these isozymes have differences in their substrate specificities and kinetic properties (1). Immunological studies indicated that rabbit reticulocyte 15-LO is specific to red cells (3), while another report showed that the 15-LOs of leukocytes, air way epithelial cells, and reticulocytes are structurally related (7). It was unkown whether the 15-LO activities detected in many human cells are due to the same enzyme or if isozymes are present. In this report we show that there are two 15-LO isozymes in human leukocytes.

MATERIAL AND METHODS

Enzyme Purification.

Routinely, 100 bags of human buffy-coat were obtained from the local blood center. The leukocytes were separated from erythrocytes by dextran sedimentation, followed by ammonium cloride lysis. The cell suspension (74 % were neutrophils, 2 % eosinophils, 23 % lymphocytes, 1% other cells) was homogenized by a sonicator, and centrifuged at 10,000 x g for 15 min. The 30-60 % ammonium sulfate fraction of the supernatant was applied to a gel filtration column, Superose 12. The active fractions were further purified by column chromatographies, on anion-exchange (Mono Q), hydroxyapatite, cation-exchange (Mono S), and chromatofocusing (Mono P) columns. The enzyme activity was assayed at 22 °C for 5 min in 0.1 ml of a standard reaction mixture which contained 0.1 M Tris-HCl pH 7.0, 160 µM arachidonic acid, 2 mM $CaCl_2$, 0.02 % Tween 20, 1mM DTT, and 0.5 nmol of 13-hydroperoxyocta-decadienoic acid as an activator. The reaction was terminated by addition of the acidic organic solvent, and after centrifugation, an aliquot of the supernatant was analyzed by reversed-phase HPLC. One unit of enzyme activity is defined as one nmol of HPETE produced during the 5-min incubation period. An aliquot of the Mono P fractions was subjected to SDS polyacrylamide gel electrophoresis, stained by silver. Another aliquot was subjected to N-terminal amino acid sequence analysis by Edman degradation.

Eosinophil-Enriched Leukocytes.

Eosinophil-enriched leukocytes were obtained from a patient with eosinophilic leukemia. The differential cell count of the leukocytes was 64 % eosinophils, 33 % neutrophil, 2 % lymphocytes, and 1% other cells. The cell suspension was sonicated, and the 15-lipoxygenase activity of 10,000 x g supernatant was absorbed by hydroxyapatite powder and eluted with 0.2 M phosphate buffer. The 30-60 % ammonium sulfate precipitate of the eluted protein was applied to the Mono S column.

Northern Blot Analysis of Leukocyte Total RNAs.

The DNA probe which encodes reticulocyte 15-LO was made using polymerase chain reaction, from cDNA library of human buffy-coat. A DNA of 521 base pair length (from 1378th to 1898th nucleotide of the reticulocyte 15-LO cDNA sequence (6)) was obtained. This DNA was cut by a restriction enzyme, Sau3A I, and the longer fragment of 372 base pairs was used as the reticulocyte 15-LO probe. Total RNAs obtained from eosinophil-enriched leukocytes and normal leukocytes were electrophoresed in formaldehyde/agorose gel and transferred onto nitrocellulose filter. The filter was hybridized to the reticulocyte 15-LO probe and washed at 60 °C in 0.1 x SSC, 0.1 % SDS for 1 hr.

RESULTS

On a Mono Q column, 15-LO activity was separated from 5-LO activity. Two peaks with 15-LO activity were observed on the hydroxyapatite chromatography, and the separation of two peaks became much clearer on a Mono S column (**FIG.1.**). The minor peak (Peak I) was eluted with 0.2 M of NaCl, while the major peak (Peak II) was eluted with 0.4 M of NaCl. The activity ratio of Peak I to Peak II was about 1 : 4.5.

Both of two peaks with 15-LO activity were purified to homogeneity

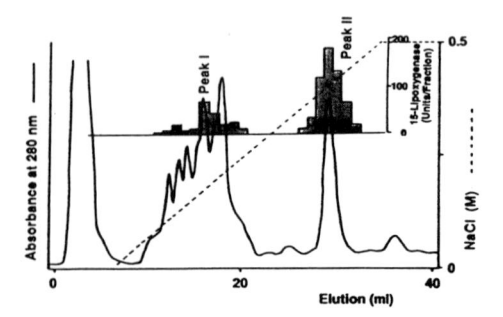

FIG.1., **Resolution of two peaks on a cation-exchange column.** The active fractions from hydroxyapatite column were applied to a Mono S column.

```
Reticulocyte     MG LYRIRVSTGASLYAGSNNQVQLWVGQHG
Eosinophil        X LYRIRVSTGASLYA
Leukocyte Peak I  X LYRIRVSTGASLYAGSNNQVQLWVGQHG
         Peak II  X LYXIX VSTGAX LYAGSN TQV
```

FIG.2., N-terminal amino acid sequence for human 15-lipoxygenase of reticulocyte (6), eosinophil (5), and leukocyte Peak I, Peak II. Sequence identity is indicated by the *bold* line. X is undetermined amino acid.

on SDS polyacrylamide gel electropholesis and had same molecular size, 74 kD. Comparison of the N-terminal amino acid sequences of Peak I and Peak II with those of the reticulocyte 15-LO (6) and eosinophil 15-LO (5) reveals that Peak I has identical N-terminal sequence to reticulocyte 15-LO and eosinophil 15-LO, but the 19th amino acid, asparagine, is changed to threonine in the major leukocyte 15-LO, Peak II (**FIG.2.**).

FIG.3. shows the cation-exchange chromatography of the leukocyte homogenates obtained from a patient with eosinophilia. In this homogenate, Peak I is the predominant peak oposite to normal leukocytes (the activity ratio of Peak I to Peak II was 1.9:1).

Northern blot analysis shows that there are two clear bands (3.0 and 4.4 kilobase) which hybridize to reticulocyte 15-LO DNA in the RNAs of eosinophil-enriched leukocytes, however RNAs of normal leukocytes did not hybridize to the probe (**FIG.4.**).

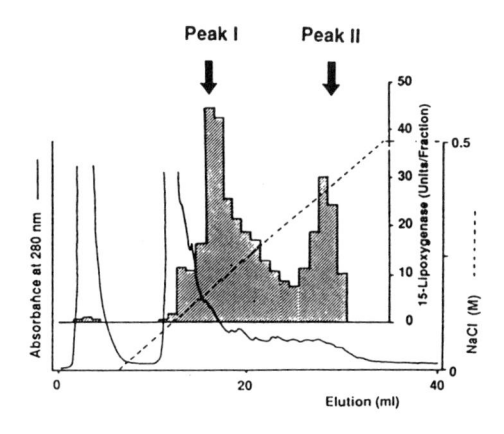

FIG.3., **Cation-exchange chromatography of the homogenates from eosinophil-enriched leukocytes.** After hydroxyapatite batch fractionation and ammonium sulfate precipitate, the 30-60% precipitates was applied to a Mono S column.

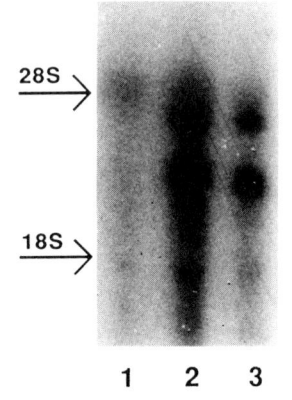

FIG.4., **Northern blotting of leukocyte total RNA probed with a reticulocyte 15-lipoxygenase cDNA.** 1) normal leukocyte RNA 15 µg, 2-3) leukocyte RNA from patient with eosinophilia: 2) 15 µg, 3) 5 µg.

DISCUSSION

Mammalian 15-lipoxygenase activity exists in leukocytes, eosinophils, reticulocytes, and airway epithelial cells. Human eosinophil 15-LO (5) and rabbit reticulocyte 15-LO (2) have been purified, and the cDNA of human reticulocyte 15-LO and rabbit reticulocyte 15-LO (2) have been isolated. An antibody against rabbit reticulocyte 15-LO can react with human reticulocyte 15-LO, but cannot with human leukocytes though human leukocytes apparently have 15-LO activity (3). On the other hand, it is reported that human leukocytes and tracheal cells have immunoreactive bands which can be detected by the antibody against the recombinant human reticulocyte 15-LO (7).

Our present study shows that there are two different proteins (isozymes) with 15-lipoxygenase activity in human leukocytes. The minor isozyme was enriched in the leukocytes from an eosinophilic patient and had the same N-terminal amino acid sequence as eosinophil 15-LO and reticulocyte 15-LO. Furthermore, the RNAs from eosinophil-enriched leukocytes hybridized to reticulocyte 15-LO cDNA. These findings indicate that the minor isozymes comes from eosinophils, and may be identical to reticulocyte 15-LO. The major isozyme is a new protein and has similar but not identical N-terminal sequence to reticulocyte 15-LO.

REFERENCES

1. Axelrod, B., Cheesbrough, T.M., and Laasko, S. (1981): In: *Methods in Enzymology: Lipoxygenase from Soybeans,* edited by Lowenstein, J. M., Vol. 71, pp. 441-451, Academic Press, San Diego
2. Fleming, J., Thiele, B. J., Chester, J., O'Prey, J., Janetzki, S., Aitken, A., Anton, I. A., Rapoport, S. M., and Harrison, P. R. (1989): *Gene,* 79: 181-188.
3. Kroschwald, P., Kroschwald, A., Kuhn, H., Ludwig, P., Thiele, B. J., Höhne, M., Schewe, T., and Rapoport, S. M. (1989): *Biochem. Biophys. Res. Commun.,* 160: 954-960.
4. Rapoport, S. M., Schewe, T., Wiesner, R., Halangk., W., Ludwig, P., Janicke-Hohne, M., Tannert, C., Hiebsch, C., and Klatt, D. (1979): *Eur. J. Biochem.,* 96: 545-561.
5. Sigal, E., Grunberger, D., Craik, C. S., Caughey, G. H., and Nadel, J. A. (1988): *J. Biol. Chem.,* 263: 5328-5332.
6. Sigal, E., Craik, C. S., Highland, E., Grunberger, D., Costello, L. L., Dixon, R. A. F., and Nadel, J. A. (1988): *Biochem. Biophys. Res. Commun.,* 157: 457-464.
7. Sigal, E., Grunberger, D., Highland, E., Gross, C., Dixon, R. A. F., and Craik, C. S. (1990): *J. Biol. Chem.,* 265: 5113-5120.

SELECTIVE INCORPORATION OF 15-HETE IN PHOSPHATIDYLINOSITOL: AGONIST-INDUCED DEACYLATION AND TRANSFORMATION OF STORED HETEs BY HUMAN NEUTROPHILS

Charles N. Serhan* and Mark E. Brezinski

Hematology Division, Department of Medicine
Brigham and Women's Hospital and Harvard Medical School
Boston, Mass. 02115

Although elevated levels of 15-HETE have been detected in various tissues, its role in inflammation and other physiologic responses remains of interest (10). Recent results indicate that 15-HETE injected into plaque lesions of psoriasis vulgaris in humans results in complete regression of the lesions (3). In addition, intraarticular administration of 15-HETE in canines with carragheenan-induced arthritis significantly reduces both the clinical severity and volume of effusates (4). 15-HETE can block both cyclooxygenase and the formation of LTB_4 (9,12), and is a substrate for lipoxin biosynthesis by human neutrophils in vitro (7); however, the biochemical bases for the observed "anti-inflammatory" actions of 15-HETE remain to be elucidated.

Stenson and Parker (11) first demonstrated that 5-HETE is incorporated into phospholipids and triglycerides of PMN, a finding which has been extended to a wide range of cell types (10). In view of recent observations with 15-HETE and its transformation products (1,5,6), the present studies were undertaken to examine the following: Is 15-HETE incorporated into human PMN lipids in a profile similar to that of either AA or 5-HETE? Second, can either esterified 15-HETE or 5-HETE be mobilized upon activation of PMN and, if so, are they subject to lipoxygenation? Third, are functional responses of PMN altered by these events?

METHODS AND MATERIALS

Radiolabeled eicosanoids were from NEN Research Products, Boston, MA. 15S-HETE and 5S-HETE were prepared by $SnCl_2$ reduction of 15S-HPETE generated with soybean lipoxygenase and 5S-HPETE from potato tubers, respectively. The identities and concentrations of 15S-HETE and 5S-HETE were confirmed by GC-MS, RP, and chiral column HPLC. PMN obtained from healthy volunteers were suspended in PBS, and contained 98 ± 1% PMN in reported experiments (<2% were permeable to trypan blue) (2). Suspensions (30 x 10^6 cells/ml) were warmed to 37°C for 5 min. 15-[^{3}H]HETE (183.5Ci/mmol) was added and incubations were stopped by addition of $MeOH/CHCl_3$ (5:2 v/v; 3.5 ml) at indicated intervals (15 sec-

*For correspondence.

20 min). In parallel incubations, PMN were exposed to either 5-[^{3}H]HETE (192.0Ci/mmol) or AA[^{14}C] (52.8mCi/mmol). Inositol phospholipids were examined as in (13). Phospholipids were separated by a modification of previously described techniques, which permitted analysis of individual phospholipid, TG, and CE from the same incubation (2). For analysis of eicosanoids, incubations were stopped with the addition of MeOH containing PGB$_2$ (100ng) and products were extracted and chromatographed as in (7). Aggregation was monitored with a four channel aggregation profiler (model PAP-4, Biodat Co., Halbow, Pa.). PMN (5 x 10^6 cells/ml) were exposed to either vehicle (0.4 vol %, EtOH) or varying concentrations of agonist.

RESULTS AND DISCUSSION

Upon exposure to 15-[^{3}H]-HETE, PMN rapidly incorporated label into phospholipids (2). Incorporation was time-dependent (nearly maximal within 5 min) and was associated with PI (approx. 20% of recovered label), while uptake into other phospholipid classes, CE, or TG represented <4-5% (Table 1). To determine if labeled 15-HETE was esterified in the sn2 position, labeled PI was isolated from PMN and incubated with snake venom PLA$_2$ (24°C, pH 6.5). Following extraction and RP-HPLC, 98.9% of the radiolabel was released from PMN-derived PI, which coeluted with 15-HETE (n=2). These findings indicate that PMN rapidly esterify 15-[^{3}H]-HETE into the sn-2 of PI. Although the incorporation of 15-HETE into PIP or PIP$_2$ represented a relatively low percentage of added material, the relative levels of 15-[^{3}H]-HETE esterified were comparable to those observed with [1-^{14}C]-labeled AA (2). Comparison of the incorporation patterns for 15-HETE, 5-HETE and AA with PMN revealed differences between the profiles (Table 1). Unlike 15-HETE, incorporation of either 5-HETE or AA was predominately associated with TG (approx. 8 and 28%, respectively). Of the lipid classes, 15-HETE was dominant in PI among the phospholipid of PMN, while both 5-HETE and AA were incorporated mainly into PC. The values obtained with both 5-HETE and AA are consistent with those reported earlier (11).

Since PMN stored 15-HETE in PI, we determined whether PMN mobilize this source upon activation. After labeling with 15-[^{3}H]-HETE, PMN were exposed to agonists or vehicle alone. PMN exposed to either FMLP (100 nM), PMA (100 nM) or A$_{23,187}$ (5 μM) each showed a significant reduction in labeled PI (>50% decrease). PMN labeled with 15-HETE also displayed an impaired ability to generate LTB$_4$ and its ω-oxidation products (not shown). In contrast, PMN incubated (20 min, 37°C) separately with either 5-HETE (30 μM) or AA (30 μM) followed by washing

TABLE 1. Comparison of 5-[^{3}H]-HETE, 15-[^{3}H]-HETE, and [1-^{14}C]-AA Incorporation into PMN Lipids

PMN lipid	15-HETE	5-HETE	AA
PI	20.0 ± 6.0	0.6 ± 0.1	4.6 ± 0.6
PC	1.0 ± 0.1	1.5 ± 0.2	6.7 ± 0.9
PE	3.0 ± 1.0	0.8 ± 0.1	2.2 ± 0.3
PS	0.6 ± 0.1	0.4 ± 0.0	0.4 ± 0.1
SP	0.5 ± 0.1	1.0 ± 0.3	0.1 ± 0.1
TG	0.0 ± 0.0	8.0 ± 1.0	28.0 ± 4.0
CE	0 ± 0	0.1 ± 0.1	0 ± 0

PMN (30 x 10^6/ml) were incubated with either [^{3}H]15-HETE, 5-[^{3}H]HETE, or [1-^{14}C]AA for 20 min at 37°C. Incubations were stopped with MeOH:CHCl$_3$ (5:2 vol/vol; 3.5 ml). The distribution of radiolabel into PMN lipids was determined after two-dimensional TLC. Values represent means ± SEM for 3-5 separate experiments.

and stimulation with ionophore (5 µM, 20 min, 37°C) generated amounts of LTB_4, 20-OH-LTB_4, and 20-COOH-LTB_4 which were not statistically different from PMN treated with vehicle alone (n=3). We next determined whether agonist-induced release of esterified HETEs also promotes their oxygenation (Table 2). In response to either $A_{23,187}$, PMA or FMLP, PMN deacylated 15-HETE and converted it to 5,15-DHETE, LXA_4 and LXB_4. In the absence of an agonist, PMN did not generate either 5,15-DHETE or lipoxins (Table 2A). PMN also released and transformed esterified 5-HETE; however, a different profile of products was obtained (Table 2B). With all three stimuli, 5-HETE was converted to both its ω-oxidation product 5,20-DHETE and 5,15-DHETE. In contrast to 15-HETE, none of the stimuli induced the formation of [^{3}H]-lipoxins from esterified 5-[^{3}H]-HETE. Together these results indicate that esterified sources of HETEs can be mobilized and transformed by PMN.

The impact of esterified 15-HETE on agonist-induced aggregation of PMN was examined. Threshold concentrations required to induce aggregation were determined in each case rather than monitoring relative changes in light transmittance since the latter may not represent an accurate value when comparing two distinct groups of cells (i.e. PMN vs. 15-HETE esterified PMN) with potentially different light scattering properties. For PMN exposed to FMLP, threshold concentration required to provoke aggregation was approx. two orders of magnitude higher for cells with esterified 15-HETE (p < 0.05). In contrast, either $A_{23,187}$ or PMA gave statistically significant differences in the threshold concentration

TABLE 2. Agonist-Induced Release and Transformation of Stored 5-HETE and 15-HETE in Human PMN*

A. 15-[^{3}H]-HETE-labeled PMN

Agonist	LXA$_4$	LXB$_4$	5,15-DHETE	15-HETE
A-23,187 (5 µM)	62	32	752	72
PMA (100 nM)	10	20	175	645
FMLP (100 nM)	15	15	45	1300
Vehicle	0	0	0	30

B. 5-[^{3}H]-HETE-labeled PMN

Agonist	LXA$_4$	5,20-DHETE	5,15-DHETE	5-HETE
A-23,187 (5 µM)	0	1225	172	1113
PMA (100 nM)	0	885	45	800
FMLP (100 nM)	0	2150	110	2220
Vehicle	0	107	0	247

*PMN (3 x 10^7 cells/ml) were labeled with either A) 15-[^{3}H]HETE and 15-HETE (30 µM) or B) 5-[^{3}H]HETE and 5-HETE (30 µM) for 20 min at 37°C. After washing in PBS to eliminate unesterified materials, cells were exposed to agonists or vehicle alone (0.4% EtOH, vol/vol) and incubated for 20 min at 37°C. Products were extracted and analyzed by RP-HPLC equipped with a photodiode array detector. Values represent the average cpm associated with PMN-derived products obtained for two representative experiments. Products were identified by both coelution with synthetic standards and characteristic UV spectra.

required to induce aggregation. Also, when PMN were incubated with either AA (30 μM) or 5-HETE (30 μM) followed by washing, the concentrations of these stimuli required to induce aggregation were not significantly altered (2).

CONCLUSIONS

The formation of lipoxins by FMLP-stimulated, 15-HETE-labeled PMN demonstrates receptor-mediated generation of these bioactive eicosanoids from stores within a single cell type. Recently, another receptor-mediated mechanism of lipoxin biosynthesis has been demonstrated during PMN-platelet interactions with FMLP and thrombin-stimulated cells (8). Since LXA_4 is reported to (i) inhibit PMN responses to LTB_4 and FMLP (6), (ii) inhibit LTB_4-induced inflammation in the hamster cheek pouch (5) and antagonize both the cellular and in vivo actions of LTD_4 in glomerular hemodynamics of rats (1), the acylation of one of its precursors (15-HETE) and agonist-induced formation described here may represent a scenario that can contribute to the production of lipoxins during complex tissue level events. This form of "priming" and/or remodeling of cell membranes to give altered profiles of eicosanoids following a second challenge of phagocytic cells may be relevant in inflammation.

In addition, the finding that PMN with esterified 15-HETE in PI show an impaired ability to generate LTB_4, and required FMLP in concentrations ≈ 2 orders above those for control PMN to aggregate (2), suggests that these events may be causally related to some of the anti-inflammatory actions observed with in vivo injections of 15-HETE (3,4). Moreover, our finding that esterified stores of HETE can be deacylated upon cell activation and are transformed suggests that cells can be primed by lipid remodeling to express new profiles of eicosanoids, the balance of which may regulate the actions of pro-inflammatory mediators.

Acknowledgments. The authors thank Kelly-Ann Sheppard for technical assistance and Mary Halm Small for skillful preparation of the manuscript. This work was supported in part by National Institutes of Health grants #AI26714 and GM38765. C.N.S. is a Pew Scholar in the Biomedical Sciences.

REFERENCES

1. Badr, K.F., DeBoer, D.K., Schwartzberg, M., and Serhan, C.N. (1989): Proc. Natl. Acad. Sci. USA **86**: 3438-3442.
2. Brezinski, M.E., and Serhan, C.N. (1990): (submitted).
3. Fogh, K., Søgaard, H., Herlin, T., and Kragballe, K. (1988): J. Am. Acad. Dermatol. **18**: 279-285.
4. Fogh, K., Hansen, E.S., Herlin, T., Knudsen, V., Henriksen, T.B., Ewald, H., Bünger, C., and Kragballe, K. (1989): Prostaglandins **37**: 213-228.
5. Hedqvist, P., Raud, J., Palmertz, U., Haeggström, J., Nicolaou, K.C., and Dahlén, S.-E. (1989): Acta Physiol. Scand. **137**: 571-574.
6. Lee, T.H., Horton, C.E., Kyan-Aung, U., Haskard, D., Crea, A.E.G., and Spur, B.W. (1989): Clin. Sci. **77**: 195-203.
7. Serhan, C.N. (1989): Biochim. Biophys. Acta **1004**: 158-168.
8. Serhan, C.N., and Sheppard, K.-A. (1990): J. Clin. Invest. **85**: 772-780.
9. Setty, B.N.Y., and Stuart, M.J. (1986): J. Clin. Invest. **77**: 202-211.
10. Spector, A.A., Gordon, J.A., and Moore, S.A. (1988): Prog. Lipid Res. **27**:271.
11. Stenson, W.F., and Parker, C.W. (1979): J. Clin. Invest. **64**: 1457-1465.
12. Vanderhoek, J.Y., Bryant, R.W., and Bailey, J.M. (1980): J. Biol. Chem. **255**: 10064-10065.
13. Van Dongen, C.J., Zwiers, H., and Gispen, W.H. (1985): Anal. Biochem. **144**: 104-109.

INHIBITION OF 5-LIPOXYGENASE: DEVELOPMENT OF HYDROXAMIC ACIDS AND HYDROXYUREAS AS POTENTIAL THERAPEUTIC AGENTS.

JOHN A. SALMON, WILLIAM P. JACKSON AND LAWRENCE G. GARLAND.

Wellcome Research Laboratories
Langley Court
Beckenham
Kent BR3 3BS
U.K.

INTRODUCTION

Leukotrienes (LTs) are implicated as mediators of several pathophysiological events; in particular they may signal the cell influx at sites of inflammation and cause bronchoconstriction in asthma. Therefore, compounds which inhibit the formation of LTs or antagonise their effects may have therapeutic potential. Previously we have described (1,2) the synthesis and activity of a series of acetohydroxamic acids which were potent and relatively selective inhibitors of the 5-lipoxygenase (5-LO) and consequently reduced the formation of all LTs. Although several of the compounds inhibited 5-LO ex vivo after oral administration they had relatively short half-lives (1-2h; eg. BW A4C). In this paper we shall describe the strategy that we adopted for developing 5-lipoxygenase (5-LO) inhibitors with longer half-lives and high oral bioavailability.

Evaluation of Inhibitors of 5-LO

Compounds were evaluated initially for their inhibitory potency against 5-LO in vitro. As described previously (2,3) we chose initially to monitor the inhibition of the synthesis of LTB_4 from exogenous arachidonic acid by human PMN.
Potent inhibitors of 5-LO in vitro were examined for their ability to reduce A23187-stimulated synthesis of LTB_4 in whole blood ex vivo. Also the concentration of unchanged compound in the plasma was determined by HPLC in the same experiments and therefore possible active metabolites would be detected. These experiments provided information on the oral bioavailability and half-life of the compounds.

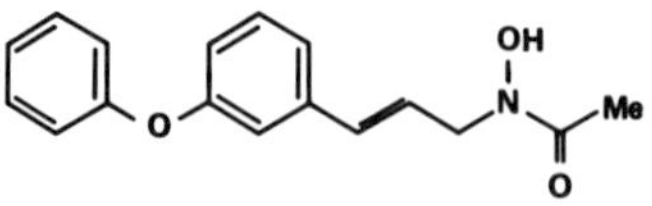

FIG. 1. Structures of 5-LO inhibitors

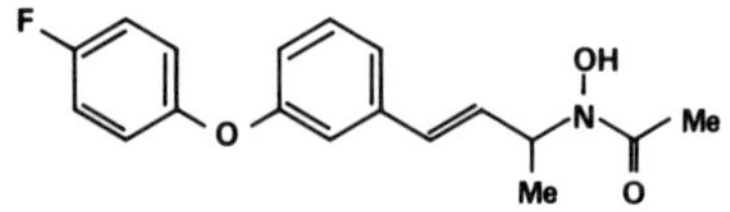

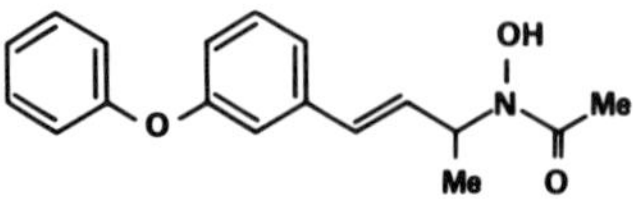

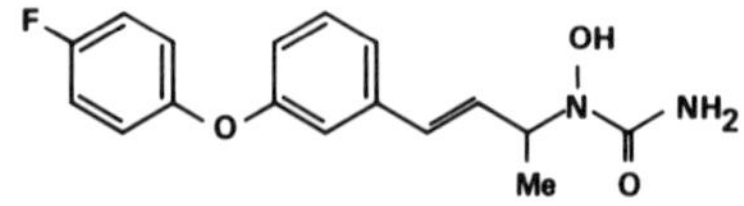

Pharmacokinetics of Acetohydroxamic acids

The major routes of metabolism of the acetohydroxamic acid BW A4C (Fig 1) have been elucidated. Three major transformations occurred (i) oxidation of the methylene adjacent to the hydroxamic acid moiety leading to the formation of the corresponding carboxylic acid (ii) glucuronidation of the N-hydroxy (iii) reduction of the N-hydroxy to form the acetamide analogue (3). None of the metabolites were inhibitors of 5-LO.

Oxidation of the methylene adjacent to the hydroxamate moiety suggested that substitution at this position may improve metabolic stability. Indeed, higher and longer lasting plasma concentrations of unchanged compound were observed after administration of the α-methyl analogue (BW B218C) than after BW A4C (see 3). The α-methyl analogue of 5-LO was a more effective inhibitor of 5-LO ex vivo and this activity was maintained for longer because of the higher plasma concentrations. No carboxylic acid metabolite was detected after administration of the α-methyl acetohydroxamic acid.

Further increases in the half-lives of acetohydroxamic acids were achieved by substitution in the 3-phenoxy group. The pharmacokinetic profile of the 4-fluorophenoxy compound (BW A360C) was one of the most suitable for a therapeutic agent.

The α-methyl analogues were studied initially as racemic mixtures but because of the potential for stereoselective metabolism the chirality of the metabolites was investigated. Unchanged compound was extracted from plasma of animals dosed (p.o) with BW B218C; purification was performed by reverse phase (RP)-HPLC and then recovered material was subjected to chiral HPLC. Also, the glucuronide of BW B218C was extracted from plasma and purified by RP-HPLC;

incubation with β-glucuronidase liberated the aglycone which was then subjected to chiral HPLC. In rats, rabbits and dogs more than 90% of the unchanged compound recovered from plasma chromatographed as the S-enantiomer but the majority of the aglycone derived from the glucuronide chromatographed as the R-enantiomer (Salmon et al; to be published). Therefore, the glucuronidation of BW B218C and similar α-methyl acetohydroxamic acids is stereoselective. The 5-LO inhibitory potency of pairs of enantiomers was identical.

Pharmacokinetics of Hydroxyureas

Hydroxyureas exhibited similar potency against 5-LO in vitro as their acetohydroxamic analogues. However, it was feasible that the two classes of compounds could be metabolised differently and therefore that they exhibit different potencies and durations of activity in vivo. It was assumed that oxidation on the carbon α to the hydroxyurea would occur as was the case with the acetohydroxamic acids (see above) and therefore all compounds evaluated contained an α-methyl substitution to block this metabolite step. Most experimental work was conducted with BW B70C which is the 4-fluorophenoxy compound, since its acetohydroxamic acid

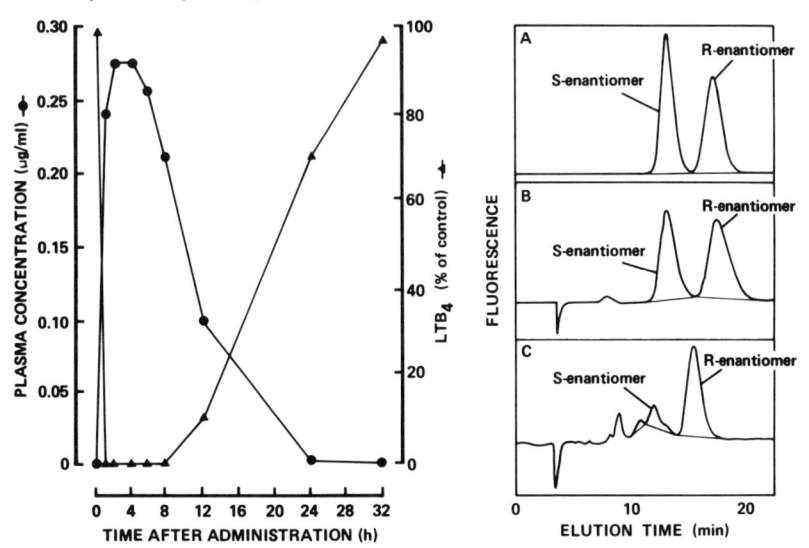

FIG. 2. Left Panel: Mean plasma concentration of unchanged compound and inhibition of LTB_4 synthesis in A23187-stimulated blood ex vivo after oral administration of 2mg/kg BW B70C to rabbits (n=3).
Right Panel: Chiral HPLC of standard racemic BW B70C (A), unchanged compound recovered from plasma 2h after oral administration to a rat (B) and to a dog (C).

counterpart (BW A360C) was one of the most effective and long lasting compounds in vivo.

Studies in animals revealed that BW B70C had a long biological half-life and high oral bioavailability; for example, synthesis of LTB_4 in A23187-stimulated blood ex vivo was inhibited completely for more than 8h after oral administration of 2mg/kg to rabbits (Fig 2). BW B70C was, relative to the acetohydroxamic acids, a poor substrate for glucuronidation. However, stereoselective metabolism of BW B70C was detected; interestingly the S-enantiomer had a higher clearance than the R-enantiomer in all these species (cf acetohydroxamic acids) but it was more marked in dogs than in rats and rabbits. The evidence for the stereoselective metabolism was obtained by comparing the duration of activity after administration of the separate enantiomers and also by chiral analysis of the unchanged drug in plasma after administration of the racemate (Fig.2).

CONCLUSIONS

Investigation of the metabolic transformation of acetohydroxamic acids and hydroxyureas has enabled the identification of potent inhibitors of 5-LO which have high oral bioavailabilies and relatively long biological half-lives. For example, (R)-BW B70C has an oral bioavailability in excess of 60% and a half-life of more than 6h in dogs. Therefore, these compounds should provide experimental tools for the investigation of the pathophysiological roles of 5-LO metabolites. It is also possible that they may offer novel therapy for the treatment of asthma, ulcerative colitis and other inflammatory conditions.

REFERENCES

1. Jackson, W.P., Islip, P.J., Kneen, G., Pugh, A. and Wates, P.J., J. Med. Chem. (1988). 31 499-500.

2. Tateson, J.E., Randall, R.W., Reynolds, C.H., Jackson, W.P., Bhattacherjee, P., Salmon, J.A. and Garland, L.G. (1988): Br. J. Pharmacol., 94, 528-539.

3. Salmon, J.A., Jackson, W.P. and Garland, L.G. (1989). In: Therapeutic Approaches to Inflammatory Disease, edited by A.J. Lewis, N.S. Doherty and N.R. Ackerman. pp. 137-146 Elseview Science, Amsterdam.

INHIBITION OF LEUKOTRIENE C₄ OUTPUT FROM RAT ISOLATED HEART AND LUNG BY THE SULPHASALAZINE DERIVATIVE Ph CL28A

Y.S. Bakhle, *M. Nakamura and J.J. Pankhania

Dept. of Pharmacology, Royal College of Surgeons,
Lincoln's Inn Fields, London WC2A 3PN, U.K
and
* Dept. of Anesthesiology, Kinki University School of Medicine,
377 – 2 Ohno – Higashi, Osakasayama, Osaka, Japan.

The azobenzene compound Ph CL28A (2 – hydroxy – 5 – [[3,5 – bis – (methoxycarbonyl) phenyl] azo] – benzene acetic acid) is a potent inhibitor of prostaglandin 15 – hydroxydehydrogenase (PGDH), the major enzyme in PG inactivation (4). Recently Ph CL28A has been ascribed important actions on eicosanoid biosynthesis. Thus, PGI_2 output from rat isolated lungs, stimulated with the calcium ionophore A23187, was increased four – fold during infusions of this compound (2). Furthermore, Ph CL28A inhibited peptido – leukotriene (LT) synthesis by rat tissues in vitro (3). Synthesis of LTs can be decreased by PGs (5,6,8) and one mechanism by which LT synthesis might be affected by Ph CL28A is via an increase in the amounts of PGs synthesized at the same time. We have examined the interactions between PGI_2 and LT synthesis in the presence of Ph CL28A, using rat isolated hearts and lungs. These tissues were chosen because peptido – LTs are potent coronary vasoconstrictors and bronchoconstrictors. Decreased synthesis of these LTs in either tissue would be a therapeutically useful effect.

MATERIALS AND METHODS

Preparation of isolated tissues

Lungs were isolated from male Wistar rats (200 – 250 g). Ph CL28A was given by i.p. injection (30 mg/kg body weight of a solution freshly made in 0.5% (w/v) Na_2CO_3). 60 min later, rats were anaesthetized, the lungs removed and perfused via the pulmonary artery with Krebs solution (gassed with 95% O_2; 5% CO_2 and warmed to 37°) at 8 ml/min (1). After a 10 min period of perfusion the assays were started. The hearts were isolated from male Wistar rats (250–300 g) as described by Yaacob & Piper (10) and perfused via the aorta with warmed and gassed Krebs solution, at a constant flow of 8 ml/min, with a coronary perfusion pressure (CPP) of 40 mmHg. Cardiac developed tension (CDT) was also measured. Hearts were allowed to beat spontaneously and perfused for at least 40 min before the assays were started. Hearts were treated with Ph CL28A by perfusing with Krebs solution containing the drug (0.3 µM) for at least 20 min before, and during, injection of ionophore.

Radioimmunoassay (RIA) of eicosanoids

Calcium ionophore A23187 (3µg) was injected into the perfusate entering the heart or lung and effluent collected for 5 min immediately following the injection. Eicosanoids in the effluent were extracted by adsorption on, and subsequent elution from, Sep–Pak C_{18}. Recoveries of $6-oxo-PGF_{1\alpha}$ and LTC_4 were at least 80%. The RIA procedures have been described previously (7,9). Cross–reactivities of the anti–sera were as follows: anti–$6-oxo-PGF_{1\alpha}$, PGE_2 = 4.8%, $PGF_{2\alpha}$ = 5.4%, 15–oxo derivatives of these PGs, 0.5%: anti–LTC_4, LTB_4 = 0.05%, LTD_4 = 29.4%, LTE_4 = 0.7%. Because there was significant cross–reaction between LTC_4 and LTD_4, we have referred to the LTs assayed here as "immunoreactive LTC_4" (ir–LTC_4). The lower limits of the RIA were for $6-oxo-PGF_{1\alpha}$, 0.2 ng/ml and LTC_4, 2.5 ng/ml.

5, 8, 9, 11, 12, 14, 15 (n)–$^3H-6-oxo-PGF_{1\alpha}$, (100 Ci/nmol) and 14, 15 (n)–$^3H-LTC_4$ (36 Ci/mmol) were obtained from New England Nuclear, Boston, Mass. U.S.A. The antiserum to $6-oxo-PGF_{1\alpha}$ was kindly donated by Dr. J.A. Salmon (Wellcome Foundation, U.K.) and that to LTC_4 was prepared in this laboratory. We thank Dr. W. Dawson (Lilly Research Centre, U.K.) for calcium ionophore A23187, Merck Sharp and Dohme (U.K.). for indomethacin and particularly Mr. H. Agback (Pharmacia, Sweden) for Ph CL28A.

RESULTS

Eicosanoid output from rat isolated lungs

Output of $6-oxo-PGF_{1\alpha}$ induced by ionophore was increased five–fold by treatment with Ph CL28A in vivo and at the same time, output of ir–LTC_4 was reduced to about 30% of that in lungs from untreated rats. In further experiments, isolated lungs were continuously perfused with Krebs solution containing indomethacin (5µg/ml). In these lungs, $6-oxo-PGF_{1\alpha}$ output, induced by ionophore, was negligible either with or without treatment with Ph CL28A. However, there was no change in ir–LTC_4 output in untreated lungs and, after Ph CL28A, this output was still inhibited to about 30% of the untreated value.

Cardiac responses and eicosanoid output in rat isolated hearts

In response to the ionophore there was a rapid increase in CPP (mean maximal increase, 13.8±3.4 mmHg; n=5). Although CPP returned to near normal levels in about 10-15 min after ionophore, an irreversible increase in CPP followed later. The initial vaso-constriction was accompanied by an equally brief increase in CDT (mean maximal effect, 0.5±0.1 g tension). Relatively more $6-oxo-PGF_{1\alpha}$ was released by ionophore from heart than from lung, the ratio of $6-oxo-PGF_{1\alpha}$: ir-LTC_4 being about 12:1 (see Table 1).

Treatment with Ph CL28A abolished the late CPP increase but not the early rise in CPP, nor the small change in CDT. Although the mean value of $6-oxo-PGF_{1\alpha}$ output was lower during Ph CL28A infusion, this effect was not statistically significant. However, the output of ir-LTC_4 was decreased by Ph CL28A (Table 1).

TABLE 1. Effects of treatment with Ph CL28A on eicosanoid release induced by calcium ionophore from rat isolated tissues.

	Eicosanoid released (ng)			
	$6-oxo-PGF_{1\alpha}$		ir-LTC_4	
	Untreated	Ph CL28A	Untreated	Ph CL28A
a. Lungs Control	10.7±1.9	53.0±10.1*	7.9±1.3	2.9±0.5*
Indomethacin (5 µg/ml)	ND	0.9±0.9	9.4±1.6	3.2±0.9*
b. Hearts	73.6±12.3	51.9±3.9	5.7±0.6	4.0±0.4*

* significantly different from untreated value; $p > 0.05$. ND = not detectable. Mean values (±s.e.mean) of the total released in the 5 min collection from 4-9 lungs in each condition are shown.

DISCUSSION

Our experiments have shown inhibition of ir-LTC_4 output in two tissues where LTs have important biological effects. In lung, the peptido-LTs are potent bronchoconstrictors and LTB_4 is important in oedema formation in airways mucosa. Although we did not assay LTB_4 specifically in this work, inhibition of 5-lipoxygenase would decrease production of all LTs. It is particularly significant that LTC_4 synthesis in lung was inhibited after in vivo treatment, amplifying results obtained in vitro with rat mast cells and gastric mucosa by Berry et al. (3), where PG levels were not measured nor was indomethacin present. So the lower LT synthesis could be due to increased PG output (5,6,8). This possibility was reinforced in our work by the marked increase in $6-oxo-PGF_{1\alpha}$ output from lung after in vivo treatment with Ph CL28A. However, our results with indomethacin showing a marked inhibition of LTC_4 output in the absence of any $6-oxo-PGF_{1\alpha}$ (PGI_2) synthesis clearly refutes this hypothesis for lung.

The results from rat heart showing, for the first time, inhibition of LTC_4 production in this tissue by Ph CL28A, also did not support a causal link between increased PGI_2 synthesis and decreased LT output. Here there was no increase in $6-oxo-PGF_{1\alpha}$ but a trend towards to *inhibition* of $6-oxo-PGF_{1\alpha}$ output, but $ir-LTC_4$ synthesis was still clearly decreased. Thus in two different tissues and with two different modes of administration of Ph CL28A, the inhibition of LTC_4 output was independent of the output of $6-oxo-PGF_{1\alpha}$, arguing strongly for a direct inhibition of LT biosynthesis, probably at the level of 5-lipoxygenase, as the major mode of action of Ph CL28A on LT output.

Our work also shows that the effects of Ph CL28A on PGI_2 synthesis will vary between different tissues. PGI_2 output in the coronary circulation may be potentiated at a higher concentrations of Ph CL28A than that effective in lung (0.3 μM). Nevertheless, further studies of the inhibition of LT synthesis by Ph CL28A in different model systems are clearly justified.

1. Bakhle, Y.S. (1979): *Br. J. Pharmacol.*, 65: 635–639.
2. Bakhle, Y.S. and Pankhania, J.J. (1987): *Br. J. Pharmacol.*, 92: 189–196.
3. Berry, C.N., Chastagnol–Hermann, D.C. and Lloyd, K.G. (1988): *Br. J. Pharmacol.*, 93: 141P.
4. Berry, C.N., Hoult, J.R.S., Phillips, J.A., McCarthy, T.M. and Agback, H. (1985): *J. Pharm. Pharmacol.*, 37: 622–628.
5. DiMarzo, V., Tippins, J.R. and Morris, H.R. (1987): *Biochem. biophys. Res. Commun.*, 147: 1213–1218.
6. Elliott, G.R., Lauwen, A.P.M. and Bonta, I.L. (1989): *Br. J. Pharmacol.*, 96: 265–270.
7. Hayes, E.C., Lombardo, D.L., Girard, Y., Maycock, A.L., Rokach, J., Rosenthal, A.S., Young, R.N., Egan, R.W. and Zweerink, H.J. (1983): *J. Immunol.*, 131: 429–433.
8. Karmazyn, M. (1987): *J. Mol. Cell. Cardiol.*, 19: 221–230.
9. Watts, I.A., Zakrzewski, J.T. and Bakhle, Y.S. (1982): *Thromb. Res.*, 28: 333–342.
10. Yaacob, H.B. and Piper, P.J. (1988): *Br. J. Pharmacol.*, 95: 1322–1328.

TRANSFORMATIONS OF α-LINOLENIC ACID IN LEAVES OF CORN (ZEA MAYS L.)

Mats Hamberg

Department of Physiological Chemistry, Karolinska Institutet, Box 60400, S-104 01 Stockholm, Sweden

ABSTRACT

Short incubation of [1-^{14}C]α-linolenic acid with whole homogenate of leaves of corn (Zea mays L.) led to the formation of 4 major lipoxygenase products, i.e. 12-oxo-13-hydroxy-9(Z),15(Z)-octadecadienoic acid, 12-oxo-10,15(Z)-phytodienoic acid (12-oxo-PDA), 9(R,S)-hydroxy-12-oxo-10(E),15(Z)-octadecadienoic acid, and 13-oxo-9,11-tridecadienoic acid. Trapping experiments demonstrated transient appearance of the unstable allene oxide, 12,13(S)-epoxy-9(Z),11,15(Z)-octadecatrienoic acid, precursor of the three first mentioned compounds. The major lipoxygenase products formed from endogenous α-linolenic acid upon homogenization of corn leaves were identified as 12-oxo-13-hydroxy-9(Z),15(Z)-octadecadienoic acid (11.4 ± 2.4 µg/g) and 12-oxo-PDA (5.8 ± 1.2 µg/g). Steric analysis showed that 12-oxo-PDA formed from endogenous α-linolenic acid was largely the natural 9(S),13(S) enantiomer. Thus, corn leaves, like seeds of corn, contain hydroperoxide dehydrase and allene oxide cyclase. However, the lipoxygenase of corn leaves specifically catalyzed oxygenation of the 13 (ω6) position of α-linolenic acid and thus differed from the previously recognized corn seed lipoxygenase which is specific for the 9 position.

INTRODUCTION

12-Oxo-10,15(Z)-phytodienoic acid (12-oxo-PDA) is a C_{18} cyclopentenone which is formed from α-linolenic acid via 13(S)-hydroperoxy-9(Z),11(E),15(Z)-octadecatrienoic acid (13(S)-HPOT) in many plants (9). Further conversion of 12-

oxo-PDA by reduction of the double bond of the five-membered ring followed by three steps of β-oxidation results in the formation of 7-iso-jasmonic acid, a C_{12} cyclopentanone with growth-regulating and senescence-promoting effects (9). The mode of formation of 12-oxo-PDA from 13(S)-HPOT has been clarified in recent work. The initial reaction is catalyzed by hydroperoxide dehydrase (4) and results in the formation of the unstable allene oxide 12,13(S)-epoxy-9(Z),11,15(Z)-octadecatrienoic acid (12,13(S)-EOT). Subsequent cyclization of the allene oxide in the presence of allene oxide cyclase (5) yields 9(S),13(S)-12-oxo-PDA, i.e. the natural stereoisomer in which the configurations of the two asymmetric carbon atoms are the same as those of the corresponding carbons of 7-iso-jasmonic acid. In the absence of allene oxide cyclase the allene oxide undergoes spontaneous chemical cyclization to produce racemic 12-oxo-PDA in 10-20% yield (1,5).

Seeds of corn (Zea mays L.) contain hydroperoxide dehydrase, allene oxide cyclase, and lipoxygenase. It is well documented that, at a physiological pH, the lipoxygenase of corn seeds catalyzes oxygenation of carbon 9 of linoleic and α-linolenic acids to produce 9(S)-HPOD and 9(S)-HPOT, respectively (2,3). Thus, in corn seed the specificity this lipoxygenase will preclude biosynthesis of 12-oxo-PDA and 7-iso-jasmonic acid from α-linolenic acid. The present paper is concerned with transformations of α-linolenic acid in leaves of young plants of corn and with the presence in corn leaves of a major lipoxygenase activity which catalyzes oxygenation of α-linolenic acid specifically into 13(S)-HPOT.

EXPERIMENTAL

Chemicals
[1-^{14}C]α-Linolenic acid obtained from Amersham, U.K., was diluted with unlabeled material (specific radioactivity, 1.8 kBq/μmol unless otherwise indicated). 13(S)-[1-^{14}C]HPOT (specific radioactivity, 16.2 kBq/μmol) was prepared by incubation of [1-^{14}C]α-linolenic acid with soybean lipoxygenase, whereas 9(S)-[1-^{14}C]HPOT (specific radioactivity, 3.9 kBq/μmol) was obtained by incubating [1-^{14}C]α-linolenic acid with tomato lipoxygenase. The chemical and radiochemical purity of the specimens was in excess of 96% as judged by radio-TLC.

[1-^{14}C]14-Oxo-15-hydroxy-5(Z),8(Z),11(Z)-eicosatrienoic acid was prepared by incubation of 15(S)-[1-^{14}C]HPETE (3.1 μmol) with a suspension of the 105,000g particle fraction (7 mg of protein) of corn seed homogenate in 60 ml of 0.1 M potassium phosphate buffer pH 6.7 (5). The pure compound (specific activity, 2.5 kBq/μmol) was obtained following purification by silicic acid chromatography and reversed phase HPLC.

The methyl esters of the following reference compounds were prepared as indicated. 9(S)-HOT and 13(S)-HOT: reduction of the corresponding hydroperoxides with $SnCl_2$ (3); 12-oxo-13-hydroxy-9(Z),15(Z)-octadecadienoic acid and 9(R,S)-hydroxy-12-oxo-10,15-octadecadienoic acid: incubation of 13(S)-HPOT with corn hydroperoxide dehydrase (4,5); 9-hydroxy-10-oxo-12(Z),15(Z)-octadecadienoic acid and 10-oxo-13-hydroxy-11,15-octadecadienoic acid: incubation of 9(S)-HPOT with corn hydroperoxide dehydrase (4,5); 12-oxo-13-methoxy-9(Z),15(Z)-octadecadienoic acid: generation of 12,13(S)-EOT from 13(S)-HPOT followed by trapping by addition of methanol (4); 9(S),13(S)-12-oxo-PDA: incubation of 13(S)-HPOT with hydroperoxide dehydrase and allene oxide cyclase from corn (5). Racemic 12-oxo-PDA was prepared by an incubation carried out in the absence of allene oxide cyclase.

$^{18}O_2$ (98.1 atom%) was purchased from Amersham, U.K.

Incubations and Treatments

Corn kernels (Bear X8632, Noble Bear Hybrid Corn, Inc., Decatur, IL) were germinated in soil. Leaves were collected from plants 14-16 days after seeding. Segments (0.5 g) were minced in 0.1 M potassium phosphate buffer pH 6.7 (5 ml, 5°C) containing either of [1-^{14}C]α-linolenic acid (210 µM), 13(S)-[1-^{14}C]HPOT (34 µM), or 9(S)-[1-^{14}C]HPOT (34 µM). The leaf tissue was homogenized at 5°C for 1 min with a Polytron. One half of the homogenate was immediately added to 10 ml of methanol whereas the other half was stirred at 22° for 10 min prior to addition of methanol. The mixtures were centrifuged at 750g for 10 min and the supernatant diluted with water, acidified and extracted with two portions of diethyl ether. The residue obtained after evaporation of the solvent (recovery of added radioactivity, 90-95%) was treated with diazomethane for 10 s and analyzed by radio-TLC.

RESULTS AND DISCUSSION

Lipoxygenase Products formed from [1-^{14}C]α-Linolenic Acid

Homogenization of corn leaves at 5°C for 1 min in the presence of 210 µM [1-^{14}C]α-linolenic acid led to the formation of 4 major labeled products as shown by radio-TLC (Fig. 1). Incubation of the homogenate at 22°C for 10 min did neither result in an increased conversion of the labeled substrate, nor in a significant change of the product composition. Because substrate was not depleted it appeared that the lipoxygenase responsible for the initial reaction was rapidly inactivated.

Compound A (Fig. 1) migrated like authentic methyl 9(R,S)-hydroxy-12-oxo-10,15-octadecadienoate (R_f 0.18). The Me_3Si derivatives of Compound A and of methyl 9(R,S)-hydroxy-12-oxo-10,15-octadecadienoate gave an identical C-

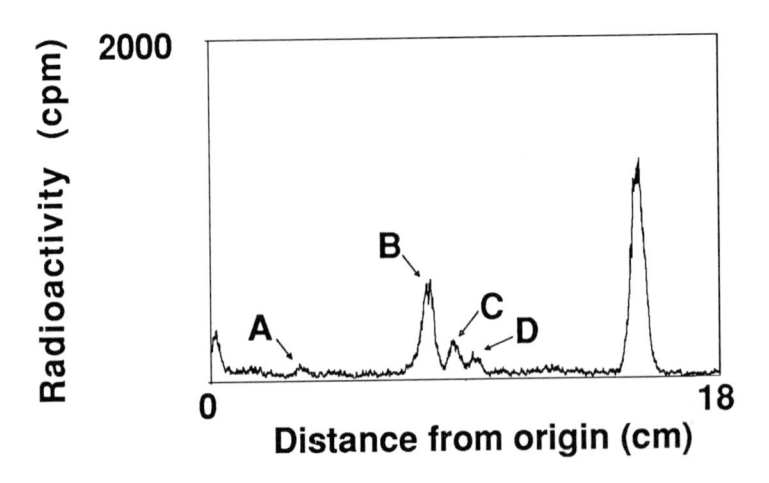

FIG. 1. Thin layer radiochromatogram of esterified product obtained following homogenization of 0.5 g of corn leaves in 5 ml of buffer containing 210 µM [1-^{14}C]α-linolenic acid. Solvent system, ethyl acetate/toluene (15/85, v/v).

value (21.56) and identical mass spectra. Further identification of Compound A as the methyl ester of the γ-ketol 9(R,S)-hydroxy-12-oxo-10,15-octadecadienoic acid was based on results of sodium borohydride reduction, and oxidative ozonolysis (5). The geometric configurations of the double bonds were not determined but were likely to be 10(E),15(Z).

Compound B (Fig. 1; R_f 0.43) was identified as the methyl ester of the α-ketol 12-oxo-13-hydroxy-9(Z),15(Z)-octadecadienoic acid by comparison with the authentic compound by GLC (C-value of Me$_3$Si derivative, 20.98) and mass spectrometry (prominent ions at m/e 381 (M-15), 327 (M-69), 299, 298 (M-98; rearrangement with loss of OHC-CH$_2$-CH=CH-C$_2$H$_5$), 270 (M-126; rearrangement with loss of ·CO-CH(O·)-CH$_2^5$-CH=CH-C$_2$H$_5$ or its equivalent), 171 (Me$_3$SiO$^+$=CH-CH$_2$-CH=CH^{2}C$_2$H$_5$), 129, 103, and 73. Treatment of Compound B with sodium borohydride yielded methyl 12,13-dihydroxy-9,15-octadecadienoate, and oxidative ozonolysis resulted in the formation of methyl hydrogen azelate (cf. ref. 4).

Compound C (Fig. 1; R_f 0.48) was identified as the methyl ester of 12-oxo-PDA by comparison with authentic material by GLC (C-value, 20.17; plus a minor peak at C-19.75 due to the trans isomer formed by thermal isomerization), and mass spectrometry. Treatment of Compound C with 0.1 M sodium hydroxide resulted in isomerization into the side chain trans isomer (6), and subsequent treatment with sodium borohydride gave two methyl 12-hydroxy-15(Z)-

phytoenoates epimeric at C-12 (side chain trans isomers)(6).
Compound D (Fig. 1; R_f 0.52) appeared with a C-value of 16.02. The mass spectrum showed prominent ions at m/e 238 (M), 206 (M-32; loss of CH_3OH), 178, 109, 95, and 81 (cf. ref. 10). The uv spectrum showed an absorption band with λ_{max} 273 nm (in ethanol). Treatment of Compound D with O-methylhydroxylamine (1 mg) in pyridine (0.1 ml) resulted in the formation of an O-methyloxime derivative, the mass spectrum of which showed ions of high intensity at m/e 267 (M), 236 (M-31), 204 (M-(31+32)), 189, 171, 110 ($[CH=CH-CH=CH-CH=NOCH_3]^+$), and 80. Further support for the presence of an aldehyde group in Compound D was provided by its conversion into methyl 13-hydroxy-9,11-tridecadienoate upon treatment with $NaBH_4$. The C-value of the Me_3Si derivative of this compound was 16.81 and the mass spectrum showed ions of high intensity at m/e 312 (M), 297 (M-15), 265 (M-(15+32), 215, 155 ($[CH=CH-CH=CH-CH_2-OSiMe_3]^+$), and 73. Finally, oxidative ozonolysis performed on Compound D yielded methyl hydrogen azelate. This finding, coupled with the uv data which indicated the presence in Compound D of a carbonyl group in conjugation with two double bonds, localized the double bonds to the Δ^9 and Δ^{11} positions. On the basis of these results Compound D was identified as methyl 13-oxo-9,11-tridecadienoate.

Lipoxygenase Products formed from 13(S)- and 9(S)-HPOT
The products obtained following homogenization of corn leaves in the presence of 13(S)-[1-^{14}C]HPOT (34 µM) were identical to those obtained from α-linolenic acid, i.e 12-oxo-13-hydroxy-9(Z),15(Z)-octadecadienoic acid, 12-oxo-PDA, 9(R,S)-hydroxy-12-oxo-10,15-octadecadienoic acid, and 13-oxo-9,11-tridecadienoic acid. Homogenization of corn leaves in the presence of 9(S)-[1-^{14}C]HPOT (34 µM) led to the formation of 9-hydroxy-10-oxo-12(Z),15(Z)-octadecadienoic acid (major product) as well as a small amount of 10-oxo-13-hydroxy-11,15-octadecadienoic acid. The C-values of the Me_3Si derivatives of the methyl esters of these compounds (20.93 and 21.72, respectively) and the mass spectra recorded on the derivatives were identical to the C-values and mass spectra of the corresponding derivatives of the authentic compounds.

Trapping Experiment
Corn leaves (0.5 g) were homogenized at 0° for 30 sec in 5 ml of buffer containing [1-^{14}C]α-linolenic acid (210 µM). Methanol (100 ml) was added and the mixture kept at room temperature for 1 h. Analysis of the esterified product by radio-TLC showed the presence of a peak of non-polar material which was not seen when addition of methanol was omitted. This material was identified as methyl 12-oxo-13-methoxy-9(Z),15(Z)-octadecadienoate by GC-MS and by its conversion into methyl 12-hydroxy-13-methoxy-9,15-

octadecadienoate upon treatment with sodium borohydride. Formation of 12-oxo-13-methoxy-9(Z),15(Z)-octadecadienoic acid in short time incubations terminated by addition of a large volume of methanol demonstrated that there was a transient appearance of the unstable allene oxide 12,13(S)-EOT (4,5)(Fig. 2).

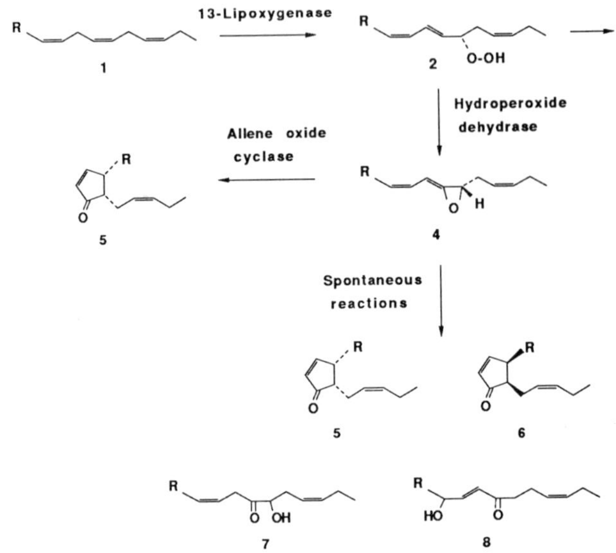

FIG. 2. Transformations of α-linolenic acid in corn leaf homogenate. 1, α-linolenic acid; 2, 13(S)-HPOT; 3, 13-oxo-9,11-tridecadienoic acid; 4, 12,13(S)-EOT; 5 and 6, 9(S),13(S) and 9(R),13(R) enantiomers of 12-oxo-PDA, respectively; 7, α-ketol; 8, γ-ketol. R, $(CH_2)_7$-COOH.

Quantitative Determination of Lipoxygenase Products

Leaves of corn (1 g) were homogenized in 10 ml of buffer at 5° for 1 min in the absence or in the presence of α-linolenic acid (210 μM). Methanol (20 ml) containing 46 nmol of [1-^{14}C]14-Oxo-15-hydroxy-5(Z),8(Z),11(Z)-eicosatrienoic acid was added. Material isolated by extraction with diethyl ether was treated with diazomethane for 10 s and subjected to TLC. A broad zone containing the compounds to be analyzed as well as the internal standard (R_f 0.36-0.63) was scraped off. Material eluted from the silica gel with methyl formate was treated with hexamethyldisilazane and trimethylchlorosilane and analyzed by GLC. The amounts of 12-oxo-PDA and the α-ketol 12-oxo-13-hydroxy-9(Z),15(Z)-octadecadienoic acid were calculated from the peak areas and from the amount of internal standard added (Table 1).

TABLE 1. Amounts of 12-oxo-PDA and α-ketol in corn leaf homogenate. Amounts given are µg per g of leaves, wet weight, in 3 exp.

Condition	Compound analyzed	Amount (µg/g)
α-Linolenic acid not added	12-oxo-PDA	5.8 ± 1.2
α-Linolenic acid not added	α-ketol	11.4 ± 2.4
210 µM α-linolenic acid added	12-oxo-PDA	54.6 ± 5.4
210 µM α-linolenic acid added	α-ketol	201.4 ± 29.2

Steric Analysis of 12-Oxo-PDA

Corn leaves (3 g) were homogenized at 5°C for 1 min in 30 ml of buffer. The methyl ester of 12-oxo-PDA, produced from endogeous α-linolenic acid, was subjected to steric analysis (6) and was found to consist of 86% of the 9($\underline{S}$),13($\underline{S}$) enantiomer and 14% of the 9($\underline{R}$),13($\underline{R}$) enantiomer. Thus, 72% of total 12-oxo-PDA was enzymatically formed. An identical result was obtained by a calculation (5) based on the ratio between the amounts of 12-oxo-PDA and α-ketol produced from endogenous α-linolenic acid (Table 1).

Search for Lipoxygenase Products in Intact Corn Leaves

The results of incubations of [1-^{14}C]α-linolenic acid (Fig. 2) and the finding that homogenization of corn leaves produced 12-oxo-PDA as well as α-ketol from endogenous α-linolenic acid (Table 1) made it of interest to examine whether lipoxygenase products are natural constituents of corn leaves. Accordingly, leaves (1 g) of corn plants were cut off and immediately placed in 10 ml of ice-cold methanol containing 46 nmol of [1-^{14}C]14-Oxo-15-hydroxy-5($\underline{Z}$),8($\underline{Z}$),11($\underline{Z}$)-eicosatrienoic acid. The tissue was minced and homogenized at 0° with a Polytron. Analysis of the esterified diethyl ether extract by GLC showed the presence of 13($\underline{S}$)-HOT (4.8 ± 0.6 µg/g of leaf tissue (wet weight)). Further identification of 13($\underline{S}$)-HOT (methyl ester) was achieved by uv spectrometry (λ_{max} 234 nm), catalytic hydrogenation (yielding methyl 13-hydroxyoctadecanoate), and oxidative ozonolysis of the MC derivative (yielding the MC derivative of $\underline{S}$-malic acid plus methyl hydrogen azelate). Ketols, 12-oxo-PDA, and hydroxy acids other than 13($\underline{S}$)-HOT were not detectable by GLC.

These experiments suggested the presence of 13($\underline{S}$)-HOT in intact leaves of corn. A control experiment was performed in which a trace amount (2 µg; 14 kBq) of [1-^{14}C]α-linolenic acid was added to the methanol solvent prior to homogenization. Conversion of the labeled α-linolenic acid induced by homogenization was less than 0.2 %. Although this experiment tended to support the idea of 13($\underline{S}$)-HOT being a real constituent of intact corn leaves, the result of another control experiment was contradictory. In this experiment 2.3 g of corn leaves were homogenized in 30 ml of methanol at 0°C under an atmosphere of $^{18}O_2$ (diluted with some air, because of technical difficulties in carrying out the homogenization in a sealed vessel). This led to the formation of $^{18}O_2$-labeled 13(S)-HOT, i.e. 33% ^{18}O molecules and 67% unlabeled molecules. Thus, part (or all) of 13(S)-HOT isolated was in fact synthesized upon homogenization of the tissue, in spite of the fact that the medium used was ice-cold methanol. It seems important that such control experiments with $^{18}O_2$ be carried out in similar situations where lipoxygenase products have been proposed to exist as endogenous constituents of tissues (7,8).

CONCLUSION

Leaves of young plants of corn were found to contain a lipoxygenase activity that catalyzed oxygenation of the C-13 (ω6) position of α-linolenic and linoleic acids. This was in contrast to the previously recognized corn seed lipoxygenase, that catalyzes oxygenation of C-9, to produce 9(S)-HPOT and 9(S)-HPOD from α-linolenic and linoleic acids, respectively (2,3). Leaves of corn plants also contained hydroperoxide dehydrase (4) and allene oxide cyclase (5), and thus possessed the enzymatic machinery needed for biosynthesis of 9(S),13(S)-12-oxo-PDA from α-linolenic acid. 13(S)-HOT was identified in methanol extracts of corn leaves. The finding that extraction of leaves carried out under $^{18}O_2$ led to the formation of ^{18}O-labeled 13(S)-HOT showed that part or all of the hydroxy acid was formed during the extraction procedure and indicated that it was not an endogenous constituent of corn leaves.

REFERENCES

1. Brash, A.R., Baertschi, S.W., Ingram, C.D., and Harris, T.M. (1988): Proc. Natl. Acad. Sci. USA, 85:3382-3386.
2. Gardner, H.W., and Weisleder, D. (1970): Lipids, 5:678-683.
3. Hamberg, M. (1971): Anal. Biochem., 43:515-526.
4. Hamberg, M. (1987): Biochim. Biophys. Acta, 920:76-84.
5. Hamberg, M., and Fahlstadius, P. (1990): Arch. Biochem. Biophys., 276:518-526.
6. Hamberg, M., Miersch, O., and Sembdner, G. (1988): Lipids, 23:521-524.
7. Kühn, H., and Brash, A.R. (1990): J. Biol. Chem., 265:1454-1458.
8. Kühn, H., Weisner, R., Alder, L., and Schewe, T. (1989): Eur. J. Biochem., 186:155-162.
9. Vick, B.A., and Zimmerman, D.C. (1987): In: The Biochemistry of Plants, edited by P.K. Stumpf. Vol. 9, pp. 53-90. Academic Press, New York.
10. Vick, B.A., and Zimmerman, D.C. (1989): Plant Physiol., 90:125-132.

Advances in Prostaglandin, Thromboxane, and Leukotriene Research, Vol. 21,
edited by B. Sameulsson et al.
Raven Press, Ltd., New York © 1990.

FORMATION OF UNIQUE BIOLOGICALLY ACTIVE PROSTAGLANDINS IN VIVO BY A NON-CYCLOOXYGENASE FREE RADICAL CATALYZED MECHANISM

Jason D. Morrow, Kristina E. Hill, Raymond F. Burk,
Tarek M. Nammour, Kamal F. Badr, and L. Jackson Roberts, II

Departments of Pharmacology and Medicine,
Vanderbilt University, Nashville, Tennessee 37232-6602

Recently we reported the discovery that a series of unique PGF_2 compounds are readily produced in vitro during storage of plasma at -20°C by a non-cyclooxygenase free radical catalyzed mechanism (4). The mechanism that was proposed to explain the formation of these prostaglandins (4) derives from previous studies which demonstrated that autoxidation of fatty acids in vitro results in the formation of bicyclic endoperoxides (6,7). Arachidonyl radicals are initially formed by abstraction of an allelic hydrogen. Subsequently, attack by molecular oxygen occurs followed by endocyclization and an additional insertion of a molecule of oxygen to yield PGG_2-like bicyclic endoperoxides. The bicyclic endoperoxides were found to be directly reduced by naturally occurring substances in plasma to PGF_2 compounds. This mechanism thus leads to the formation of the 4 PGF_2 regioisomers shown in Figure 1, each of which can theoretically be comprised of 8 racemic diastereomers.

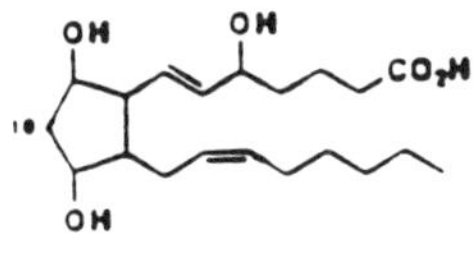

I

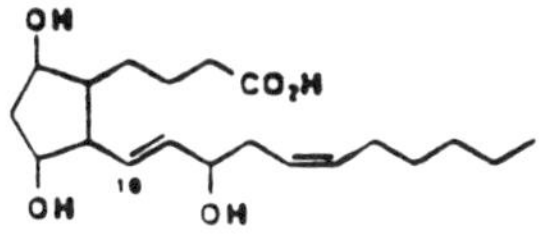

II

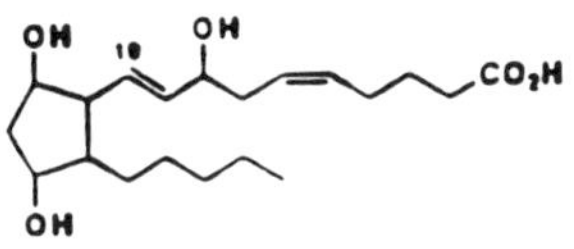

III

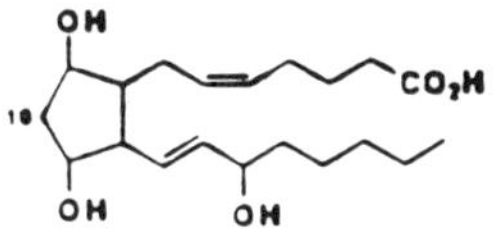

IV

Figure 1

Since the formation of these prostanoids in vitro appeared to be a very facile process, we explored the possibility that they may also be produced in vivo by a similar free radical catalyzed mechanism independent of the cyclooxygenase enzyme.

RESULTS

PGF$_2$ compounds were analyzed by capillary gas chromatography negative ion chemical ionization mass spectrometry (4). Analysis of fresh human plasma revealed a series of peaks presumably representing PGF$_2$ compounds ranging from approximately 5-50 pg/ml. The pattern of these peaks in fresh plasma was very similar to the pattern of peaks that were documented to represent PGF$_2$ compounds generated in vitro in plasma during storage (4). Analysis of fresh human urine was then carried out which again revealed an almost identical series of presumed PGF$_2$ peaks ranging from approximately 500-3000 pg/ml.

The close similarity of the pattern of these peaks in fresh plasma and urine with PGF$_2$ compounds generated in vitro from oxidation of plasma arachidonic acid suggested that these peaks also represented PGF$_2$ compounds. However, several lines of additional supporting evidence were also obtained. First, the presumed PGF$_2$ compounds in fresh plasma and urine were found to co-chromatograph on capillary GC with PGF$_2$ compounds generated in vitro during storage of plasma. Further employing deuterated silyl ether derivatives, the compounds were found to have 3 hydroxyls and catalytic hydrogenation indicated they contained 2 double bonds. Finally, analysis of 1 liter of urine by electron ionization mass spectrometry revealed multiple mass spectra eluting from the capillary GC-column over a 20-25 second period similar to the mass spectra that were obtained of the PGF$_2$ compounds generated in vitro during storage of plasma (4). Interpretation of these mass spectra revealed fragmentation ions consistent with the presence of each of the four PGF$_2$ regioisomers shown in Figure 1, suggesting that they were formed by the same free radical catalyzed mechanism.

The above data provided strong evidence that these compounds detected in fresh plasma and urine are, in fact, PGF$_2$ compounds. We then addressed the question whether these compounds are produced in vivo or whether they arise from ex vivo formation. Several lines of evidence were obtained which argued against the possibility that these compounds are formed ex vivo. First, although the antioxidant BHT markedly inhibits the formation of these compounds in vitro by greater than 90% (4), BHT did not suppress levels detected in fresh plasma and urine. In addition, unlike plasma, incubation of urine for 7 days at 37°C, and storage for 6 months at -20°C, did not increase the levels of these compounds. The possibility that the origin of these compounds may be from dietary lipid intake was then considered. However, the levels measured in urine in 4 volunteers on an ad lib diet were unchanged from the levels measured following 4 days on a diet consisting solely of glucose polymers. Levels measured in each of the above paired groups varied by a mean of 10% or less. Collectively, these results provided strong evidence that these prostaglandins are, in fact, produced in vivo.

We then examined whether the cyclooxygenase enzyme is involved in their formation. For this, 3 normal volunteers were administered high doses of the cyclooxygenase inhibitors, indomethacin (200 mg/day), ibuprofen (4000 mg/day) and naproxen (4000 mg/day). These drugs failed to suppress the levels of these compounds measured in both plasma and urine indicating that their formation occurs independent of cyclooxygenase activity.

To further substantiate that the formation of these compounds in vivo occurs by the proposed mechanism of arachidonate peroxidation, we assessed their production in 2 well defined animal models of free radical catalyzed lipid peroxidation. The first model involves the administration of diquat to selenium-deficient rats. Diquat undergoes redox cycling in vivo producing superoxide anions which lead to marked lipid peroxidation in these animals (2). Following administration of diquat, plasma was obtained 1½ hours later and analyzed for PGF_2 compounds. The levels were found to be dramatically elevated 27-200 fold above levels measured in control rats. The second model employed the administration of CCl_4 to normal rats. CCl_4 is metabolized in vivo by P-450 to $CCl_3\cdot$ radicals which induce lipid peroxidation (3). Circulating levels of these PGF_2 compounds were found also to be markedly elevated in blood drawn 1½ hours after administration of CCl_4 by 10-30 fold above normal and their formation was not inhibited by indomethacin pretreatment.

It was then considered of interest to examine whether these novel F-type prostaglandins may exert biological activity. Others have previously shown that autoxidation of fatty acids in vitro results in the formation of bicyclic endoperoxides in which the side chains are predominantly oriented cis (5). Thus, one of the PGF_2 compounds whose formation would be favored by the proposed mechanism would be 8-epi-$PGF_{2\alpha}$. It is of considerable interest to note that the levels of these compounds in normal human plasma and urine are approximately an order of magnitude higher than levels of cyclooxygenase derived prostaglandins. Because the levels of these compounds in urine are quite high, and may derive in part from local production in the kidney, we examined the effects of 8-epi-$PGF_{2\alpha}$ on renal function. Initially, 8-epi-$PGF_{2\alpha}$ was infused into a systemic vein in 5 rats at a dose of 5 µg/kg/min. This resulted in marked reductions in both glomerular filtration rate and renal blood flow by 40-45% that were unaccompanied by changes in systemic blood pressure. 8-epi-$PGF_{2\alpha}$ was then infused intrarenally. This also caused a marked parallel reduction in glomerular filtration rate and renal plasma flow in a dose dependent fashion over a range of infusion rates of 0.5-2.0 µg/kg/min. At the highest dose, 2 µg/kg/min, glomerular filtration rate and renal blood flow fell to zero, urine flow ceased, and the kidney took on a pale and mottled appearance indicative of severe vasoconstriction. At similar doses, intrarenal infusion of cyclooxygenase derived $PGF_{2\alpha}$ and $9\alpha,11\beta$-PGF_2 have no significant effects on renal blood flow. Interestingly, 8-epi-$PGF_{2\alpha}$ is approximately an order of magnitude more potent than leukotriene D_4, the most potent renal vasoconstricting eicosanoid known (1).

CONCLUSIONS

In summary, although the catalytic activity of the cyclooxygenase has been assumed obligatory for endogenous prostaglandin biosynthesis, these studies have elucidated that a series of novel biologically active prostaglandins are produced in vivo independent of cyclooxygenase activity. The discovery that the formation of these compounds is catalyzed by free radicals and that they can exert potent biological activity provides the background and rationale for a new area for investigation into the possibility that these prostanoids may participate as mediators in the pathophysiology of oxidative stress and injury. It is well recognized that problems exist regarding the specificity and sensitivity of existing methods to assess oxidant stress in vivo (8). Thus, the possibility that quantification of these prostanoids may provide a new non-invasive approach for the assessment of oxidant status in humans merits further investigation. Finally, in view of the fact that prostaglandins can be produced in vivo by a non-cyclooxygenase mechanism, it is important to recognize that limitations at times, may exist, regarding the reliability of the use of cyclooxygenase inhibitors to assess the role of prostaglandins in certain pathophysiological processes.

ACKNOWLEDGMENTS

This work was supported by NIH grant GM 42056.

REFERENCES

1. Badr, K. F., DeBoer, D. K., Schwartzberg, M., and Serhan, C. N. (1989): Proc. Natl. Acad. Sci. U.S.A., 86:3483-3442.
2. Burk, R. F., Lawrence, R. A., and Lane, J. M. (1980): J. Clin. Invest., 65:1024-1031.
3. Burk, R. F., Reiter, R., and Lane, J. M. (1986): Gastroenterology, 90:812-818.
4. Morrow, J. D., Harris, T. M., and Roberts, L. J., II. (1990): Anal. Biochem., 184:1-10.
5. O'connor, D. E., Mihelich, E. D., and Coleman, M. C. (1984): J. Amer. Chem. Soc., 106: 3577-3584.
6. Porter, N.A., and Funk, M.O. (1975): J. Org. Chem., 40:3614-3615.
7. Pryor, W. A., and Stanley, J.P. (1975) J. Org. Chem., 40:3615-3617.
8. Pryor, W. A. (1989): Free Rad. Biol. Med., 3:177-178.

A NOVEL PROSTAGLANDIN METABOLIC PATHWAY FROM A MARINE MOLLUSC: PROSTAGLANDIN-1,15-LACTONES.

Vincenzo Di Marzo, Guido Cimino, Guido Sodano, Aldo Spinella and Guido Villani.

C.N.R.-Istituto per la Chimica di Molecole d'Interesse Biologico, Via Toiano 6, 80072, Arco Felice, (NA), Italy.

Prostaglandins (PG's) and other eicosanoids have been suggested to participate in many aspects of marine and freshwater invertebrate physiology (2). However, only in a few cases, as in the gorgonian coral *Plexaura homomalla* (3), the structures of the prostanoids involved and their biosynthesis have been completely elucidated (2). We have recently isolated novel PG-derivatives, PG-1,15-lactones, of the E (PGEL's) and A series, in both the mantle and the dorso-lateral appendices (cerata) of the opisthobranch mollusc *Tethys fimbria* (1). The occurrence, in the same species, of PG-1,15-lactones of the F series (PGFL's) as well as preliminary data about the tissue distribution, biosynthesis and metabolism of PG-1,15-lactones will be briefly described herein.

MATERIALS AND METHODS

The molluscs were caught in the bay of Naples. Mantle and cerata were separately homogenated with 5% CH_3COOH+ 15 μM indomethacine. Supernatants from a 10000 rpm centrifugation of the homogenates were pre-purified by means of Sep-pak C-18 cartridges eluted with CH_3OH, and the eluates submitted to RP-HPLC (Spherisorb ODS-2 C-18 column; 90 min gradient from 30 to 70% CH_3CN/0.1% CF_3COOH in H_2O/0.1% CF_3COOH, flow rate=1 ml/min, UV absorbance monitored at 205 nm). This method allowed the purification and quantitation (detection limit =1 μg) of both PG's and PG-lactones. PGFL-fatty acyl esters were isolated by means of acetone extraction, diethyl ether extraction and SiO_2 t.l.c developed with C_6H_6/diethyl ether 8/2.

Structure characterization was achieved mainly by means of proton nuclear magnetic resonance (N.M.R.) for PGFL's and of proton N.M.R., electron impact mass spectrometry (EIMS) and gas chromatography (GC) following methanolysis for PGFL-fatty acyl esters.

In vivo conversion experiments were conducted by injecting 5 μCi [3-H]-PGE2 or -PGF2α (200 Ci/mmol, Amersham) into the mantle of *T. fimbria* and using specimens of comparable size for each experiment.

RESULTS AND DISCUSSION

HPLC of extracts from both the mantle and cerata of *T. fimbria* showed the presence of peaks co-eluting with PGE2 and PGE3 standards as well as of the previously described PGEL's. Two new components were also present whose structures were identified as those of PGF2α- and PGF3α-1,15-lactone-11-acetates from the comparison of their proton NMR spectra with those of PGEL's (1) and of synthetic PGF2α -1,15-lactone. The amounts of PG's and PG-1,15-lactones in *T. fimbria* mantle (M) and cerata (C), expressed in μg/wet tissue weight ± s.e. (n=3), are shown in Table 1.

TABLE 1.

	PGE3	PGE2	PGE3-lact.	PGE2-lact.	PGF3α-lact.ac.	PGF2α-lact.ac.	PGA3-lact.
C	98±11	37±8	245±46	221±43	139±56	30±20	124±30
M	75±20	20±8	89±16	99±7	199±10	60±20	97±7

When [3-H]-PGE2 was injected into the mollusc mantle high incorporation of label was observed for PGE2-1,15-lactone only, whereas upon injection of [3-H]-PGF2α highly labelled PGE2-1,15-lactone and PGF2α -1,15-lactone-11-acetate were found (Table 2). This showed that: 1) PG-lactones are synthesized *in vivo* from the corresponding acids; 2) an unusual oxidation from PGF2α to PGE2 free acids and/or lactones occurs *in vivo*. Although PGF2α -1,15-lactone was absent from both mantle and cerata extracts, high incorporation of label was observed in the HPLC fractions corresponding to this compound which might be a short lived

TABLE 2. Radioactivity [cpm and (cpm/mg pure compound)] incorporated *in vivo* into PG-lactones using [3H]-PGE2 (*) and [3H]-PGF2α

		MANTLE			CERATA	
Days	PGE2 lactone	PGF2α lactone	PGF2α lact.ac.	PGE2 lactone	PGF2α lactone	PGF2α lact.ac.
1	63900 (127000) 161177* (179086*)	99470	15000 (150000)	61170 (120000) 89100* (89100*)	N.D.	1410 (27000)
2	132020 (132020) 47440* (79077*)	31650	60000 (580263)	194600 (870000) 194810* (243513*)	3120	6040 (110545)

intermediary in the biosynthesis of PGF2α -1,15 lactone-11-acetate and PGE2-1,15-lactone.

The specific radioactivity incorporated in PGE2-lactone decreased in the mantle and increased in the cerata with longer incubation periods, thus suggesting that this metabolite might be mainly synthesized in the mantle and then transported and accumulated into the cerata. This finding and the lack of an analogous effect for PGFL's parallel the data reported in Table 1 about the tissue distribution of PG-lactones.

The next experiments were aimed at investigating the possible role of PGE2- and PGE3-1,15-lactones after their transfer to the cerata. Spontaneous detachment of the cerata, during T. fimbria typical defense behaviour, was induced and the appendices, in triplicate, were either immediately frozen or kept contracting in sea water and at room temperature for different periods of time. The tissue was then extracted and PG's and PG-lactones purified and quantitated. As shown in Table 3, the amounts of PG's were higher, while the quantities of PG-lactones were correspondingly lower, the longer the time of contraction of the cerata after their detachment. In order to confirm that the newly formed PG's originated from the corresponding lactones and not from de novo biosynthesis, radiolabelled PGE2-1,15-lactone (15000 cpm, obtained pure from the previous in vivo conversion experiments) was injected into cerata which were then treated as above. This resulted in the production of tritiated PGE2, purified by HPLC, and in the corresponding decrease of the radioactivity in HPLC fractions containing PGE2-lactone (Table 3).

TABLE 3. *In vivo* conversion of PG-lactones to PG's.

Time	PGE2(%)	TOT	PGE3(%)	TOT	PGE2	PGE2-lact.
0	13.5+11.1	69+24	35.9+10.0	39+9	540	5500
15'	42.2+5.4*	84+3	67.9+11.0	23+3	3200	1800
4 h	46.0+4.1**	70+22	69.3+7.6*	22+4	5325	1300

Quantitative data[a] (% of TOT in μg + s.e., n=3) | Experiments with [3H]-PGE2-lactone (cpm)

[a]Statistical analysis was carried out using the unpaired Student's T test; *=P<0.05, **=P<0.005. TOT=PG+lactone

Thus, lactonization of PGE2 and, conceivably, PGE3 might represent the first mechanism ever reported by which PG's, as structurally related compounds, are stored *in vivo* ready to be released upon a physiological stimulus, such as a defensive reaction, to effect their biological action. It is not clear, however, what is this action. Histological analyses of *T. fimbria* cerata have revealed the presence of several contractile fibers similar to mammalian smooth muscle which is usually potently contracted or relaxed by PGE₂. Lactone-derived PG's might be responsible for the irregular and prolonged contractions occurring in the cerata upon detachment.

Other possible biological roles for PG-lactones in *T. fimbria* physiology must be taken into account. PGEL's, but not PG's or PGFL's, are in fact secreted in the mollusc defensive secretion and might be used as defense allomones. More interestingly, we have isolated high amounts of a mixture of PGFL-11- and -9- fatty acyl esters from the mollusc reproductive gland (0.95 mg/g dry weight tissue) and eggmass (1.6 mg/g dry weight tissue). Methanolysis of the mixture yielded PGF₂α- and PGF₃α-methyl esters and a series of saturated and unsaturated fatty acid methyl esters which included, as revealed by GC, mainly palmitoyl, arachidonyl and cis-5,8,11,14,17-eicosapentenoyl methyl esters. EIMS of the mixture confirmed the presence, among the others, of 9-arachidonyl-PGF₂α -1,15-lactone and of 9-eicosapentenoyl-PGF₃α -1,15-lactone, e.g. of PG-derivatives esterified with their own precursors. Further studies are needed to clarify the physiological significance of this finding in *T. fimbria* reproduction. Preliminary data suggest that these metabolites are derived from the mantle PGFL's.

In conclusion, we have described here the finding of a novel and, possibly, multi-functional metabolic pathway concerning unprecedented PG-derivatives. The extremely high espression of the PG branch of the arachidonate cascade in *T. fimbria*, apart from having facilitated the study of PG-lactone structure and *in vivo* synthesis, promotes the future use of this mollusc as a model for research on the control of PG biosynthesis. It will be also interesting to determine, by means of techniques more sensitive than the ones used in this study, whether the PG-lactone pathway is also present in other organisms.

ACKNOWLEDGEMENTS

The authors wish to thank Mr. A. Crispino, Ms. C. Minardi and Mr. A. Trabucco for precious assistance and Dr. G.L. Bundy, Upjohn Co., Kalamazoo, USA, for the gift of synthetic PGF₂α-1,15-lactone.

REFERENCES

1. Cimino, G., Spinella, A. and Sodano, G., (1989), *Tetrahedron Lett.*, 30:3589-3592.
2. Stanley-Samuelson, (1987), *Biol. Bull.*, 173:92-109.
3. Weinheimer, A.J. and Spraggins, R.L., (1969), *Tetrahedron Lett.*, 59:5185-5188.

LEUKOTRIENE A₄ HYDROLASE IN THE B-LYMPHOCYTIC CELL LINE *RAJI*

Björn Odlander, Jesper Haeggström, Tomas Bergman, Olof Rådmark, Anders Wetterholm and Hans-Erik Claesson

Dept. of Physiological Chemistry, Karolinska Institutet, S-104 01 Stockholm, Sweden

INTRODUCTION

Leukotrienes (LT) are formed from arachidonic acid in several types of leukocytes, and exert profound biological effects (10). The introduction of molecular oxygen at position C-5, yielding 5(S)-hydroperoxy-eicosatetraenoic acid (5-HPETE), is catalyzed by the 5-lipoxygenase. This enzyme also forms the next intermediate in leukotriene biosynthesis (10), the unstable allylic epoxide leukotriene A₄ (LTA₄). Lymphocytes do not have the ability to form this compound (5,7), but these cells do have enzymatic capacity to further metabolize LTA₄ into LTB₄ (5), a reaction catalyzed by the LTA₄ hydrolase.

LTB4 influences cellular activation, cell growth and immunoglobulin production in B-lymphocytes (11). Several other effects of LTB₄ on the immunological system has been described (2). In a previous study, we found that the monoclonal B-lymphocytic cell line *Raji* (5) possessed a higher capacity to convert LTA₄ into LTB₄, than other lymphocytic cells. We have thus purified LTA₄ hydrolase from *Raji* cells and investigated its properties.

EXPERIMENTAL PROCEDURES

Enzyme purification: *Raji* cells (8) were homogenized and LTA₄ hydrolase was purified by means of streptomycin and ammonium-sulphate precipitations followed by fast protein liquid chromatography (FPLC) using anion exchange, hydrophobic interaction and molecular exclusion columns, which will be described in more detail elsewhere (Odlander et al, 1990, to be published). Assay of enzyme activity: LTA₄ was kindly provided by Dr. A. Ford-Hutchinson, (Merck-Frosst, Canada). Analysis of LT was performed on reverse phase (RP) high performance liquid chromatography (HPLC) as described (4). Heat-treatment: LTA₄ hydrolase was kept at 60°C in a sealed vial from which aliquots were removed at indicated times of treatment and immediately put on ice. Enzymatic activity was assayed using an LTA₄ concentration of 50 µM (10s, 0°C). Electrophoresis: Sodium dodecyl sulphate - polyacrylamide gel electrophoresis (SDS-PAGE, 10-15 % gradient gels) and isoelectric focusing (pH-interval 4-6.5) were performed on a PHAST-system (Pharmacia AB, Sweden). Gels were stained with Coomassie brilliant blue. Amino acid analysis and N-terminal sequence analysis was performed as described (3).

RESULTS AND DISCUSSION

The 10.000g supernatant of homogenized *Raji* cells was assayed for LTA$_4$ hydrolase activity giving 27.9 nmol LTB$_4$/10^9 cells in the preparation. The corresponding figure for human leukocytes is 14.6 (9). This difference is in accordance with our previously reported data, which showed that *Raji* has a high capacity to convert LTA$_4$ into LTB$_4$ (5). When high-speed centrifugation was performed, enzyme activity was almost completely recovered in the 105.000g supernatant (data not shown). Leukotriene A$_4$ hydrolase was purified from *Raji* using ammonium-sulphate precipitations and FPLC with anion exchange, hydrophobic interaction (HIC) and molecular exclusion techniques. This resulted in an apparently homogeneous enzyme preparation (Fig 1), with an overall purification which was more than 1400-fold, and a yield of approximately 25% (Table 1).

Physical properties: SDS-PAGE indicated an M$_r$ of 68.000 for *Raji* LTA$_4$ hydrolase (fig 1, right), but the M$_r$ according to molecular exclusion chromatography was 51.000, suggesting a non-globular behaviour during this chromatography. Stokes radius was determined and was found to be 3.1 nm, and isoelectric focusing indicated a pI of 5.0 (Fig 1, left). Treatment with the reducing agent dithiothreitol (DTT, 2 mM, 30 min) did not alter pI. The amino acid composition was found to be similar to the one of LTA$_4$-hydrolase in human leukocytes. The N-terminal amino acid sequence was PEIVDTXSLASPASVXRTKHL, which is identical to the one in human peripheral leukocytes (9) and human lung (6).

TABLE 1. Purification of LTA$_4$ hydrolase from *Raji* cells. Aliquots from each purification step was assayed for enzymatic activity (1 min, 20°C, 45μM LTA$_4$). Data are presented as mean ± SD.

	Specific activity (nmol LTB$_4$/mg protein)	Yield (%)	Purification (-fold)	(n)
10.000g supernatant	0.25±0.08	100	-	5
Precipitations	0.64±0.1	72±15	2.6	4
Mono-Q	17.4±6.7	58±18	69.6	6
HIC	123.4±47	35±17	494	4
Superose-12	354.8±69	26±15	1419	6

Enzyme kinetics: Enzymatic activity of *Raji* LTA$_4$ hydrolase persisted for approx. 40 seconds. A second addition of LTA$_4$ did not lead to further formation of LTB$_4$ (data not shown). At 20°C, using 1 min incubations (Table 1), the specific activity was found to be 355 nmol LTB$_4$/mg/min ± 69 (mean ± SD, n=6). When incubations were performed at 37°C, the amount of LTB$_4$ formed in 1 min incubations decreased slightly. This was probably due to reduced substrate stability, since initial enzyme velocities at 37°C were increased (data not shown). Treatment of enzyme with DTT (2 mM, 30 min), did not significantly alter enzyme activity.

In order to minimize the influence of substrate instability and self-inactivation, apparent kinetic constants were determined in short-time incubations at low temperature (10s, 0°C). The catalysis obeyed Michaelis-Menten kinetics (fig 2A).

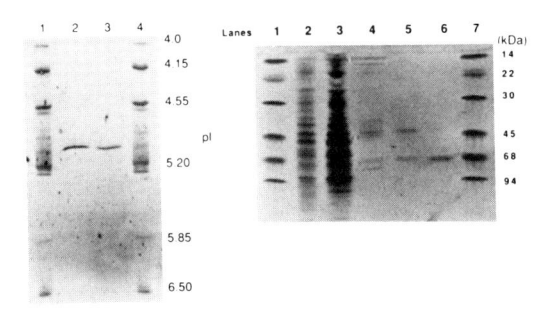

FIG 1. Isoelectric focusing (left) of *Raji* LTA4 hydrolase (Lanes 1 and 4: standard, 2: untreated enzyme, 3: enzyme treated with DTT)   SDS-PAGE (right) of the various steps of purification (1 and 7: standards, 2: 10.000g supernat., 3: precipitations, 4: Mono-Q, 5: HIC, 6: Superose-12)

Data were plotted according to Eadie and Hofstee and apparent kinetic constants were determined. V_{max} was found to be 1095 nmol/mg/min $\pm$ 199 and K_m was 12.3 µM $\pm$ 3.7 (mean $\pm$ SD). The turn-over number at 0°C was found to be 79 min^{-1}. This gives an apparent second-order rate constant at 0°C of 1.1 x10^5 M^{-1}s^{-1}. The corresponding constant for LTA4 hydrolase in human peripheral leukocytes (9) was 5 x10^4, suggesting a higher catalytic efficiency for the *Raji* enzyme. However, two preparations of *Raji* LTA4 hydrolase showed an altered behaviour where saturation kinetics did not conform to the Michaelis-Menten equation (fig 2B). This was not due to the reductive state of the enzyme, since neither catalyzis nor pI was altered by treatment with DTT. In preparations not obeying Michaelis-Menten kinetics, V_{max} was 1976 and 2215 nmol/mg/min, respectively, and K_m was 2.16 and 2.77 µM, respectively. In these preparations the turn-over number was approx. 138 min^{-1}.

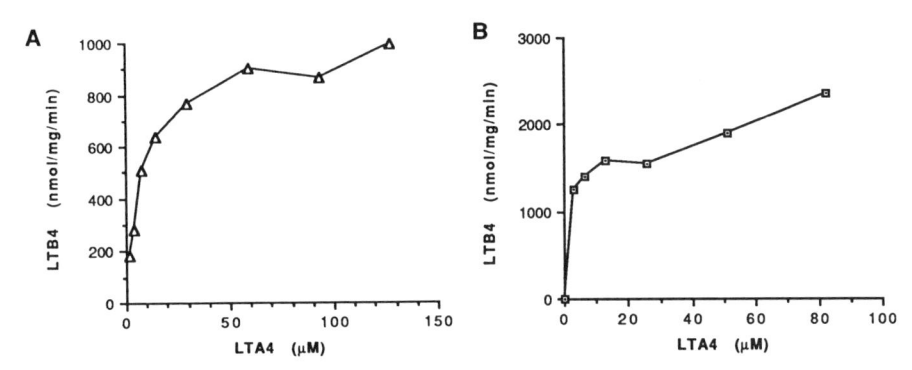

FIG 2. Saturation kinetics of two preparations of *Raji* LTA4 hydrolase

Heat-inactivation: Heat-treatment (60°C) inactivated the enzyme, and the time-course for this inactivation was studied. The pattern of inactivation varied between enzyme batches. Fig 3A shows a linear correlation between ln for specific activity (0°C, 10s incubations) and time of heat-treatment. This inactivation pattern was obtained in several independent experiments. However, in two preparations of *Raji* LTA4 hydrolase, which both exhibited one single band at M_W 68.000 on

SDS-PAGE, a non-linear inactivation pattern was found (Fig 3B). Out of this pattern, two independent linear inactivation curves could be deduced, suggesting the presence of two enzymes with different temperature stabilities.

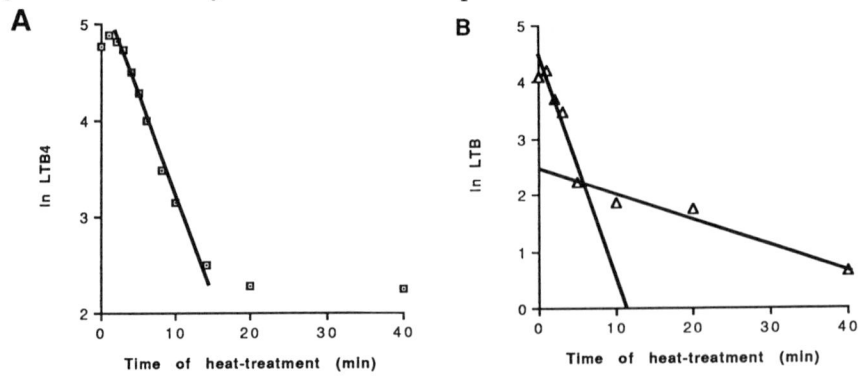

FIG 3. Heat-inactivation (60°C) of two preparations of *Raji* LTA4 hydrolase.

Regarding structural parameters, *Raji* LTA4 hydrolase is similar to this enzyme from other sources (1,3,6,9). The *Raji* cell has a higher capacity than human peripheral leukocytes (9), as well as normal lymphocytes (5), to convert LTA4 into LTB4. The catalytic efficiency of *Raji* LTA4 hydrolase was found to be higher than the one in human peripheral leukocytes (9). LTB4 is a growth factor in B-lymphocytes (11) and an efficient LTA4 hydrolase in *Raji* might thus provide this Burkittlymphoma derived cell with a growth-promoting agent. Some preparations of *Raji* LTA4 hydrolase did not conform to Michaelis-Menten kinetics and showed an altered temperature sensitivity. These observations might be due to post-translational modification of the LTA4 hydrolase. Another possibility is that subclones of *Raji* contain an enzyme with a slightly modified primary structure, having a further increased catalytic efficiency.

ACKNOWLEDGEMENTS

This work was supported by grants from The Swedish Medical Research Council (03X-217, 03X-07467, 03X-3532 and 03X-07135) and the Swedish Cancer Society (2 801-B90-01XA).

REFERENCES

1. Bito, H., Ohishi, N., Miki I., Minami M., Tanabe T., Shimizu T., and Seyama, Y. (1989): J. Biochem., 105:261-264.
2. Ford-Hutchinson, A.W. (1990): Critical Reviews in Immunology, 10:1-12.
3. Haeggström, J, Bergman T, Jörnvall H, and Rådmark,O.(1988): Eur.J.Biochem,174:717-724.
4. Odlander, B., and Claesson, H-E. (1987): Biomed. Chrom., 2:145-147.
5. Odlander, B., Jakobsson P.J., Medina J.F., Rådmark O., Yamaoka K.A., Rosén A., and Claesson, H-E. (1989): Int. J. Tissue React., 11:277-289.
6. Ohishi, N., Izumi T., Minami M., Kitamura S., Seyama Y., Ohkawa S., Terao S., Yotsumoto H., Takaku F., and Shimizu, T. (1987): J. Biol. Chem., 262:10200-10205.
7. Poubelle, P.A., Borgeat P., and Rola-Pleszczynski, M. (1987): J. Immunology, 139:1273-1277.
8. Pulverthaft, R.J.V. (1966): J. Clin. Pathol., 18:261-273.
9. Rådmark, O, Shimizu T, Jörnvall H, and Samuelsson, B. (1984): J.Biol. Chem., 259:12339-
10. Samuelsson, B., Dahlén, S-E., Lindgren, J.Å., Rouzer, C.A. and Serhan, C.N. (1987): Science, 237:1171-1176.
11. Yamaoka, K.A., Claesson H-E., and Rosén, A. (1989): J. Immunol., 143:1996-2000.

PGH SYNTHASE: INTERACTION WITH HYDROPEROXIDES AND INDOMETHACIN

Richard J. Kulmacz[1], Yong Ren[1], Ah-Lim Tsai[2], and Graham Palmer[3]

[1]Department of Biochemistry, Univ. of Illinois at Chicago, Chicago, IL 60612; [2]Div. of Hematology and Oncology, Univ. of Texas Health Sci. Center, Houston, TX 77030; [3]Dept. of Biochemistry and Cell Biology, Rice Univ., Houston, TX 77251

Prostaglandin H (PGH) synthase has two catalytic activities: a cyclooxygenase activity that produces PGG_2 from arachidonate and oxygen, and a heme-dependent peroxidase activity that reduces hydroperoxides like PGG_2 to the corresponding alcohols (e.g., PGH_2). The cyclooxygenase reaction is thought to be a free radical chain reaction that is initiated by oxidized intermediates in the peroxidase reaction cycle (2,3). Studies of the interaction of hydroperoxides with the synthase has led to the discovery of a hydroperoxide-induced free radical whose electron paramagnetic resonance (EPR) spectrum is similar to that of the tyrosyl radical in ribonucleotide reductase (reviewed in Ref. 7). Better characterization of the hydroperoxide-induced free radical is needed to establish its structure and its relation to catalysis by the synthase.

We have examined the kinetics of free radical formation with both ethyl hydroperoxide (EtOOH) and 15-hydroperoxyeicosatetraenoic acid (15-HPETE) and pure ovine PGH synthase. Because the hydroperoxide-induced free radical in the synthase is not stable at room temperature the reactions were conducted at -14 °C. Both hydroperoxides generated within a few seconds a free radical species whose EPR spectrum was dominated by a doublet at g=2.005, with splitting of 16 G and a peak-trough width of 35 G (Fig. 1); this doublet was observed previously in reactions with HOOH (4) and has been attributed to a tyrosyl radical (1). Over the next 20 s or so of reaction with 15-HPETE (120 s with EtOOH) the doublet signal gave way to a singlet with similar peak-trough width (Fig. 1); a similar singlet was observed previously for reactions with 15-HPETE at higher temperatures (4). Thus, two related but distinct radicals were produced in series by both EtOOH and the lipid hydroperoxide.

The intensity of the doublet / singlet combination (obtained by double integration of the $g = 2$ EPR signal) peaked at 0.6 spins / heme after about 120 s of reaction with EtOOH, and at 0.3 spins / heme after about 20 s of reaction with 15-HPETE; the intensity declined slowly in reactions with EtOOH, more rapidly in reactions with 15-HPETE. Inclusion of 15-HETE (5-fold excess over heme) with EtOOH resulted in a more rapid decrease of the radical signal intensity than with EtOOH alone, indicating that some group in the polyunsaturated fatty acid was capable of acting as a reductant for the radicals. This reduction might plausibly occur by abstraction of an allylic hydrogen from the fatty acid back bone by the radical; just such a hydrogen abstraction constitutes the rate-determining step in the proposed mechanism of the cyclooygenase reaction.

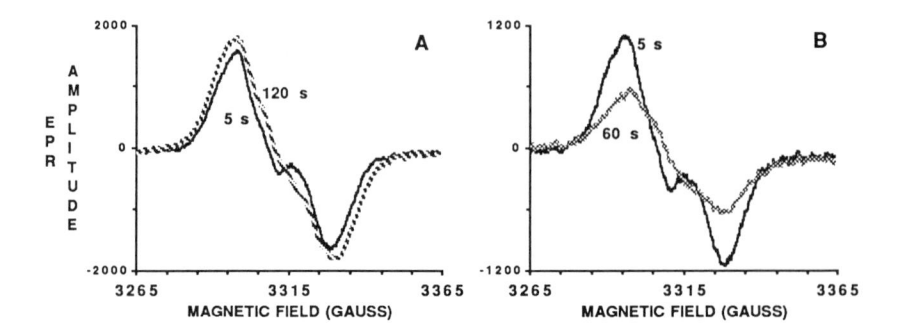

FIG. 1. EPR spectra of PGH synthase during reaction with hydroperoxides. The synthase holoenzyme (16 μM heme) was mixed with a 10-fold excess of either EtOOH (Panel A) or 15-HPETE (Panel B) at -14°C, and then frozen in Dry Ice / acetone at the indicated times. The spectrum in the g = 2 region was recorded at 11 K with a power level of 10 μW, a frequency of 9.29 GHz, and a modulation amplitude of 2 G.

Tetranitromethane (TNM) has been reported to react selectively with tyrosyl groups in protein, converting them to nitrotyrosyl residues (6). When the synthase holoenzyme was reacted with 1 mM TNM at room temperature, the cyclooxygenase activity was lost in an exponential fashion (Fig. 2); the peroxidase activity was lost more slowly than the cyclooxygenase activity. Removal of the synthase heme to form the apoenzyme, or addition of anti-cyclooxygenase agents (indomethacin or ibuprofen) before reaction with TNM decreased the rate of loss of the cyclooxygenase activity by about 20-fold. A similar destruction of the cyclooxygenase activity by TNM, and protection by anti-cyclooxygenase agents, has been found very recently by Smith and his colleagues (5). Amino acid analysis of holoenzyme reacted with TNM indicated formation of 2 nitrotyrosyl residues / subunit at the point where >90% of the cyclooxygenase activity was lost; the apoenzyme reacted with TNM under the same conditions had only 1 nitrotyrosyl residue / subunit. Addition of a stoichiometric amount of indomethacin (1 indomethacin / synthase dimer) before reaction of holoenzyme with TNM was found to block the loss of the residual cyclooxygenase activity (4% of uninhibited velocity) and to decrease the formation of nitrotyrosine by about 1 residue / subunit. These results suggest that the specific nitration of a single tyrosine residue near the cyclooxygenase active site (of the 27 tyrosine residues in the synthase) was responsible for the loss of cyclooxygenase activity.

Treatment with TNM was found to change the EPR spectrum of the synthase little. However, upon reaction of the TNM-treated synthase with EtOOH only a singlet radical signal was produced (Fig. 3); this singlet had a peak-trough width of about 24 G, much narrower than the singlet observed with the native synthase. The intensity of the EtOOH-induced radical singlet in the TNM-treated synthase peaked at 0.3 spins / heme after 60 s. Thus, treatment of the synthase with TNM resulted in nitration of one or two tyrosine residues, perturbation of the hydroperoxide-induced radical, and differential loss of cyclooxygenase activity; removal of the heme or addition of anti-cyclooxygenase agents prevented loss of cyclooxygenase and decreased nitration of tyrosine. This provides strong evidence that the hydroperoxide-induced radicals are indeed tyrosyl radicals, and that the tyrosyl radicals are important to cyclooxygenase catalysis.

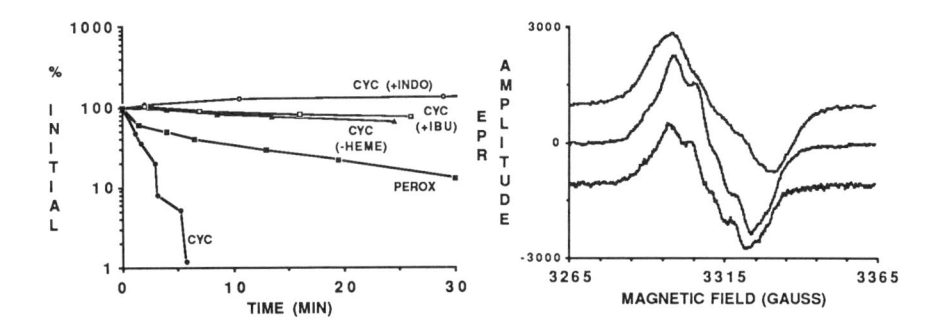

FIG. 2. Effects of incubation with TNM on the cyclooxygenase (CYC) and peroxidase (PEROX) activities of PGH synthase. The synthase holoenzyme was preincubated with either indomethacin (INDO; 1 / dimer), with ibuprofen (IBU; 200 µM), or with no addition before incubation with 1 mM TNM in pH 8.0 buffer at room temperature. In one experiment (- HEME) apoenzyme was substituted for the holoenzyme. Aliquots were removed at the indicated times for assay of cyclooxygenase or peroxidase activity (2).

FIG. 3. EPR spectra of the synthase (upper trace), the TNM-treated synthase (lower trace), and the indomethacin-synthase complex (middle trace) after reaction with EtOOH. The TNM-treated synthase (7 µM heme) and the indomethacin-synthase complex (19 µM heme; 1 mol indomethacin / subunit) were mixed with a 10-fold excess of EtOOH (over heme) for 60 s (TNM-synthase) or 320 s (Indomethacin-synthase) at -14°C, and then frozen in Dry Ice / acetone. The spectrum of the EtOOH adduct of the untreated synthase at 120 s was taken from Fig. 1. The spectra in the g = 2 region were recorded at 11 K with a power level of 10 µW, a frequency of 9.29 GHz, and a modulation amplitude of 2 G. The amplitudes in the two spectra are scaled to represent contributions from equal concentrations of synthase heme.

The EPR spectrum of the resting synthase was also found to be little changed upon formation of the complex with indomethacin. Just as observed with the TNM-treated synthase, however, only a narrow singlet was produced upon reaction of the indomethacin-synthase complex with EtOOH (Fig. 3); in fact the shape of the singlet was almost identical with that seen with the TNM-treated enzyme. The parallels between indomethacin and TNM in their alteration of the EPR signals from the hydroperoxide-reacted synthase, and in their differential inhibition of the cyclooxygenase activity, suggests that in both cases the cyclooxygenase activity is impaired by perturbation of a catalytically-important tyrosyl residue.

Acknowledgements: This work was supported in part by National Institutes of Health grants GM30509 (RJK) and GM21337 (GP), and Welch Foundation grant C636 (GP).

REFERENCES

1. Karthein, R., Dietz, R., Nastainczyk, W., and Ruf, H.H. (1988): *Eur. J. Biochem.*, 171: 313-320.
2. Kulmacz, R.J. (1986): *Arch. Biochem. Biophys.*, 249: 273-285.
3. Kulmacz, R.J., Miller, J.F., Jr., and Lands, W.E.M. (1985): *Biochem. Biophys. Res. Commun.*, 130:918-923.
4. Kulmacz, R.J., Tsai, A.-L., and Palmer, G. (1987): *J. Biol. Chem.*, 263: 10524-10531.
5. Smith, W.L., DeWitt, D.L., Kraemer, S.A., Andrews, M.J., Hla, T., Maciag, T., and Shimokawa, T. (1990): In: *Advances in Prostaglandin, Thromboxane, and Leukotriene Research*, edited by P. Hedqvist and S.-E. Dahlen, in press, Raven Press, New York.
6. Sokolovsky, M., Riordan, J.F., and Vallee, B.L. (1966): *Biochemistry*, 5: 3582-3589.
7. Stubbe, J.A. (1989): *Annu. Rev. Biochem.*, 58: 257-285.

EVIDENCE FOR TWO POOLS OF PROSTAGLANDIN H SYNTHASE IN HUMAN ENDOTHELIAL CELLS

Ah-Lim Tsai, R. Sanduja and Kenneth K. Wu

Department of Medicine,
Division of Hematology-Oncology,
University of Texas Medical School
at Houston, Texas 77030 USA

Prostaglandin H (PGH) synthase occupies a crucial position in eicosanoid biosynthesis. It has 2 enzymic activities; the cyclooxygenase catalyzes the conversion of arachidonic acid to PGG_2 and the peroxidase, PGG_2 to PGH_2. The cyclooxygenase undergoes rapid inactivation following the conversion PGG_2 to PGH_2 (1,2). Hence, this enzyme is a major limiting step in eicosanoid biosynthesis. Recent studies have confirmed that PGH synthase has a rapid turnover rate with the T1/2 estimated to be less than 10 min in one study (3). However, detailed characterization of the kinetics of its turnover has not been done. In the present study, we performed kinetic analysis of the degradation and synthesis of PGH synthase in quiescent and stimulated cultured human umbilical vein endothelial cells (HUVEC).

A reverse immunoblot technique described previously (4) was used to quantitate the kinetics of PGH synthase degradation. Monolayers of confluent HUVEC in T-25 flasks (2×10^6 cells per flask) were pulse-labeled with L-(^{35}S) methionine for 45 min followed by chase with unlabeled methionine. At specified time points, cells were lysed and radiolabeled PGH synthase was measured by reverse immunoblot. As shown in Fig. 1a, the radiolabeled PGH synthase declined rapidly in the quiescent cells as well as in the IL-1 stimulated cells with a rate constant of 0.1 min^{-1}, T1/2 5 min). There was no apparent difference in the T1/2 between the IL-1 (10 u/ml) and medium-treated cells. However, a fraction of the newly synthesized enzymes (50% for medium-treated cells and 30% for IL-1 treated cells) remained undegraded. When the time period was extended to 180 min as shown in Fig. 1b, the degradation curve fit a biphasic model for cells treated with medium alone as well as for cells treated with 20 nM phorbol 12-myristate 13-acetate (PMA). In addition to a initial rapid phase of decline which exhibited rate constants similar to those shown in Fig. 1a, there was a second phase of slow degradation. The rate constants for the slow-phase were 0.0043 min^{-1} and 0.0057 min^{-1} for PMA- and medium-treated cells respectively. The T1/2 for this slow-phase of degradation was approximately 120 min. These results indicate that degradation of PGH synthase in quiescent HUVEC is biphasic and neither IL-1 nor PMA causes any significant change in either phase of degradation.

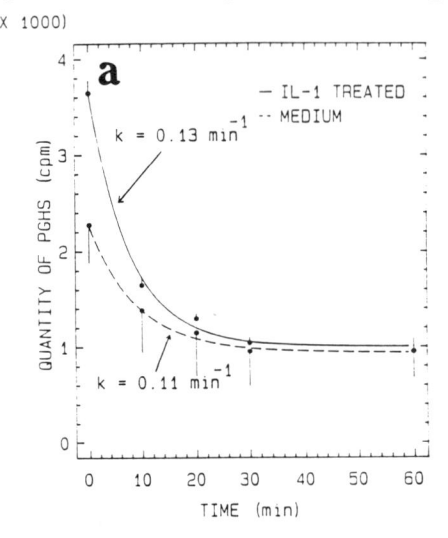

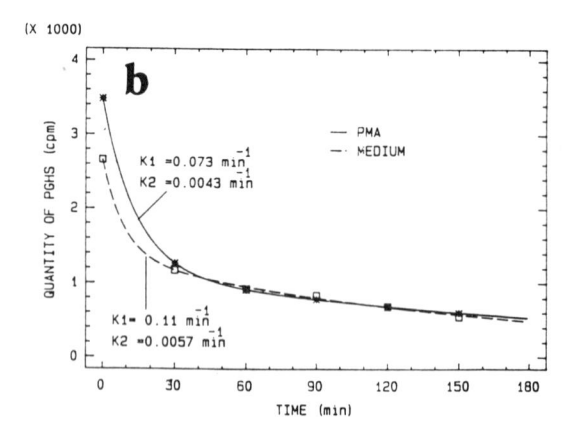

FIG. 1. Kinetics of HUVEC PGH synthase degradation. a. Cells were treated with medium or recombinant IL-1ß (10 u/ml). b. PMA- or medium treated cells. The curves fit a biphasic model. K_1 refers to the rate constant of the rapid phase while K_2 the slow phase of degradation.

Both IL-1 and PMA have been shown to increase the steady-state level of PGH synthase and consequently the steady biosynthesis of eicosanoids in endothelial cells and fibroblasts (5). Since neither stimuli accelerate the degradation rate of the enzyme, their stimulating effect must reside in their enhancement of de novo enzyme synthesis. We, therefore, compared the synthetic rate of PGH synthase in HUVEC stimulated with PMA with that in the medium control cells. Monolayers of confluent HUVEC were pulse-labeled with L-[^{35}S] methionine for a specified time-period, the cells were lysed and the radiolabeled PGH synthase was measured by reverse immunoblot. Data were fitted by one-compartment model of Schimke (6) assuming a constant rate of protein synthesis (V) and a first order rate constant for degradation (Kd). Synthesis of PGH synthase in quiescent HUVEC appeared biphasic and was fitted by two-species one-compartment model. The synthetic rates for the rapid- and the slow-phase of methionine incorporation were 13 and 2 cpm/min respectively (Table 1). PMA (20nM) significantly enhanced the methionine incorporation (Table 1). Fitting of the kinetic data by two-species, one-compartment model revealed that the enhancement was primarily due to a rapid increase in the initial phase of synthesis. The rate constant was increased by 3-fold. PMA did not influence the slow phase of methionine incorporation (V= 2, similar to medium control). IL-1 at 10 u/ml also enhanced the rapid phase of incorporation only and its enhancing effect appeared to be greater than PMA.

In summary, the kinetic analysis of the experimental data clearly indicates that both synthesis and degradation of PGH synthase in unstimulated HUVEC are biphasic, an initial rapid phase followed by a slow phase (kinetic data are summarized in Table 1). These results imply that there exist 2 pools of enzymes. One pool is rapidly synthesized and degraded while the other is much more stable. The exact nature of these 2 pools of enzyme is unknown but there are several possibilities. It may represent 2 separate physical compartments, 2 biochemically different enzymes, i.e.

TABLE 1. Kinetic analysis of the synthetic and degradation rates of PGH synthase in cultured endothelial cells

	Medium	PMA-treated	IL-1 treated
FAST PHASE			
SYNTHESIS (cpm/min)	13	32-45	-
DEGRADATION (1/min)	0.13	0.08	0.11
SLOW PHASE			
SYNTHESIS (cpm/min)	2-3	1.5-2	-
DEGRADATION (1/min)	0.004	.002-.004	0.004

isozymes or enzymes with and without hemes. Stimuli which upregulate the enzyme mass do so primarily by increasing the rapid phase of synthesis. Hence, at least conceptually the rapid-phase may represent the exitable pool of PGH synthase while the steady phase, the constitutive pool. Further experiments are underway to unravel this complex mechanism of PGH synthase synthesis and degradation.

ACKNOWLEDGEMENTS

The authors wish to thank Xiao-ming Xu for excellent technical assistance and Gay Fullerton for secretarial assistance. The work was supported by grants from the National Institutes of Health (NS-23327 and HL-35387).

REFERENCES

1. Hemler, M.E. and Lands, W.E.M. (1980): J. Biol. Chem., 255:6253-6261.
2. Egan, R.W., Paxton, J. and Kuehl, F.A. Jr. (1976): J. biol. Chem., 251, 7325-7335.
3. Fagan, J.M., and Golberg, A.L. (1986): Proc. Natl. Acad. Sci., 83:2771-2775.
4. Wu, K.K., Hatzakis, H., Lo, S.s., Seong, D.C., Sanduja, S.K., and Tai, H-H. (1988): J. Biol. Chem., 263:19043-19047.
5. Raz, A., Wyche, A. and Needleman P. (1989): Proc. Natl. Acad. Sci., 86:1657-1661.
6. Schimke, R.T. and Doyle, D. (1970): Annu. Rev. Biochem., 39:929-976.

PROSTACYCLIN SECRETION AND SPECIFIC INTRACELLULAR PROTEIN PHOSPHORYLATION

J.H. Grose, L. Caron, M. Lebel and J. Landry

Department of Medicine, Faculty of Medicine, Laval University and Laval University Research Center, L'Hôtel-Dieu de Québec, Québec, P.Q., Canada G1R 2J6.

Prostacyclin (PGI_2) is a major prostaglandin (PG) secreted by bovine endothelial cells (2). The regulation of PGI_2 secretion is complex, and numerous mechanisms have been proposed to account for the various agonist-mediated stimulation of this prostanoid. Phosphorylation of specific intracellular proteins is considered an important mechanism for signal transmission in various types of stimulus-response coupling (3). The balance between phosphorylation-dephosphorylation of unique cellular proteins represents the means by which extracellular and intracellular information are integrated to determine the precise activity of an in vivo metabolic pathway. The steady-state levels of phosphorylation are closely related to the relative activities of the protein kinases and phosphatases that catalyse the interconversion process. The present study was designed to investigate the possible variations in the phosphorylation patterns of specific intracellular proteins during modulation of PGI_2 secretion in cultured bovine aortic endothelial cells, and to attempt to establish some relationship between the two events.

MATERIALS AND METHODS

CPA-47 cells (American Type Culture Collection) were routinely grown until confluency and subcultured in 6 well culture plates at a density of 10^5 cells/well in Eagle's minimal essential medium supplemented with 10% fetal calf serum. All cell cultures were grown at 37°C in a controlled humidified incubator under 95% air and 5% CO_2. The cells were used 48 h after subculture. In phosphorylation experiments, the cells were rinced twice with 5 ml of phosphate and serum-free Earle's balanced salt solution containing pyruvate (100 mg/l)) and glutamine (290 mg/l), and then incubated in 1 ml of the same solution containing ^{32}P-orthophosphate (25 µCi/ml) for a total period of 125 min. During this interval,

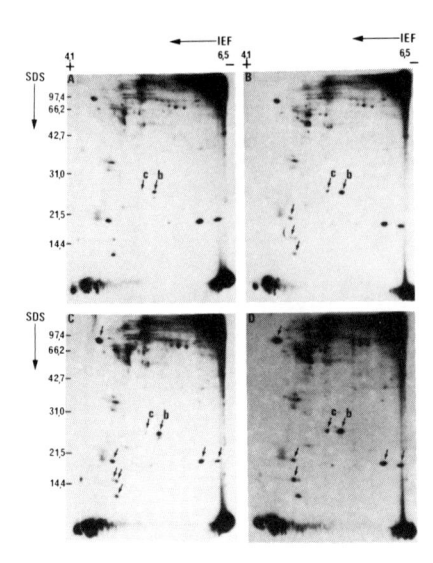

Fig.1. Two-dimensional gel analysis of protein phosphorylation in control (panel A) and in BK (panel B), PMA (panel C) and PMA + BK (panel D) treated cells.

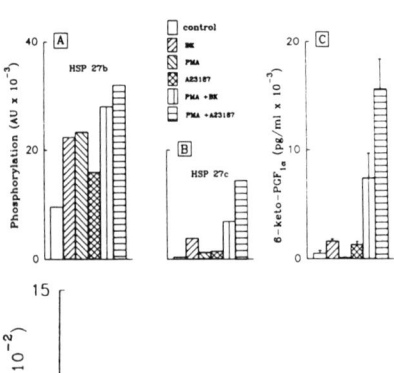

Fig.2. Quantitative ^{32}P-uptake in the b (panel A) and c (panel B) forms of 27 kDa proteins and changes in PGI$_2$ secretion (panel C) under various treatments.

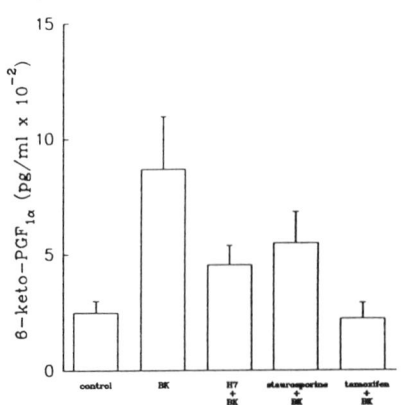

Fig.3. Effect of different PKC inhibitors on PGI$_2$ secretion in BK treated cells.

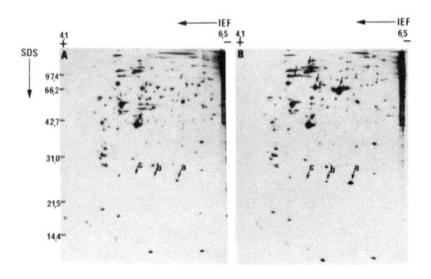

Fig.4. Two-dimensional gel analysis of ^{3}H-labeled proteins in control (panel A) and in heat-shocked (panel B) cells.

substances such as bradykinin (BK, 10^{-7}M; 5 min), the protein kinase activator phorbol 12-myristate 13-acetate (PMA, 10^{-7}M; 60 min), the ionophore A23187 (10^{-6}M; 60 min) or their combinations were added at the indicated time periods before the end of the total incubation periods. In the experiments in which the different protein kinase inhibitors were tested, H-7 (100 μM), staurosporine (20 nM) and tamoxifen (5 μM) were preincubated with the cells for 1 h before the addition of BK. The cells were then washed, and the cellular proteins extracted in the lysis buffer containing 9.5 M urea, 0.5% CHAPS, 2% (1.4% pH 5-7, 0.4% pH 3-10, 0.2% pH 2.5-4) ampholytes, 5% β-mercaptoethanol, 20 mM NaF and 1 mM phenyl methyl sulfonyl fluoride. The samples (20μg) were analysed by two-dimensional gel electrophoresis (7). Specific spots on the autoradiograms were quantitated by densitometric scanning. Similar protocols were used in the PGI$_2$ secretion studies; PGI$_2$ was quantitated as 6-keto-PGF$_{1\alpha}$ by a specific radioimmunoassay (6). The 6-keto-PGF$_{1\alpha}$ values are the means of triplicate experiments. The conditions for the heat-shock experiments were similar, except that the cells were exposed to 44°C for 20 min prior to subsequent manipulations.

RESULTS

Typical two-dimensional gel electrophoresis phosphoprotein profiles under different conditions are shown in Fig. 1. Compared to the control (Fig. 1A), variations in phosphorylation patterns are evident in the treated samples, particularly in the 27 kDa regions. The 27 kDa proteins exist as variants (a, b and c forms) between pI 5.5-6.0, but only the b and c forms show varying degrees of ^{32}P-incorporation. Fig. 2 illustrates the quantitative estimation of the phosphorylation levels of the b (Panel A, HSP27b) and c (Panel B, HSP27c) isoforms with the corresponding changes in PGI$_2$ secretion (Panel C). Under all conditions, the phosphorylation densities are higher in the b variants than in the c forms. Although PMA alone did not modify PGI$_2$ secretion in the presence of increased phosphorylation of the 27 kDa isoforms, subsequent addition of BK to the PMA treated cells resulted in a more pronounced PGI$_2$ response associated with further increased phosphorylation of the same proteins. Incubation of the cells with BK, the ionophore A23187 or its combination with PMA increased ^{32}P incorporation into the 27 kDa variants with proportional increases in PGI$_2$ production. The highest increments are indicated in the experiments which included the combinations of PMA and BK, and PMA plus the ionophore. The BK induced augmentation of PGI$_2$ secretion was suppressed by the different PKC inhibitors H-7, staurosporine and tamoxifen (Fig. 3), in the presence of proportional phosphorylation inhibition of the 27 kDa isomers (data not shown). Exposure of the cells at 44°C for 20 min also induced the increased phosphorylation of the identical 27 kDa variants (data not shown) as documented (5). Further proof that the 27 kDa proteins are related to the heat shock protein (HSP) family was indicated in ^{3}H-leucine (100 μCi/ml) uptake experiments showing increased synthesis of the same proteins 5 h after heat-shock treatment of the cells, using two-dimensional gel electrophoresis of the cell extracts (Fig. 4); the synthesis of the non-phosphorylated ^{3}H-a form is clearly evident on the autoradiogram (Fig. 4,B).

DISCUSSION

The results of the present study are in agreement with a previous report (4) that BK, PMA and the ionophore A23187 can modify the phosphorylation states of numerous specific intracellular proteins in bovine aortic endothelial cells. These observations have been further extended to indicate a close relationship between the degree of phosphorylation of the 27 kDa variants and enhancement of PGI_2 secretion. Through the use of established criteria (1,5), these proteins are identified as members of the low molecular heat-shock proteins, HSP27, which have been well-characterized in thermotolerance studies (1,5) using other cell types. There are no reports relating these substances to PG metabolism. Evidence provided in the present study thus represents the first report implicating the HSP family in the modulation of PGI_2 secretion, possibly through the dynamic equilibrium of the phosphorylation states of the preexisting proteins within the cell. In some instances, enhanced HSP27 phosphorylation alone may not necessarily modulate PGI_2 secretion. Optimal PGI_2 resonsiveness to agonists probably requires a combination of adequate phosphorylation levels in the presence of sufficient concentrations of other intracellular mediators, such as Ca^{++}. The secretion of PGI_2 is modulated by different PKC sensitive mechanisms, as suggested in the experiments in which the different PKC inhibitors diminished the BK stimulated PGI_2 secretion with proportional suppression of phosphorylation levels of the HSP27 variants. These studies suggest a possible novel function for the heat-shock proteins.

ACKNOWLEDGEMENTS

The authors wish to thank Mrs E. Lemay for her secretarial assistance. These studies were supported by grants from the Medical Research Council of Canada.

REFERENCES

1. Arrigo, A.P., and Welch, W.J. (1987): J. Biol. Chem., 262: 15359-15369.
2. Clark, M.A., Littlejohn, D., Mong, S., and Crooke, S.T. (1986): Prostaglandins, 31: 157-165.
3. Cohen, P. (1985): Eur. J. Biochem., 151: 439-448.
4. Demolle, D., Lecomte, M., and Boeynaems, J.M. (1988): J. Biol. Chem., 263: 18459-18465.
5. Landry, J., Chrétien, P., Lambert, H., Hickey, E., and Weber, L.A. (1989): J. Cell Biol., 109: 7-15.
6. Lebel, M., Grose, J.H., and Falardeau, P. (1989): Prostaglandins Leuk. Essen. Fatty Acids, 35: 41-49.
7. O'Farrell, P.H. (1975): J. Biol. Chem., 250: 4007-4021.

INHIBITION OF DE NOVO SYNTHESIS AND MESSAGE EXPRESSION OF PROSTAGLANDIN H SYNTHASE BY SALICYLATES

R. Sanduja, D. Loose-Mitchell and K.K. Wu

Departments of Medicine and Pharmacology, University of Texas Medical School at Houston
Houston, TX 77030, USA

It is generally believed that the action of nonsteroidal anti-inflammatory drugs (NSAIDS) is mediated by inhibiting the cyclooxygenase activity of prostaglandin H (PGH) synthase thereby blocking the biosynthesis of inflammatory eicosanoids. Aspirin causes irreversible inhibition of cyclooxygenase activity by acetylating a specific serine residue of PGH synthase (1) while indomethacin, ibuprofen and naproxen inhibit the cylooxygenase activity by different mechanisms but the exact biochemical mechanism is not fully elucidated. It is intriguing to note that despite a very weak anti-cyclooxygenase activity, sodium salicylate exhibits anti-inflammatory actions equipotent to aspirin (2). Moreover, the action of aspirin cannot be explained entirely by its acetylation capacity because of its rapid deacetylation in vivo (3). It is, therefore, possible that the salicylate may exert its anti-inflammatory activity by mechanism distinct from inhibition of the cylooxygenase activity. In this paper, we present evidence to indicate that the salicylate inhibits de novo synthesis and the mRNA levels of PGH synthase in cultured human umbilical vein endothelial cells (HUVEC).

PGH synthase is a membrane-associated hemeprotein widely distributed in mammalian cells and tissues. The protein has 2 catalytic sites; the cyclooxygenase catalyzes the conversion of arachidonic acid to PGG_2 and the peroxidase, the conversion of PGG_2 to PGH_2. The cyclooxygenase activity undergoes rapid inactivation after the conversion of PGG_2 to PGH_2 and has very short half-life. Autoinactivation of cyclooxygenase is a key limiting step in prostanoid synthesis. Inflammatory mediators, i.e. interleukin-1 (IL-1) and growth factors are capable of circumventing this limitation by inducing de novo synthesis of PGH synthase and consequently causing sustained synthesis of PGE_2 and PGI_2. Recombinant IL-1ß (rIL-1ß) increased the PGH synthase mass as measured by the Western blot analysis in a concentration- and time-dependent manner (4). The 70-kDa band reached plateau after HUVEC had been treated with 25-50 u/ml of rIL-1ß for 4-6 h. Using a 2.1 Kb cDNA recently cloned from a HUVEC cDNA library, we performed experiments to determine whether IL-1 increased the PGH synthase mRNA levels in HUVEC. Northern blot analysis revealed that rIL-1ß increased the 2.7 Kb mRNA levels in a concentration- and time-dependent manner similar to that of the 70-kDa band on the Western blot. The mRNA levels reached plateau after HUVEC had been treated with rIL-1ß at 25-50 u/ml for 4-6 h. Blotting of the gels with a ß tubulin cDNA showed that IL-1 had no effect on the ß-tubulin mRNA expression. These data indicate that IL-1 stimulates the expression of PGH synthase gene with a subsequent increase in the de novo synthesis of PGH synthase. Continuous synthesis of the enzymes provides new cyclooxygenase activity needed for the sustained synthesis of PGE_2 and a PGI_2.

Cytokines (IL-1 and IL-6) and prostaglandins (PGE_2 and PGI_2) are important inflammatory mediators (5). Since IL-1 induces sustained PGE_2 and PGI_2 formation, we reasoned that the salicylates may achieve their antiinflammatory action by suppressing the de novo synthesis of PGH synthase. To test this hypothesis, we incubated monolayers of HUVEC in T-75 flasks with aspirin, sodium salicylate or medium alone at 37°C for 30 min. After washing, cells were incubated with fresh culture media in the presence or absence of rIL-1ß (10 u/ml). At 2 h, cells were lysed and the 70-kDa band was analyzed by Western blot (6). Aspirin or sodium salicylate at 25 ug/ml abolished the 70-kDa band in quiescent cells and in IL-1 treated cells. Acetaminophen (25 ug/ml) and naproxen (30 ug/ml) also decreased the 70-kDa while indomethacin (50 uM) did not. We then carried out a series of experiments to determine the IC_{50} for the active compounds. The results are summarized in Table 1.

TABLE 1. <u>Comparison of the potency of aspirin for inhibition of the synthesis of PGH synthase with its anti-cyclooxygenase activity</u>

	IC_{50} (uM) Aspirin	Na Salicylate
PGH synthase protein	0.06	0.06
PGH synthase mRNA	0.06	
Anti-cyclooxygenase activity	35-10,000	weak

The IC_{50} of aspirin and salicylate was equivalent, i.e. approximately 60 nM. These results are very interesting for two reasons. First, sodium salicylate is equipotent to aspirin in reducing the enzyme mass in HUVEC. Secondly, the IC_{50} of aspirin for inhibiting the enzyme synthesis is several orders of magnitude lower than that required to inhibit the enzyme activity (7,8). Based on these published data, we conclude that aspirin is at least three orders of magnitude more potent in blocking the synthesis of PGH synthase than in direct inhibition of its activity.

To elucidate the mechanism by which the salicylate inhibits the synthesis of PGH synthase, we evaluated the effect of aspirin on the PGH synthase mRNA levels. Asprin inhibited the HUVEC PGH synthase mRNA levels both in quiescent cells and IL-1 stimulated cells. The IC_{50} of aspirin in reducing the mRNA levels in HUVEC treated with 10 u/ml of rIL-1ß for 4 h was approximately 60 nM which is comparable to that of inhibiting the 70-kDa band. Moreover, the duration of asprin effect on blocking the mRNA level was also 4 h. These data strongly suggest that salicylates inhibit the transcription of PGH synthase. The exact mechanism by which this occurs is being investigated in our laboratory.

In summary, we have presented a novel mechanism by which salicylates inhibit eicosanoid biosynthesis and consequently achieves anti-inflammatory action. A schematic view is shown in Fig. 1. The inflammatory mediator, IL-1, causes a sustained stimulation of PGE_2 and PGI_2 synthesis not only by activating phospholipase A_2 but also by inducing de novo synthesis of PGH synthase. IL-1 appears to increase the PGH synthase gene transcription with subsequent enhancement of enzyme synthesis. This action is dependent on protein kinase C activation (9). The salicylate reduces the enzyme mass by downregulating the expression of PGH synthase. This novel mechanism provides a plausible explanation for the anti-inflammatory action of sodium salicylate and other salicylate compounds. Furthermore, these studies shed light on the molecular regulation of arachidonic acid metabolism. Further studies will provide valuable information concerning the molecular mechanisms by which NSAIDS work.

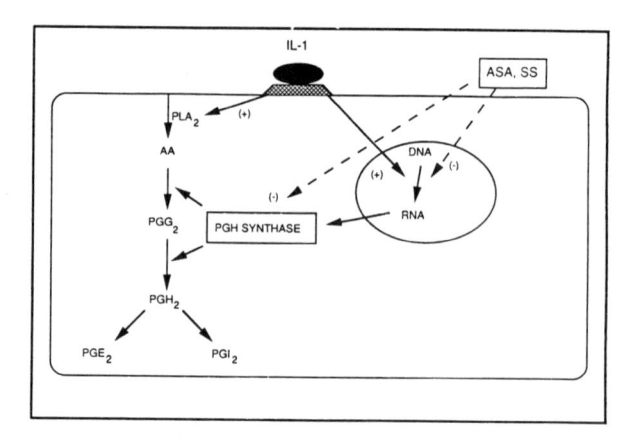

FIG. 1. Schematic illustration of the mechanisms by which IL-1 and salicylates regulate PGH synthase formation.

ACKNOWLEDGEMENTS

The authors wish to thank Xiao-Ming Xu for technical assistance and Nancy Fernandez and Gay Fullerton for typing the manuscript. The work was supported by grants from the National Institutes of Health (NS-23327 and HL-35387).

REFERENCES

1. Roth, G.J., Sanford, N., and Majerus, P.W. (1975): Proc. Natl. Acad. Sci., USA 72:3073-3076.
2. Vane, J., and Botting, R. (1987): FASEB J. 1:89-96.
3. Higgs, G.A., Salmon, J.A., Henderson, B., and Vane, J.R. (1987): Proc. Natl. Acad. Sci. USA 84:1417-1420.
4. Raz, A., Wyche, A., Siegel, N., and Needleman, P. (1988): J. Biol. Chem. 263:3022-3028.
5. Dinarello, C.A. (1988): FASEB J. 2:108-115.
6. Wu, K.K., Hatzakis, H., Lo, S.S., Seong, D.C., and Sanduja, S.K. (1988): J. Biol. Chem. 263:19043-19047.
7. Flower, R.J. (1974): Pharmacol. Rev. 26:33-67.
8. Burch, J.W., Baenziger, N.L., Sanford, H., and Majerus, P.W. (1978): Proc. Natl. Acad. Sci. USA 75:5181-5184.
9. Raz, A., Wyche, A., and Needleman, P. (1989): Proc. Natl. Acad. Sci., USA 86, 1657-1661.

EFFECTS OF NON-STEROIDAL ANTI-INFLAMMATORY DRUGS ON THE IN VIVO SYNTHESIS OF THROMBOXANE AND PROSTACYCLIN IN HUMANS

Viktor Drvota, Ole Vesterqvist and Krister Gréen

Department of Clinical Chemistry and Blood Coagulation, Karolinska Hospital
S-104 01 Stockholm, Sweden

Considerable interest has been focused on the role of thromboxane A_2 (TxA_2) and prostacyclin (PGI_2) in cardiovascular disease in humans (5,11). Measurement of urinary metabolites represents one way to obtain reliable information on the in vivo synthesis of TxA_2 and PGI_2 (7). Since 1983, we have studied the in vivo synthesis of these two eicosanoids by measurement of two of the major urinary metabolites, 2,3-dinor-TxB_2 and 2,3-dinor-6-keto-$PGF_{1\alpha}$ (12,15). The methods are based on gas chromatography - mass spectrometry and deuterated internal standards.

For an adequate design of studies in humans and for the interpretation of obtained data it is of importance to know how different drugs affect the in vivo synthesis of TxA_2 and PGI_2. Of particular interest is those drugs belonging to the group called non-steroidal anti-inflammatory drugs (NSAIDs). We have therefore in a number of investigations studied the effects of various NSAIDs on the in vivo synthesis of TxA_2 and PGI_2 in healthy humans (3,6,10, 12,13,14). In this article, our most important findings will be discussed.

ASPIRIN

A single oral dose of 500 mg of aspirin causes a substantial inhibition of TxA_2 synthesis for 2-3 days, whereafter the synthesis slowly recovers to normal rate within 8-10 days (13). However, the inhibition of PGI_2 production is shortlasting (3-4 h) (10). The rapid recovery of PGI_2 synthesis is due to the fact that endothelial cells, which are nucleated, soon can resynthesize new cyclooxygenase (4) in contrast to platelets, which lack nuclei, and thus are not capable of producing new enzyme. The results suggest that a single dose of aspirin, of the order of 500 mg every third day, should be an alternative to daily low dose aspirin for long term inhibition of TxA_2 synthesis without inhibition of PGI_2 for more than a few hours following dosing. This dose regimen efficiently inhibits the enhanced TxA_2 formation in patients with acute myocardial infarction without significantly reducing PGI_2 formation (8).

NAPROXEN

500 mg naproxen causes a marked reduction of both TxA_2 and PGI_2 synthesis for about two days (14). The reduction of TxA_2 was somewhat more pronounced than the reduction of PGI_2.

INDOMETHACIN

50 mg of indomethacin inhibits both TxA_2 and PGI_2 synthesis for about 20-24 hours (13). This inhibition was thus not so protracted as for naproxen. This is not unexpected since indomethacin has a shorter plasma half life (1).

PIROXICAM

20 mg of piroxicam seems to reduce both TxA_2 and PGI_2 synthesis for 3-4 days (3). The maximal inhibition was not so pronounced as it was for the other drugs presented here. The recovery of TxA_2 synthesis to normal levels was somewhat more protracted than for PGI_2.

The fact that naproxen, indomethacin and piroxicam seem to inhibit both TxA_2 and PGI_2 synthesis as long as they are present in the blood, indicates that these drugs are reversible inhibitors of cyclo-oxygenase (9).

PARACETAMOL

500 mg paracetamol (Acetaminophen) does not affect TxA_2 synthesis (13), but very unexpectedly causes a

marked reduction of PGI_2 synthesis for 6-8 h (6). Paracetamol is a widely used analgetic/antipyretic drug with no or little antiinflammatory effect (1). It does not affect platelet aggregation (2) and bleeding time (1) probably because of the lack of effect on TxA_2 synthesis. The fact that paracetamol only inhibits PGI_2 production could theoretically be disadvantageous for patients suffering from cardiovascular disease.

SUMMARY

Most NSAIDs seem to have inhibitory effects on the in vivo synthesis of both TxA_2 and PGI_2. However there are large differences in the duration of the inhibitory effects as shown in the table below. Aspirin, indomethacin, naproxen and piroxicam inhibit the second wave of platelet aggregation (2). This effect on platelet aggregation persists as long as each drug causes inhibition of TxA_2 synthesis. Thus, inhibition of TxA_2 synthesis is likely to be the reason for the effect of NSAIDs on platelet function. The lack of effect of paracetamol on TxA_2 synthesis together with the lack of effect on platelet aggregation by paracetamol are in further support of this.

Drug	Inhibition of TxA_2	PGI_2
Aspirin	10 days	3-4 h
Naproxen	2 days	2 days
Indomethacin	24 h	24 h
Piroxicam	3-4 days	3-4 days
Paracetamol (Acetaminophen)	-	6-8 hours

REFERENCES

1. Brogden R.N. (1986). Drugs 32:27-45.
2. Cronberg S., Wallmark E. and Söderberg I. (1984). Scand. J. Haematol., 33:155-159.

3. Drvota V., Gréen K. and Vesterqvist O. (to be published).
4. Fagan J.M. and Goldberg A.L. (1986). Proc. Natl. Acad. Sci. USA. 83: 2771-2775.
5. Fitzgerald G.A., Catella F. and Oates J.A. (1987). Hum. Pathol., 18:248-252.
6. Gréen K., Drvota V. and Vesterqvist O. (1989). Prostaglandins, 37:311-315.
7. Gréen K., and Vesterqvist O. (1986). Advances in Prostaglandin, Thromboxane and Leukotriene Res., vol 16:309-324.
8. Rasmanis G., Vesterqvist O., Gréen K., Edhag O. and Henriksson P. (1988). The Lancet, ii: 245-247.
9. Stanford N., Roth G.J., Shen T.Y. and Majerus P.W. (1977). Prostaglandins, 13:669-675.
10. Vesterqvist O. (1986). Eur. J. Clin. Pharmacol., 30:69-73.
11. Vesterqvist O. (1988). Scand. J. Clin. Lab. Invest., 48:401-407
12. Vesterqvist O. and Gréen K. (1984). Prostaglandins, 28:139-154.
13. Vesterqvist O. and Gréen K. (1984). Prostaglandins, 27:627-644.
14. Vesterqvist O. and Gréen K. (1989) Eur. J. Clin. Pharmacol., 37:563-565.
15. Vesterqvist O., Gréen K., Lincoln F.H. and Sebek O.K. (1983). Thromb. Res., 33:39-49.

REBOUND ELEVATION IN URINARY THROMBOXANE B_2 AND 6-KETO-$PGF_{1\alpha}$ EXCRETION AFTER ASPIRIN WITHDRAWAL

J H Vial L J McLeod *M S Roberts

Departments of Medicine and Physiology, University of Tasmania, PO Box 252C, Tasmania 7001, Australia and *Department of Medicine, University of Queensland, Australia

INTRODUCTION

The time taken for recovery to normal of urinary metabolites of prostacyclin (PGI_2) and thromboxane A_2 (TXA_2) and for platelet function after aspirin dosing is well established. Prostacyclin metabolites return to normal within about 3 days with those of TXA_2 and platelet function recovering in about 7-10 days reflecting the need for production of new platelets for cyclooxygenase recovery (1,3,4). There is, however, little information as to what happens after prostanoid metabolites first return to normal. Therefore, in a study in which we measured the immunoreactive urinary hydrolysis products of PGF_2 and TXA_2, respectively 6-keto-$PGF_{1\alpha}$ (6 keto) and thromboxane B_2 (TXB_2), with different doses and formulations of aspirin, we followed the recovery of these hydrolysis products for 14 days after withdrawal from aspirin and the response following subsequent re-exposure to aspirin.

METHODS
Subjects and design

The subjects were 6 male and 6 female healthy volunteers aged 20-26 years who gave informed consent and had not taken non-steroidal anti-inflammatory drugs for at least 2 weeks. The study was approved by the University of Tasmania Ethics Committee (Human Experimentation).

The study design was a randomised cross-over using 3 treatment groups in 2 phases. In the first phase the 12 subjects were allocated randomly to 1 of 3 doses; controlled release aspirin (Ecotrin, SK&F, Sydney) in doses of 325 and 1300mg and 300mg aspirin (Aspro Clear, Nicholas) which were taken as a single daily dose for 7 days. In the second phase 2 weeks after the first phase, each subject was randomly re-allocated to 1 of the dosage regimens not taken in the initial phase.

Twenty-four hour urine samples were collected prior to dosing, after 7 days of aspirin, 3, 7 and 14 days after aspirin withdrawal in the first phase and for 3 and 7 days after aspirin withdrawal in the second phase.

Urinary immunoreactive(i) 6-keto-PGF$_{1\alpha}$ and TXB$_2$

Urinary 6 keto and TXB$_2$ levels were determined using a ^{125}I radioimmunoassay kit (New England Nuclear). The kit workup procedure was followed. The minimum level of detection for these assays was 20pg/ml of urine. The 6 keto workup was validated by using reverse phase HPLC with ^{3}H 6-keto-PGF$_{1\alpha}$ as an internal standard to measure recovery and to identify the 6 keto containing fraction prior to radioimmunoassay.

RESULTS

For both urinary 6 keto and TXB$_2$ the percentage depression of excretion rates at the end of 7 days treatment compared to control was the same for the different doses of aspirin. Similarly, the absolute excretion rates at 0 and 7 days were the same for the different doses and for that reason it was considered reasonable to combine the results from the different doses.

Urinary i 6 keto

Prior to aspirin treatment the 6 keto excretion was 7.99±0.82ng/hr (n=12) and this fell to 5.30±0.76ng/hr (n=12) (p<0.003) after 7 days of aspirin treatment. Three days after cessation of aspirin the excretion rate had risen to 13.12±4.20ng/hr (n=12) and this was not statistically significantly elevated compared to the control excretion rate. Seven days and 14 days after cessation of aspirin the excretion rates were 19.86±4.14ng/hr (n=12) and 16.80±3.17ng/hr (n=12) which were both significantly elevated (p<0.02 and p<0.01 respectively) compared to control. At the end of the second period of aspirin dosing the excretion rate fell to 7.18±1.35 (n=12) Three days and 7 days after withdrawal from the second aspirin dosing the excretion rates were 12.53±3.32ng/hr (n=12) and 20.41±5.51ng/hr (n=12) respectively. These were not significantly different from the levels at these times after the first aspirin withdrawal phase. The excretion rate 7 days after the second aspirin withdrawal was statistically significantly greater (p<0.05) than the control excretion rate but not greater than the excretion rate just before the commencement of the second dose of aspirin.

Urinary i TXB$_2$

Prior to aspirin treatment the TXB$_2$ excretion rate was 7.91±0.75ng/hr (n=12) and fell to 3.67±0.49ng/hr (n=12) (p<0.001)at the end of the first 7 days of aspirin treatment.Three and 7 days after cessation of aspirin the excretion rates were respectively 5.05±0.64ng/hr (n=12) and 10.02±1.20ng/hr (n=12). The excretion rate 3 days after aspirin was less (p<0.002) than control and 7 days after aspirin was not significantly different than control. Fourteen days after the first aspirin treatment the excretion rate was 14.45±1.41ng/hr (n=12) and thus was significantly greater than the control excretion rate (p<0.003).

At the end of the second period of aspirin treatment the urinary TXB$_2$ rate fell to 5.93+0.87ng/hr (n=12) Three and 7 days after aspirin withdrawal the excretion rates were respectively 7.12±1.41ng/hr (n=12) and 12.78±1.41ng/hr (n=12).

The 3 day withdrawal excretion rate was a little higher for the second withdrawal, compared to the first (p<0.01) but the 7 day excretion rates were not different. The second 7 day withdrawal TXB_2 excretion rate, however, was statistically significantly greater than the original control rate (p<0.0008).

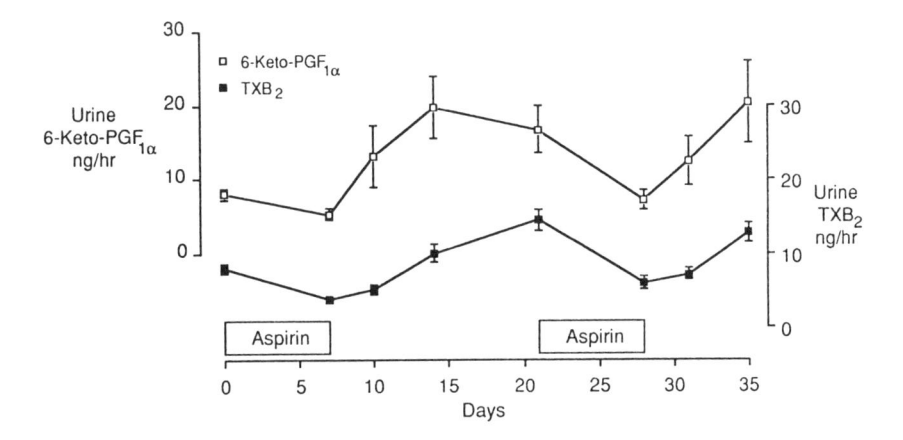

Fig.1 Urinary TXB_2 and 6-keto-$PGF_{1\alpha}$ excretion rates (ng/hr±SE) - before, at the end of 7 days aspirin, 3, 7 and 14 days after aspirin withdrawal, and at the end of a second 7 day aspirin treatment, and 3 and 7 days after the second aspirin withdrawal.

DISCUSSION :

These results show that urinary 6 keto excretion rates rebounded above control rates after aspirin withdrawal reaching a peak 7 days after withdrawal but were still elevated at 14 days. The rebound of urinary TXB_2 excretion was delayed until 14 days after aspirin withdrawal. The excretion rates for both 6 keto and TXB_2 were elevated at the commencement of the second aspirin dosing period. However, the excretion rates overall at the end and after withdrawal from the second period of aspirin were not different compared to those after the first period of aspirin treatment except for TXB_2 3 days after the second aspirin withdrawal which was a little higher.

The delay in the urinary TXB_2 rebound is consistent with irreversible inhibition of platelet and megakaryocyte cyclooxygenase by aspirin which means that new platelets have to be generated and released for platelet cyclooxygenase recovery (5) and is suggestive that the TXB_2 rebound originates in the platelets. If the rebound in 6 keto reflects increased endothelial PGI_2 release one might expect that as the 6 keto excretion rate was still above normal at the time of the TXB_2 rebound, the increased PGI_2 release might partially offset any tendency to increased platelet activation and TXA_2 generation.

In many studies including this one 14 days is considered an adequate time for subjects to be free of non-steroidal anti-inflammatory agents before making control prostaglandin measurements. This study suggests that 14 days after ceasing aspirin there may still be a carry-over rebound effect which could lead to over-estimation of baseline prostaglandin production.

This rebound has even more important potential clinical implications. As a result of the extensive evidence of the value of aspirin as an antiplatelet agent in the secondary prevention of thrombosis and emboli in cardiovascular disease (2) it is in now widespread clinical use for these clinical indications. A rebound increase in platelet activity following cessation of aspirin in these patients could represent a thrombotic risk in individuals already predisposed to thrombotic events. In patients who are receiving aspirin as an anti-inflammatory a rebound in prostanoid inflammatory medication could result in disease exacerbation. Further studies in the appropriate clinical settings are necessary to determine the clinical significance of prostanoid rebound.

REFERENCES

1. Ali, M., McDonald, J.W.D., Thiesen, J.J., Coates, P.E. (1980): *Stroke*, 11:9-13.

2. Antiplatelet Triallists Collaboration (1988): Secondary prevention of vascular disease by prolonged antiplatelet treatment. Br Med J, 196:320-331.

3. Fitzgerald, G.A., Oates, J.A., Hawinger, J., Maas, R.L., Roberts, L.HJ., Lawson, J.A., Brash, A.R. (1983): *J Clin Invest* 71:678-686.

4. Roberts, M.S., McLeod, L.J., Cossum, P.A., Vial, J.H. (1984): *Eur J Clin Pharmacol* 27:67-74.

5. Roth, G.J., Stanford, N., Majerus, P.W. (1975) *Proc Natl Acad Sci USA* 72:3073-3076.

MECHANISM-BASED INACTIVATION OF THROMBOXANE A_2 SYNTHASE

F.A. Fitzpatrick, D. Jones, S. Winitz and H.T. Fish

Department of Pharmacology C236
University of Colorado Health Sciences Center
4200 East Ninth Avenue
Denver, Colorado 80262 USA

INTRODUCTION

Several chemically reactive substances participate in the biosynthesis of eicosanoids. Their catalytic transformation has been characterized according to conventional enzymological models; however, 'suicide' inactivation, a feature associated with many of these enzymes has been neglected. This process, or related auto-inactivation processes have been described for prostaglandin H (PGH) synthase (3,12); 5-lipoxygenase (11); 15-lipoxygenase (1,13); PGI_2 synthase (2) and leukotriene (LT)A_4 hydrolase (4,7,8). Compared to other biosynthetic pathways the arachidonic acid cascade contains abundant examples of 'suicide' inactivation which is often defined as a partition between enzymatic inactivation and enzymatic turnover during catalysis (10,14). 'Suicide' inactivation is probably significant from three perspectives including: i) rate limitations in eicosanoid formation ii) irreversible inactivation and chemical modification of biosynthetic enzymes or other macromolecules iii) substrate redistribution among alternate biosynthetic pathways. We have investigated the mechanism based inactivation of thromboxane synthase in platelets. This model system is attractive for several reasons. First, others have reported contradictory findings on the inactivation of this enzyme (5,6); however, it seemed more likely that Hall et al. (5) were correct considering the chemically reactive nature of the substrate PGH_2 and its product thromboxane (Tx) A_2. Second, mechanism-based inactivation during eicosanoid biosynthesis has rarely been reported for intact cells. We report that suicide inactivation of thromoxane synthase occurs in intact platelets. Consideration of this trait may clarify the role of thromboxanes in the cell biology of thrombosis or other disorders involving TxA_2.

EXPERIMENTAL

Human whole blood (45 ml) collected over 3.8% trisodium citrate (5 ml) was centrifuged for 20 min at 200x g and the platelet rich plasma was removed. Suspensions of human washed platelets in Hanks balanced salt solution containing 0.05 M HEPES buffer pH 7.4 were prepared as described (9). Washed platelets were incubated for 1 minute at 37°C then transferred to an aggregometer cuvet containing PGH_2. Samples (50 ul) were withdrawn after 3 minutes for determination of their TxB_2 content by immunoassay. The residual platelet suspension was incubated with a second, successive aliquot of PGH_2 to determine any change in the thromboxane synthase activity. The platelet suspensions contained a 0.5 uM LY655,240 a TxA_2 receptor antagonist, or 0.3 uM PGI_2 an agent which elevates intracellular cyclic AMP in order to prevent aggregation without inhibiting thromboxane biosynthesis. This procedure assured that differences in TxB$_2$ biosynthesis were not attributable to presentation of PGH$_2$ to suspended platelets during the first incubation, compared to platelet aggregates during the second incubation. For the experiments presented the number of consecutive incubations with PGH$_2$ was varied from 2 to 8. This assured that decay of substrate did not account for the effects described. To determine the kinetics of 'suicide' inactivation platelet suspensions were incubated with PGH$_2$ as described. At 15 second intervals, for 2 minutes, portions were removed incubated with a second aliquot of PGH$_2$ to monitor the remaining Tx synthase activity as a function of time. To determine if inactivation was reversible or irreversible platelet suspensions were incubated with PGH$_2$ then washed with 5 volumes of Ca^{++} free Hanks buffer containing 10 mg/ml of bovine serum albumin (BSA) to sequester any enymatic or non-enzymatic products of PGH$_2$. After centrifugation platelets were resuspended to their original concentration and incubated with a second aliquot of PGH$_2$. Control platelets were washed and resuspended analogously to monitor any loss of Tx synthase activity attributable to the procedure rather than the initial exposure to PGH$_2$.

RESULTS

Multiple, consecutive incubations between PGH$_2$ (1-3 ug/ml) and platelet suspensions (2-4 x 10^7 cells/ml) showed that product formation approached an asymptote by the fourth incubation [Figure 1].

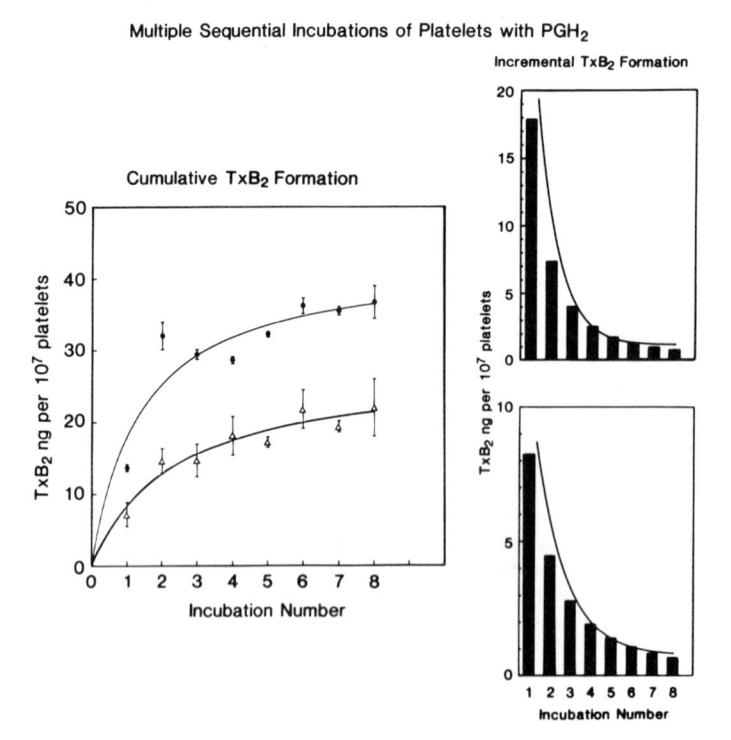

FIGURE 1. Cumulative TxB$_2$ Formation [left] and Incremental TxB$_2$ Formation [Right] During 8 Consecutive Incubations between PGH$_2$ and Washed Platelets. Closed circles are 3 ug PGH$_2$/ml; triangles are 1 ug PGH$_2$/ml.

These results indicate that there is a loss of Tx synthase enzymatic activity accompanying catalysis. The asymptote does not represent saturation of the catalytic process because the substrate was consumed completely before replenishment during the next incubation. The right hand panels depict incremental TxB_2 formation during each incubation for different quantities of PGH_2 [3 ug/ml upper; 1 ug/ml lower]. Incremental formation approached zero in each case. The decline in incremental formation was quantitatively associated with the amount of TxB_2 formed. For instance, the upper panel shows a drop from 18 ng TxB_2 (incubation 1) to 7 ng TxB_2 (incubation 2) or a decline of 61%; the lower panel showed a drop from 8.2 ng TxB_2 (incubation 1) to 4.5 ng TxB_2 (incubation 2) or a decline of 45%. In other words the decline in Tx synthase activity was greater when more TxB_2 was produced. Inactivation, not inhibition by stable end products, accounts for the results. TxB_2 in concentrations up to 100 uM did not inhibit the Tx synthase in intact platelets. Furthermore, the effect was irreversible: washing and resuspension did not restore Tx synthase activity. Platelets which were incubated with PGH_2 (3 ug/ml), washed, resuspended, and incubated with a second aliquot of PGH_2 produced 33.8 $\pm$ 4.9 ng TxB_2 per 10^7 cells (mean $\pm$ SE, n=3). This was significantly different, p<.05, from control platelets which produced 51.8 $\pm$ 6.9 ng TxB_2 per 10^7 cells after they were washed, resuspended and incubated with PGH_2 (3 ug/ml).

The results indicate that Tx synthase in intact platelets is susceptible to suicide inactivation. This corresponds with findings by Hall et al. (5) who reported that Tx synthase isolated from platelets was inactivated during catalysis. It differs from reports by Ullrich and colleagues (6). The process described here is interesting in several contexts. First, it may represent a naturally occurring equivalent to selective enzymatic inhibition, permitting diversion of substrate from one biosynthetic pathway into another. Second, it may provide a basis for developing improved models to understand the role of eicosanoids in chronic disorders, in contrast to acute disorders. For instance, modification of cellular macromolecules leading to the formation of autoantibodies is plausible. Third, it may provide a basis to design substrates with no intrinsic biological activity which might be mechanism based inhibitors of the Tx synthase enzyme.

ACKNOWLEDGMENTS

This work was supported by a grant from the National Institutes of Allergy and Infectious Diseases R01 AI 26730.

REFERENCES

1. Corey, E.J., and Park, H. (1982): J. Am. Chem. Soc., 104: 1750-1751
2. DeWitt, D. and Smith, W. (1983): J. Biol. Chem., 258: 3285-3293
3. Egan, R., Paxton, J., and Kuehl, F. (1976): J. Biol. Chem., 251: 7329-7335
4. Evans, J., Nathaniel, D., Zamboni, R., Ford-Hutchinson, A.W. (1985): J. Biol. Chem., 260: 10966-10970
5. Hall, E., Tuan, W., and Venton, D. (1986): Biochem J., 233: 637-641
6. Hecker, M. and Ullrich, V. (1989): J. Biol. Chem., 264: 141-150
7. McGee, J. and Fitzpatrick, F.A. (1985): J. Biol. Chem., 260: 12832-12837
8. Ohishi, N., Izumi, T., Minami, M., Kitamura, S., Seyama, Y., Ohkawa, S., Terao, S., Yotsumoto, H., Takaku, F., and Shimizu, T. (1987): J. Biol. Chem., 262: 10200-10205
9. Patscheke, H. and Worner, P. (1978): Thrombosis. Res., 12: 485-496
10. Rando, R. (1984): Pharmacological Rev., 36:111-142
11. Rouzer, C. and Kargman, S. (1988): J. Biol. Chem., 263: 20980-20988
12. Smith, W. and Lands, W.E.M. (1972): Biochemistry, 11: 3276-3285
13. Smith, W. and Lands, W.E.M. (1972): J. Biol. Chem., 247: 1038-1047
14. Walsh, C. (1984): Ann. Rev. Biochem., 53: 494-535

SELECTIVE THROMBOXANE SYNTHASE INHIBITION DOES NOT INCREASE IN VIVO SYNTHESIS OF PROSTACYCLIN IN HEALTHY HUMANS

Ole Vesterqvist*, Krister Gréen*, Peter Henriksson**, Gundars Rasmanis** and Olof Edhag**

*Department of Clinical Chemistry and Blood Coagulation, Karolinska Hospital, S-104 01 Stockholm, Sweden.
**Department of Medicine, Huddinge Hospital, S-141 86 Stockholm, Sweden.

A number of thromboxane synthase inhibitors have been developed during the last few years. The rationale behind this development is a desire to specifically inhibit the synthesis of thromboxane A_2 (TxA_2) without interfering with the synthesis of prostacyclin. It has even been suggested that a specific inhibition of thromboxane synthase would cause a redirection of platelet-derived endoperoxides into synthesis of prostacyclin in the endothelial cells (5). There is however conflicting evidence in the literature whether such an "endoperoxide shunt" exists in vivo or not.

We have earlier studied the effect of U-63,557A [5-(3'-pyridinylmethyl)benzo-furan-2-carboxylate] on the urinary excretion of 2,3-dinor-TxB_2 and 2,3-dinor-6-keto-$PGF_{1\alpha}$, two major urinary metabolites of thromboxane B_2 and prostacyclin in humans (2). A single oral dose of 200 mg U-63,557A caused a more than 60 % reduction of TxA_2 formation and the duration of the effect was about 8 h. There was however no obvious effect on the excretion of 2,3-dinor-6-keto-$PGF_{1\alpha}$ (2). In the present study the effects of an intravenous infusion of the thromboxane synthase inhibitor CGS 13080 [imidazo-(1,5-2)pyridine-5-hexanoic acid] were studied on the in vivo synthesis of TxA_2 and prostacyclin in healthy volunteers (4).

SUBJECTS AND METHODS

Six healthy male volunteers participated and they refrained from all physical exercise from the evening before the study until all urine collections were completed. All received constant 6-hours intravenous infusions of CGS 13080 at 0.08 and 0.25 mg/kg x h. Each dose was given at two different occasions at least two weeks apart and the volunteers were put to bed one h before the start of infusion and they stayed in bed throughout the infusion period.
The in vivo synthesis of TxA_2 and prostacyclin was studied by measurements of the urinary excretion of $2,3$-dinor-TxB_2 and $2,3$-dinor-6-keto-$PGF_{1\alpha}$, respectively, using deuterated internal standards and gas chromatography - mass spectrometry (10).

RESULTS

The plasma levels of CGS 13080 reached steady state concentrations within one hour at both infusion rates. Infusion of CGS 13080 caused a significant inhibition ($p < 0.0001$) of the excretion of the TxA_2 metabolite at both doses (Fig 1). However, infusion of the thromboxane synthase inhibitor did not alter the excretion of the prostacyclin metabolite (Fig 1). The inhibitory effect of CGS 13080 on TxA_2 biosynthesis seemed to last for quite a long time since the excretion of the metabolite was still 6-14 h after infusion stop significantly lower than preinfusion rate, low dose: 217 (35) vs 360 (90) pg/mg creatinine and high dose: 222 (36) vs 385 (84) pg/mg creatinine. This despite a rapid drop in the plasma drug level after cessation of the infusion.

DISCUSSION

The biosynthesis of TxA_2 and prostacyclin shows some special features that have to be considered when studies are designed and interpreted. Firstly, there is a diurnal variation in the excretion of the TxA_2 metabolite in that the excretion is somewhat higher during 2-3 h after awakening (7). Secondly, physical exercise increases the excretion of the prostacyclin metabolite (8). Careful studies of prostacyclin should therefore be done in humans at complete rest and urine collected during the sleep could preferably be used for reference (9). This effect of physical activity on prostacyclin biosynthesis may have

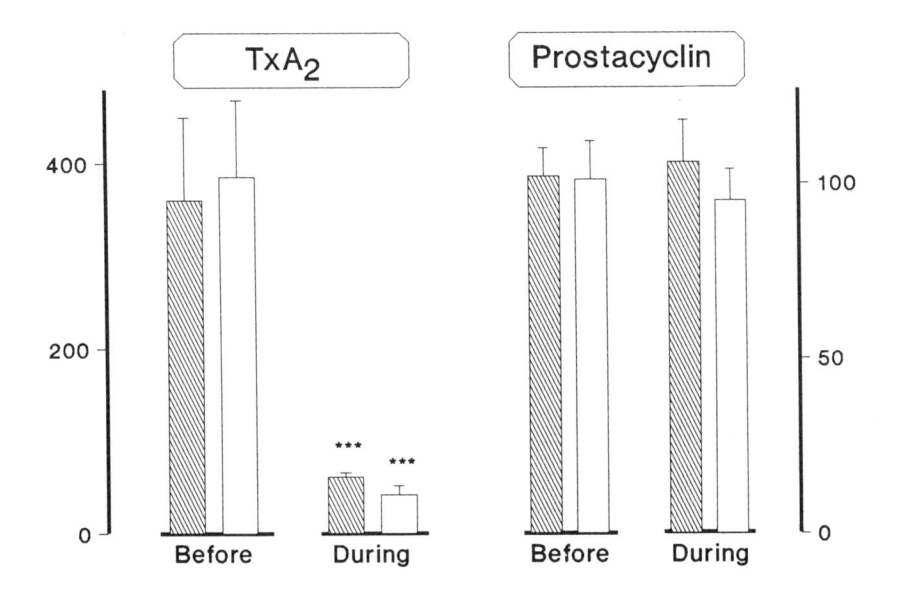

Fig 1. Urinary excretion of the TxA$_2$ and prostacyclin metabolites, 2,3-dinor-TxB$_2$ and 2,3-dinor-6-keto-PGF$_{1\alpha}$ (pg/mg creatinine), in healthy volunteers before and during intravenous infusion of the thromboxane synthase inhibitor CGS 13080. Infusion rates: 0.08 mg/kg x h (hatched bars) and 0.25 mg/kg x h (open bars). Mean ± SEM, *** p< 0.0001.

confounded earlier studies of the effects of various thromboxane synthase inhibitors on the biosynthesis of prostacyclin.

The present study demonstrates that CGS 13080 is a powerful reversible inhibitor of TxA$_2$ biosynthesis in humans. The inhibition was obvious already during the first two hours of infusion with about 35 % reduction of the urinary excretion of 2,3-dinor-TxB$_2$ in the urine collected between 0-2 h (4). After 2 hours of infusion the inhibition seemed to be maximal with an 80-90 % reduction in the urinary excretion of the TxA$_2$ metabolite. Both doses had similar effects. Although the biosynthesis of TxA$_2$ was inhibited by more than 80 %, infusion of CGS 13080 did not affect the excretion of the prostacyclin metabolite (Fig 1). These data are in obvious conflict with an earlier study where the excretion of 2,3-dinor-6-keto-PGF$_{1\alpha}$ was measured in five healthy males after an oral dose of 100 and 200 mg of CGS 13080 and where it was stated that the larger dose increased prostacyclin production by almost 100 % (1). However, at the time of that study it was not known that physical activity stimulates prostacyclin production (8). It is important to keep in mind that in the present study the volunteers were in a supine position under physical inactivity throughout the study. The present study does not however exclude a possible increase in prostacyclin biosynthesis caused by selective inhibition of thromboxane synthase in a situation with increased formation of both TxA_2 and prostacyclin.

The present study demonstrates that CGS 13080 is a potent and selective inhibitor of the in vivo synthesis of TxA_2 in humans. Our results also demonstrate that this inhibition of TxA_2 is not associated with any transfer of endoperoxides to prostacyclin synthesizing cells in vivo in healthy humans.

ACKNOWLEDGEMENTS

These studies were supported by The Swedish Medical Research Council (no 07134 and 08120).

REFERENCES

1. FitzGerald G.A. and Oates J.A. (1984). Clin. Pharmacol. Ther., 35: 633-640.
2. Gréen K. and Vesterqvist O. (1986). In: Adv. in Prostaglandin, Thromboxane, and Leukotriene Res Vol 16, edited by U. Zor, Z. Naor, and F. Kohen. pp 309-324. Raven Press, New York.
3. Henriksson P., Wennmalm Å., Edhag O., Vesterqvist O. and Gréen K. (1986). Br. Heart. J., 55: 543-548.
4. Henriksson P., Rasmanis G., Edhag O., Vesterqvist O. and Gréen K. (1990). Prostaglandins, 39: 99-107.
5. Marcus A.J., Weksler B.B., Jaffe E.A. and Broekinan M.J. (1980). J. Clin. Invest., 66: 979-986.
6. Rasmanis G., Vesterqvist O., Gréen K., Edhag O. and Henriksson P. (1988). Lancet, ii: 245-247.
7. Vesterqvist O. and Gréen K. (1984): Prostaglandins, 27: 627-644.
8. Vesterqvist O. and Gréen K. (1984): Prostaglandins, 28: 139-154.
9. Vesterqvist O. (1988). Scand. J. Clin. Lab. Invest., 48: 401-407.
10. Vesterqvist O. and Gréen K. (1989). Eur. J. Clin. Pharmacol., 37: 563-565.

EICOSANOID SYNTHESIS IN MURINE MACROPHAGES
CAN BE SHIFTED FROM PROSTAGLANDINS TO LEUKOTRIENES
BUT NOT *VICE VERSA* BY SPECIFIC INHIBITORS
OF CYCLOOXYGENASE OR 5'-LIPOXYGENASE ACTIVITY

Volkhard Kaever and Klaus Resch

Institute of Molecular Pharmacology, Medical School Hannover, D-3000 Hannover 61, Federal Republic of Germany

In an experimental model system resident mouse peritoneal macrophages were treated with zymosan or combinations of direct protein kinase C activators plus calcium ionophores for 1 hr and eicosanoid production was determined. At a marginally enhanced intracellular calcium level, which was measured by the Fura-2 technique, only a rise in prostaglandin E_2 synthesis was detected. At a high intracellular calcium level and concomitant arachidonate 5-lipoxygenase activation released arachidonic acid was preferentially converted to leukotriene C_4, whereas prostaglandin E_2 secretion was even diminished. By inclusion of the prostaglandin endoperoxide synthase inhibitor indomethacin the observed shift from prostaglandin to leukotriene synthesis became obvious at lower increases in the intracellular free calcium concentration. On the other hand, specific inhibition of the arachidonate 5-lipoxygenase activity by the translocation inhibitor L-663,536 (3-[1-(4-chlorobenzyl)-3-t-butyl-thio-t-isopropylindol-2-yl]-2-2-dimethylpropanoic acid) resulted in a total prevention of calcium ionophore plus protein kinase C or zymosan-induced leukotriene C_4 synthesis but did only negligibly enhance prostaglandin E_2 production. From these data the assumption that arachidonic acid from different pools is accessible as substrate to prostaglandin endoperoxide synthase and arachidonate 5-lipoxygenase, respectively, is further strengthened.

INTRODUCTION

Besides their antimicrobial and tumoricidal activities macrophages exert potent regulatory functions within the immune system. Numerous soluble and particulate stimuli not only induce the synthesis and secretion of various enzymes and cytokines, but moreover the production of biologically highly active eicosanoids, which are deeply involved in the regulation of inflammatory and allergic reactions (6). The explicite spectrum of eicosanoids produced by a defined macrophage subpopulation depends on the tissue origin of the cells, their differentiation and activation stage and the nature of the stimulus used.

We have shown previously that in resident mouse peritoneal macrophages the activation of the calcium- and phospholipid-dependent protein kinase C (PKC) leads to an increase in free arachidonic acid (AA) available for PG synthesis within minutes (3,7). We then investigated in more detail by which factors the ratio of PG and LT synthesis may be controlled within this cell type.

In this report the effects of indomethacin and the specific AA 5-lipoxygenase translocation inhibitor L-663,536 (1) on macrophage eicosanoid synthesis are shown.

MATERIALS AND METHODS

Resident macrophages were achieved by peritoneal lavage from untreated DBA/2 mice and maintained in serumfree medium as described recently (7) in 24 or 96-well plates at a cell density of 5×10^5 cells/ml. After a preincubation time of 2 hrs non-adherent cells were removed by washing and the adherent macrophages (about 50 % of the peritoneal exsudate cells) were used in the individual experiments. Eicosanoids were determined from the cellular supernatants by specific radioimmunoassay (2) or enzyme-linked immunosorbent assay using monoclonal anti PGE_2 or LTC_4 antibodies (kindly provided by Prof. K. Brune, Erlangen, FRG) in accordance to a described method (8). PGE_2 was obtained from Paesel, Frankfurt, FRG. LTC_4 and L-663,536 were kindly provided by Hoechst, Frankfurt, FRG, and Merck Frosst, Point Claire-Dorval, Canada, respectively. Data are means of duplicate cell incubations and quadruplicate eicosanoid determinations.

RESULTS

We were interested to determine whether at different intracellular calcium levels the specific inhibition of AA metabolizing enzymes such as PG endoperoxide synthase or AA 5-lipoxygenase would result in a shift in eicosanoid production. Fig. 1 shows the effect of indomethacin on LTC_4 synthesis induced by various concentrations of the calcium ionophore A23187 in the presence of a suboptimal concentration of the direkt PKC activator 12-O-tetradecanoylphorbol 13-acetate (TPA). Blockade of the PG endoperoxide synthase activity by 100 nM indomethacin largely inhibited PGE_2 synthesis. Under this condition LTC_4 synthesis was induced at lower concentrations of A23187, although the maximal ionophore-induced LTC_4 production was not enhanced.

Using the same experimental design the effects of the specific AA 5-lipoxygenase translocation inhibitor L-663,536 on PGE_2 and LTc_4 synthesis were investigated (Fig. 2). TPA on its own (10 nM) resulted in a strong increase in PGE_2 but not LTC_4 production. At low ionophore concentrations (in the nanomolar range) in the presence of TPA AA release was synergistically enhanced and free AA was predominantly metabolized into PGE_2. In contrast, LTC_4 was synergistically increased only at higher concentrations of A23187, which represent the condition for AA 5-lipoxygenase

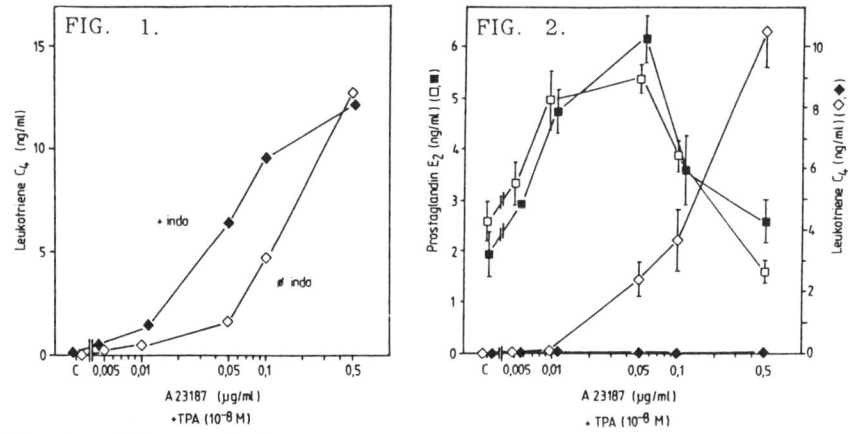

FIG. 1. Effect of indomethacin on A23187/TPA-induced LTC₄ synthesis. Mouse peritoneal macrophages were stimulated for 60 min with A23187 in the indicated concentrations plus TPA (10 nM) after a preincubation time of 20 min in the absence (open symbols) or presence (closed symbols) of indomethacin (100 nM). LTC₄ was determined in the supernatants by specific immunoassay.
(c), controls in the absence (◊) or presence (♦) of TPA alone; indo, indomethacin

FIG. 2. Effect of L-663,536 on A23187/TPA-induced eicosanoid synthesis. Mouse peritoneal macrophages were stimulated for 60 min with A23187 in the indicated concentrations plus TPA (10 nM) after a preincubation time of 20 min in the absence (open symbols) or presence (closed symbols) of L-663,536 (100 nM). PGE₂ (□,■) and LTC₄ (◊,♦) were determined in the supernatants by specific immunoassay.
(c), controls in the absence (□, ◊) or presence (■,♦) of TPA alone.

activation. Although L663,536 used in a concentration of 100 nM totally inhibited LTC₄ production PGE₂ synthesis was not essentially influenced (Fig. 2).

Similar data were obtained when zymosan was added as stimulus. LTC₄ synthesis could be totally blocked by L663,536 (halfmaximal inhibition at about 10 nM) although PGE₂ production at the same time was nearly unchanged (data not shown).

DISCUSSION

One important cofactor for PKC, different phospholipases, and AA 5-lipoxygenase activities is the intracellular calcium. Many physiological stimuli induce eicosanoid synthesis by an increase of phosphoinositide turnover and thus lead to the activation of PKC (via diacylglycerols) and an enhanced calcium level (via inositol 1,4,5-trisphosphate). Taken together, our results obtained with a model system using calcium ionophores and PKC activators as stimuli of eicosanoid synthesis supposed that PKC activation is necessary for AA elevation and the intracellular calcium level then determines the ratio of PG and LT formation (4,5).

Interestingly, at high LTC$_4$ production PGE$_2$ synthesis was even diminished. This may simply be due to the limitation of the common substrate AA. Alternatively, elevation of the intracellular calcium level might induce the liberation of AA from distinct lipid pools or cellular compartments only accessible for the AA 5-lipoxygenase.

From the data obtained by addition of indomethacin to A23187 plus TPA-stimulated cells it can be speculated that AA released at low intracellular calcium levels and not metabolized by the inactivated AA endoperoxide synthase is accessible as substrate for a partially activated AA 5-lipoxygenase. On the other hand, inhibition of AA 5-lipoxygenase activity by L-663,536 did not clearly enhance PGE$_2$ production in zymosan or A23187 plus TPA-stimulated macrophages. This makes likely that AA as substrate accessible for PG endoperoxide synthase or AA 5-lipoxygenase, respectively, is released from different lipid pools or cellular compartments.

ACKNOWLEDGEMENTS

We wish to thank Dr. C.B. Pickett, Merck Frosst, Pointe Claire-Dorval, Canada, and Prof. K. Brune, Erlangen, FRG, for generously providing us with L-663,536 and anti PGE$_2$ or LTC$_4$ monoclonal antibodies, respectively. This work was supported by grants Ka730/1-3 from the Deutsche Forschungsgemeinschaft and 01KC89087 from the Bundesminister für Forschung und Technologie.

REFERENCES

1. Gillard, J., Ford-Hutchinson, A.W., Chan, C., Charleson, S., Denis, D., Foster, A., Fortin, R., Leger, S., McFarlane, C.S., Morton, H., Piechuta, H., Riendeau, D., Rouzer, C.A., Rokach, J., Young, R., MacIntyre, D.E., Peterson, L., Bach, T., Eiermann, G., Hopple, S., Humes, J., Hupe, L., Luell, S., Metzger, J., Meurer, R., Miller, D.K., Opas, E., and Pacholok, S. (1989): *Can. J. Physiol. Pharmacol.*, 67:456-464.
2. Kaever, V., Goppelt-Strübe, M., and Resch, K. (1988): *Prostaglandins*, 35:885-902.
3. Kaever, V., Pfannkuche, H.-J., Wessel, K., and Resch, K. (1989): *Agents and Actions*, 26:175-177.
4. Kaever, V., Pfannkuche, H.-J., and Resch, K. (1989): In: *Progress in Clinical and Biological Research, vol. 301, Prostaglandins in Clinical Research-Cardiovascular System*, edited by K. Schrör and H. Sinzinger. pp. 535-539, Alan R. Liss, New York.
5. Kaever, V., Pfannkuche, H.-J., Wessel, K., and Resch, K. (1990): *Biochem. Pharmacol.*, 39:1313-1319.
6. Nathan, C.F. (1987): *J. Clin. Invest.*, 79:319-326.
7. Pfannkuche, H.-J., Kaever, V., Gemsa, D., and Resch, K. (1989): *Biochem. J.*, 260:471-478 (1989).
8. Reinke, M., Piller, M., and Brune, K. (1989): *Prostaglandins*, 37:577-586.

SYNTHESIS AND BIOLOGICAL EVALUATION OF 2,3,5-TRIMETHYL-6-(3-PYRIDYLMETHYL)-1,4-BENZOQUINONE (CV-6504), A DUAL INHIBITOR OF TXA$_2$ SYNTHASE AND 5-LIPOXYGENASE WITH SCAVENGING ACTIVITY OF ACTIVE OXYGEN SPECIES (AOS)

Shinji Terao, Sigenori Ohkawa, Zen-ichi Terashita, Yumiko Shibouta and Kohei Nishikawa

Chemistry Research Laboratories and Biology Research Laboratories, Takeda Chemical Industries, Ltd, Osaka, Japan

INTRODUCTION

In our continuous efforts of new drug evaluation we have designed and synthesized novel types of compounds effective in the arachidonic acid (AA) cascade and also against active oxygen species (AOS). These are individually selective enzyme inhibitors for 5-lipoxygenase (5-LO)[1] and TXA$_2$ synthase,[2] TXA$_2$ receptor antagonists;[3] and scavengers of AOS.[4]

In this paper, we describe the synthesis and biological effects of 2,3,5-trimethyl-6-(3-pyridylmethyl)-1,4-benzoquinone (CV-6504) and its derivatives, which are intended to have the dual function of inhibiting TXA$_2$ synthase and 5-LO, and scavenging AOS. There are increasing reports suggesting that noxious mediators such as TXA$_2$ and LTs and AOS generating systems act together or sometimes synergistically in many disease states including stroke, myocardial infarction, inflammation, rheumatoid arthritis, etc. It was thought that compounds inhibiting such enzymes and AOS generation might be more effective and something different than individually selective enzyme inhibitors,[1-2] receptor antagonists,[3] and or specific AOS scavengers.[4]

MOLECULAR DESIGN AND SYNTHESIS

We designed and synthesized four types of molecules (Type 1 compounds to Type 4 compounds),[5] all of which contain para-quinonyl and 3-pyridyl moieties that are required for inhibition of 5-LO and TXA$_2$ synthase. These were also expected to have

Type 1   Type 2   Type 3

Type 4   CV-6504

antioxidant activity because of the redox nature of the quinone moiety in the living system.

BIOLOGICAL RESULTS AND DISCUSSION[5-6]

Three in vitro tests and one ex vivo assay for inhibition of TXB_2 and LTB_4 production, and of lipid peroxidation (LP) were examined. Compound 7 exhibited the most potent activity for inhibition of TXB_2 production in vitro. The short alkyl chain compounds and CV-6504 also exhibited potent activities both in vitro and ex vivo. The compounds having hydroxyl and phenyl groups had rather weak activities.

In the 5-LO inhibition test, CV-6504 was highly effective. However, compounds having carboxyl groups were very weak. The substitution of methyl groups by methoxy groups on the quinone ring abolished this activity. As shown in the Table, it was found that the relationship between structure and LP inhibition was similar to that of the 5-LO inhibition activity. Since CV-6504 showed the most potent and well-balanced inhibitory activities on TXA_2 synthase and 5-LO as well as inhibitory activity on LP, this compound was chosen for further biological investigation.

Effects of CV-6504 on the production of TXB_2, LTB_4, and 6-keto $PGF_{1\alpha}$ were examined in human whole blood in vitro. It was found that production of both TXB_2 and LTB_4 was inhibited in a dose dependent manner, whereas the amount of 6-keto $PGF_{1\alpha}$ was increased significantly in the ex vivo experiments.

Recently, it has been suggested that various chemical mediators, including TXA_2, LTs, and AOS might be involved in the

Summary of Screening Results of 3-Pyridylmethyl-1,4-benzoquinones

Compound	R	type	% inhibition of TXB$_2$ Production in vitro[1] 10^{-6}M	ex vivo[2] 10mg/kg	Inhibition of LTB$_4$ Production[3] IC$_{50}$ (×10^{-8}M)	% inhibition of Lipid Peroxidation[4] 10^{-6}M
1	-Me	1	89	90	950	93
2	-CH$_2$Me	1	76	75	66	83
3	-(CH$_2$)$_3$Me	1	46	70	7.3	83
4	-(CH$_2$)$_3$OH	1	61	72	10	83
5	-(CH$_2$)$_4$COOH	1	90	64	6000	34
6	-(CH$_2$)$_5$COOH	1	86	90	930	49
7	-(CH$_2$)$_6$COOH	1	90	97	700	52
8	-CH=CHCOOH	2	22	nd[5]	8700	39
9(CV-6504)	-Me	3	60	86	6.2	80
10	-(CH=CH)$_2$-	3	57	92	8.2	42
11	-OMe	3	40	74	520	39
12	-CH=CHCOOH	4	79	90	880	14

[1] Percent inhibition of the amount of TXB$_2$ formed by incubating PGH$_2$ with horse platelet microsomes. Values are the mean of duplicate experiments.

[3] The molar concentration of test compound required to reduce by 50% the amount of LTB$_4$ formed by RBL-1 cells.

[4] Inhibition of lipid peroxidation in rat brain homogenates.

[5] not determined

pathogenesis of renal glomerular diseases. It was reported that increases in urinary protein excretion, plasma malondialdehyde level, and renal cortical TXB$_2$ and LTs production were observed in puromycin aminonucleoside (PAN, 100mg/kg, i.p.) treated rats. Oral continuous administration of CV-6504 to PAN treated rats for 2 weeks markedly reduced their plasma and urinary MDA. In this experiment the urine volume was not affected by administration of CV-6504. The antiproteinuric effect of CV-6504 was observed at doses of more than 3mg/kg (p.o.) in the PAN treated rats. The effect of CV-6504 (10 mg/kg/day, p.o., for 1-2 weeks) was also examined on the production of TXB$_2$ and LTs using exogenous AA and cortical slices of the kidney, isolated from PAN treated rats. The amounts of TXB$_2$ and LTs were markedly decreased.

In order to explain the mode of action of CV-6504, we examined effects of individual or of combinations of various selective inhibitors and/or AOS scavengers in PAN treated rats. It was found that the combination of CV-4151 (a TXA$_2$ synthase inhibitor), AA-861 (a 5-LO inhibitor) and CV-3611 (an AOS scavenger) at maximum doses was more effective than individual administration of each drug or of any combination of two drugs alone. These results indicate that compounds such as CV-6504 which inhibit TXA$_2$ synthase, 5-LO, and AOS generation are superior to individual enzyme inhibitors and AOS scavengers in

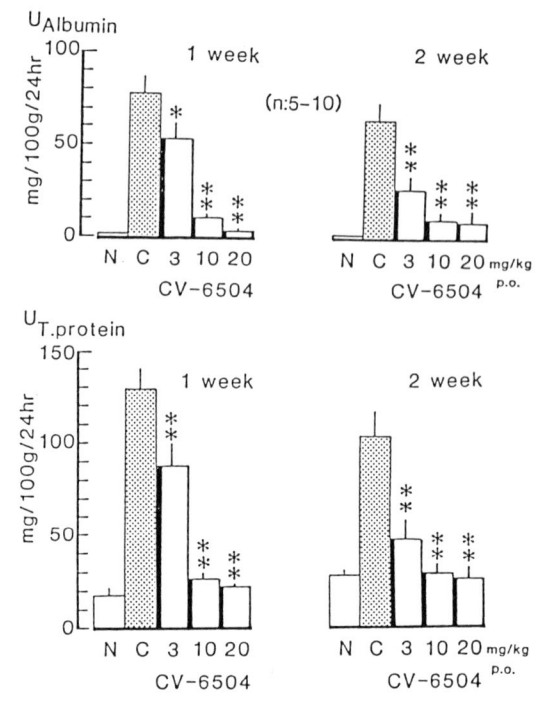

Antiproteinuric effect of CV-6504 in puromycin aminonucleoside nephrotic rats

the PAN treated rat model system. Therefore, CV-6504 might be useful for the treatment of renal and other complex diseases in humans. Accordingly, this compound is now under clinical investigation.

REFERENCE

1. Terao,S.,Shiraishi,M.,Kato,K.,Ohkawa,S.,Ashida,Y.,Maki,Y. (1982): J. Chem. Soc. Perkin Trans. 1, 2909.
2. Kato,K.,Ohkawa,S.,Terao,S.,Ashida,Y.,Terashita,Z.,Nishikawa,K. (1985): J. Med. Chem., 28: 287.
3. Shiraishi,M.,Kato,K.,Terao,S.,Ashida,Y.,Terashita,Z.,Kito,G. (1989): J. Med. Chem., 32: 2214
4. Kato,K.,Terao,S.,Shimamoto,N.,Hirata,M.(1988): J. Med. Chem., 31: 793.
5. Ohkawa,S.,Terao,S.,Terashita,Z.,Shibouta,Y.,Nishikawa,K. (1990): J. Med. Chem., 33: in press.
6. Shibouta,Y.,Terashita,Z.,Imura,Y.,Shino,A.,Nishikawa,K., Fujiwara,Y.(1990): XIth International congress of Nephrology: July 15-20, Tokyo, Japan, P3-379.

METABOLISM OF RADIOISOTOPIC VARIANTS OF LTE$_4$ IN HUMAN SUBJECTS AND EXCRETION OF URINARY METABOLITES

*A. Sala, +N. Voelkel, #J. Maclouf, and *R.C. Murphy

*National Jewish Center for Immunology and Respiratory Medicine
1400 Jackson Street, Denver, CO 80206
+University of Colorado HSC, Cardiovascular Pulmonary Division,
4200 E. 9th Ave., Denver, CO 80262
#INSERM, U150, Hopital Lariboisiere
6, rue Guy-Patin, 75475 Paris Cedex 10, FRANCE

INTRODUCTION

LTC$_4$ is derived from arachidonic acid following the action of the enzyme 5-lipoxygenase with the intermediate formation of leukotriene A$_4$ (9). This reactive intermediate is conjugated to the sulphydryl in the tripeptide glutathione catalyzed by the enzyme LTC$_4$ synthase. LTC$_4$ is synthesized by a variety of cells (3) such as mast cells, eosinophils, and macrophages as well as by transcellular biosynthetic mechanisms involving the formation of LTA$_4$ in one cell such as the neutrophil followed by a successful glutathione conjugation taking place in other cells such as a platelet (4). Much less is known about subsequent biotransformation of this active sulfidopeptide leukotriene in animals including man. Enzymes are known to be present in plasma which rapidly metabolize LTC$_4$ to the cysteinyl leukotriene E$_4$ (LTE$_4$) through the intermediate formation of the cysteinylglycine derivative LTD$_4$ (2). The metabolic fate of LTE$_4$ has been the subject of several investigations. In the rat it is rapidly converted into N-acetyl-LTE$_4$ (1) and subsequently subjected to ω-oxidation and several rounds of β-oxidation from the ω-terminus (10). These resulting metabolites have been observed in rat bile and in minor amounts in urine (7). In humans, infusion with [14,15-^{3}H]LTC$_4$ resulted in 12-20% recovery of label in excreted urine (5). When [^{3}H$_8$]LTC$_4$ was infused in man, more than 40% of the radioactivity appeared in urine (6). The present study was designed to assess the influence of the position of the radiolabeled in the sulfidopeptide leukotriene on the observed pattern of radioactive metabolites excreted in urine.

METHODS

Three differently labeled LTE$_4$ radioisotopic variants ([^{3}H]LTE$_4$, [^{14}C]LTE$_4$, and [^{35}S]LTE$_4$) (Fig. 1) were diluted in 10 ml sterile saline and infused into the right hand dorsal digital vein over a period of 10 min. Urines were collected at 2, 5, 8, 15, 24 hr following infusion. The urines were acidified to pH 4 with formic acid and applied to a 100 ml XAD-8 open column. After washing with water (2 volumes), the material retained was eluted with 2 vol of methanol. This eluate was dried under reduced pressure, reconstituted in 1 ml of 15% methanol/water and injected onto a reverse phase HPLC column using a linear gradient from 16 mM ammonium formate (pH 4.8) to methanol/water/acetic acid (90/10/0.1, v/v/v) over 55 min. The effluent was analyzed with an on-line radioactive HPLC monitor.

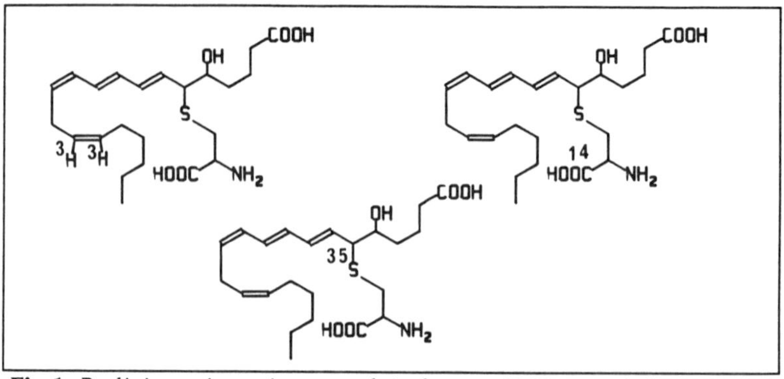

Fig.1 *Radioisotopic variants used in human LTE$_4$ metabolism studies: [14,15-^{3}H]LTE$_4$, [cys-^{14}CO]LTE$_4$, [^{35}S]LTE$_4$.*

RESULTS AND DISCUSSION

Infusion with [14,15-^{3}H]LTE$_4$ (2.1 μCi) resulted in a total excretion of radioactivity during the first 24 hr of 9.9% of the infused LTE$_4$ (Table 1). Most of the radioactivity coeluted with authentic LTE$_4$ (Fig. 2), but a minor amount of N-acetyl-LTE$_4$ was detectable during the first urine collection (0-2 hr). This data is in agreement with previous studies that reported the lack of any detectable major metabolites except LTE$_4$ after infusion with [14,15-^{3}H]LTC$_4$ (5).

TABLE 1: Radioactivity in timed urine collection

	^{3}H	^{14}C	^{35}S
0-2h	7.3	10	13.6
2-5h	1.8	9	12
5-8h	0.8	4.7	9.7
8-15h	n.d.	5.6	7
15-24h	n.d.	1.6[1]	6
	9.9	30.9	44.3

n.d. = not detectable
[1] The low number of counts in this sample make it possibly inaccurate.

Infusion with [cys-^{14}CO]LTE$_4$ (0.36 μCi) resulted in a 3-fold increase in the radioactivity excreted into urine during the first 24 hr. A major difference was observed at the 2-5 hr urine collection period and this fraction revealed two new radioactive metabolites (Fig. 2) less lipophilic than LTE$_4$ and eluting earlier on the reverse phase-HPLC system. These metabolites, identified as 16-COOH-Δ^{13}-LTE$_4$ and 14-COOH-LTE$_3$ (8), were maximally excreted in the 2-5 hr fraction, but were detectable in the excreted urine even 15 hr following the infusion. Infusion with [^{35}S]LTE$_4$ (4 μCi) revealed the excretion of identical metabolites as that observed following infusion with [cys-^{14}CO]LTE$_4$ even though the amount of radioactivity used for this latter experiment was 10 times less. With the [^{35}S]LTE$_4$ experiment, the signal-to-noise in the radioactive monitor was substantially increased allowing the detection of other metabolites, as well as 16- and 14-COOH-LTE$_4$ metabolites in the first urine collection (0-2 hr, Fig. 2). The urinary metabolites of LTE$_4$ accounted for approximately 7.35% of the total injected [^{35}S]LTE$_4$ (Table 2).

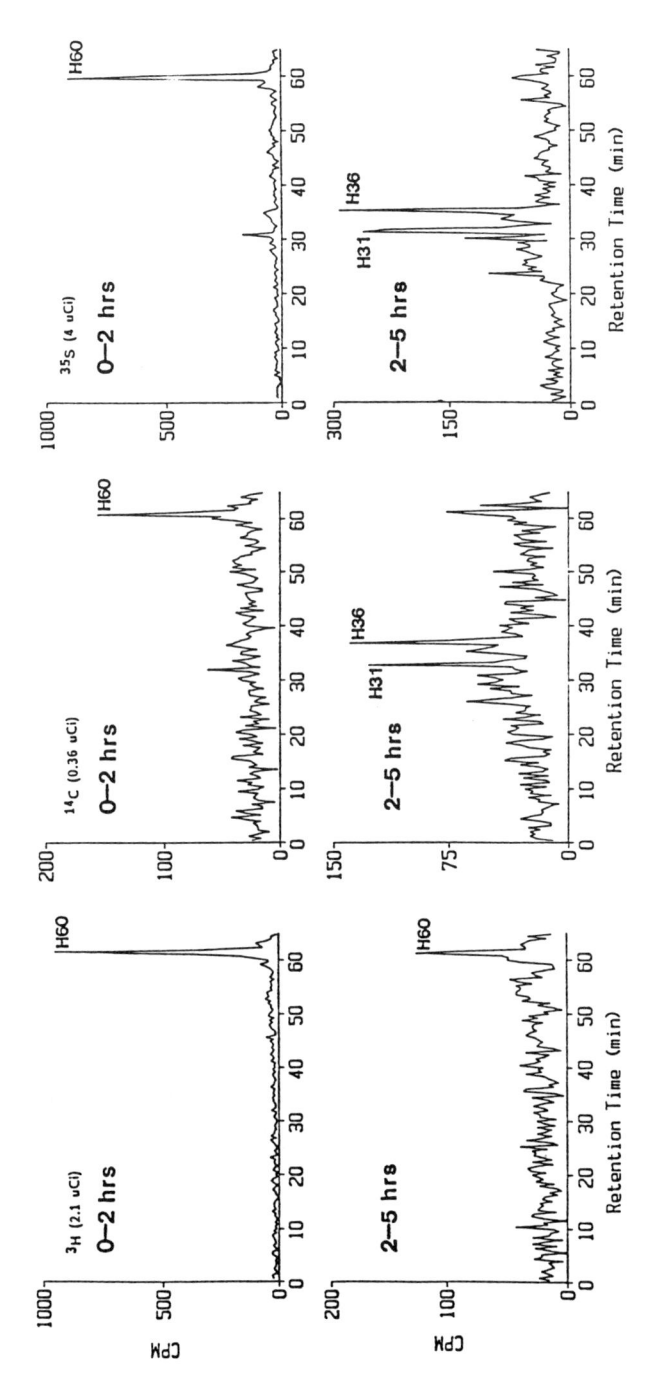

Fig. 2 *Reverse phase HPLC separation of urine extracts following infusion of human volunteers with the three differently radiolabeled LTE$_4$ tracers.*

TABLE 2: Human metabolites in timed urine samples

% of ^{35}S-LTE$_4$ injected

	LTE$_4$	NAc-LTE$_4$	14-COOH LTE$_3$	16-COOH-Δ^{13} LTE$_4$
0-2h	7.3	0.55	1.3	0.55
2-5h	0.52	n.d.	2.1	1.35
5-8h	n.d.	n.d.	0.6	0.55
8-15h	n.d.	n.d.	0.9	0.4
	7.82	0.55	4.5	2.85

Results of this work illustrate the importance of the position of the radiolabeled tracer in following of the metabolic fate of these biologically relevant molecules. For example, it is interesting to note that both of these newly described LTE$_4$ metabolites do not retain the [^{3}H] atoms carried in the 14 and 15 carbon positions of LTE$_4$. While it is obvious that all tritium atoms would be lost in the 14-carboxy-LTE$_4$, the exact mechanism responsible for the loss of all tritium atoms in the 16-carboxy-Δ^{13}-LTE$_4$ metabolite is less clear. One possibility might involve the peroxisomal acyl CoA oxidase acting upon 16-carboxy-LTE$_3$ followed by the action of *cis-trans*-2,3-enoyl-CoA isomerase working reversibly. In such a mechanism, the hydrogen atoms carbons 14 and 15 would equilibrate with water, thereby loosing the radiolabel tracer from the metabolite. It is also important to point out that the position of the ^{14}C- and ^{35}S- labels on the cysteine residue of LTE$_4$ focus attention on LTE$_4$ metabolites which still retain this structural feature. Other metabolites of LTE$_4$, which loose both the cyteine moiety and the tritium atoms at carbon 14 and 15, would not be detected by this multilabel approach.

ACKNOWLEDGEMENT
This work was supported, in part, by a grant from the NIH (HL25785).

REFERENCES
1. Hagerman, W., Dewslinger, C., and Keppler, D. (1985). *FEBS Lett.*, 180:309-313.
2. Heavey, J.D., Soberman, R.J., Lewis, R.A., Spur, B., and Austen, K.F. (1987): *Prostaglandins*, 33:693-708.
3. Lewis, R.A. and Austen, K.F. (1984): *J. Clin. Invest.*, 73:889-897.
4. Maclouf, J. and Murphy, R.C. (1988): *J. Biol. Chem.*, 263:174-181.
5. Maltby, N.H., Taylor G.W., Ritter, J.M., Moore, K., Fuller, R.W., and Dollery, C.T. (1990): *J. Allergy Clin. Immunol.*, 85:3-9.
6. Orning, L., Kaisjer, L., and Hammarstrom, S. (1985): *Biochem. Biophys. Res. Commun.*, 130:214-220.
7. Perrin, P., Zirrolli, J., Stene, D., Lellouche, J.P., Beaucourt, J.P., and Murphy, R.C. (1988): *Prostaglandins*, 37:53-60.
8. Sala, A., Voelkel, N., Maclouf, J., and Murphy, R.C. (1990): *J. Clin. Invest.*, submitted.
9. Samuelsson, B. (1983): *Science*, 220:568-575.
10. Stene, D.O. and Murphy, R.C. (1988): *J. Biol. Chem.*, 263:2773-2778.

BIOSYNTHESIS AND METABOLISM OF LEUKOTRIENE B$_4$ BY RAT POLYMORPHONUCLEAR LEUKOCYTES

William S. Powell and Francine Gravelle

Endocrine Laboratory, Royal Victoria Hospital, 687 Pine Avenue West, Montreal, Quebec, Canada H3A 1A1

Leukotriene B$_4$ (LTB$_4$) is metabolized by polymorphonuclear leukocytes (PMNL) by three pathways, initiated by LTB$_4$ 20-hydroxylase (2), a 19-hydroxylase (4), and a combination of a 12-hydroxy dehydrogenase and a 10,11-reductase (6). Human PMNL metabolize LTB$_4$ principally to its 20-hydroxy derivative, which is further converted to 20-oxo (7) and omega-carboxy (1) metabolites by these cells. Porcine PMNL exhibit little LTB$_4$ omega-oxidation activity, and instead convert this substance to 10,11-dihydro-LTB$_4$ and 10,11-dihydro-12-oxo-LTB$_4$ (6).

RESULTS

Stimulation of carragenan-elicited rat pleural PMNL (9) with A23187 (5 µM) for 30 min resulted in the formation of a large number of products which absorbed in the UV at either 235 nm or 280 nm. Quantitation of these products by precolumn extraction/reversed phase-high pressure liquid chromatography (RP-HPLC) (3) using PGB$_2$ as an internal standard indicated that at this time the major products were 10,11-dihydro-LTB$_4$ > 5-HETE > 10,11-dihydro-12-oxo-LTB$_4$ > 19-hydroxy-LTB$_4$ > HHT > LTB$_4$. Further analysis of the 10,11-dihydro-LTB$_4$ by normal phase-HPLC revealed that the stereochemistry of the 12-hydroxyl group had been inverted in about 15 to 20% of this material, resulting in the formation of 12-epi-10,11-dihydro-LTB$_4$. We have previously shown that porcine PMNL can interconvert 10,11-dihydro-LTB$_4$, 12-epi-10,11-dihydro-LTB$_4$, and 12-oxo-10,11-dihydro-LTB$_4$ in a reversible manner (8). Although only small amounts of LTB$_4$ were detected after incubation of PMNL with A23187 for 30 min, LTB$_4$ was the major arachidonic acid metabolite formed after 5 min.

Identification of polar metabolites of arachidonic acid

In addition to 19-hydroxy-LTB$_4$ (**product 1**), which we had previously identified after incubating LTB$_4$ with rat PMNL, endogenous arachidonic acid was converted to at least 5 other polar metabolites absorbing at either 235 or 280 nm. All of these products were also formed after incubation of PMNL with LTB$_4$ (2 µM) for 30 min (Fig. 1). Products 1 (i.e. 19-hydroxy-LTB$_4$) and 3 exhibited

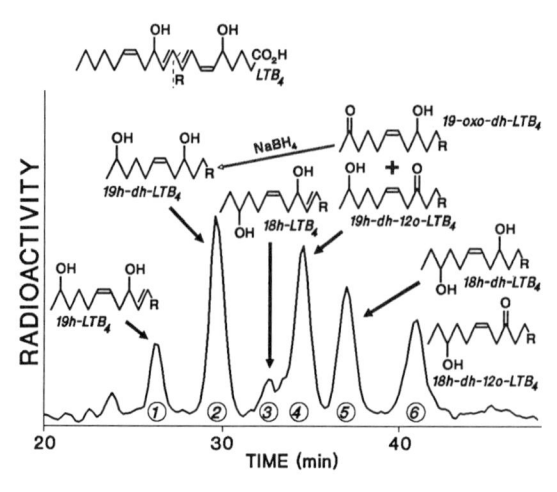

FIG. 1. RP-HPLC of the polar products formed after incubation of rat pleural PMNL (30 x 10^6 cells/ml) with LTB_4 (2 μM) for 30 min.

typical leukotriene UV spectra with absorption maxima at 261, 270, and 282 nm, whereas the remaining products exhibited absorption maxima at 230 nm, suggesting that one of the three conjugated double bonds of the substrate had been reduced.

The methyl ester, trimethylsilyl ether derivative of the major product (**product 2**) has a mass spectrum very similar to that of 10,11-dihydro-LTB_4, except that ions containing the omega end of the molecule were shifted upwards by 88 mass units, demonstrating the presence of a hydroxyl group in this region of the molecule. This hydroxyl group is clearly in the 19-position as indicated by the intense ion at m/z 117 (CH_3-CH=$^+OSiMe_3$), showing that this compound is identical to 19-hydroxy-10,11-dihydro-LTB_4.

Product 3 had a retention time very similar, but not identical, to that of 20-hydroxy-LTB_4. The mass spectrum of the methyl ester, trimethylsilyl ether derivative of this compound is very similar to that of 19-hydroxy-LTB_4 except that the intense ion at m/z 117 (CH_3-CH=$^+OSiMe_3$) in the latter was replaced by an ion at m/z 131 (CH_3-CH_2-CH=$^+OSiMe_3$), indicating that the omega-hydroxyl group is present at the 18-position instead of the 19-position. Thus product 3 is identical to 18-hydroxy-LTB_4.

The mass spectrum of the major component of **peak 4**, both before and after hydrogenation, indicated that an oxo group was present between carbons 13 and 20. Reduction of this compound with sodium borohyride (Fig. 1) resulted in the formation of a product which cochromatographed with 19-hydroxy-10,11-dihydro-LTB_4, suggesting that it compound is identical to 19-oxo-10,11-dihydro-LTB_4.

Peak 4 also contained a second component which has a mass spectrum similar to that of 10,11-dihydro-12-oxo-LTB_4, except that a hydroxyl group was present in the 19-position, as indicated by an intense ion at m/z 117. Peak 4 therefore also contains 19-hydroxy-10,11-dihydro-12-oxo-LTB_4.

The methyl ester, trimethylsilyl ether derivative of **product 5** has a mass spectrum similar to that of product 2, except that the intense ion at m/z 117 was replaced by an ion at m/z 131 (CH_3-CH_2-CH = $^+OSiMe_3$; base peak), indicating that a hydroxyl group was present in the 18-position, and that product 5 is 18-hydroxy-10,11-dihydro-LTB_4.

The mass spectrum of **product 6** is similar to that of 19-hydroxy-10,11-dihydro-12-oxo-LTB_4 except that the ion at m/z 117 was replaced by an ion at 131 (base peak), and there was an ion at M-29 due to the loss of an ethyl group from the omega end of the molecule. This indicates that product 6 is 18-hydroxy-10,11-dihydro-12-oxo-LTB_4.

Metabolism of arachidonic acid by elicited and peripheral PMNL

The experiments described above were all done with PMNL obtained 4 hours after intrapleural injection of carrageenan into rats. We also performed experiments in which arachidonic acid in the presence of A23187 was incubated with peripheral PMNL obtained from the blood (Fig. 2). The amounts of products formed by all of the enzymes involved in the biosynthesis and metabolism of LTB_4 were elevated in the elicited cells. 5-Lipoxygenase activity was about twice as high in the elicited cells, whereas the amounts of LTA hydrolase, 18-hydroxylase, and 19-hydroxylase products were about three times higher in these cells. The greatest difference was observed for 10,11-reductase products, which were about 8 times higher in the carrageenan-elicited cells. In contrast, nearly identical amounts of HHT were formed by elicited and peripheral PMNL (Fig. 2).

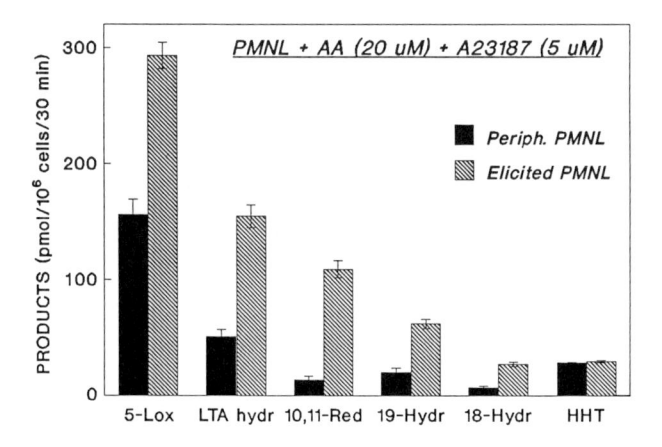

FIG. 2. The total amounts of metabolites formed by pathways involved in the biosynthesis and metabolism of LTB_4 by rat PMNL. PMNL obtained either from the blood (periph. PMNL) or the pleural cavity 4 h after injection of carrageenan (elicited PMNL) were incubated with arachidonic acid (20 µM) in the presence of A23187 (5 µM) for 30 min and the products analyzed by RP-HPLC. 5-Lox, 5-lipoxygenase; LTA hydr, LTA hydrolase; 10,11-red, 10,11-reductase; 19-hydr, 19-hydroxylase; 18-hydr, 18-hydroxylase; HHT, 12-hydroxy-5,8,10-heptadecatrienoic acid.

TABLE 1. *Major pathways for the metabolism of hydroxy-eicosanoids by PMNL.*

STRUCTURAL REQUIREMENTS	PATHWAY	SUBSTRATES	SPECIES
OH OH (on CO₂H chain)	20-hydroxylase	LTB_4 LTB_5 6-trans-LTB_4 12-epi-6-trans-LTB_4 12-epi-8-cis-6-trans-LTB_4 12-HETE	HUMAN
	19-hydroxylase	LTB_4 10,11-dh-LTB_4 10,11-dh-12o-LTB_4	RAT
	18-hydroxylase	LTB_4 10,11-dh-LTB_4 10,11-dh-12o-LTB_4	RAT
OH OH (on CO₂H chain)	10,11-reductase 12-dehydrogenase	LTB_4 LTB_5 6-trans-LTB_4 12-epi-6-trans-LTB_4 12-epi-8-cis-6-trans-LTB_4 12-HETE 13-HODE	PIG RAT
OH (on CO₂H chain, HO)	reductase-2 5-dehydrogenase	6-trans-LTB_4 12-epi-6-trans-LTB_4 12-epi-8-cis-6-trans-LTB_4	PIG HUMAN

DISCUSSION

The major metabolite of arachidonic acid formed after incubation of rat PMNL with A23187 is LTB_4. However, this substance is rapidly metabolized by these cells by 3 major pathways: (i) the 12-hydroxy dehydrogenase/10,11-reductase pathway, resulting in the formation of 10,11-dihydro-12-oxo-LTB_4 and 10,11-dihydro-LTB_4, (ii) the 19-hydroxylase pathway, and (iii) the 18-hydroxylase pathway (Table 1). Combination of the dehydrogenase/reductase pathway with the omega-hydroxylase pathways results in the formation of most of the polar metabolites shown in Fig. 1. In contrast to rat PMNL, human PMNL metabolize LTB_4 almost exclusively by the 20-hydroxylase pathway, which is not very significant in rat PMNL. Human PMNL also contain a dehydrogenase/reductase pathway which converts 6-trans isomers of LTB_4 (but not LTB_4 itself) to dihydro products via 5-oxo intermediates (5). Porcine PMNL also contain the latter pathway, as well as the 12-hydroxy dehydrogenase/10,11-reductase pathway, but exhibit very little omega-oxidation activity.

REFERENCES

1. Jubiz, W., Radmark, O, Malmsten, C., Hansson, G., Lindgren, J.A., Palmblad, J., Uden, A.-M., and Samuelsson, B. (1982) *J. Biol. Chem.* **257**: 6106-6110.
2. Lindgren, J.A., Hansson, G., and Samuelsson, B. (1981) *FEBS Lett.* **128**: 329-335.
3. Powell, W.S. (1987) *Anal. Biochem.* **164**: 117-131.
4. Powell, W.S. (1987) *Biochem. Biophys. Res. Commun.* **145**: 991-998.
5. Powell, W.S., and Gravelle, F., (1988) *J. Biol. Chem.* **263**: 2170-2177.
6. Powell, W.S., and Gravelle, F., (1989) *J. Biol. Chem.* **264**: 5364-5369.
7. Soberman, R.J., Sutyak, J.P., Okita, R.T., Wendelborn, D.F., Roberts, L.J., and Austen, K.F. (1988) *J. Biol. Chem.* **263**: 7996-8002.
8. Wainwright, S., Falck, C., Yadagiri, P. and Powell, W.S. (1990) *Biochemistry* **29**: 1180-1185.
9. Yue, T.L., Varma, D.R., and Powell, W.S. (1983) *Biochim. Biophys. Acta* **751**: 332-339.

THE CYTOCHROME P450 METABOLIC PATHWAY OF ARACHIDONIC ACID IN THE CORNEA

Michal Laniado Schwartzman, Karen L. Davis, Motonobu Nishimura, Nader G. Abraham and Robert C. Murphy

Departments of Pharmacology and Medicine, New York Medical College, Valhalla, New York and Department of Pediatrics, National Jewish Center, Denver, Colorado.

Cytochrome P450 (P450) represents a unique family of hemoproteins that serve as the terminal acceptor in the NADPH-dependent mixed function oxidase system which catalyzes the oxidative transformation of a large number of endogenous and exogenous substrates. It is comprised of three components: (i) P450 as the hemoprotein; (ii) a flavoprotein reductase [NADPH P450 (c) reductase]; (iii) phosphatidylcholine. P450 exists in multiple forms which differ in substrate specificity, positional specificity and stereospecificity (11). In the presence of NADPH and molecular oxygen it metabolizes arachidonic acid (AA) to several oxygenated metabolites including: 1) four regioisomeric epoxides (5,6; 8,9; 11,12; 14,15 EETs), which can be hydrolyzed by epoxide hydrolase to the corresponding diol derivatives (DHTs); 2) six regioisomeric cis-trans conjugated mono-hydroxy-eicosatetraenoic acids (HETEs); and 3) ω and ω-1 alcohols (6). Although the biological role of the third metabolic pathway of AA is just beginning to be understood, there is strong evidence that certain products will affect cellular functions. Recent studies have demonstrated that the EETs and their hydrolytic metabolites, DHTs, possess a wide range of biological activities. These include stimulation of peptide hormone release, inhibition of Na,K-ATPase, vasodilatation, mobilization of Ca^{+2} and inhibition of platelets aggregation (6). The ω and ω-1 alcohols of AA are also biologically active; 20-HETE is a potent vasoconstrictor (10) and 19-HETE is a stimulator of Na,K-ATPase activity (5). The biological effects together with the demonstration that some of these metabolites appear in urine and tissues (9) implicate a role for these compounds in physiological and pathophysiological processes.

P450 SYSTEM IN OCULAR TISSUES

The P450 system is present in several ocular tissues. Shichi et al. (20) demonstrated the existence of aryl hydrocarbon hydroxylase in bovine retina, lens, cornea, iris, retinal pigment epithelium (RPE) and ciliary body epithelium (CBE). The highest activity was found in the CBE and RPE, the two ocular tissues adjacent to rich blood supplies. Thus, the CBE and RPE are the site of metabolism and detoxification of drugs and chemicals that are carried to ocular tissues via the circulating blood. Our studies confirmed these findings of a high concentration of drug metabolizing enzymes in the CBE and RPE. We anticipated that where the P450-dependent monooxygenase activities were high, the metabolism of AA via this pathway would be high as well. However, we observed the opposite. The tissues that had the highest level of P450 and its components, CBE and RPE, had the lowest capability of metabolizing AA via P450 and exogenous AA was mainly converted into PGs (17). Thus, these two tissues are lacking (not expressing) the P450 species that catalyzes the conversion of AA into oxygenated metabolites. However, the corneal epithelium, which has low activity of the P450 drug metabolizing system and its components, possesses the highest activity of a P450 species capable of metabolizing AA to biologically active compounds (17). Such a specific P450 isozyme has been purified in our laboratory and designated as P450-AA epoxygenase (19). Western blot analysis of microsomal preparations from corneal epithelium with antibodies raised against human liver P450-AA epoxygenase clearly demonstrated the existence of a corneal protein that cross-reacted with antibodies to this isozyme (Figure 1).

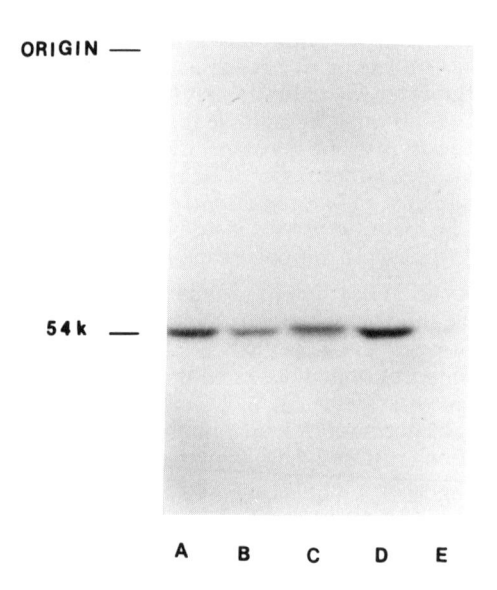

Figure 1: Western Blot Analysis of P450 Epoxygenase in Various Tissues. A-Human liver P450-AA epoxygenase, B-Rat liver, C-Rat kidney, D-Rabbit cornea, E-Rabbit heart.

The corneal epithelium metabolizes AA to PGs, thromboxane and prostacyclin (8) and following injury or addition of Ca^{+2} ionophore, 5-, 12(S)-HETE, LTB4 and LTC4 are generated (1). However, under certain conditions such as increased cofactor availability (altered redox state), AA may be directed to the P450 pathway in the corneal epithelium rather than to the cyclooxygenase and/or lipoxygenase pathways.

P450 ARACHIDONATE METABOLISM IN CORNEAL EPITHELIUM

Our studies over the past 3 years have uncovered a novel metabolic pathway for AA, the P450-dependent monooxygenase system, in the corneal epithelium of the human, rabbit and bovine eye. In broken cell preparations (homogenates or microsomes) this pathway is expressed upon addition of NADPH and molecular oxygen, whereas in intact tissue (cell suspension or culture and intact corneal epithelium) an appropriate stimulus is needed (vide infra). The formation of these metabolites is not inhibited by aspirin, indomethacin, BW755C or NDGA but is abolished by any intervention to the P450 system (inhibitors such as SKF-525A and carbon monoxide, and antibodies to P450-AA epoxygenase or P450 (c) reductase) (18). The P450-AA metabolites of the corneal epithelium include four major compounds initially designated according to their elution times on reverse-phase HPLC as compound A, B, C and D (18). The structure of two compounds, C and D, have been identified using the following paradigm: synthesis from AA in bovine corneal microsomes, isolation and purification to homogeneity, chemical modification and GC/MS analysis, chemical synthesis of the identified structure and its possible isomers, and comparison of the biological properties of the synthetic material to that derived from biological sources.

Biosynthesis and Biological Properties of Compound C

Compound C is 12(R)-hydroxy-5,8,10,14-eicosatetraenoic acid, **12(R)-HETE** (18). It is a potent inhibitor of partially purified Na,K-ATPase from different tissues (Table 1).

TABLE 1. Effect of 12(R)HETE and 12(S)HETE on ouabain-sensitive Na,K-ATPase[a]

Na,K-ATPase activity (µmol Pi/hr/mg)

Source	Vehicle	12(R)HETE	12(S)HETE
Rat renal cortex	91.9±10.2	39.4±4.7*	91.3±8.7
Rat heart ventricle	22.7±3.5	10.0±2.3*	20.5±1.9
Bovine corneal epithelium	24.5±2.9	11.6±2.4*	23.7±4.6

[a]Test compounds (10^{-6}M) were added to the assay mixture 10 min before starting the reaction with the addition of ATP (15). Values are means±SE, n=6-24. *p<0.005 from the vehicle control.

Its inhibitory effect is stereospecific (12(S)HETE is inactive) and exclusive for Na,K-ATPase, since it lacked an effect on other ATPases. However, the mechanism by which 12(R)HETE inhibits Na,K-ATPase and its effectiveness in in vivo situations remains uncertain. Masferrer and Mullane (12) demonstrated that 12(R)HETE inhibited K+-induced relaxation of the rabbit aorta; the relaxant response to [K+], following exposure to zero K+ buffer is considered a functional measure of the electrogenic pumping of Na+ and K+, and can be attenuated by ouabain (23). Furthermore, 12(R)HETE has been shown to increase urine volume and electrolyte excretion in the isolated perfused rat kidney (22); effects consistent with inhibition of Na,K-ATPase activity. Evidence for a link between pump inhibition by 12(R)HETE and the function of specialized transport epithelia has also been found in the cornea. Infusion of 12(R)HETE into the endothelial side of the isolated perfused rabbit cornea produced a dose-dependent increase in corneal thickness, an effect characteristic of ouabain and other inhibitors of corneal endothelial Na,K-ATPase activity (3). An inhibitor of Na,K-ATPase may have fundamental importance in ocular-transporting epithelial functions that rely on this pump activity. Deturgescence of the cornea mediated by the corneal endothelium and secretion of aqueous humor by the ciliary body are examples of basic physiological functions which are dependent upon metabolic pumps and are readily inhibited by ouabain. If indeed the P450 products function in the modulation of aqueous humor secretion, then manipulation of the pathway might be useful in the management of ocular hypertension (glaucoma). Ocular hypertension can be monitored by measuring the pressure in the anterior chamber of the eye (IOP). In measuring the effect of topically applied 12(R)HETE on IOP of rabbit eyes we clearly demonstrated that a low dose (0.5µg) of 12(R)HETE lowers IOP by as much as 7 mmHg. Furthermore, this effect is maintained for several days, without causing ocular side effects such as conjunctival hyperemia, aqueous flare and miosis (14). This investigation did not examine the mechanism by which 12(R)HETE reduces IOP. However, being a potent inhibitor of Na,K-ATPase activity suggests that 12(R)HETE mediates a decrease in the rate of aqueous humor secretion via a possible inhibition of the ciliary epithelial Na,K-ATPase (21).

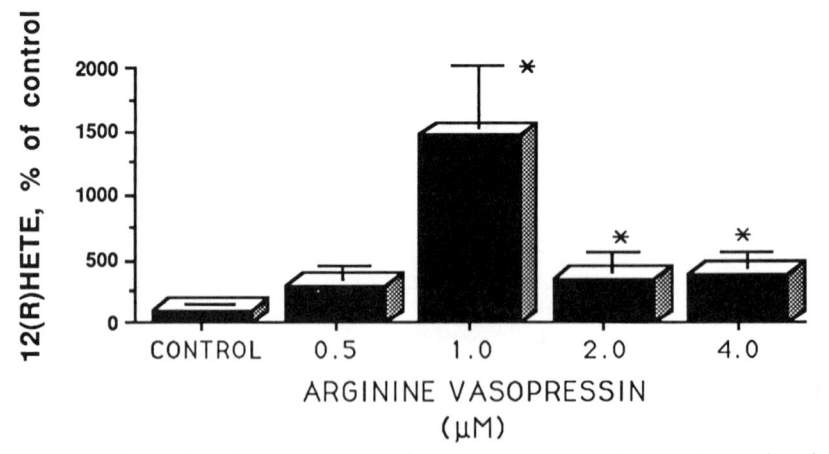

Figure 2: Effect of arginine vasopressin (AVP) on 12(R)HETE formation in corneal epithelial sheets.

The formation of 12(R)HETE can be regulated by physiological and pathophysiological interventions. Incubation of 14C-AA-labeled corneal epithelial sheets with arginine vasopressin (AVP), a hormone known to lower IOP, resulted in the formation of labeled 12(R)HETE suggesting its production from endogenous AA. The maximal response was obtained with 1µM AVP and represents a 15-fold increase in 12(R)HETE formation compared with that of control tissue (Figure 2). Digitonin, a detergent which causes a mild keratitis of the cornea also stimulated the release of endogenous 12(R)HETE.

Our findings, including enantiomer specific biological and enzymatic effects, strongly suggest that endogenous levels of 12(R)HETE may serve a variety of physiological and/or pathological functions in vivo. 12(R)HETE derived from one or more ocular tissues may be a potent endogenous modulator of IOP. Further studies are needed to elucidate the mechanism of 12(R)HETE effects on Na,K-ATPase and IOP, as well as to determine the therapeutic potential of this novel compound.

Biosynthesis and Biological Properties of Compound D

Compound D is 12(R)-hydroxy-5,8,14-eicosatrienoic acid, **12(R)-DH-HETE** (16). Although, its structure is similar to that of 12(R)HETE (it lacks the 11,12 double bond), its biological properties are much different. 12(R)DH-HETE dilates blood vessels including the conjunctival capillaries with a potency 4-8 times greater than acetylcholine (13). In doses as low as 5 ng, it increases the aqueous humor protein concentration by 7 fold indicating that it is at least 20-fold more potent than PGE2 in producing the breakdown of the blood-aqueous barrier (13). These properties suggest that it is a pro-inflammatory agent. Several studies have indicated that corneal vascularization is usually a manifestation of a chronic inflammatory response, and that leukocytic infiltration of the corneal stroma precedes and accompanies the corneal vascularization. 12(R)DH-HETE (0.5 µg) induced an extensive neovascularization within 4 days following slow release from an inert polymer implant. As the implant was depleted of this compound, blood flow through the new vessels ceased, suggesting that the presence of functioning new vessels in the cornea may be dependent on the presence of 12(R)DH-HETE (13). The direct chemotactic property of this compound was tested in human neutrophils and found to be more potent but less efficacious than LTB4. Thus, 12(R)DH-HETE may be an indirect angiogenic factor, i.e. a molecule which stimulates the release of a primary angiogenic factor from other cells present in the biological system (7). The angiogenic effect of 12(R)DH-HETE could be due to its ability to attract neutrophils, lymphocytes or macrophages into the cornea. These blood elements may alone, or in combination with 12(R)DH-HETE, elicit neovascularization. However, we can not exclude the possibility that 12(R)DH-HETE is a direct angiogenic factor as well, i.e., a molecule which acts primarily on endothelial cells. Indeed, in recent experiments, we found that 12(R)DH-HETE (10^{-10}M) increases ^{3}H-thymidine incorporation into the DNA of cultured bovine pulmonary artery endothelial cells by 2-3 fold. The latter finding suggests that this compound is mitogenic to endothelial cells and strengthens its possible direct role in angiogenesis. Eliason and Elliott (4) recently demonstrated that corneal epithelial homogenates contain heat stable factor(s) which stimulate the proliferation of endothelial cells in vitro and vascularization of the cornea in vivo. These authors concluded that the corneal epithelium is the source of a secreted stimulant(s) for the growth of vascular endothelial cells. 12(R)DH-HETE, which is an endogenous metabolite of AA in the corneal epithelium, has the characteristics of such a factor; it not only possesses pro-inflammatory properties, but also has very potent angiogenic capabilities. Thus, 12(R)DH-HETE may qualify as that intrinsic corneal angiogenic factor and may, in association with other inflammatory mediators, account for the growth of new vessels in the cornea which frequently appears in chronic inflammation or in the reparative stages of an acute injury.

Experiments to mimic acute and chronic inflammation were performed by placing a gas-impermeable contact lens on the rabbit eye and measuring endogenous 12(R)DH-HETE formation. Hypoxic and inflamed corneas had a much higher capacity of generating this compound. In fact, a 27-fold increase in 12(R)DH-HETE formation over the untreated corneas was noted with a corresponding progression of the inflammatory response: from edema and vasodilation (red eye) to massive neovascularization of the avascular cornea.

THE BIOSYNTHETIC PATHWAY OF 12(R)HETE AND 12(R)DH-HETE

The metabolites described herein are structurally similar except for the absolute stereochemistry at C-12 and the presence of a saturated bond at C-10,11. Designation of the stereochemistry of the hydroxy group at C-12 for both 12(R)HETE and 12(R)DH-HETE is a consequence of the nomenclature priority rules and, in fact, these metabolites have opposite absolute stereochemistries.

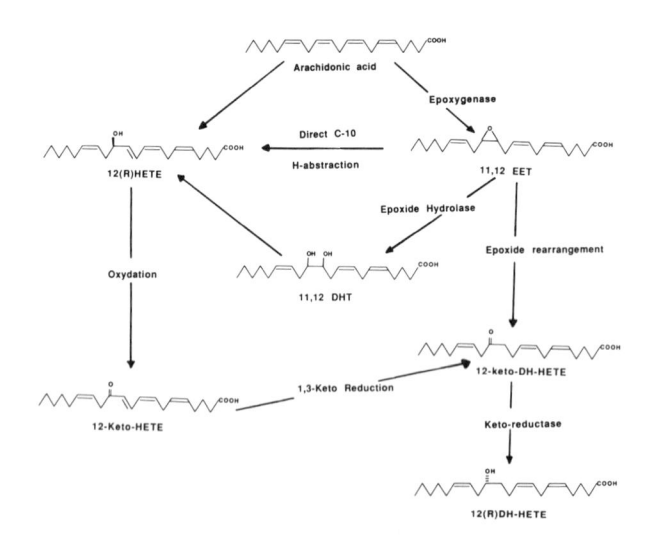

Figure 3: Possible enzymatic steps for the formation of 12(R)HETE and 12(R)DH-HETE.

The possible biochemical/enzymatic steps for the formation of both compounds in the cornea are presented in Figure 3. The action of corneal microsomal P450 could result in the direct formation of 12(R)HETE from AA by a lipoxygenase-like reaction without an intermediate epoxide (2). Alternatively, 11,12EET formed by P450 epoxygenase could serve as a common intermediate for the formation of both 12(R)HETE and 12(R)DH-HETE. 12(R)HETE can be obtained by either removal of a water molecule from the diol derivative of 11,12EET or by a direct hydrogen abstraction at C-10 of 11,12EET. The formation of 12(R)DH-HETE would require the activity of a keto-reductase and the formation of a keto intermediate. Corneal epithelial microsomes are able to generate 12(R)DH-HETE from 12(R)HETE in the presence of both NAD/NADPH and a 12-keto-DH-HETE intermediate (HPLC) can be detected. The keto intermediate can also be detected when AA is incubated with corneal microsomes in the presence of these cofactors.

In summary, our studies over the past three years clearly show that in the cornea, and possibly in other ocular tissues, AA derivatives other than the classical PGs or the more recently discovered LTs can be formed, and that at least some of the AA metabolites produced via the P450 system have potent biological activities. In fact, two of these metabolites, 12(R)HETE and 12(R)DH-HETE appear to be of greater potency than classical PGs with respect to their effect on active ion transport systems, vasodilatation, or the breakdown of the blood-aqueous barrier. The fact that 12(R)HETE was found to be a potent inhibitor of Na,K-ATPase activity without appreciable vascular effects or effects on barrier permeability, while the other compound 12(R)DH-HETE was found to have a potent effect on the last two parameters without an influence on the first, suggests that products of the P450 system are capable of inducing or modulating highly specific cellular functions.

REFERENCES

1. Bazan, H.E.P., Birkle, D.L., Beuerman, R.W., Bazan, N.G. (1985): *Cur. Eye. Res.* 4:175-179.
2. Capdevila, J., Yadagiri, S., Manna, S., Falck, J.R. (1986):*Biochem. Biophys. Res. Commun.*, 141:1007-10011.
3. Edelhauser H.F., Geroski, D.H., Woods,W., Hollet, G. and Schwartzman, M.L. (1990): *Invest. Ophthalmol. Vis.* Sci. 31:474.
4. Eliason, A.J., Elliot, J.P. (1987): *Invest. Ophthalmol. Vis. Sci.* 28:1963-1969.
5. Escalante, B, Falck, J.R., Yadagiri, P., Sun, L. and Schwartzman, M.L. (1988): *Biochem. Biophys. Res. Comm.* 152:1259-1274.
6. Fitzpatrick, F.A. and Murphy, R.C. (1989): *Pharmacol. Rev.* 40:229-241 and references therein.
7. Folkman, J, and Klagsbum M. (1987): *Science* 235:442-447.
8. Kulkarni, P.S., Fleisher, L., Srinivanan, B.D. (1984): *Cur. Eye. Res.* 3:447-452.
9. Karara, A. Dishman, E., Blair, I., Falck, J.R. and Capdevila, J.H. (1989): *J. Biol. Chem.* 264:19822-19827.

10. Laniado Schwartzman, M., Falck, J.R., Yadagiri, P. and Escalante, B. (1989): *J. Biol Chem.* 264:11658-11662
11. Lu, A.Y. H. and West, S.B. (1980): *Pharmacol. Rev.* , 31:277-295.
12. Masferrer, J.L., Mullane, K.M. (1988): *Eur. J. Pharmacol.* , 151:487-490.
13. Masferrer, J., Murphy, R.C., Pagano, P.J., Dunn, M.W. and Schwartzman, M.L.(1989) *Invest. Ophthalmol. Vis. Sci.*30:454-460.
14. Masferrer, J.L., Dunn, M.W. and Laniado Schwartzman, M. (1990): *Invest. Ophthalmol. Vis. Sci.* 31:535-539.
15. Masferrer, J.L., Rios, A.P. and Schwartzman, M.L. (1989) *Biochem. Pharmacol.* In press.
16. Murphy, R.C., Falck, J.R., Lumin, S., Yadagiri, P., Zirrolli, J.A., Balazy, M., Masferrer, J.L., Abraham, N.G. and Schwartzman, M.L. (1988): *J. Biol. Chem.* 263:17197-17202.
17. Schwartzman, M.L., Masferrer, J., Dunn, M.W., McGiff, J.C. and Abraham, N.G. (1987) *Cur. Eye Res.* 6:623-629.
18. Schwartzman, M.L., Masferrer, J., Abraham, N.G., McGiff, J.C. and Murphy, R.C. (1987): *Proc. Natl. Acad. Sci. USA,* 84:8125-8129.
19. Schwartzman, M.L., Davis, K.L., McGiff, J.C., Levere, R.D. and Abraham, N.G. (1988): *J. Biol. Chem.* 263:2536-2542.
20. Shichi, H., Atlas, S.A. & Nebert, W. (1975): *Exp. Eye Res.* 21:557-567.
21. Socci, R.R, Bhattacherjee, P. and Delamere, N. (1989): *Invest. Ophthalmol. Vis. Sci.* 30 (Suppl): 447, 1989.
22. Takahashi, K., Capdevila, J., Falck, J.R., Jacobson, H.B., Badr, J.F.(1988) *FASEB J.* 2:5620.
23. Webb, R.C. and Bohr, D.F. (1987): *Blood Vessels* . 15:198-207.

BIOSYNTHESIS OF P450 PRODUCTS OF ARACHIDONIC ACID IN HUMANS: INCREASED FORMATION IN CARDIOVASCULAR DISEASE

Francesca Catella, John Lawson, Greg Braden, Desmond J. Fitzgerald, Elizabeth Shipp and Garret A. FitzGerald.

The Division of Clinical Pharmacology, Vanderbilt University, Nashville, Tennessee 37232, USA.

INTRODUCTION.

The recognition of the biological properties of P450-derived metabolites of arachidonic acid (1) has excited much interest in their possible role in human disease. To facilitate our ability to address this hypothesis we developed sensitive and specific quantitative assays for several epoxyeicosatrienoic acids (EETs) and their dihydroxy derivatives (DHETs) in human urine.

METHODS.

To assess the biosynthesis of EETs in human urine we synthesized deuterated internal standards for the 8,9-, 11,12- and 14,15- regioisomers and developed an extraction procedure based on that reported by Turk et al (2). This reduced any EETs present to DHETs which were then derivatized as their pentafluorobenzyl ester, trimethylsilyl (TMS) ether derivatives for quantitation by selected ion monitoring employing capillary gas chromatography negative ion, chemical ionization mass spectrometry.

This approach (3) resulted in clearly defined peaks corresponding to the authentic material and the internal standard respectively (Figure 1). Delayed analysis of the sample or the presence of the antioxidant (Fig 2) did not alter the values measured, making the contribution of ex vivo autoxidation of arachidonic acid in urine to the measured DHETs unlikely.

Address correspondence to Dr. FitzGerald.

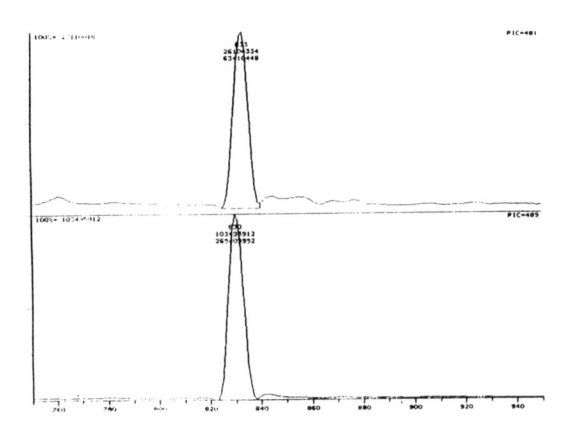

Figure 1. Representative selected ion monitoring traces of the pentafluorbenzyl ester, bis TMS derivative of 14,15-DHET. The peak corresponding to the endogenous material is shown in the upper panel monitoring, mass/charge (m/z) 481 and that corresponding to the octadeuterated internal standard, monitored at m/z 489 in the lower panel.

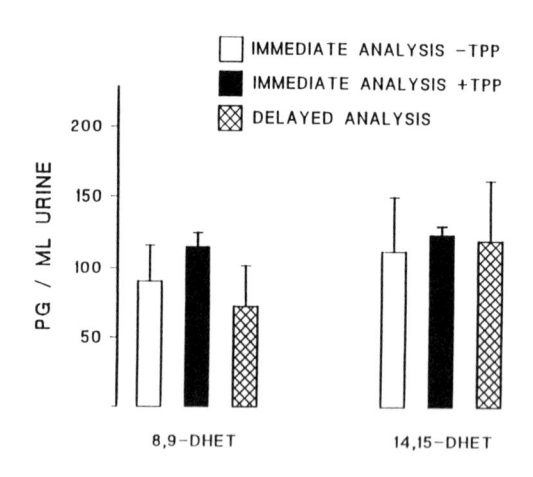

Figure 2. Quantitative analysis of 8,9- and 14,15-DHET in human urine. No significant differences were observed when the samples were collected in the absence (□) or presence (■) of the antioxidant triphenylphosphine (TPP) or when analysis of samples without the antioxidant was delayed while they stood at room temperature for 24 hours (▨).

RESULTS AND DISCUSSION.

Given the in vitro effects of EETs and DHETs on renal tubular ion flux, vascular tone and platelet function we investigated their biosynthesis in normal pregnancy and in patients with pregnancy induced hypertension, a disease characterized by alterations in volume homeostasis, vascular tone and platelet function.

Excretion of 8,9- but not 11,12- or 14,15-DHET was increased in normal pregnancy. By contrast, there was a further increase in excretion of 11,12- and 14,15-DHET in patients with pregnancy induced hypertension. This was particularly marked in the case of the latter isomer, which has been tentatively identified as the major P450 product of arachidonic acid in human reproductive tissues (4).

High concentrations of EETs inhibit platelet function. While some are cyclooxygenase inhibitors, 14,15-EET has a differential effect on aggregation induced by the prostaglandin endoperoxide analog, U 46619, which it inhibits and thrombin, which it does not (1). We found that 14,15 - EET does not compete at the binding site for U 46619 in human platelets. Stimulation of adenylate cyclase in platelets activates a specific phosphodiesterase which can confound attempts to detect a rise in cyclic AMP (5). In the presence of the phosphodiesterase inhibitor, IBMX, we found that 14,15 - EET caused a small (roughly 20%), but reproducible maximal increment in cyclic AMP. To assess the functional importance of this increment, we characterized the dose response relationship between the diterpine analog, forskolin and cyclic AMP in human platelets and between forskolin and the aggregation response to U 46619 and thrombin. Pretreatment of platelets with forskolin sufficient to increase cyclic AMP by 20% inhibited aggregation induced by U 46619. Thrombin required much greater increments in cyclic AMP to be inhibited. Thus, cyclic AMP may contribute to the inhibitory effects of 14,15-EET on platelet function.

Unstable angina is a syndrome of platelet activation in which biosynthesis of the predominantly platelet-and vascular derived eicosanoids, thromboxane (Tx) A_2 and prostacyclin (PGI_2), respectively, is increased. Similarly, coronary angioplasty is a marked, albeit transient, stimulus to formation of these eicosanoids. We found that excretion of 11,12- and 14,15- DHET is increased in patients with unstable coronary disease compared with age and sex matched controls and that there is a further marked increase in DHET excretion coinciding with coronary angioplasty.

The origin of EETs and DHETs in human urine remains to be defined. It seems likely that at least under physiological circumstances, the kidney is a major source of these compounds in urine. Thus, administration of [^{3}H]-14,15-EET to dogs resulted in a marked increase in its DHET in plasma but negligible radioactivity was recovered in urine. Whether the increase in urinary DHETs which we observed during coronary angioplasty resulted from renal production in response to the angiographic dye load or from other tissue sources remains to be determined.

ACKNOWLEDGEMENTS

Supported by grants from the National Institutes of Health(HL 30400 and GM 15431) and Daiichi Seiyaku. Dr. Catella held a Faculty Development Award from the Pharmaceutical Manufacturers' Award Foundation. Dr. FitzGerald is an Established Investigator of the American Heart Association and the William Stokes Professor of Experimental Therapeutics.

REFERENCES.

1. Fitzpatrick F. and Murphy R. (1989) Pharm Rev 40:229-241.

2. Turk J., Wolf B.A., Comens P.G., Colca J., Jakshik B. and McDaniel M.L. (1985) Biochim Biophys Acta 835:1-17.

3. Catella F., Lawson J.A., Fitzgerald D.J. and FitzGerald G.A. (1990) Proc Natl Acad Sci (USA) in press.

4. Patel L., Sullivan M.H.F. and Elder M.G. (1989) Prostaglandins 38: 615-624.

5. Grant, P.G., Mannarino, A.F., Colman, R.W. (1988) Proc. Natl. Acad. Sci. USA. 85: 9071-9075.

A NOVEL ARACHIDONIC ACID 18(R)-HYDROXYLASE AND EICOSAPENTAENOIC ACID W3-EPOXYGENASE OF SEMINAL VESICLES

Ernst H. Oliw

Department of Pharmacology,
Uppsala Biomedicinska Centrum,
Box 591, S-751 24 Uppsala, Sweden

Seminal fluids of primates and sheep contain prostaglandins (PGs) and cytochrome P-450 (P-450) metabolites of PGs. PGE_1 and PGE_2 are metabolized to 19(R)-hydroxy-PGE_1 and 19(R)-hydroxy-PGE_2 by P-450 of primate seminal vesicles (7). The capacity to hydroxylate PGE, as judged from the PGE_1/19-hydroxy-PGE_1 and PGE_2/19-hydroxy-PGE_2 ratios of seminal fluid, varies considerably between different men (about 23% are slow and 77% are rapid hydroxylators (6)). P-450 enzymes of genital glands and endocrine organs are often substrate and product specific in contrast to many hepatic P-450 (1,4,5). It therefore seemed of interest to determine whether polyunsaturated fatty acids (PUFAs) could be metabolized to tissue specific metabolites by P-450 of genital glands. The microsomal fractions of seminal vesicles of the cynomolgus monkey (Macaca fascicularis) were found to contain a P-450 with a unique w3-hydroxylase and w3-epoxygenase activity (3).

ARACHIDONIC ACID 18(R)-HYDROXYLASE

In the presence of NADPH, $[^{14}C]$ arachidonic acid (20:4) was converted by microsomes of seminal vesicles to PGs (about 50% of recovered radioactivity) and to 18(R)-hydroxy-5,8,11,14-eicosatetraenoic acid (18(R)-HETE; about 13%). The latter was identified by capillary GC-MS and by comparison with authentic material, which was obtained from 20:4 by fungal biosynthesis (Gaeumannomyces graminis (3,10)). The seminal biosynthesis of 18(R)-HETE was further investigated in the presence of diclofenac sodium, which completely inhibited the PG biosynthesis.

The biosynthesis of 18(R)-HETE required NADPH and it was only partly supported by NADH. The biosynthesis was reduced by well-known P-450 inhibitors (proadifen and CO). Significant biosynthesis of any other monooxygenase metabolites of 20:4 could not be detected. Finally, results from an incubation under an atmosphere of oxygen-18 showed that the hydroxyl oxygen of 18-HETE was derived from the atmosphere. These results suggested that 18(R)-HETE was formed by a P-450 (designated P-450$_{w3}$) of seminal vesicles (3).

The geometry of the hydroxyl of 18-HETE methyl ester was determined by capillary GC-MS analysis of diastereoisomeric 2(S)-phenylpropionic acid derivatives of the monodeuterated 18(R,S)-HETE standard and of the seminal metabolite (2,3). The analysis showed that the seminal 18-HETE mainly consisted of the 18(R) enantiomer (about 95%). The fungal 18-HETE metabolite was also almost optically pure and it had the same geometrical configuration. Fungal biosynthesis could thus be used to generate 18(R)-HETE in mg amounts for biological studies.

18(R)-HETE contracted the guinea pig lung strip and relaxed isolated guinea pig arteries (Oliw and Dahlén, unpublished). These effects might be due to direct actions on the smooth muscle cells, since 18(R)-HETE is only slowly metabolized to 18-hydroxy-PGs by cyclooxygenase (10). A structurally related compound, 19(R)-HETE, was also biologically active in these test systems. It will therefore be of interest to determine whether 18(R)-HETE exerts any specific biological actions, e.g. in reproduction.

Some other ^{14}C-labeled fatty acids were also investigated as substrates of P-450$_{w3}$ and/or related microsomal enzyme(s). Stearic acid was not metabolized, while linoleic acid (18:2) was monohydroxylated at the w3 position (80%) or at the w2 position (20%). 20:4 was thus metabolized with greater product specificity than 18:2.

Microsomes of monkey liver, renal cortex and lung were also investigated for arachidonic acid 18(R)-hydroxylase, but significant amounts of the enzyme could not be detected. Hepatic microsomes metabolized 20:4 extensively to epoxides/diols and renal cortical microsomes converted 20:4 to 20-HETE and to 12(S)-HETE.

W3-EPOXIDATION OF EICOSAPENTAENOIC ACID

Incubation of ^{14}C-labeled eicosapentaenoic acid (20:5) with microsomes of monkey seminal vesicles, NADPH and diclofenac yielded a major polar product, which was purified by RP-HPLC and identified as 17,18-

dihydroxy-5,8,11,14-eicosatetraenoic acid by GC-MS (3). Other monooxygenase metabolites of 20:5 could not be detected. The 17,18-diol was also synthesized from 20:5 by the fungus G. graminis. It seemed likely in both cases that 17,18-dihydroxy-5,8,11,14-eicosatetraenoic acid was formed by enzymatic hydrolysis of 17(18)epoxy-5,8,11,14-eicosatetraenoic acid. This epoxide could be isolated with help of an epoxide hydrolase inhibitor, 1(2)epoxy-3,3,3-trichloropropane (TCPO; (8)).

Incubation of [^{14}C]20:5 with seminal microsomes, NADPH, diclofenac and TCPO yielded little 17,18-dihydroxyeicosatetraenoic acid as judged from RP-HPLC, but large amounts of a considerably less polar metabolite. This metabolite was most likely the epoxide since it had the same elution volume as the authentic 17(18)epoxide of 20:5 on RP-HPLC and since it was only formed in small amounts without TCPO. This inhibitor thus increased the epoxide/diol ratio about 14 times (cf. Fig. 1).

Two other ^{14}C-labeled fatty acids of the n-3 series, linolenic acid (18:3) and docosahexaenoic acid (22:6), were also investigated as substrates of P-450$_{w3}$. 18:3 was metabolized to 15,16-dihydroxy-9,12-octadecadienoic acid (chromatogram in Fig. 1A), while the 15(16)epoxide could be isolated in the presence of TCPO (Fig. 1B). This biological product had the elution volume as authentic 15(16)epoxy-9,12-octadecadienoic acid on RP-HPLC. As shown in Fig. 1, seminal microsomes also metabolized 18:3 to a metabolite (marked II in Fig. 1), which eluted between the diol and the epoxide on RP-HPLC. This product has not yet been fully characterized, but it required NADPH for biosynthesis and it was not inhibited by TCPO. In contrast, 22:6 was only slowly metabolized by seminal microsomes and NADPH to one major product, which was identified as 19,20-dihydroxy-4,7,10,13,16-docosapentaenoic acid. The mass spectra of the dihydroxy metabolites of 18:3 and 22:6 were identical with published mass spectra (9).

The w3-epoxygenation of 20:5 and the 18(R)-hydroxylation of 20:4 were both inhibited by proadifen and by CO in a parallel fashion (3). The question whether w3-epoxidation of n-3 fatty acids and w3-hydroxylation of n-6 fatty acids are catalyzed by one enzyme, which seems likely, or by two different ones can presumably not be settled until P-450$_{w3}$ has been purified.

n-3 PUFAs are of increasing importance in health and disease. It will therefore be interesting to investigate the tissue and species distribution of P-450$_{w3}$ and possible biological actions of w3-epoxides.

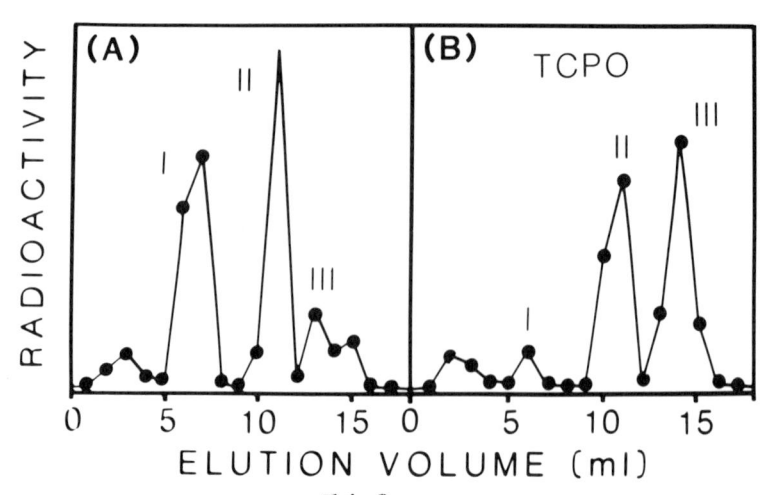

FIG. 1. Metabolism of [^{14}C]18:3 by microsomes of monkey seminal vesicles. A, RP-HPLC of metabolites (control). B, as in A but in the presence of 2 mM TCPO, an epoxide hydrolase inhibitor. Peak I in A marks 15,16-dihydroxy-9,12-octadecadienoic acid, peak III in B marks 15(16)epoxy-9,12-octadecadienoic acid.

ACKNOWLEDGMENTS

Supported by MFR (grant 06523). I wish to thank Dr. M. Hamberg for generous help and advice.

REFERENCES

1. Fitzpatrick, F.A. and Murphy, R.C. (1989): Pharmacol. Rev., 40:229-241.
2. Hammarström, S. and Hamberg, M. (1973): Anal. Biochem., 52:169-179.
3. Oliw, E.H. (1989): J. Biol. Chem., 264:17845-17853.
4. Oliw, E.H. (1989): Biochim. Biophys. Acta, 1001:107-110.
5. Oliw, E.H. and Hamberg, M. (1986): Biochim. Biophys. Acta, 879:113-119
6. Oliw, E.H. and Johnsen, O. (1988): Biochim. Biophys. Acta, 963:295-301
7. Oliw, E.H., Kinn, A-C and Kvist, U. (1988): J. Biol. Chem., 263:7222-7227.
8. Oliw, E.H., Oates, J.A. and Guengerich, F.P. (1982) J. Biol. Chem., 257:3771-3781.
9. Pace-Asciak, C.R. (1989): Adv. Prostaglandin, Thromboxane Leukotriene Res., 18:1-565.
10. Sih, C.J., Ambrus, G., Foss, P. and Lai, C.J. (1969): J. Am. Chem. Soc., 91:3685-3687.

BRAIN SYNTHESIS AND CEREBROVASCULAR ACTION OF CYTOCHROME P-450 / MONOOXYGENASE METABOLITES OF ARACHIDONIC ACID

E. F. Ellis, S. C. Amruthesh, R. J. Police and L. M. Yancey

Department of Pharmacology and Toxicology,
Medical College of Virginia,
Richmond, Virginia 23298 USA

We and others have previously reported that brain metabolizes arachidonic acid (AA) via the cyclooxygenase and lipoxygenase pathways. However it is presently unknown whether whole brain metabolizes AA by the NADPH-dependent cytochrome P-450 / monooxygenase pathway. The purpose of this investigation was to examine whether this pathway exists in brain and if so whether the metabolites are vasoactive on the cerebral microcirculation. Our results indicate that 5,6-epoxyeicosatrienoic acid (5,6-EET) is formed and that it causes dilation of in vivo cerebral arterioles via its metabolism by cyclooxygenase and production of dilator oxygen free radicals.

METHODS

Mouse brains were perfused in situ, removed and slices incubated in 20 ml of Krebs-Ringer bicarbonate containing 0.2 µCi/ml ^{3}H-AA and 16 µg/ml unlabeled AA for 20 min. The buffer was extracted with ethyl acetate, the extract washed with water and then evaporated. The sample was then redissolved in ethanol and injected onto a C_{18} reverse-phase Radialpak A HPLC system. Using a programmable gradient wherein the concentration of methanol was increased in steps, prostaglandins, HETEs, leukotrienes and EETs were separated from arachidonic acid in a 120 min HPLC program. Various radioactive peaks were identified by radiolabeled standards or by GC/MS.

Anesthetized New Zealand White rabbits were used to study the effect of AA metabolites on cerebral arteriolar diameter using the acute cranial window technique and in vivo microscopy as previously described (2). Blood pressure was monitored and blood gases were controlled by regulation of the ventilator rate and volume. A round metal cranial window was implanted on the midline just caudal to the suture connecting the frontal and parietal bones. Two openings in the cranial window allowed for filling the space under the cranial window with test solutions. Two to four vessels were studied in each animal using a Vickers image-splitting device which enables the precise measurement of arteriolar diameter. Various compounds and peaks synthesized by the mouse brain were diluted in artificial CSF and their effects on diameter were examined. In addition, the effects of authentic EETs (Biomol, Plymouth Meeting, PA) were examined. In some experiments we also analyzed by RIA (Advanced Magnetics, Cambridge, MA) the CSF effluent from under the cranial window following the application of various EETs in order to determine whether the EETs stimulated formation of PGs by the cortical brain tissue.

RESULTS

Table 1 shows the average distribution of radioactivity obtained by HPLC analysis. While several of the peaks co-chromatographed with authentic prostaglandin standards and were identified as such using GC/MS, a number of the peaks did not chromatograph with known products. We especially concentrated on peak X, which co-chromatographs with radiolabeled authentic 5,6-EET. Assuming that peak X was 5,6-EET, it was converted to the respective DHET, derivatized and analyzed by GC/MS. Figure 1 shows the total ion current and the mass fragmentogram obtained by GC/MS analysis of peak X and is consistent with peak X being 5,6-EET.

In order to examine the vasoactivity of the various compounds formed by mouse brain selected peaks including X, V and III were dried with nitrogen and redissolved in acetone and placed in artificial CSF. Application of the vehicle had no effect on diameter however peak X produced transient vasodilation of the cerebral arterioles (figure 2A). Other metabolites including metabolites III and V had little vasoactivity. In this same series of experiments we also examined the effect of authentic 5,6-EET. We found that both authentic 5,6-EET and compound X produced identical patterns of transient vasodilation.

In another series of experiments, we compared the effects of the four synthetic EETs (figure 2B) and found that of these four EETs 5,6-EET was the most vasoactive, 8,9-EET had less vasoactivity and 11,12- and 14,15-EET were virtually inactive. Since it is known that 5,6-EET can be metabolized by

Table 1. Percentage distribution of products formed from [^{3}H]-AA by blood-free mouse brain slices.[a]

Peak number	HPLC retention (min)	% Radioactivity
I	9.5	3.0 ± 0.3
II (PGs and TxB$_2$)	22.2	4.7 ± 1.1
III	37.8	3.1 ± 1.0
IV (LTB$_4$)	43.7	1.2 ± 0.2
V	48.3	2.2 ± 0.2
VI	53.6	1.6 ± 0.2
VII (15-HETE)	59.4	1.6 ± 0.0
VIII (12-HETE)	67.3	3.7 ± 0.3
IX (5-HETE)	74.9	1.6 ± 0.2
X	85.0	2.3 ± 0.2
AA	111.8	75.0 ± 3.1

[a]Based on their HPLC retention time, GC retention time and mass spectra assignment of the following previously reported brain metabolites was made: II (6-keto-PGF$_{1\alpha}$, TxB$_2$, PGD$_2$, PGE$_2$ and PGF$_{2\alpha}$); IV (LTB$_4$); VII (15-HETE); VIII (12-HETE) and IX (5-HETE). Percent radioactivity values are mean ± SEM of 6 experiments.

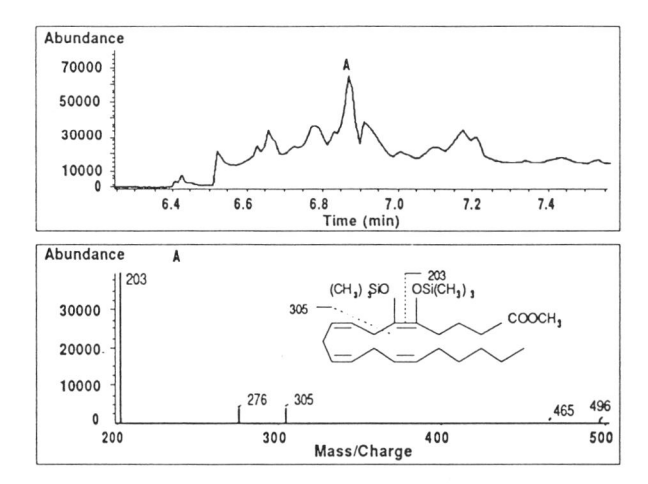

Figure 1. Mass Fragmentogram Obtained by Gas Chromatographic - Mass Spectrometric Analysis of Peak X

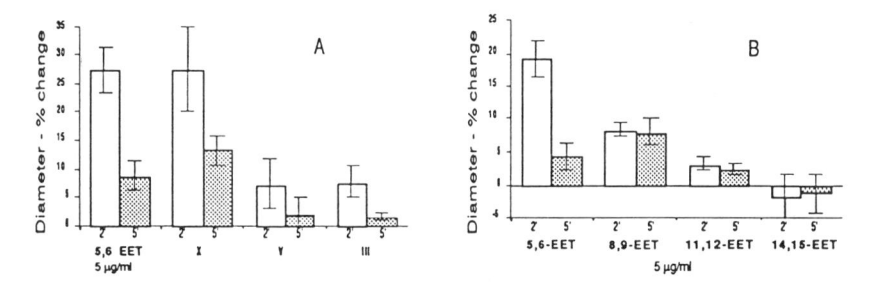

Figure 2. The effect of mouse brain slice metabolites of arachidonic acid and authentic EETs on in vivo cerebral arteriolar diameter.

cyclooxygenase we next determined whether indomethacin, a cyclooxygenase inhibitor, would prevent vasoactivity of 5,6-EET. As shown in figure 3A, indomethacin inhibited 5,6-EET-induced vasodilation. Also, we have previously shown that arachidonic acid-induced dilation of rabbit cerebral arterioles is due to dilator free radicals formed during cyclooxygenase metabolism of AA. We therefore examined the effect of the radical scavengers superoxide dismutase (SOD) and catalase on the arteriolar response to 5,6-EET. As can be seen in figure 3B, SOD plus catalase significantly reduced the dilator response, implying that 5,6-EET-induced dilation is via free radicals formed subsequent to metabolism of 5,6-EET by prostaglandin synthase. Additionally, we found that 5,6-EET did not induce formation of PGE_2 or 6-keto-$PGF_{1\alpha}$ by the brain. This implies 5,6-EET is not stimulating formation of prostaglandins from endogenous arachidonate. However application of arachidonic acid to the brain surface produced large increases in these two prostanoids. These prostaglandin analytic results further strengthen the conclusion that 5,6-EET is metabolized by brain cyclooxygenase.

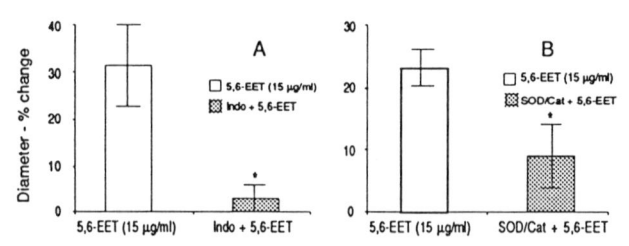

Figure 3. The effect of indomethacin and SOD plus catalase on 5,6-EET-induced cerebral arteriolar dilation in rabbits.

DISCUSSION

Our results indicate that mouse brain slices are capable of forming at least one EET, that being the 5,6 species. Evidence supporting this conclusion includes that peak X co-chromatographs with authentic radiolabeled 5,6-EET standard and that peak X gives a mass fragmentogram identical to that described for authentic 5,6-EET.

In addition to formation of 5,6-EET it appears quite clear that brain blood vessels are influenced by this compound. This conclusion is supported by the fact that peak X produced a transient dilation similar to that produced by the synthetic 5,6-EET. It is known that 5,6-EET is a substrate for cyclooxygenase whereas the other EETs are not well metabolized by cyclooxygenase (1). Our data show that the dilation induced by 5,6-EET is due to metabolism of this compound by brain cyclooxygenase. This is supported by our results showing that indomethacin, a known cyclooxygenase inhibitor, prevented the vasoactivity produced by 5,6-EET. The results showing that superoxide dismutase plus catalase also inhibit dilation indicate that free radicals produced subsequent to metabolism of 5,6-EET are responsible for dilation. This is similar to previous investigations in which we and others have shown that arachidonic acid application causes dilation which is also inhibited by indomethacin or SOD plus catalase (3). Other agonist-induced mechanisms appear to operate in the same manner since bradykinin-induced dilation is also inhibited by indomethacin and the same free radial scavengers, indicating that an endogenous arachidonic acid cascade can be triggered by receptor-mediated mechanisms.

In past studies where indomethacin affected some experimental paradigm in the brain the obvious conclusion was that its only effect was on the formation of the 2-series of prostanoids from arachidonic acid via PG synthase. The implication of our current work is that indomethacin and similar agents may also be inhibiting cyclooxygenase metabolism of cytochrome P-450 / monooxygenase metabolites of AA. Together these chemical and biological findings indicate that P-450 / monooxygenase metabolites, with their subsequent metabolism by cyclooxygenase, may be important mediators of normal physiologic responses of cerebral vessels, as well as potential mediators of pathophysiological phenomena.

REFERENCES

1. Fitzpatrick, F.A., and Murphy, R.C. (1989): *Pharmacol. Rev.* 40:229-241.
2. Kamitani, T., Little, M.H., and Ellis, E.F. (1985): *Circ. Res.* 57, 545-552.
3. Kontos, H.A., Wei, E.P., Povlishock, J.T., and Christman, C.W. (1984) *Circ. Res.* 55, 295-303

AN EPOXYGENASE METABOLITE OF ARACHIDONIC ACID 5,6 EPOXY-EICOSATRIENOIC ACID MEDIATES ANGIOTENSIN-INDUCED NATRIURESIS IN PROXIMAL TUBULAR EPITHELIUM

Michael F. Romero, Zuhayr T. Madhun, Ulrich Hopfer and Janice G. Douglas

Division of Endocrinology and Hypertension,
Department of Medicine and Departments of Genetics and Physiology and Biophysics, University Hospitals of Cleveland,
Case Western Reserve University School of Medicine,
Cleveland, Ohio 44106, USA

ABSTRACT

Several laboratories have documented that angiotensin II (AII) induces natriuresis in proximal tubular epithelium by a mechanism that has as yet not been disclosed. The present studies were designed to test the hypothesis that cytochrome P450-dependent metabolites of arachidonic acid mediate this effect. In cultured rabbit proximal tubule a ketoconazole-sensitive product comigrating with 5,6-epoxy-eicosatrienoic acid (5,6-EET) on reverse phase and normal phase HPLC was stimulated two-fold by AII. We employed cultures of early S1 segments on a modified Ussing chamber as a bioassay to evaluate the effects of AII and 5,6-EET on unidirectional ^{22}Na (apical to basolateral) flux (J_{Na}). AII inhibited J_{Na}, an effect that was abolished by ketoconazole. Furthermore, 5,6-EET decreased J_{Na} in a manner analogous to AII, and the effect was potentiated by inhibition of endogenous 5,6-EET production. Employing the Ca^{2+}-sensitive fluorescent probe, Fura 2, we observed a dose-dependent increase in $[Ca^{2+}]_i$ with nM to μM 5,6-EET, effects that were abolished by depletion of extracellular Ca^{2+} and voltage-sensitive Ca-channel blockers. These observations support the hypothesis that 5,6-EET represents the second messenger that mediates AII-induced natriuresis via stimulation of Ca^{2+} influx through voltage-sensitive channels.

CYTOCHROME P450-DEPENDENT METABOLISM OF ARACHIDONIC ACID

Attempts to discern the signal transduction pathway that mediates AII-induced natriuresis confirmed the lack of involvement of adenylate cyclase or phospholipase C but implicated phospholipase A_2 (3,4,11). This pathway mediates release of arachidonic acid and lysophosphatidylcholine from phosphatidylcholine and is stimulated by nM concentrations of AII and greater (3). Employing [^{14}C]-arachidonic acid-labeled epithelial cells maintained short-term in culture, we observed that the major product comigrated on reverse phase and normal phase HPLC with 5,6-EET. GC/mass spectrometric analysis of the pentafluorobenzyl ester verified that the product was an epoxide (Aubrey Morrison, personal communications). Product formation was stimulated from 17 ± 4% (n=7) of the total free counts recovered to 28 ± 3% with 10 nM AII and inhibited by ketoconazole. Despite the fact that P450 isozymes have been documented in proximal tubular epithelium, their importance has not been appreciated (5). This is the first documentation that a P450 isozyme, epoxygenase, metabolizes arachidonic acid in this nephron segment.

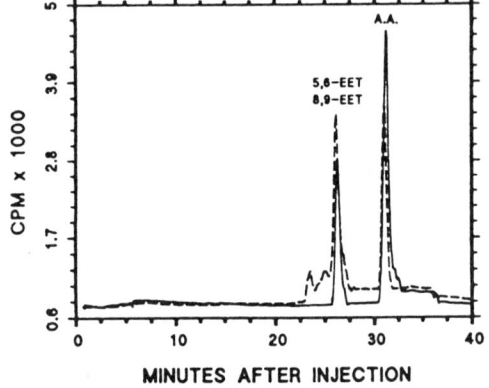

FIG. 1. HPLC analysis of ethylacetate extracts of Percoll gradient isolated proximal tubular cells (11) grown to confluence on 75 cm^2 flasks and labeled for 4 hours with [^{14}C]-arachidonic acid (24 μCi/mmole). Reverse phase HPLC employed a Bandapak C18 column and elution with a linear gradient of acetonitrile: water from 1:1 to 1:0 with 0.1% acetic acid (1). EET standards were generated by the method of Corey (2). AA = arachidonic acid; solidline = control; broken line = AII-stimulated.

ELECTROLYTE TRANSPORT

The physiological relevance of this epoxygenase metabolite was evaluated employing a monolayer of microdissected S$_1$ cultures grown to confluence on a porous membrane support (8,9). Table 1 illustrates that monolayers respond to 50 nM AII with a 12% decrease in J$_{Na}$ analogous to previous reports employing microperfused tubules and micropuncture techniques (6,10). Ketoconazole diminished the AII-mediated response to -4% consistent in its ability to inhibit AII-induced 5,6-EET production. Under basal conditions, 5,6-EET inhibited J$_{Na}$ by 11%. However, this effect was augmented to -25% following pretreatment of monolayers with ketoconazole. Our presumption is that by inhibiting endogenous 5,6-EET production, as confirmed biochemically, the contribution of exogenous 5,6-EET was more apparent. Thus, we have demonstrated that both AII and 5,6-EET decrease apical-to-basolateral Na fluxes. AII's effect is abolished by ketoconazole while that of 5,6-EET is amplified consistent with 5,6-EET as the second messenger mediating AII's effect on Na transport.

TABLE 1. J_{Na} (Apical to Basolateral)

Stimulus	% Change (mean ± SE)	n
AII (50 nM)	-12 ± 2	4
+ketoconazole	- 4 ± 2	4
5,6-EET (2µM)	-11 ± 5	7
+ketoconazole	-25 ± 6	3

THE MECHANISM OF 5,6-EET-INDUCED INHIBITION OF TRANSCELLULAR NA FLUX

The precise mechanism whereby 5,6-EET inhibits Na transport of proximal tubule is not known. We observed that 5,6-EET inhibits Na-K-ATPase of cultured proximal tubule by 53% but only at µM concentration. Alternatively, we have proposed that 5,6-EET may increase cytosolic Ca^{2+}, an effect that has been known to inhibit Na reabsorption in epithelial cells by an undisclosed mechanism. To address this question we conducted fluorescence measurements of Fura 2-loaded epithelial cells and observed a dose-dependent increase in $[Ca^{2+}]_i$ from 10^{-8} to 10^{-6}M 5,6-EET (7). The rise in $[Ca^{2+}]_i$ were blocked by La^{3+}, voltage-sensitive Ca^{2+} channel blockers, and acute depletion of extracellular Ca^{2+}.

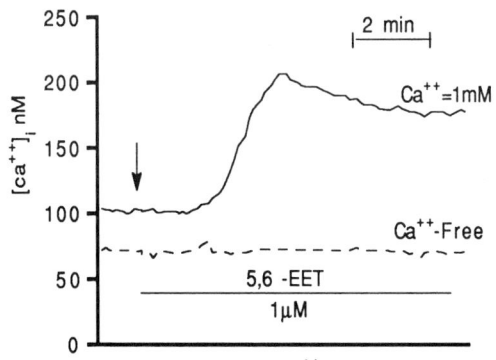

FIG. 2. 5,6-EET-induced rise in $[Ca^{++}]_i$ is blocked by depletion of extracellular Ca^{2+}.

Small increments in $[Ca^{2+}]_i$ were observed with 8,9-and 14,15-EET but not with 11,12-EET consistent with a specific receptor mediated effect. Thus, 5,6-EET blocks Na entry in proximal tubular epithelial cells by initiating Ca^{2+} influx through voltage-sensitive channels and, in turn, facilitating Ca^{2+}-calmodulin dependent inhibition of Na^+/H^+ exchanger of the luminal cell membrane. The extent to which other mechanisms are involved has as yet to be determined. A model which integrates AII-induced signal transduction and the steps involved in mediating natriuresis in proximal tubular epithelium is included below:

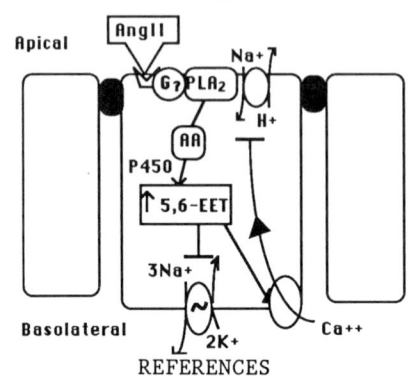

REFERENCES

1. Capdevila, J., Marnett, L.J., Chacos, N., Prough, R.A., and Estabrook, R.W. (1982): Proc. Natl. Acad. Sci. Ital., 79:767-770.
2. Corey, E.J., Marfat, A., Falck, J.R., and Albright, J.O. (1984): J. Am. Chem. Soc., 102:1433-1435.
3. Douglas, J.G., Romero, M., and Hopfer, U. (1990): Kidney Int., (in press).
4. Douglas, J.G. (1987): Am. J. Physiol., 253:F1-F7.
5. Finlayson, M.J., Dees, J.H., Masters, B.S.S., and Johnson, (1987): Arch. Biochem. Biophys., 252:113-120.
6. Harris, P.J. and Young, J.A. (1977): Pflügers Arch., 367:295-297.
7. Madhun, Z, Goldthwait, D.A., Hopfer, U., and Douglas, J. (1990): Clin. Res., 38:314.
8. Romero, M.F., Douglas, J.G., and Hopfer, U. (1989): J. Cell. Biol., 109(4):210.
9. Romero, M.F., Hopfer, U., and Douglas, J.G. (1990): Kidney Int., 37:350.
10. Schuster, V.L., Kokko, J.P., and Jacobson, H.R. (1984): J. Clin. Invest., 73:507-515.
11. Welsh, C., Dubyak, G., and Douglas, J.G. (1988): J. Clin. Invest., 81:710-719.

ACKNOWLEDGEMENTS

The authors wish to thank Janice Carpenter and Florence Stewart for expert secretarial assistance and C. Erhart, J. Harris, P. Finesilver and J. Preston for expert technical assistance. Grant support was from NIH:DK27651, HL22990, HL39012, HL41618 (JGD) and HL07415 (MFR).

ION TRANSPORT INHIBITION IN THE MEDULLARY
THICK ASCENDING LIMB OF HENLE'S LOOP
BY CYTOCHROME P450-ARACHIDONIC ACID METABOLITES

B. Escalante, D. Erlij,[*]
J.R. Falck[**] and J.C. McGiff

Departments of Pharmacology,
New York Medical College,
Valhalla, NY 10595,
Physiology, State University
of New York,[*] Downstate Medical Center,
Brooklyn, NY, 11203, and Molecular Genetics,
University of Texas,[**] Health Science Center, Dallas, TX 75235

Introduction

The medullary thick ascending limb of Henle's loop (mTALH) contributes to the regulation of extracellular fluid volume by establishing the renomedullary solute gradient. We have shown that mTALH cells metabolize arachidonic acid (AA) primarily via cytochrome P450 monooxygenases (4), to several metabolites (P450-AA), which, when separated by reverse-phase, high-performance liquid chromatography (HPLC), segregated into two peaks designated P_1 and P_2 (3,7). P_2, the more polar peak, is associated with one or more P450-AA metabolites capable of inhibiting Na^+-K^+-ATPase in concentrations estimated to be less than 0.1μM (7). This effect suggests that P450-AA metabolites (P_2) may play a role in the regulation of fluid and electrolyte metabolism in the mTALH segment. This interpretation, however, requires further support, as previous observations indicate that substances that have marked inhibitory effects on the isolated Na^+-K^+-ATPase do not always have an equivalent effect when they are given to intact cells or injected into the whole organism (2). Therefore, we examined the effects of P450-AA metabolites (P_2) on ion transport of intact mTALH cells using two indices of ion transport: [86]Rb uptake in isolated cells, and O_2 consumption in cultured cells.

Methods

Freshly isolated or primary cultured mTALH cells were used. The mTALH cells were isolated from rabbits by using an immunodissection method described (1). [86]Rb uptake: [86]Rb uptake was measured according to methods previously used in other cell preparations (8), with small modifications. Freshly isolated cells (40-80 μg protein) were incubated on ice for 20 min in 1 ml K^+-free Hank's balanced-salt solution. Uptake was initiated by adding [86]Rb (1 μCi) (specific activity 0.3 μg Ci) and 5 mM K^+ to 1 ml cell aliquots in the shaking water bath at 37°C. Isotope uptake was terminated at 5 min. The cells were centrifuged immediately at 13,000 g for 30 s, and the radioactivity of the pellet determined. ^{86}Rb was normalized by the amount of Rb uptake/µg protein for each sample. To assess the effect of P_2 (1µM) on mTALH cell ion transport, P_2 was added 10 min prior to addition of ^{86}Rb.

Oxygen Consumption: Primary cultures of mTALH cells were prepared following isolation of mTALH cells (1). After 7 to 8 days, the cells formed confluent monolayers and exhibited cell contact inhibition. Cultured cells (5x10^6 cells) were suspended in phosphate buffer saline (PBS). O_2 consumption was monitored with a Clark-type electrode. O_2 consumption was recorded for 15 min, then P_2 (0.01 to 1µM) was added to the chamber and O_2 consumption recorded for experimental periods of 15 min.

Results

Incubation of mTALH cells with ^{14}C-labeled AA resulted in the formation of two oxygenated metabolites, identified as P_1 and P_2 by HPLC retention times of 18 and 16 min, respectively (3). Formation of these metabolites was not affected by indomethacin (3µM). P_2 was separated and purified by HPLC and tested on ^{86}Rb uptake and O_2 consumption in mTALH cells.

Effect of P450-AA metabolite P_2 on mTALH cell ^{86}Rb uptake: using freshly isolated mTALH cells, P_2 (1µM) had an inhibitory effect on ^{86}Rb uptake (Fig 1). Moreover, when ^{86}Rb uptake was inhibited by ouabain (1mM), addition of P_2 had no further inhibitory effect on ^{86}Rb uptake, suggesting that the inhibitory effect of P_2 on ion transport was via an ouabain-sensitive mechanism.

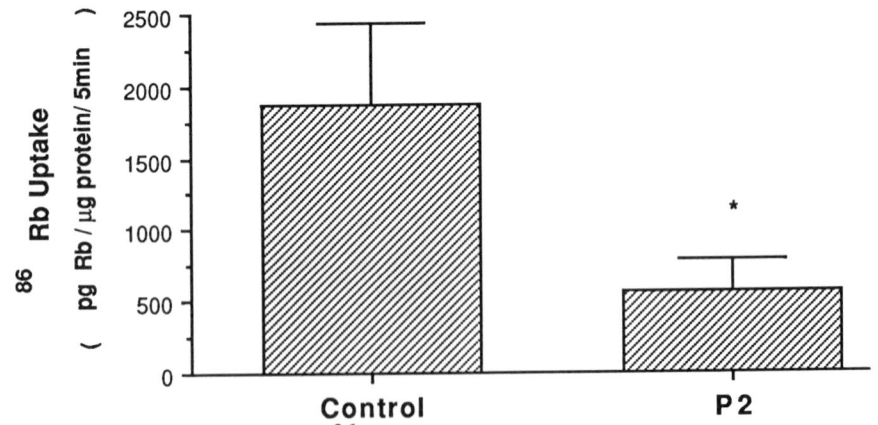

FIG. 1. EFFECT OF P_2 ON ^{86}Rb UPTAKE. Immunodissected mTALH cells were preincubated with the P450-AA metabolite (P_2) (1µM) or solvent for 10 min. ^{86}Rb uptake was initiated by adding ^{86}Rb (1 µCi) and uptake stopped at 5 min. Each bar represents the mean ± SEM of 4 experiments. *=p<0.05

Effect of P450-AA metabolite P_2 on O_2 consumption by primary cultured mTALH cells: O_2 consumption by cultured mTALH cells is dependent to a large extent on the activity of Na^+-K^+-ATPase activity, driven by Na^+ entry through the NaCl cotransport system. Oxygen consumption by 7 day old cultured mTALH cells (5×10^6 cells) was inhibited by both ouabain (1mM), from 289 ± 20 to 181 ± 24, nmol $O_2/5 \times 10^6$ cells/min, and furosemide (1mM) from 220 ± 5 to 158 ± 4 nmol $O_2/5 \times 10^6$ cells/min, providing further evidence that O_2 consumption in this cell preparation was in part mediated by Na^+-K^+-ATPase activity. The putative Na^+-K^+-ATPase inhibitor, P_2, (0.01 to 1 μM), inhibited O_2 consumption in a dose-dependent manner (Fig. 2). The inhibitory effect of P_2 was abolished when O_2 consumption was previously inhibited by ouabain, supporting the idea that the effect of P_2 was mediated via an ouabain-sensitive mechanism. Recently, we have found that the synthetic standard 20-carboxy arachidonic acid (20-COOH-AA) comigrates with P_2 on reverse-phase HPLC. Therefore, we tested 20-COOH-AA on ^{86}Rb uptake and O_2 consumption. 20-COOH-AA (1μM) inhibited ^{86}Rb uptake from a control value of 1292 ± 240 to 718 ± 95 pg ^{86}Rb/mg protein/2 min, and O_2 consumption from a control value of 260 ± 8 to 190 ± 9 nmol $O_2/5 \times 10^6$ cell/min, respectively.

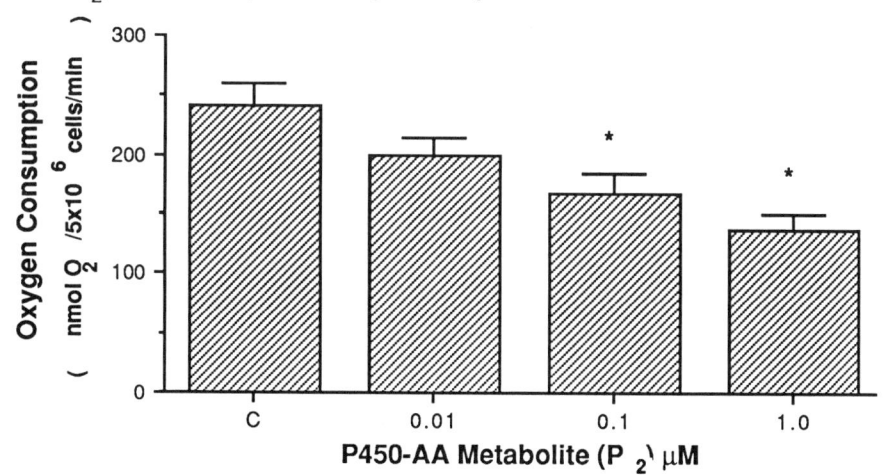

FIG. 2. DOSE-RESPONSE EFFECT OF P_2 ON O_2 CONSUMPTION OF CULTURED mTALH CELLS. 7-day-old cultured mTALH cells were exposed to increasing concentrations of P_2 (0.01 to 1 μM) and O_2 consumption measured for 15 min periods. Results are expressed as nmol of $O_2/5 \times 10^6$ cells/min. Each bar represents the mean $\pm$ SEM of 5 experiments. P_2 characterized initially in 1985 (7) refers to a P450-AA product(s) possessing primarily Na^+-K^+-ATPase inhibitory activity. *=$p<0.05$

Discussion

P_2 and 20-COOH-AA inhibited both ^{86}Rb uptake and O_2 consumption in mTALH cells, supporting our initial observation that a P450-AA metabolite (P_2) inhibited Na^+-K^+-ATPase activity (7). Further, this effect was, presumably, mediated via an ouabain-sensitive mechanism, since under conditions of inhibition of ion transport by ouabain, neither the P450-AA metabolite (P_2), nor synthetic 20-COOH-AA, further affected ^{86}Rb uptake or O_2 consumption, suggesting that the mechanism of action was associated either primarily or secondarily with a Na^+-K^+-ATPase effect. Thus, a P450-AA metabolite (20-COOH-AA) that inhibits K fluxes and NaCl transport in the mTALH cells supports this hypothesis: stimulation of AA metabolism in the mTALH segment contributes to the regulation of Na^+ reabsorption, and, thereby, extracellular fluid volume. Several authors have reported that other P450-AA metabolites can affect epithelial function either by a direct effect on ion transport (6) or by interfering with the action of vasopressin (5).

ACKNOWLEDGEMENTS

The authors wish to thank J. Jones and P. Blank for typing the manuscript and M. Steinberg for editing. This work was supported by NIH Program Project Grant HL34300, R01 HL 25394 (JCM) and R01 DK 33612 (DE).

REFERENCES

1. Allen, M.L., Nakao, A., Sonnenburg, W.K., Burnatowska-Hledin, M., Spielman, W.S., Smith, W.L., (1988): Am. J. Physiol. 255:F704-F710.
2. Beauwens, R., Crabbe, J., Rentmeesters, M. J. Physiol. (London) (1981): 310:293-305.
3. Carroll, M.A., Schwartzman, M., Baba, M., Miller, M.J.S., McGiff, J.C. (1988): Am. J. Physiol. 255:F151-F157.
4. Ferreri, N.R., Schwartzman, M., Ibraham, N.G., Chander, P.N., McGiff, J.C. (1984): J. Pharmacol. Exp. Ther. 231:441-448.
5. Hirt, D.L., Capdevila, J., Falck, J.R., Breyer, M.D., Jacobson, H.R. (1989): J. Clin. Invest. 84:1805-1812.
6. Jacobson, H.R., Corona, S., Capdevila, J.,Chacos, N., Manna, S., Womack, A., Falck, J.R. (1984): In: Prostaglandins and Membrane Ion Transport, edited by P. Braquet et al., New York, Raven Press, pp. 311-318.
7. Schwartzman, M., Ferreri, N.R., Carroll, M.A., Songu-Mize, E., McGiff, J.C. (1985): Nature, 314:620-622.
8. Seri, I., Kone, B.C., Gullans, S.R., Aperia, A., Brenner, B.M., Ballermann, B.J. (1988): Am. J. Physiol. 255:F666-F673.

SYNTHESIS AND BIOLOGICAL ACTIVITY OF EPOXYEICOSATRIENOIC ACIDS (EETS) BY CULTURED BOVINE CORONARY ARTERY ENDOTHELIAL CELLS

M. Rosolowsky, J.R. Falck*, W.B. Campbell

Departments of Pharmacology and Molecular Genetics*
University of Texas Southwestern Medical Center
5323 Harry Hines Boulevard
Dallas, Texas USA 75235

INTRODUCTION

A previous study in our laboratory demonstrated that prostacyclin (PGI_2), PGE_2 and 12-, 15-, and 11-hydroxyeicosatetraenoic acids (HETEs) were released by cultured bovine coronary artery endothelial cells (11). In 1987, Pinto and coworkers (8) reported a cytochrome P_{450}-dependent relaxation of dog coronary arteries by arachidonic acid. However, the compound(s) promoting relaxation was not identified. Preliminary evidence from our laboratory suggested that epoxyeicosatrienoic acids (EETs) may be synthesized by cultured bovine coronary artery and human umbilical endothelial cells (11,12). Therefore, the aims of this study are to determine if cultured endothelial cells synthesize EETs and to test their effects on vascular tone of bovine coronary arteries.

METHODS

Endothelial cells were isolated from large epicardial bovine coronary arteries by a procedure previously described (11). Experiments were performed on cells upon reaching approximately 95% confluency at either second or third passage. Cells were incubated in a 10 mM HEPES balanced salts solution and stimulated with ^{14}C-arachidonic acid (1 Ci/mmol), 10 µM unlabelled arachidonic acid and 5 µM A23187 for 30 minutes at 37°C in 95% air and 5% CO_2. Media and cells were then scraped into a tube, and the supernatant was extracted over octadecylsilyl extraction columns as previously described (11). Extracts were chromatographed on a reverse phase HPLC. Solvent A was distilled water and solvent B contained acetonitrile/ glacial acetic acid (999:1). A linear gradient from 50% solvent B in solvent A to 100% solvent B over 40 minutes was used at a flow rate of 1 ml/min. The EET fraction was collected, extracted with ethyl acetate/ cyclohexane (1/1) and chromatographed on a normal phase HPLC. An isocratic mobile phase of hexane/isopropanol/glacial acetic acid (995:4:1) with a flow rate of 2 ml/min was used to resolve the EET fraction.

Bovine circumflex coronary arteries were dissected from hearts obtained from the slaughterhouse. Rings (5 mm long) were suspended at optimal resting tension of 8 gm in an organ chamber filled with a Krebs bicarbonate solution. Vessels were then contracted with U46619 (20 nM) before receiving a concentration range of EET regioisomers or PGI$_2$.

RESULTS AND DISCUSSION

The radioactive profile of a typical incubation of cultured bovine endothelial cells is shown in figure 1. Previous studies have characterized the radiolabelled peaks in the PG fraction by mass spectrometry as 6-keto PGF$_{1\alpha}$, a stable metabolite of PGI$_2$, and PGE$_2$ (11). It appears that 6-keto PGF$_{1\alpha}$ is the major prostaglandin released by endothelial cells of large blood vessels of a variety of species. Endothelial cells from human umbilical artery and vein (12), human pulmonary artery and vein (6), bovine (4) and porcine (4) aorta also synthesize PGI$_2$. On the other hand, endothelial cells from microvessels of rabbit heart synthesize PGE$_2$ as the major PG metabolite (3).

Previously, we showed by using mass spectrometry that 12-, 15-, and 11-HETEs were synthesized by bovine coronary artery endothelial cells (11) and human umbilical endothelial cells (12). In the present study, radioactive peaks comigrating with 9-, 8-, and 5-HETEs were also noted in the incubation media from 20 pooled flasks of cells. The production of HETEs by cultured endothelial cells has also been reported by several laboratories (5,7,14).

The EET fraction was rechromatographed on normal phase HPLC (figure 2). Five radioactive peaks were identified and four migrated with 14,15-EET, 11,12-EET, 8,9-EET and 5,6-EET. These were further identified as EETs by mass spectrometry. The synthesis of EETs by cultured endothelial cells has only been reported in preliminary studies from our laboratory (11) and that of Pritchard and coworkers (9). We found and confirmed by mass spectrometry that EETs were also synthesized by canine coronary arteries, and that stenosed endothelially injured vessels produced substantially more EETs than normal arteries (13).

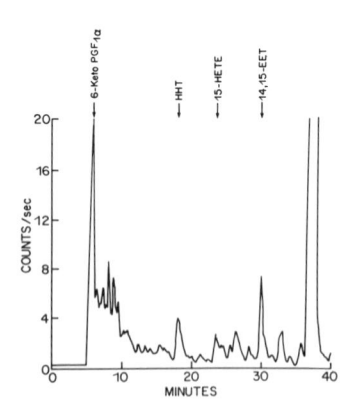

FIG. 1. Separation of ^{14}C-arachidonic acid metabolites from cultured endothelial cells of bovine coronary arteries. Migration times of known standards are shown above the chromatogram.

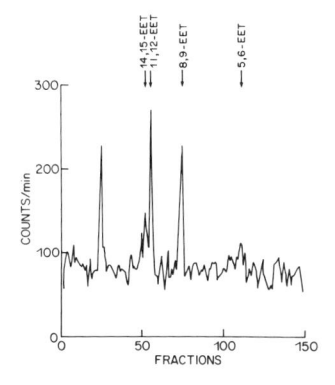

FIG. 2. Separation of ^{14}C-metabolites of the EET fraction of bovine coronary artery endothelial cells.

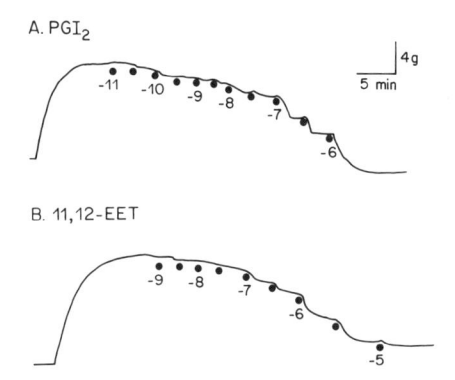

FIG. 3. Relaxation of bovine coronary arteries *in vitro* by PGI$_2$ (A) and 11,12-EET (B). Vessels were pre-contracted with 20 nM U46619. A concentration range of PGI$_2$ (10^{-11}-10^{-6} M) or 11,12-EET (10^{-9}-10^{-5}) was added in a cumulative fashion.

We tested the effects of synthetic EETs on vascular tone of isolated bovine coronary arteries. The four EET regioisomers had no effect on basal vascular tone. However, when the vessels were contracted with U46619, all four isomers caused relaxations. The results with 11,12-EET are shown in figure 3B. This EET relaxed vessels in concentrations between 10^{-9} and 10^{-5} M. Similar results were obtained with PGI$_2$ (Figure 3A). PGI$_2$ was at least 10-fold more potent than 11,12-EET. The other EET regioisomers also produced similar concentration related-relaxations (data not shown). This finding is consistent with our previous report in dog coronary arteries (13). Along these lines, 11,12-, and 8,9-EETs were reported to dilate microvessels of rat intestine (10), and 5,6-EET was found to dilate isolated, perfused rat tail artery (1). We also tested the EETs on platelet aggregation using canine platelet-rich-plasma. The EETs did not affect aggregation of unstimulated platelets, nor did they affect collagen-induced aggregation over a concentration range of

10^{-9} through 10^{-4} M (data not shown). The lack of effect of EETs on platelet aggregation are at odds with the findings of Fitzpatrick and coworkers (2) who found that all EET regioisomers at concentrations from 1 to 10 µM inhibited human platelet aggregation. However, these studies used washed platelets. In fact, when human platelet-rich plasma was used by these workers (2), much greater concentrations of EETs (50- 200 µM) were required to inhibit platelet aggregation.

In conclusion, we report that endothelial cells of the bovine coronary artery release 14,15-, 11,12-, 8,9- and 5,6-EETs. These compounds relax isolated bovine coronary arteries but are at least 10-fold less potent than PGI_2. The EETs have no effect on aggregation of canine platelet-rich plasma. The physiological significance of the EETs is not clear, but it is possible that they may act, along with PGI_2, to reduce coronary vascular tone.

ACKNOWLEDGEMENTS

The authors thank Mr. Scott Breeding for his technical assistance and Mrs. Juanita Coley for her secretarial assistance. This work was supported by grants from the National Institutes of Health (Ischemic Heart Specialized Center of Research, HL-17669 and DK-38226).

REFERENCES

1. Carroll, M.A., Schwartzman, M., Capdevila, J., Falck, J.R., and McGiff, J.C. (1987): *Eur. J. Pharm.*, 138:281-283.
2. Fitzpatrick, F.A., Ennis, M.D., Baze, M.E., Wynalda, M.A., McGee, J.E., and Liggett, W.F. (1986): *J. Biol. Chem.*, 261:15334-15338.
3. Gerritsen, M.E. and Cheli, C.D. (1983): *J. Clin. Invest.*, 72:1658-1671.
4. Hong, S.L. (1980): *Thromb. Res.*, 18:787-791.
5. Hopkins, N.K., Oglesby, T.D., Bundy, G.L., and Gorman, R.R. (1984): *J. Biol. Chem.*, 259:14048-14053.
6. Johnson, A.R. (1980): *J. Clin. Invest.*, 65:841-850.
7. Mayer, B., Moser, R., Gleispach, H., and Kukovetz, W.R. (1986): *Biochim. Biophys. Acta*, 875:641-653.
8. Pinto, A., Abraham, N.G., and Mullane, K.M. (1987): *J. Pharmacol. Exp. Ther.*, 240:856-863.
9. Pritchard, K.A., Tota, R.R., Stemerman, M.B., and Wong, P.Y-K. (1990): *Biochem. Biophys. Res. Commun.*, 167:137-142.
10. Proctor, K.G., Falck, J.R., and Capdevila, J. (1987): *Circ. Res.*, 60:50-59.
11. Revtyak, G.E., Johnson, A.R., and Campbell, W.B. (1988): *Am. J. Physiol.*, 254:C8-C19.
12. Revtyak, G.E., Johnson, A.R., and Campbell, W.B. (1988): *Am. J. Physiol.*, 255:C214-C225.
13. Rosolowsky, M., Falck, J.R., Willerson, J.T., and Campbell, W.B. (1990): *Circ. Res.*, 66:608-621.
14. Takayama, H., Gimbrone, M.A., and Shafer, A.I. (1987): *Thromb Res*, 45:803-816.

MODIFICATION OF THE EICOSANOID SYSTEM AND CELL SIGNALLING BY PRECURSOR FATTY ACIDS.

P. C. Weber and Alois Sellmayer
Universität München, Institut für Prophylaxe und Epidemiologie der Kreislaufkrankheiten, Pettenkofer Str. 9, 8000 München 2.

Introduction

Physiological and pathophysiological reactions like vascular resistance, thrombosis, wound healing, inflammation and allergy are modulated by oxygenated metabolites of arachidonic acid (AA; 20:4n-6 or 20:4w-6) and related polyunsaturated fatty acids that are collectively termed eicosanoids. These compounds include prostaglandins, prostacyclin, thromboxane, leukotrienes and hydroxylated derivatives of arachidonic acid.
Precursors of cellular eicosanoids are essential fatty acids which must be provided from the diet. Synthesis of eicosanoids is under the control of specific cellular enzymes mediating the uptake, release and oxygenation of the precursor fatty acid.
Mammalian cell membranes consist of a lipid bilayer composed primarily of phospholipids and cholesterol. Proteins that have important cellular signalling functions such as receptors, transporters and enzymes are embedded in the lipid bilayer. Although the following review will focus on the modification of the eicosanoid system and other mediator compounds by dietary fatty acids, it is clear that some of the resulting changes in cell signalling might be more directly related to the modifications in the fatty acid composition of membrane phospholipids and their effects on those proteins embedded in the lipid bilayer.
The following review describes briefly some of the important factors involved in the pathogenesis of atherosclerosis and chronic inflammation/cell proliferation and how n-3 fatty acids interfere at several sites with this process.

Eicosanoids and Cell Signalling

As shown in Figure 1, eicosanoids and related lipid mediators, such as 1,2 diacylglycerol (DAG) or platelet activating factor (PAF), exert a modulatory role in coupling cellular responses to various stimuli and in mediating cell-to-cell interactions. Thus some eicosanoids like thromboxane A_2, leukotriene B_4 cytochrome P450 products may amplify an initial (Ca^{++}-related) signal for cell activation by stimulating specific membrane receptors coupled to phospholipase C, thereby further increasing intracellular Ca^{++} concentrations. In contrast, other eicosanoids, such as PGI_2 or PGD_2 may blunt an initial signal for cell activation by decreasing i. c. Ca^{++} release via an increase of cAMP. For details see Ref. 1.

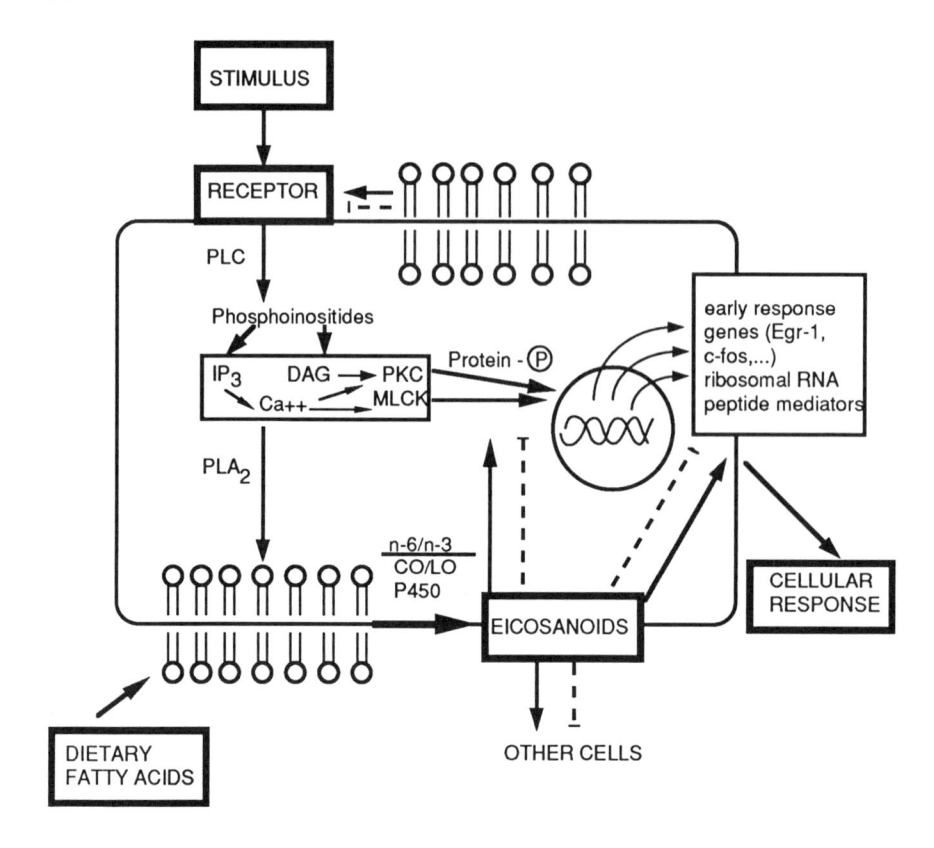

Figure 1: Scheme of the putative role of n-3 and n-6 eicosanoid precursor fatty acids (FA) in cell membrane phospholipids as determined by dietary fatty acid intake for the modulation of stimulus response coupling.
PLC, phospholipase C; IP3, inositol trisphosphate; DAG, 1,2 diacylglycerol; PKC, protein kinase C; MLCK, myosine light chain kinase; PLA2, phospholipase A2; CO, cyclooxygenase; LO, lipoxygenase; CP450, cytochrome P450; protein-P, phosphorylated proteins; peptide mediators, e.g. IL-1, TNF, PDGF. (inhibition---᛫; stimulation ⟶).

Dietary Modification of the Eicosanoid System

Interference with eicosanoid synthesis is characteristic for antiinflammatory drugs and antithrombotic agents, antihypertensives and diuretics, suggesting that eicosanoids are involved in a broad spectrum of prevailing diseases. A change of eicosanoid production and eicosanoid-dependent cellular function may, however, also be achieved by altering eicosanoid precursor availability.
Under our "Western" dietary conditions, arachidonic acid is by far the dominant precursor fatty acid of biologically highly active eicosanoids of the two-series (Figure 2). The major primary source of AA in our food chain is

linoleic acid(18:2n-6). At variance to the fatty acids of the linoleic- or n-6-family in terrestrial animals and in most plant seeds - which are the major sources of our eicosanoid precursor fatty acids - the fatty acids of the a-linolenic- or n-3-family predominate in green leaves and especially in marine lipids. Here, eicosapentaenoic acid (EPA; 20:5n-3) and docosahexaenoic acid (DHA; 22:6n-3) are the major polyunsaturated fatty acids. The desaturation step from the n-6 fatty acids to the n-3 fatty acids seems to be carried out exclusively in green leaves and phytoplankton to form a-linolenic acid (18:3n-3) from linoleic acid (18:2n-6).

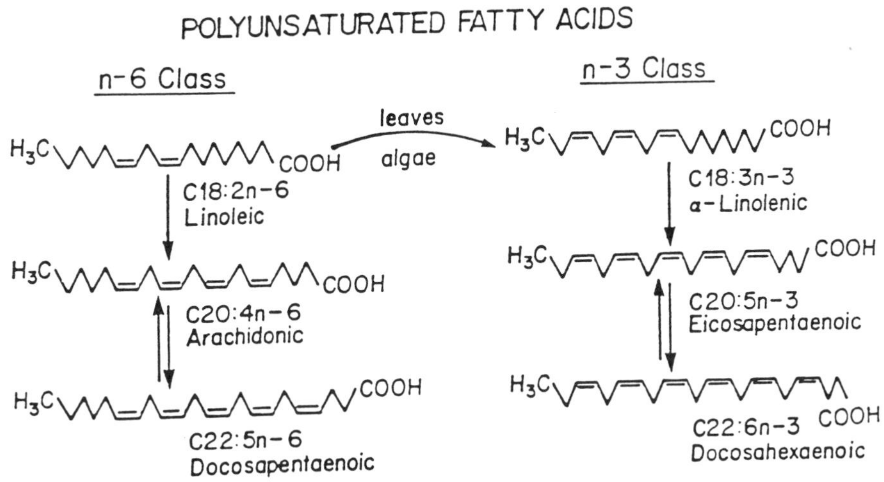

POLYUNSATURATED FATTY ACIDS

n-6 Class

C18:2n-6
Linoleic

C20:4n-6
Arachidonic

C22:5n-6
Docosapentaenoic

n-3 Class

C18:3n-3
a-Linolenic

C20:5n-3
Eicosapentaenoic

C22:6n-3
Docosahexaenoic

Figure 2: Relation of Important Polyunsaturated Fatty Acids of the n-6 and n-3 Classes.
The transformations depicted by the arrows incorporate two or more reaction steps. The arching arrow indicates that only in leaves and algae is n-6 linoleic acid desaturated to form n-3 alpha-linolenic acid, the progenitor of the n-3 class of fatty acids.

In the mammalian organism fatty acids belonging to different families such as n-3 and n-6 fatty acids cannot be interconverted. Therefore, nutritional intake determines the fatty acid composition of phospholipids in plasma and in cell membranes to a great extent.
In this respect "we are what we eat."

Several independent lines of evidence suggest that changes in the natural history of hypertensive, atherothrombotic and inflammatory disorders may be achieved by altering the eicosanoid precursor availability.
Table1 summarizes observations on the functional effects of n-3 fatty acids in the diet on mechanisms involved in cardio-vascular disorders.

Table 1: Some Functional Effects of n-3 Fatty Acids

- Reduce Platelet Aggregation
- Increase Platelet Survival
- Increase Bleeding Time
- Reduce Blood Pressure
- Reduce Vasospastic Response to Vasoconstrictors
- Increase Vascular (Arterial) Compliance
- Decrease Blood Viscosity
- Reduce Albumin Leakage in Type 1 Diabetes mellitus
- Reduce Cardiac Arrhythmias
- Increase Cardiac ß-Receptor Function
- Increase Postischemic Coronary Blood Flow
- Reduce Vascular Intimal Hyperplasia

Biochemical Effects of n-3 Fatty Acids

Arachidonic Acid

In the mammalian organism, linoleic acid (LA, C18:2n-6), the parent fatty acid of the n-6 fatty acid family, is slowly desaturated and elongated to arachidonic acid (AA, C20:4n-6) the dominant precursor fatty acid of eicosanoids under our Western dietary conditions. AA is a potent aggregator of platelets in vitro. After infusion or dietary intake of AA, in vivo animal and human studies show that platelets are more sticky and lead to thrombus formation. Recently, a new role of AA and some of its metabolites in the intracellular signalling pathway associated with cell proliferation and gene expression has been suggested (3). Such a function would place AA into a strategic position to modulate key cellular events in atherosclerotic and chronic inflammatory disorders.
n-3 Fatty acids do not only replace AA and LA in certain cellular phospholipids (especially PC, PE) but they redistribute these n-6 fatty acids from the phospholipid fraction into cholesterol esters and triacylglycerols (4, 5, 6). Together with the high affinity of n-3 fatty acids to the etherlipid fraction of phospholipids this may have important implications for the composition of specific intracellular lipid pools and the formation of lipid mediators from AA or EPA.

Thromboxane

Due to the early findings on fish oils and platelet aggregation and the potential role of eicosapentaenoic acid (EPA, C20:5n-3) as an eicosanoid precursor, the effects of fish oil on eicosanoids were the first to be studied (7). At least two prostanoids, thromboxane and prostacyclin, are involved in atherogenesis. Thromboxane, produced in platelets from AA, is of the 2-series (TXA$_2$) and promotes platelet aggregation, an important early stage in blood clot formation and in atherogenesis. It also is a potent constrictor of arteries. n-3 fatty acids inhibit the formation of TXA$_2$ and lead to the formation of small quantities of inactive TXA$_3$ (8).

Prostacyclin

Prostacyclin, produced by endothelial cells - exerts opposite actions to thromboxanes. It prevents platelets from aggregating and dilates arteries; its actions are anti-atherogenic. Whereas thromboxane formed from EPA, unlike that from AA, has very little physiologic activity, prostacyclin (PGI$_3$) formed from EPA (9) - and DHA after retroconversion to EPA (10) - is fully active, increasing the total anti-atherogenic prostacyclin activity. Thus, the presence of EPA from fish oil in the phospholipids of membranes of platelets and endothelial cell and in plasma tips the balance in the blood vessels away from atherosclerosis (11).

Leukotrienes

Leukotrienes are potent proinflammatory and immunoactive factors. LTB$_4$, produced from AA, is a chemoattractant for neutrophils and monocytes/macrophages. These circulating white blood cells are important elements in inflammation and characterized major cellular constituents of early atherosclerotic lesions. LTB$_4$ also leads to the activation of neutrophils and macrophages. LTB$_5$ produced from EPA, on the other hand, has little physiologic effects, so that replacement of AA by EPA in cell membrane phospholipids, the inflammatory component of atherosclerosis is diminished (12,13).
Disturbances of the cell signalling process are thought to play a major role in diseases like atherosclerosis and chronic inflammation. Arachidonic acid and its metabolites formed via the cyclooxygenase, lipoxygenase or the cytochrome P450 - pathways may be important modulators of this process. The mechanisms involved include also the formation or release of messenger molecules such as inositolphosphates (e. g. IP$_3$), Ca^{++} and diglycerides. n-3 Fatty acids have been found to interfere at several sites in this signalling process (14).

Platelet Activating Factor

Platelet activating factor, PAF, is a phospholipid-like molecule now known to possess many widespread and largely adverse physiological effects. At least some of these, the activation of platelets (as its name indicates) and of monocytes/ macrophages, contribute to atherogenesis and inflammation. PAF can be synthesized by several different cell types. It has been shown in humans, that the production of PAF is markedly inhibited when the n-3 fatty acids are incorporated in their membrane phospholipids replacing AA as the precursor molecules for PAF formation (15).

Platelet Derived Growth Factor

Once platelets aggregate, as they will at a site of injury to the endothelial cells, they release several factors including platelet derived growth factor (PDGF), a potent chemoattractant and mitogen responsible, in part, for the migration of smooth muscle cells from deeper layers of the arterial wall to the site of endothelial injury or dysfunction where they multiply. PDGF, along with other factors, causes circulating monocytes, another type of white blood cells, to migrate also to the site of endothelial injury, to multiply and to change into macrophages which are scavenger cells in the developing atherosclerotic process.
Not only platelets, but also the other cell types that participate in the development of atherosclerosis, i. e. endothelial cells, monocytes/macrophages, and smooth muscle cells, produce PDGF-like proteins which stimulate cell growth in the arterial wall. When the low density lipoprotein (LDL) cholesterol level in the blood is elevated and oxidized after trapping in the vascular intima, it is the macrophages and smooth muscle cells that ingest the cholesterol to form foam cells which contribute to the atherosclerotic plaques. Recently, it has been shown that incorporating EPA into cultured aortic endothelial cells markedly reduces their production of PDGF-like proteins (16).

Oxygen Free Radicals

An important means by which neutrophils and monocytes fight infection is to attack invading bacteria or foreign cells with lethal oxygen free radicals. These highly reactive oxygen species, however, can damage normal cells and, in fact, are thought to be responsible for the cellular debris component of the atherosclerotic plaque. It has been demonstrated that feeding fish oils results in a large reduction in oxygen free radical formation by neurophils and monocytes when these cells are activated (17).
Furthermore, the formation of lipid hydroperoxides in plasma is reduced after dietary fish oil (18).

Interleukin-1 and Tumor Necrosis Factor

Interleukin-1 (IL-1), a peptide molecule produced by several of the cell types discussed here that are incriminated in the development of atherosclerosis, has been shown to cause most of the physiologic effects associated with infections: fever, malaise, sleepiness, etc. In concert with another peptide, tumor necrosis factor (TNF), it is also responsible for several effects that are atherogenic: it stimulates synthesis of adhesion molecules (proteins which cause monocytes to adhere to endothelial cells), stimulates production of cytotoxic oxygen free radicals by neutrophils and monocytes and activates platelets, neutrophils and monocytes. Again, it has been shown that feeding fish oil supplements to humans reduces the production of both IL-1 and TNF (19).

These actions of fish oils may be protective not only against atherosclerosis, but they may have beneficial effects on modulating the excessive or misdirected activity of the immune system as well, which is thought to be responsible for the so-called autoimmune diseases like lupus (20), rheumatoid arthritis (21) or colitis (22). So far, there has been no report suggesting that such damping down of the immune system by fish oils creates an increased risk of infections or cancer.

Endothelial Derived Relaxation Factor

Endothelial cell derived relaxing factor, EDRF, as its name implies, promotes relaxation of arterial smooth muscle cells and diminishes constriction of arteries when exposed to several physiologic and pharmacologic vasoconstrictor agents. These actions of EDRF are enhanced by supplementing diets of experimental animals with fish oils (23). In addition, it has been found that these potentially anti-atherosclerotic actions persist even after exposure of arteries to anoxic conditions, as may occur with decreased blood flow during and following a heart attack (24).

Conclusion

At present we do not know the biological significance and the cause of the fact that AA constitutes by far the major precursor fatty acid of eicosanoids and related lipid mediators under our Western dietary conditions. One reason might be the increasingly uniform supply of saturated and n-6 unsaturated fatty acids in our food chain, i. e. in vegetable oils and in livestock fattened with grain rich in C18:2n-6, which is slowly desaturated and elongated to AA in the mammalian organism. The further evaluation of the relationship of n-6 versus n-3 fatty acids and their eicosanoids to membrane receptor function, the modulation of transmembrane signalling mechanisms, phospholipase activation, formation of 1,2-DAG and PAF, Ca^{++}-release, inositol phosphate turnover and gene expression should contribute to a better understanding of the role of these fatty acids in cell function. It may thus open the development of new approaches to the therapy and prevention of disorders in which cellular responses to injury (such as inflammation and exaggerated cell proliferation) are a hallmark of the disease process (25, 26, 27).

References:

1) Weber P C. Aberrations in Membrane Structure and Function 1988 (Editors: Karnovski, Leaf, Bolli), p. 263-274.

2) Siess W, Weber P C, Lapetina E. Prostaglandins, Leukotriens, and Lipoxins 1985, p. 387-392.

3) Sellmayer A, Weber P C, Bonventre J V. Kidney Int. 1990, 37:351.

4) von Schacky C, Fischer S, Weber P C. J. Clin. Invest. 1985, 76:1626-1631.
5) von Schacky C, Siess W, Fischer S, Weber P C. J. Lipid. Res. 1985, 26:457-464.
6) Garg M L, Wiezbicki A A, Thomson A B, Clandinin M T. Biochem. J. 1989, 261:11-15.
7) Weber P C, Fischer S, v. Schacky C, Lorenz R, Strasser T. Prog. Lipid. Res. 1985, 25:273-276.
8) Fischer S, Weber P C. Biochem. Biophys. Res. Commun. 1983, 116:1091-1099.
9) Fischer S, Weber P C. Nature 1984, 307:165-168.
10) Fischer S, Vischer A, Praec-Mursic V, Weber P C. Prostaglandins 1987, 34:367-373.
11) Weber P C. J. Intern. Med. 1989, 225, Suppl. 1:61-68.
12) Strasser T, Fischer S, Weber P C. Proc. Natl. Acad. Sci., USA, 1985, 82:1540-1543.
13) Lee T H, Hoover R L, Williams J D, Sperling R I, Ravalese J, Spur B W, Robinson D R, Corey E J, Lewis R A, Austen K F. N. Engl. J. Med. 1985, 312:1217-1224.
14) Weber P C. Beobachtung, Experiment und Theorie in Naturwissenschaft und Medizin. Verhandlungen der Gesellschaft Deutscher Naturforscher und Ärzte. 114. Versammlung, (München 1986), Wissenschaftliche Verlagsgesellschaft mbH, Stuttgart.
15) Sperling R I, Robin J L, Kylander K A, Lee T H, Lewis R A, Austen K F. J. Immunol. 1987, 139:4186-4191.
16) Fox P L, DiCorleto P E. Science 1988, 241:453-456.
17) Fisher M, Upchurch K S, Levine P H, Johnson M H, Vaudreuil C H, Natale A, Hoogasian J J. Inflammation 1986, 34:367-373.
18) Lands W E, Miller J F, Rich S. Advances in Prostaglandin, Tromboxane, and Leukotriene Research. Raven Press 1987, 17:876-879.
19) Endres S, Ghorbani R, Kelley V E, Georgilis K, Lonnemann G, van der Meer J W, Cannon J G, Rogers T S, Klempner M S, Weber P C, Schaefer E J, Wolff S M, Dinarello C A. N. Engl. J. Med. 1989, 320:265-271.
20) Prickett J D, Robinson D R, Steinberg A D. J. Clin. Invest. 1981, 68:556-559.
21) Kremer J M, Jubiz W, Michalek A, Rynes R I, Bartholomew L, Bigaouette J, Timchalk M, Beeler D, Lininger L. Annals of Internal Medicine 1987, 106:497- 502.
22) Lorenz R, Weber P C, Szimnau P, Heldwein W, Strasser T, Loeschke K. J. Int. Med. 1989, 225:225-232.
23) Shimokawa H, Lam J Y, Chesebro J H, Bowie E J W, Vanhoutte P M. Circulation 1987, 76:898-905.
24) Malis C, Varadarajan G S, Force T, Weber P C, Leaf A. J. Am. Heart Assoc. 1988, Abstract No. 860.
25) Bonaa K H, Bjerve K S, Straume B, Gram I T, Thelle D. N. Engl. J. Med. 1990, 322:795-801.
26) Jensen T, Stender S, Goldstein K, Golmer G, Deckert T. N. Engl. J. Med. 1989, 321:1572-1577.
27) Burr M L, Gilbert J F, Holliday R M, Elwood P C, Fehily A M, Rogers S, Sweetnam P M, Deadman N M. Lancet 1989 ii:757-761.

DIETARY FISH AND PROSTANOID FORMATION IN MAN

G. Hornstra [1], A.C. van Houwelingen [1], G.A.A. Kivits [2], S. Fischer [3] and W. Uedelhoven [4]

Department of [1] Human Biology, Limburg University P.O. Box 616, 6200 MD Maastricht, the Netherlands; [2] Department of Biosciences, Nutrition and Safety, Unilever Research Vlaardingen, the Netherlands; [3] Klinikum Grosshadern, Ludwig-Maximilians-Universität München, Munich, Federal Republic of Germany, and [4] Institut für Prophylaxe der Kreislaufkrankheiten der Universität München, Munich, Federal Republic of Germany.

INTRODUCTION

The effect of dietary fish(oil) on eicosanoid formation and metabolism has been repeatedly been investigated and there is fair agreement -but no unanimity- that the formation of thromboxane A_2 (TxA_2) is reduced, due to a lower availability of the precursor fatty acid arachidonic acid (20:4(n-6), AA). In vitro studies also demonstrated the prostacyclin (PGI_2) formation to be reduced upon fish(oil) consumption, but the limited in-vivo data indicate that the total PGI_2 turnover is not decreased and may be even enhanced. Prostanoids formed from timnodonic acid (eicosapentaenoic acid, 20:5(n-3), TA) increase upon fish oil consumption. From urinary analysis it was concluded that the PGI_3 formation is considerable, but the TxB_3 production has been shown to be very limited indeed (For a review see ref. 1). Many of the studies performed so far were based on the administration of large amounts of fish(oils) and no measures have ever been taken to correct for individual differences in fish(oil) compliance. In this paper we describe a well-controlled study with a reasonable amount of dietary mackerel, administered to healthy male volunteers.

METHODS

The study design has been published in detail elsewhere (2). Briefly, in Tromsø (Norway) and in Maastricht and Zeist (the Netherlands) 80 volunteers were given one tin (135 g) of meat- or mackerel paste for a period of 6 weeks as a dietary supplement. During a 3 week run-in period, all volunteers were given the meat paste. Individual compliance was calculated on the basis of the urinary excretion of a standard, sub-therapeutic, amount of lithium, added to the supplements. Urine was also used to measure the major metabolites of PGI_2 and PGI_3 and the tetranor metabolites of the 'classical' prostaglandins. Blood was collected at weeks 0 (start of the experimental period), 3, and 6, and used to prepare platelet rich in plasma (PRP) and washed platelets for measuring prostanoid formation upon activation with collagen, and the fatty acid profile of platelet phospholipid (PL) fatty acid classes, respectively. TxB_2 and TxB_3 were measured by GC/MS and the cyclo-oxygenase-derived hydroxy fatty acids 12-HHT (ex AA) and 12-HHTE (ex TA) by HPLC. Fatty acids were measured by GC/FID after lipid extraction, TLC separation of the PL classes, PL-saponification, and methylation of the fatty acids. In addition, platelet aggregation in response to collagen was measured in citrated whole blood, using impedance aggregometry (Maastricht only). In the plasma, obtained by centrifugation after completion of the aggregation measurements, immunoreactive (ir)TxB$_2$ was measured by a commercial radioimmunoassay kit. Finally, a blood sample was allowed to clot under standard conditions for the measurement of the potential of blood platelets to produce irTxB$_2$. All measuring procedures have been described in detail before (3).

RESULTS AND DISCUSSION

The average compliance, calculated on the basis of the urinary recovery of the lithium added to the supplements, was 85 ± 4.3 % for the control group and 78 ± 3.9 % for the mackerel group. The average intake of fish fatty acids in the mackerel group was 1.3 g TA and 2.3 g cervonic acid (docosahexaenoic acid, 22:6(n-3), CA). Although in all platelets phospholipid classes of the mackerel group, the contents of TA and CA increased at the expense of AA (Fig. 1), this did not result in significant changes in the unsaturation index. In the sphingomyelin fraction, however, a significant increase in the unsaturation index was observed, which was caused by a partly replacement of most saturated fatty acids by nervonic acid (24:1(n-9)). Since sphingomyelin is mainly located at the outer leaflet of the platelet membrane (4) this change in unsaturation -and, consequently, in membrane fluidity- is likely to affect ligand-receptor interactions.

As a result of these changes in fatty acid composition, collagen-activation of PRP resulted in less eicosanoids from AA and more from TA. However, the

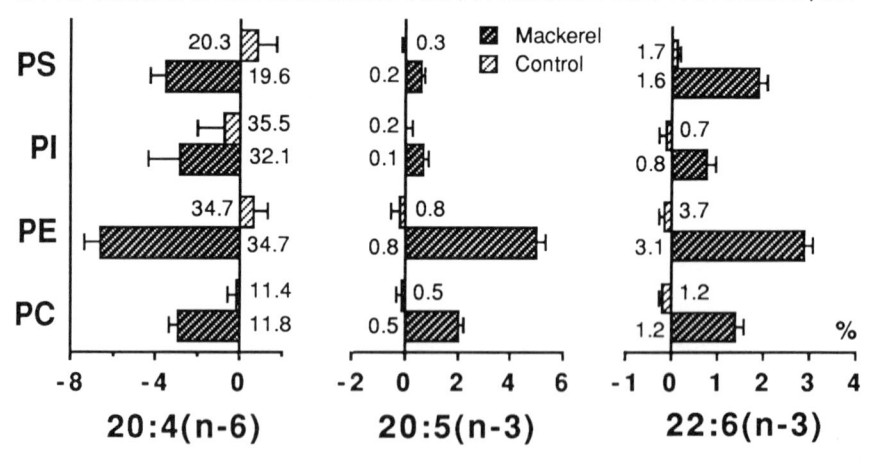

FIG. 1., EFFECT OF DIETARY MACKEREL ON THE FATTY ACID COMPOSITION (% OF TOTAL FATTY ACIDS) IN PLATELET PHOSPHOLIPID CLASSES. SMALL NUMBERS REFER TO CONCENTRATIONS AT WEEK 0. ALL DIFFERENCES BETWEEN THE GROUPS ARE SIGNIFICANT, P < 0.001, EXCEPT FOR 20:4(N-6) IN PI (P > 0.05).

reduction observed for the AA-derived products was much larger than the increase observed for the TA-derived substances. This was particularly true for TxB_2 and TxB_3. A significant correlation was observed between the results of the Tx-measurements, performed by GC/MS, and the amounts of cyclo-oxygenase-related mono hydroxy fatty acids, measured by HPLC, both for AA- as well as for TA-derived products. Although the potential of platelets to produce $irTxB_2$ was highly reduced upon mackerel consumption -as reflected by a ca. 30 % reduction of $irTxB_2$ in serum- only a tendency for such a reduction was found in collagen-activated whole blood. In the mackerel group, the dietary compliance was strongly correlation with the Tx-response (Fig. 2) which implies that a higher fish consumption than could be achieved in our study is likely to lower TxB_2 formation in collagen-activated whole blood.

The dietary compliance was also strongly correlated with the ATP release of the activated platelets (5), and since a strong correlation was also observed between $irTxB_2$ formation and various aspects of platelet function, measured in the same blood samples, it is highly likely that the reduced platelet responses following mackerel consumption are explained by the lower TxB_2 formation.

No significant differences between the groups were observed for the urinary concentration of the tetranor prostaglandin metabolites, measured as tetranor prostane dioic acid. This is in agreement with earlier results obtained for traditionally living Eskimos (6). The urinary content of 2,3-dinor-Δ17-6-keto-$PGF_{1\alpha}$, the major metabolite of PGI_3, (PGI_3-M) was strikingly increased in the volunteers of the mackerel group. Such an increase is understandable, since precursor availability (TA) is greatly improved upon fish intake. The results with respect to PGI_2 were inconsistent. In a first set of analyses, the urinary content of 2,3 dinor-6-keto-$PGF_{1\alpha}$, the major metabolite of PGI_2 was increased in the mackerel group, and strongly correlated with the urinary PGI_3-M content (Fig. 3). In a second series of analyses, however, this could not be reproduced. For none of the volunteers of the fish group a reduction in PGI_2-M was observed, which is difficult to reconcile with the lower availability of the precursor fatty acid, AA. Whether or not these effects of the mackerel supplement on the urina-

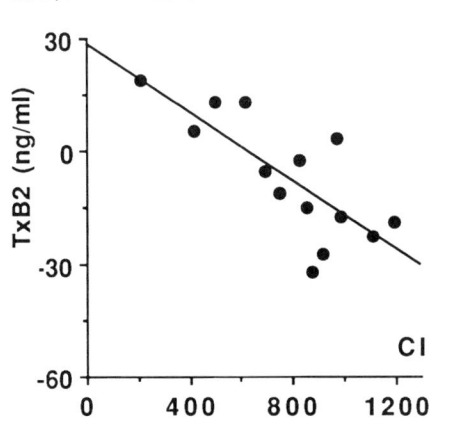

FIG. 2., RELATIONSHIP BETWEEN DIETARY COMPLIANCE (CI) AND THE CHANGE IN TXB_2 FORMATION AFTER 6 WEEKS.
$Y = 28.6 - 0.045X$; $r = -0.77$; $p < 0.001$

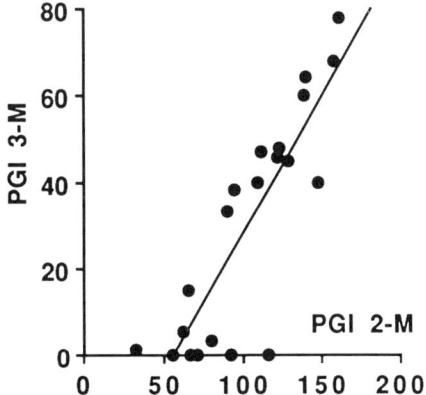

FIG. 3., RELATIONSHIP BETWEEN THE URINARY CONTENTS OF PGI_2-M AND PGI_3-M (FIRST SERIES).
$Y = -0.36 + 0.6X$; $r = 0.86$; $p < 0.001$

ry contents of PGI$_2$-M and PGI$_3$-M are of physiological relevance is not easy to decide, since increasing amounts of PGI-M in urine do not necessarily reflect an increased *vascular* PGI production. Moreover, an influence of dietary mackerel on the metabolic pathway of prostaglandins, leading to enhanced b oxidation observed before in rats (7), cannot be excluded. Finally, the pathophysiological interpretation of an enhanced PGI turnover is complicated by the higher values found for heavy smokers (8) and in severe atherosclerosis (9).

SUMMARY

Dietary mackerel causes the increase of timnodonic acid (eicosapentaenoic acid) in all platelet phospholipid classes, at the expense of arachidonic acid. Because of these fatty acid changes, the potency of platelets to produce cyclo oxygenase products from the 2-series is greatly reduced. However, upon mild platelet friggering, changes in TxB$_2$ formation are hardly significant, strongly depend on dietary compliance and require a high fish intake. The reduced formation of 2-series prostanoids is only partly compensated for by the increased formation of timnodonic acid-derived products. Urinary PGI metabolites suggest that dietary fish is associated with the enhanced turnover of PGI$_3$ without a concomitant reduction in PGI$_2$ formation. Since the site of PGI formation is not known, and an effect of dietary fish on the prostanoid metabolic routes cannot be excluded, the physiological relevance of these results is uncertain.

REFERENCES

1. Hornstra, G.(1989): In: *The role of fats in human nutrition II*, edited by M. Crawford, and A.J. Vergroesen, pp. 152-235. Academic Press, London.

2. Houwelingen, A.C. van, Nordøy, A., Beek, E. van der, Houtsmuller, U.M.T., Metz, M de, and Hornstra, G. (1987): *Am. J. Clin. Nutr.*, 46:871-875.

3. Hornstra, G., van Houwelingen, A.C., Kivits, G.A.A., Fischer, S., and Uedelhoven, W. (1991): *Prostaglandins*, accepted for publication.

4. Bevers, E.M., Comfurius, P., and Zwaal, R.F.A. (1983): *Biochim. Biophys. Acta*, 736: 57-66.

5. Houwelingen, A.C. van, Kester, A.D., and Hornstra, G. (1989): *Nutr. Res.*, 9: 1187-1196.

6. Zuccato, E., Hornstra, G., and Dyerberg, J. (1985): *Prostaglandins*, 30:465-478.

7. Hornstra, G., and Stegen, J.C.H.C. (1989): *Eicosanoids*, 2:145-149.

8. Nowak, J., Murray, J.J., FitzGerald, G.A.,.Wehr, C.J., Hammon, J.W., and Oates, J.A. (1987): *Prost. Thrombox. Leukotr. Res.*, 17:20-24.

9. FitzGerald, G.A., Smith, B., Pedersen, A.K., and Brash, A.R. (1984): *New. Engl. J. Med.*, 310:1065-1068.

THE EFFECT OF FISH OIL ON PLASMA LIPIDS, PLATELET AND NEUTROPHIL FUNCTION IN PATIENTS WITH VASCULAR DISEASE

Trevor A.Mori, Robert Vandongen, Fariba Mahanian and Andrea Douglas.

University Department of Medicine, School of Medicine, Royal Perth Hospital, Perth, Western Australia, 6000.

Epidemiologic observations and investigations of the effects of fish oils rich in ω3 polyunsaturated fatty acids (PUFAs), have drawn considerable attention because of their potential protective effect against the development of atherosclerotic vascular and coronary disease (1,3,6). Ingestion of the two major ω3 fatty acids present in fish oil, eicosapentaenoic acid (EPA) and docosahexaenoic acid (DHA) has been associated with a reduced incidence of myocardial infarction (8), beneficial alterations in plasma lipoproteins (12) and altered prostanoid metabolism (1,6). Dietary fish oil has increased bleeding time in normal persons, most likely due to a mild inhibition of platelet aggregation (4). A fall in blood pressure has been demonstrated in both normotensive (15) and hypertensive subjects (7). Altered immune and inflammatory responses have been ascribed to fish oils (1). Since hyperactivity of platelets and leukocytes, and excessive formation of thromboxane A_2 (TXA_2) and leukotriene B_4 (LTB_4), have been implicated in atherogenesis and its manifestations, it has been postulated that metabolic alterations caused by ω3 PUFAs may retard progression of thrombosis and atherosclerosis (1,3,6). The purpose of this study was to examine the effect of a fish oil supplement on plasma lipids, platelet and neutrophil function in patients with peripheral vascular disease (PVD).

METHODS

Thirty two males aged 47-71 yr, with symptomatic and angiographically demonstrated PVD, were recruited. All patients were screened and asked to maintain their medication with the exception of aspirin which was withdrawn at least 14 days prior to the start of the study. Participants were asked to maintain normal dietary patterns and physical activities. All participants were informed of the purpose of the study which was approved by the Hospital's Human Rights Committee. Patients were matched for age and body mass index, and randomly allocated to take either 15 g/day fish oil (Max EPA) or olive oil, with meals for 4 weeks. The fish oil supplement provided a daily intake of 2.8g EPA, 1.8g DHA and a total of 5.2g of ω3 fatty acids. The olive oil supplement consisted of 11.2g oleic acid. Following 2 baseline visits, patients were seen on 2 occasions after 2 and 4 weeks, and at 2 and 6 weeks post intervention. Patients abstained from food, smoking and alcohol for at least 3 hr prior to their visits. Compliance was assessed by capsule count and body weight was recorded at each visit.

Aggregation experiments were performed with 0.5 and 1.0 µg/ml collagen, and 0.05 and 0.50 µM PAF, according to methods previously described (9). Serum lipids and platelet phospholipid fatty acids were analyzed by established methods (11). Leukotrienes from calcium ionophore A23187 stimulated leukocytes were measured by HPLC (2). Serum TXB_2 was determined by RIA (9). Data was analyzed using two way analysis of variance for repeated measures. Differences between the two groups at each visit were tested using Duncan's modified t-test.

RESULTS

Baseline characteristics of the 2 groups were comparable for age, body mass index, plasma creatinine and glucose, and number of smokers. The 29 patients who commenced the study completed the 10 week trial. No changes in body weight, plasma creatinine, haematological profile, or medication were seen throughout the study.

Fish oil increased EPA (3.72 ± 0.08 to 6.59 ± 0.30 %, p <0.001) and DHA (5.33 ± 0.22 to 7.90 ± 0.32 %, p <0.001), and reduced arachidonic acid (25.10 ± 0.31 to 21.58 ± 0.33 %, p <0.001), in platelet phospholipids. Olive oil did not alter platelet phospholipid fatty acids.

Changes in serum lipids are shown in Table 1. Total cholesterol, LDL- and HDL_2-C were significantly increased following fish oil. The increase in HDL_2-C was approximately 17%. Serum triglycerides were decreased by 26% (p <0.05). Olive oil reduced total cholesterol and LDL-C (p <0.01). HDL_2-C was only moderately affected, while triglycerides remained unchanged.

After 4 weeks fish oil, LTB_4 was reduced from 2.68 ± 0.44 to 1.79 ± 0.21 ng/10^7 leukocytes (p <0.05), and LTB_5 increased from 0.28 ± 0.03 to 0.53 ± 0.04 ng/10^7 leukocytes (p <0.001). Leukotrienes were unaffected by olive oil.

Platelet aggregation to collagen and PAF was reduced following fish oil. Aggregation to 0.5 and 1.0 µg/ml collagen was reduced by 39% and 10%, respectively (p <0.05), and using 0.05 and 0.50 µM PAF, by 39% and 6%, respectively (p <0.05). Olive oil enhanced platelet aggregation to both collagen and PAF, with increases of 46% and 13% (p <0.05) using 0.5 and 1.0 µg/ml collagen, and 86% and 6% using 0.05 and 0.50 µM PAF. Serum TXB_2 increased in this group from 84.5 ± 11.8 to 116.4 ± 12.2 ng/ml (p <0.01).

DISCUSSION

We have shown that 15g/day of fish oil for 4 weeks, leads to significant changes in patients with peripheral vascular disease. Following the supplement, platelet phospholipid EPA and DHA were significantly increased at the expense of arachidonic acid. These findings are consistent with most

TABLE 1. The effect of fish oil and olive oil on lipid profiles in patients with vascular disease.

	Baseline (mM)	End of 4 wk intervention (mM)	6 wk post-intervention (mM)	Significance[a]
Total cholesterol				
Fish oil	6.1 ± 0.3	6.4 ± 0.3	6.1 ± 0.3	$p < 0.01$
Olive oil	6.1 ± 0.4	5.9 ± 0.3	6.3 ± 0.4	
LDL-C				
Fish oil	3.77 ± 0.27	4.40 ± 0.27	3.96 ± 0.32	$p < 0.01$
Olive oil	3.66 ± 0.29	3.39 ± 0.23	3.88 ± 0.36	
HDL$_2$-C				
Fish oil	0.52 ± 0.06	0.61 ± 0.06	0.56 ± 0.04	$p < 0.05$
Olive oil	0.52 ± 0.05	0.56 ± 0.06	0.53 ± 0.05	
Triglycerides				
Fish oil	2.3 ± 0.4	1.7 ± 0.2	2.3 ± 0.4	$p < 0.05$
Olive oil	2.8 ± 0.4	3.0 ± 0.4	2.8 ± 0.4	

[a] Treatment x time interaction. Results expressed as mean ± SEM

other fish oil trials (1,3,6). Dietary fish oil has been shown to prolong bleeding time in normal subjects (4), which is probably due to inhibition of platelet aggregation. This trial shows that following fish oil, platelet aggregation to collagen and PAF was significantly reduced. This was more pronounced at the lowest doses in each case. In patients taking olive oil, platelet aggregation was increased to collagen and PAF at the end of the supplementation period. This effect of olive oil has not been previously reported and remains unexplained. A significant increase in serum TXB$_2$ was observed following supplementation with olive oil. This finding has not been observed in other trials. It is not immediately apparent how olive oil, which is predominently oleic acid (18:1 ω9), could induce this alteration in serum TXB$_2$. It is tempting to speculate that the increase in TXB$_2$ is related to the increase in platelet aggregation. Alternatively, the change in platelet aggregation may be independent of serum TXB$_2$ and may just reflect changes in platelet membrane fluidity induced by oleic acid. However, this seems unlikely as no change in oleic acid content of platelet phospholipids was observed.

Leukocytes, particularly neutrophils, macrophages and monocytes, play a critical role in the evolution of the atherosclerotic plaque (14). Dietary fish oil inhibits LTB$_4$, while the analogous EPA derived metabolite LTB$_5$, which has markedly attenuated chemotactic and aggregating activities for neutrophils, is increased (13). Our observations are in accordance with these findings.

Fish oil significantly increased total cholesterol in our trial. This was accounted for by a significant rise in both LDL- and HDL$_2$-C. We have previously shown a rise in HDL$_2$-C in insulin-dependent diabetics with 15g/day fish oil for 3 weeks (11). This increase in HDL$_2$-C (equivalent to an average of 0.09 mM) is substantial and could be expected to have a marked impact on the incidence of cardiovascular disease (10). The potential benefit of the increase in HDL$_2$-C, however, needs to be assessed against the rise in

LDL-C. Dosages comparable to that used in our study, have increased total cholesterol and LDL-C, with HDL-C either unchanged or slightly increased (1,6). Serum triglycerides were significantly reduced by the fish oil in our study, which confirms that ω3 PUFAs are powerful triglyceride lowering agents (1,6). In our trial, olive oil significantly reduced total cholesterol and LDL-C. These findings agree with studies where a high monounsaturated fat diet, principally in the form of oleic acid has been used (5).

Experimental atherosclerosis has been shown to be inhibited by fish oil without changes in lipids (3). Therefore, it may be the ability of fish oils to reduce platelet and leukocyte interactions with the vessel wall, that contributes to the inhibition of atherogenesis. In summary, this study shows that dietary fish oil in patients with peripheral vascular disease exerts beneficial effects on platelet and leukocyte activity even in the presence of existing medication.

ACKNOWLEDGEMENTS

This work was supported by the Australian National Heart Foundation. We thank Ms Lynette Kelly for technical assistance. Max EPA and olive oil capsules were donated by Reckitt & Colman Pharmaceuticals, Australia.

REFERENCES

1. Budowski, P. (1988): In: *Aspects of Human Nutrition - World Review of Nutrition and Dietetics*. Vol. 57. edited by G.H. Bourne. pp. 214-274. S. Karger AG, Basel.
2. Croft, K.D., Codde, J.P., Barden, A., Vandongen, R., and Beilin, L.J. (1988): *Clin. Exp. Pharmacol. Physiol.*, 15: 517-525.
3. Goodnight, S.H., Fisher, M., FitzGerald, G.A., and Levine, P.H. (1989): *Chest*, 95:19S-25S, Supplement.
4. Goodnight, S.H., Harris, W.S., and Connor, W.E. (1981): *Blood*, 58: 880-885.
5. Grundy, S.M., Florentin, L., Nix, D., and Whelan, MF. (1988): *Am. J. Clin. Nutr.*, 47: 965-969.
6. Herold, P.M., and Kinsella, J.E. (1986): *Am. J. Clin. Nutr.*, 43: 566-598.
7. Knapp, H.R., and FitzGerald, G.A. (1989): *N. Engl. J. Med.*, 320: 1037-1043.
8. Kromhout, D., Bosschieter, E.B., and deLezenne Coulander, C. (1985): *N. Engl. J. Med.*, 312: 1205-1209.
9. McCulloch, R.K., Summers, J., Vandongen, R., and Rouse, I.L. (1989): *Clin. Sci.*, 77: 99-103.
10. Miller, N.E., Hammett, F., Saltissi, S., Rao, S., van Zeller, H., Coltart, J., and Lewis, B. (1981): *Br. Med. J.*, 282: 1741-1744.
11. Mori, T.A., Vandongen, R., Masarei, J.R.L., Stanton, K.G., and Dunbar, D. (1989): *Metabolism*, 38: 404-409.
12. Phillipson, B.E., Rothrock, D.W., Connor, W.E., Harris, W.S., and Illingworth, D.R. (1985): *N. Engl. J. Med.*, 312: 1210-1216.
13. Prescott, S.M. (1984): *J. Biol. Chem.*, 259: 7615-7621.
14. Ross, R. (1986): *N. Engl. J. Med.*, 314: 488-500.
15. Singer, P., Jaeger, W., Wirth, M., Voigt, S., Naumann, E., Zimontkowski, S., Hajdu, I., and Goedicke, W. (1983): *Atherosclerosis*, 49: 99-108.

EFFECTS OF EPA AND DHA ETHYLESTERS ON PLASMA FATTY ACIDS AND ON PLATELETS, PMN AND MONOCYTES IN HEALTHY VOLUNTEERS

E. Tremoli, C. Mosconi, P. Maderna, S. Colli, E. Stragliotto, C.R. Sirtori, and C. Galli

Institute of Pharmacological Sciences and E. Grossi Paoletti Center, University of Milan, Via Balzaretti 9, 20133 Milano, Italy

The intake of long chain polyunsaturated fatty acids (PUFA) of the n-3 series has been shown in several studies to influence plasma lipids and/or lipoproteins and to affect the function and biochemistry of blood cells, thus possibly influencing the initiation and development of pathological conditions, such as thrombosis, inflammatory disease and even atherosclerosis (3, 5). High doses of n-3 FA containing oils, given for relatively long periods of time, are generally required to obtain appreciable effects. Recently the availability of formula selectively enriched in eicosapentaenoic acid (EPA) and docosahexaenoic acid (DHA) has allowed to reduce the amount of capsules to be given, and to obtain a better compliance to the treatment. In this study we have evaluated the effects of the supplementation of a purified preparation of n-3 ethylesters, selectively enriched in EPA and DHA, to healthy male volunteers on plasma and circulating cells.

MATERIALS AND METHODS

Five healthy male volunteers (age range 25-51) free from any drug treatment were administered 1 g capsules of an EPA/DHA ethylester preparation (Norsk Hydro, Porsgrum, Norway). Each capsule contained 465 mg EPA and 283 mg DHA. Each subject received 6 capsules/day for 6 weeks. Before and at the end of the treatment blood was drawn while fasting and the following determinations were carried out: fatty acid analysis of plasma and cell lipids by gas chromatography on capillary columns; aggregation of platelet rich plasma induced by collagen, by the turbidimetric technique; thromboxane B_2 (TXB_2) levels in PRP stimulated with collagen by RIA; O_2^- production by monocytes and polymorphonuclear leukocytes (PMN) by the spectrophotometric procedure described by Babior et al (1).

RESULTS AND DISCUSSION

The intake of n-3 FA resulted in consistent changes in the levels of both n-3 and n-6 FA in all the lipid compartments evaluated. In particular arachidonic acid (AA) content of platelet and leukocyte phospholipids (PL) was reduced by the treatment, whereas the levels of AA in plasma remained unchanged. Concomitantly, levels of both EPA and DHA were significantly increased in plasma and cells. Fig. 1 shows the mean EPA/AA ratios determined in the different compartments. The major increment of the EPA/AA ratios occurred in plasma and changes of the ratios were less pronounced in cells. The EPA/AA ratio both before and after treatment were higher in PMN than in platelets and monocytes.

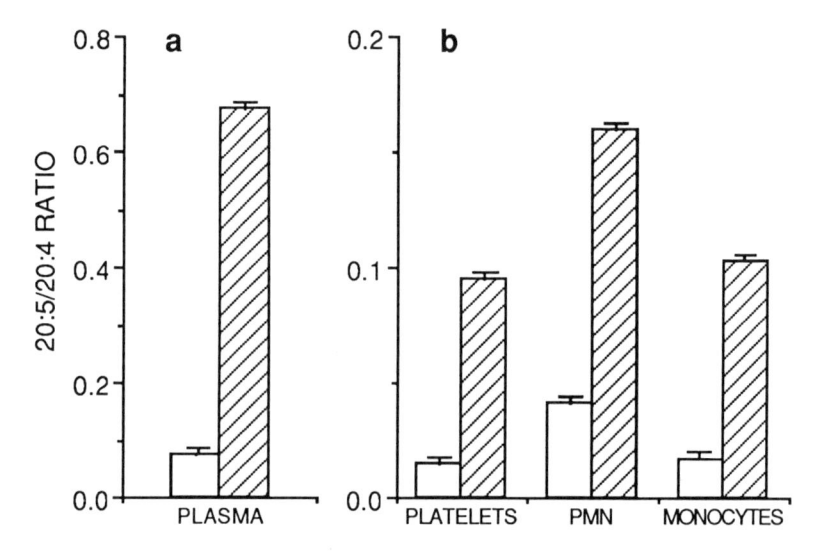

FIG. 1. EPA/AA ratio in plasma (panel a) and in platelet, PMN and monocyte (panel b) lipids. Data are the means ± SEM of ratios evaluated for each subject before (□) and after 6 week (▨) n-3 supplementation.

The modifications in cellular lipid composition were accompanied by changes in the response of cells to agonists. Indeed, following n-3 supplementation, platelet aggregation was significantly reduced, as shown by an increase in the amount of collagen required to achieve 50% irreversible aggregation (AC_{50}) (Fig. 2). In addition, the levels of TXB_2 in PRP samples stimulated with collagen were significantly reduced by the treatment (Fig. 2). These data are in accordance with most data reported by other Authors following supplementation with cod liver oil. However, the administration of fish oil concentrates with the same amount of EPA and DHA and for the same duration as in our study did not result in a significant modification of platelet aggregation, and only in a slight prolongation of bleeding time was recorded (4). On the other hand, in the above study, EPA accumulation in platelets following treatment was even higher than in our subjects.

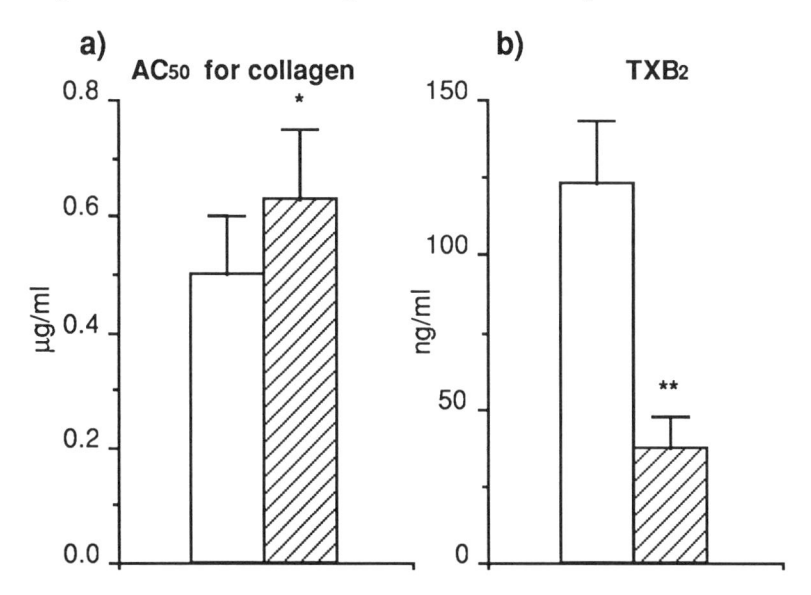

FIG. 2. Effect of n-3 supplementation on aggregation (panel a) and TXB$_2$ formation (panel b) by PRP stimulated with collagen. Data are the means ± SEM before (☐) and after (▨) n-3 supplementation. * $p < 0.05$; ** $p < 0.001$ versus before.

In consideration of the emerging role of leukocytes (polymorphonuclear leukocytes and monocytes) in myocardial ischemic events and in the early stages of atherosclerosis, the effects of n-3 supplementation on these cells were also evaluated.

As shown in Fig. 3, n-3 supplementation significantly inhibited O$_2^-$ generation by monocytes stimulated with both serum treated zymosan (STZ) and the chemotactic peptide fMLP. This effect was specific for monocytes, since O$_2^-$ generation by PMN was unaffected by the treatment.

These data confirm those previously reported by Fisher et al (2) who showed a similar impairment in O$_2^-$ generation by monocytes following n-3 supplementation. The Authors showed however that n-3 fatty acids were also capable to inhibit superoxide anion by PMN. It should be noted that the increment in the EPA content of PMN reported by these Authors was far greater than that found in our study.

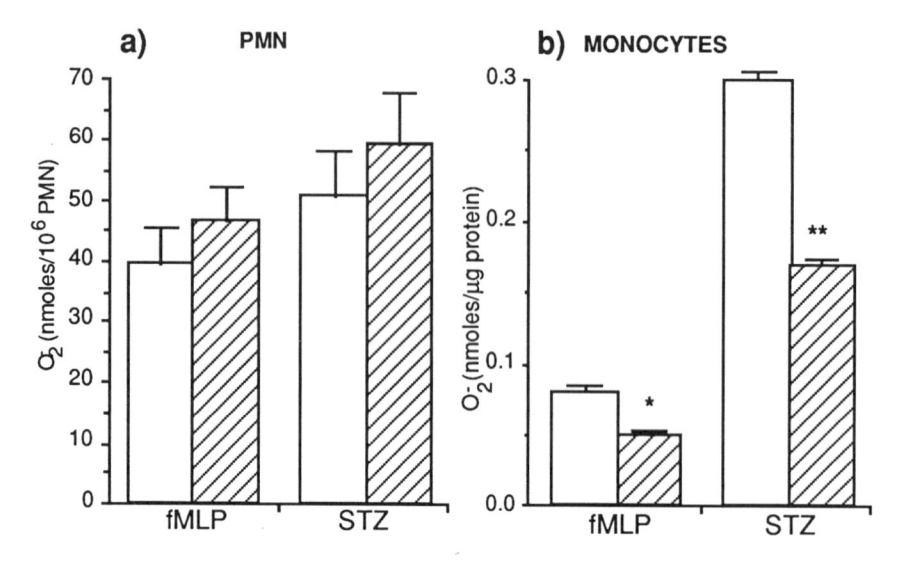

FIG. 3. Superoxide anion generation by PMN (panel a) and adherent monocytes (panel b) before (□) and after (▨) n-3 supplementation. fMLP: N-formyl-methionyl-leucyl-phenylalanine, 10^{-6} M; STZ serum treated zymosan, 1 mg/ml. * $p < 0.05$; ** $p < 0.005$ versus before.

In conclusion this study shows that the administration of a preparation highly enriched in n-3 ethylesters to healthy volunteers effectively impairs not only the function of platelets but also that of blood cells, such as monocytes, which play a role in the atherosclerotic process.

REFERENCES

1. Babior, B.M., Kipnes, R.S., and Curnutte, J.T. (1973): *J. Clin. Invest.*, 51: 741-744.

2. Fisher, M., Upchurch, K.S., Levine, P.H., Johnson, M.H., Vandrenil, C.H., Natale, A., and Hoogasian, J.J. (1986): *Inflammation*, 10: 387-392.

3. Lee, T.H., Hoover, R.L., Williams, J.D., Sperling, R.I., Ravalese, J., Spur, B.V., Robinson, D.R., Corey, E.J., Lewis, R.A., and Austen, K.F. (1985): *N. Engl. J. Med.*, 312 (19): 1217-1224.

4. Schmidt, E.B., Warming, K., Madsen, E.P., and Dyerberg, J. (1990): *Thromb. Haemost.*, 63: 1-5.

5. Von Schacky, C., Fischer, S., and Weber, P.C. (1985): *J. Clin. Invest.*, 76: 1626-1631.

EICOSANOID PRODUCTION AND MEMBRANE RELATED PROPERTIES OF ENDOTHELIAL CELLS AFTER FATTY ACID MODIFICATION IN VITRO

R. C. R. M. Vossen*, M. C. E. van Dam-Mieras**, G. Hornstra*** and R. F. A. Zwaal*

* Departments of Biochemistry and *** Human Biology, Limburg University, P. O. Box 616, 6200 MD Maastricht and ** Open university of The Netherlands, P. O. Box 2960, 6401 DL Heerlen, The Netherlands.

INTRODUCTION

Atherosclerosis affects mainly the tunica intima and the atherosclerotic lesion is characterized by the presence of deposits of lipid materials, remnants of thrombi, phagocytes, lymphocytes, smooth muscle cells and elements of connective tissue such as collagen, elastin and glycosaminoglycans within the intima (4, 10). This composition of the atherosclerotic plaque points to a local activation of the vascular wall by stimuli of an inflammatory and immunological character during its genesis (5).

The endothelial cell layer that covers the luminal side of the vessel wall actively participates in the regulation of haemostatic, inflammatory and immunologic processes that take place in or near the vascular wall (1, 15). Stimulation of the endothelial cells with for instance thrombin, IL-1, TNF and LPS induces a procoagulant response, increases the adhesivity for other cells and decreases the fibrinolytic capacity (3, 8, 11). The eicosanoids formed during endothelial cell stimulation will modulate cell-cell interaction and influence vascular permeability (2, 9).

The biomembrane is the source of substrates from which local mediators are formed upon cellular activation. As, in the in vivo situation, the lipid composition of cellular membranes will reflect that of the diet, we thought it worthwhile to develop an *in vitro* system that would enable us to study the effect of changes in biomembrane lipid composition upon endothelial cell reactivity. In this *in vitro* system, endothelial cells were grown for several passages in different fatty acid supplemented media (14). The effect of lipid modification on membrane related parameters such as endothelial cell procoagulant activity, polymorphonuclear monocyte adhesion and eicosanoid formation was studied. In this report attention is focussed on eicosanoid formation.

MATERIALS AND METHODS

Culture medium consisted of M199 (Flow lab.)/RPMI1640 (Flow lab.) (v/v) supplemented with L-glutamine (2mM), gentamicin (50 mg/ml), NaHCO$_3$ (11.9 mM)and endothelial cell growth supplement (500 µg protein/ml, prepared according to Maciag et al. (7)).Tissue culture dishes were obtained from Falcon, trypsin solution (2.5% w/v) from Flow lab. , thrombin from Roche. Human fibronectin was a gift from Dr. J. van Mourik (Central Laboratory for Blood Transfusion, Amsterdam). All chemicals used were of the purest grade available.

Endothelial cells were obtained from human umbilical veins and cultured and identified according to Vossen et al. (14). Fatty acid analyses and eicosanoid determinations were carried out as described before (14).

RESULTS AND DISCUSSION

We have shown previously (13) that the fatty acid composition of endothelial cells can be extensively modified *in vitro* in a standardized way by culturing the cells in different lipid-modified media. In the present study the fatty acyl modification is brought about by culturing the cells in culture media supplemented with the sodium salt of different fatty acids. To investigate the effect of fatty acid supplementation per se, endothelial cells were cultured in standard culture medium supplemented with a mixture of fatty acids (200 μM, consisting of 16:0 (34%), 18:0 (12%), 18:1 (34%) and 18:2 (20%)), which is comparable to the free fatty acid composition of human serum. These cells were compared to control cells grown in standard culture medium without fatty acid supplementation. The fatty acyl contents in the cells of both cultures were highly similar, as were growth characteristics, cellular morphology and reactivity.

The fatty acyl content of endothelial cell membranes was subsequently varied by culturing the cells in various fatty acid supplemented media (200 μM fatty acid). All cells showed normal morphologic appearance and normal von Willebrand factor staining. The growth rate of most manipulated cells was the same as that of the control

TABLE 1. Fatty acid composition of fatty acid-modified endothelial cells

fatty acid	control	FAmix	16:0	18:0	18:1	18:2	20:4	20:5	22:6
16:0	19.9	21.3	24.6	16.9	15.3	18.4	22.7	22.4	22.0
18:0	12.7	12.9	12.5	19.1	10.3	11.4	12.6	13.5	13.7
18:1(n-9)	17.8	18.4	13.9	13.8	40.4	10.2	14.1	18.4	17.2
18:2(n-6)	13.2	14.7	10.2	12.2	7.3	32.3	7.9	10.3	11.5
20:2(n-6)	1.0	0.9	0.6	0.7	0.7	5.2	0.6	0.3	0.1
20:3(n-6)	1.5	1.8	1.7	2.5	0.8	1.0	0.9	0.6	1.1
20:4(n-6)	10.8	10.7	14.7	15.7	6.1	5.5	17.4	3.2	7.8
20:5(n-3)	0.6	0.5	0.6	0.8	0.3	0.6	0.1	10.6	0.9
22:4(n-6)	3.8	3.9	4.3	2.5	3.5	3.4	13.1	0.6	1.1
22:5(n-3)/ 24:2(n-6)	1.1	2.6	2.3	2.4	3.2	3.9	0.6	11.8	0.6
22:6(n-3)	3.3	3.2	3.7	3.0	2.3	1.8	0.4	0.6	13.5

Values (means of at least three separate cultures) are expressed as percentage of total fatty acids. Standard errors varied from 0.1 to 1.2. for respectively small and large values.

cells, only cells grown in 20:5(n-3) and in 22:6(n-3) supplemented media exhibited occasionally a slightly reduced growth rate. Fatty acid modifications were not accompanied by significant changes in membrane phospholipid, cholesterol and protein content (data not shown).

Table 1 summarizes the effect of endothelial cell culture in different fatty acid supplemented media on the fatty acyl content of the cells. It can be concluded from table 1 that supplementation of the culture medium with a specific fatty acid resulted in an increase of that specific fatty acid and its elongation product in the cell membrane, while compensatory changes in the level of other fatty acids were observed.

Not all fatty acids could be increased to the same extent; supplementation with saturated fatty acids increased the specific fatty acyl content to only a limited extent while unsaturated fatty acids were increased to a larger extent. However, the total amount of saturated and unsaturated fatty acids in the membrane remained rather constant.

Generally speaking saturated fatty acids replace saturated fatty acids at the sn-1 position while unsaturated fatty acids are replaced by unsaturated fatty acids at the sn-2 position. Oleic acid behaved slightly different in that an increase in 18:1 was accompanied by a decrease in both polyunsaturated as well as saturated fatty acids. We might therefore speculate that 18:1 can be bound to both the sn-1 and the sn-2 position of the phospholipids, which may of course have implications for the modulation of cellular responses by local mediators.

The arachidonic acid content of endothelial cells could be increased by supplementation of arachidonic acid to the culture medium, but was also increased upon enrichment with saturated fatty acids. This latter phenomenon was also described by Heemskerk et al. for platelets obtained from dietary manipulated rats (6).

Variations in the polyunsaturated fatty acid content of endothelial cells could be important in the modulation of cellular responses. We therefore investigated their effect on the cellular procoagulant response, polymorphonuclear leucocyte (PMN) adhesion and the production of tissue plasminogen activator (tPA) and plasminogen activator inhibitor type 1 (PAI-1) (data not shown); the fatty acid composition of the membranes had only a very limited influence on these parameters (14).

As the biomembrane is the source of substrates for local mediators, eicosanoid production by the differently modified endothelial cells after stimulation with thrombin was studied. In the absence of thrombin stimulation, eicosanoid production was extremely low. The absolute amount of eicosanoids formed after thrombin stimulation differed somewhat for the different batches of endothelial cells, but the eicosanoid spectrum was always similar. The main products were 6-ketoprostaglandin $F_{1\alpha}$, and prostaglandin $F_{2\alpha}$, and small amounts of prostaglandin E_2, 12-hydroxy-5, 8, 10-heptadecatrienoic acid, 15-hydroxyeicosatetraenoic acid and thromboxane B_2 were measured also.

Generaly speaking, there was a positive correlation between the endogenous arachidonic acid content in the endothelial cell membranes and the total amount of eicosanoids produced upon thrombin stimulation of the cells. However, when the increase in membrane arachidonic acid content of the endothelial cells was obtained by supplementation of the culture medium with arachidonic acid, a decreased eicosanoid formation was found. Spector et al.(12) also describe a reduced PGI_2 production after a 24 hours incubation of confluent endothelial cell monolayers with arachidonic acid. The authors tentatively explain their observation by an inactivation of cyclooxygenase during the supplementation period. The enzyme probably is inactivated during catalysis by the hydroperoxides generated during the reaction. Another explanation may be a reduced availability of this arachidonic acid pool for eicosanoid synthesis. Further studies are necessary to gain more insight into this phenomenon.

In conclusion we can say that important changes in endothelial cell fatty acid content have no effect on growth characteristics, morphology, the procoagulant response, PMN adhesion and tPA and PAI-1 secretion but that the effect on eicosanoid production after cellular stimulation is evident.

REFERENCES

1. Ashida, E. R. , Johnson, A. R. and Lipsky, P. E. (1981): J. Clin. Invest. , 67:.1490-1499.
2. Austen, K. F. (1987): Drugs, 33 (suppl. 1): 10-17.
3. Brevario, F. , Bertocchi, F. , Dejana, E. and Bussolina, F. (1988): J. Immunol. , 141: 3391-3397.
4. Bendit, E. P. (1988): Arch. Pathol. Lab. Med. , 112: 997-1001.
5. Bruggeman, C. A. and van Dam-Mieras, M. C. E. , Prog. Med. Virol. , 38: in press.
6. Heemskerk, J. W. M. , Feijge, M. A. H. , Kalafusz, R. and Hornstra, G. (1989): Biochim. Biophys. Acta, 1004: 252-260.
7. Maciag, T. , Cerundole, I. , Istey, S. , Kelly, P. R. and Foriand, R. (1979): Proc. Natl. Acad. Sci. USA, 76: 5674-5678.
8. Nawroth, P. , Kisiel, W. and Stern, D. (1985): Clin. Haemat. , 14: 531-546.
9. Pottmeyer, E. , Vassar, M. J. and Holcraft, J. W. (1986): Crit. Care C. , 2: 683-703.
10. Ross, R. (1986): New. Eng. J. Med. ,314: 488-500.
11. Schleef, R. R. , Bevilacqua, M. P. , Sawdey, M. , Gimbrone, M. A. and Loskutoff, P. J. (1988): J. Biol. J. Biol. Chem. , 263: 5797-5803.
12. Spector, A. A. , Kaduce, T. L. , Hoak, J. C. and Czervionke, R. L. (1983): Arteriosclerosis, 3: 323-331.
13. Vossen, R. C. R. M. , van Dam-Mieras, M. C. E. ,Hornstra, G. and Zwaal, R. F. A. (1989): Thromb. Haem. , 62: 578.
14. Vossen, C. R. M. , van Dam-Mieras, M. C. E. , Hornstra, G. and Zwaal, R. F. A. , manuscript submitted for publication.
15. Wehrmacher, W. H. (1988): Sem. Thromb. , 14(suppl): 1-11.

EFFECT OF INGESTION OF EICOSAPENTAENOIC ACID ETHYL-ESTER ON THE SCAVENGER ACTIVITY FOR ACETYLATED LDL AND THE PRODUCTION OF PLATELET-DERIVED GROWTH FACTOR IN RAT PERITONEAL MACROPHAGES

Hiroyuki Saito, Ichiro Saito, Ke-Jian Chang, Yasushi Tamura and Sho Yoshida

The Second Department of Internal Medicine, School of Medicine, Chiba University, 1-8-1 Inohana, Chiba 280, Japan

It was found that the ingestion of highly purified eicosapentaenoic acid-ethyl ester (EPA-E) significantly and dose-dependently decreased the accumulation of cholesterol ester and the proteolytic degradation in rat peritoneal macrophages when incubated with acetylated low density lipoprotein (AcLDL). Another new important finding in the present study was that the production of platelet-derived growth factor (PDGF) was also significantly reduced by the ingestion of EPA-E in a dose-dependent manner. The present finding may indicate that the prophylactic effect of EPA on the development of atherosclerosis can be, at least in part, ascribed to its inhibitory effect on the formation of foam cells and on the production of PDGF in macrophages.

INTRODUCTION

In a very early stage of atherosclerosis circulating blood monocytes have been shown to invade into subendothelial space [1]. These cells have been shown to become lipid-laden macrophages, so called foam cells, after phagocytosing deposited lipids through the scavenger pathway [1,2]. These foam cells are considered to mediate a role in the development of atherosclerosis by secreting various kinds of inflammatory mediators including platelet-derived growth factor (PDGF) [3], which has been suggested to be one of potent growth factors of smooth muscle cells (SMC) [4].
Eicosapentaenoic acid (EPA), rich in marine fish oil, has been elucidated to have prophylactic effect on the development of atherosclerosis in human subjects and experimental animal models [5,6]. The beneficial effect of EPA has been partly ascribed to its anti-hyperlipidemic action and anti-platelet aggregatory action [7,8]. However, it still remained to be elucidated how EPA exerts its anti-atherosclerotic action in the vessel walls.
Accordingly the present investigation was performed to investigate the effect of administration of highly purified EPA ethyl ester on the foam cell formation and on the production of PDGF in rat peritoneal macrophages.

MATERIALS AND METHODS

Reagents
EPA ethyl ester (EPA-E) was a gift from Nippon Suisan Co., Ltd. (Tokyo, Japan). PDGF RIA kit was obtained from Amersham

International Plc. (Backinghamshire, England). Sodium [^{125}I] iodide (carrier free in diluted NaOH, pH 7-11, s.a.: 15 mCi/μg of iodine) was purchased from the Radiochemical Centre (Amersham, UK). Iodine monochloride (ICI) was a kind gift from Dr. Seijiro Mori. Trichloroacetic acid (TCA), AgNO$_3$ and glycine were from Wako Pure Chemical Industries, Ltd. (Osaka, Japan). RPMI 1640 medium was from GIBCO (NY, USA). Highly purified bovine serum albumin (HP-BSA) was from Sigma Chemical Co., Ltd. (MO, USA).

Preparation of macrophages
    Six-week-old male Wistar rats were administered 30, 60, 100, 300 mg/kg/day of EPA-E emulsion (EPA rats) or vehicle alone (control rats) during four weeks by using metal stomach catheter. Peritoneal macrophages were cultured for 1 day at 37°C in 5% CO$_2$ 95% air before using in the following experiments.

Preparation of ^{125}I-labeled acetylated low density lipoprotein (^{125}I-AcLDL)
    LDL (density 1.019-1.063 g/ml) was separated by sequential ultracentrifugation and then acetylated according to the method of Basu et al.[9]. Acetylated LDL (AcLDL) was labeled with Na ^{125}I in the presence of ICI. Final specific activities of ^{125}I-labeled AcLDL (^{125}I-AcLDL) were 70-100 cpm/ng protein.

Degradation of ^{125}I-AcLDL in macrophages
    Proteolytic degradation of ^{125}I-AcLDL in macrophages (10^6 cells) was measured by determining the amount of ^{125}I-labeled acid-soluble (non-iodide) materials, formed and released into the medium during 24 hr incubation with various concentrations of ^{125}I-AcLDL, according to the method as previously reported [10].

Accumulation of cholesteryl ester (CE) in macrophages
    CE accumulation in macrophages (10^6 cells) during 24 hr incubation with various concentrations of AcLDL was determined by the method of Heider et al.[11].

Induction and separation of PDGF in macrophages
    Macrophages (2x10^7 cells) in 150 ml of RPMI-1640 containing 10% HP-BSA were incubated for 24 hr at 37°C in 5% CO$_2$ 95% air. After the incubation, the culture medium was concentrated by using Centriprep 10 (Amicon, MA, USA) by 100 times. PDGF was separated from α$_2$-macroglobulin by the method of Kurmar et al.[12]. Briefly, the concentrated medium was acidified with 2 M glacial acetic acid and kept for 1 hr at room temperature. Then the sample was applied to Superose 12 HR 30/10 column (Pharmacia, NJ, USA), eluted with 1 M acetic acid at a flow rate of 0.5 ml/min. Each 1 ml of fraction was collected into tube containing 25 μl of 20% HP-BSA and neutralized with 0.5 ml of 2.0 M Tris base, and dialyzed overnight against RPMI-1640 at 4°C.

Assay of PDGF
    The amounts of PDGF in the eluants were determined by using Amersham PDGF RIA kit. Antiserum to PDGF used in the present study was specific to PDGF and had no cross reactivity for TGFβ,

EGF, FGF, β-thromboglobulin and platelet-factor 4 (Amersham in--house assessment).

Analysis of data
Statistical significance was determined by using Student's t test and each value represents mean ± SEM.

RESULTS AND DISCUSSION

In the present study, it was found that both the accumulation of cholesterol ester derived from AcLDL and the proteolytic degradation of ^{125}I-AcLDL in rat peritoneal macrophages were significantly decreased by the ingestion of EPA-E in a dose-dependent manner (Fig. 1, and Fig. 2). The mechanism of the inhibitory action of EPA is still unclear, but it is conceivable that EPA exerted its effect on the site of the scavenger receptor and/or lysosomal enzymes.

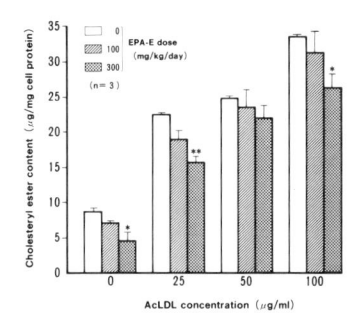

Fig.1. Effect of EPA-E ingestion on the accumulation of cholersteryl ester. Each value was represented as mean ±SEM. *:p<0.05, **:p<0.01

Fig.2. Effect of EPA-E ingestion on the proteolytic degradation of ^{125}I-AcLDL. Each value was represented as mean ±SEM. *:p<0.05, **:p<0.01

The present study also newly revealed that the production of PDGF was also significantly and dose-dependently inhibited by the ingestion of EPA-E (Fig. 3). The inhibitory mechanism of EPA still remained to elucidated in the present study. The production of PDGF is reported to be dependant on protein kinase C (PKC)[13]. Therefore, further study should be required to reveal the effect of EPA on the activity of PKC.

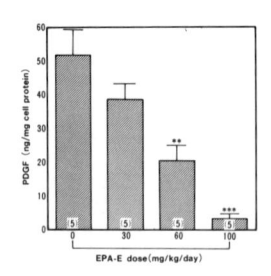

Fig. 3 Effect of EPA-E ingestion on the production of PDGF. Each value was represented as mean ± SEM.
**: P<0.01, ***: p<0.001 (n=5)

Even in these days, the role of monocytes and PDGF in the pathogenesis of atherosclerosis is still controversial [14]. However, the inhibitory effects of EPA on the formation of foam cells and PDGF are considered to, at least in part, account for the prophylactic effect of EPA on the development of atherosclerosis. Further study should be required to elucidate the effect of EPA on other function of macrophages, and on other cell type such as smooth muscle cells should also be clarified before defining the beneficial effect of EPA in atherosclerosis.

ACKNOWLEDGEMENT

This study was supported by Grant-in-Aid for Scientific Research of The Ministry of Education, Science and Culture of Japan (grant No. 02454505).

REFERENCES

1. Gerrity, R.G. (1981): Am. J. Path., 103: 181-190.
2. Brown, M.S. and Goldstein, J.L. (1983): Annu. Rev. Biochem., 52: 223-261.
3. Nathan, C.F. (1987): J. Clin. Invest., 79: 319-326.
4. Ross, R. (1983): Harvey Lect., 77: 161-182.
5. Kromhout, D., Bosschieter, E.B. and Coulander, C.L. (1985) New Engl. J. Med., 312: 1205-1209.
6. Herold, P.M. and Kinsella, J.E. (1986): Am. J. Clin. Nutr., 43: 566-598.
7. Kim, D.N., Ho, H.T., Lowrence, D.A., Schmee, J. and Thomas, W.A. (1989): Atherosclerosis, 76: 35-54.
8. Hirai, A., Terano, T., Hamazaki, T., Sajiki, J., Kondo, S., Ozawa, A., Fujita, T., Miyamoto, T., Tamura, Y. and Kumagai, A. (1982): Thromb. Res., 28: 285-298.
9. Basu, S.K., Goldstein, J.L., Anderson, R.G. and Brown, M.S. (1976): Proc. Natl. Acad. Sci. USA, 73: 3178-3182.
10. Frostegård, J., Hamsten, A., Gidlund, M. and Nilsson, J. (1990): J. Lipid Res., 31: 37-44.
11. Heider, J.G. and Boyett, R.L. (1978): J. Lipid Res., 19: 514-518.
12. Kurmar, R.K., Bennett, R.A. and Brody, A.R. (1988): FASEB J., 2: 2272-2277.
13. Ross, R., Raines, E.W. and Bowen-Pope, D.F. (1986): Cell, 46: 155-169.

EFFECT OF ORAL N-3 FATTY ACID SUPPLEMENTATION ON THE IMMUNE RESPONSE OF YOUNG AND OLDER WOMEN

Simin Nikbin Meydani, Stefan Endres, Margo M. Woods, Barry R. Goldin, Cynthia Soo, Ann Morrill-Labrode, Charles A. Dinarello, and Sherwood L. Gorbach

Animal experiments and clinical trials have indicated a potentially beneficial effect of n-3 fatty acid (FA) supplementaion on atherosclerosis and atherothrombotic disorders, autoimmune, and inflammatory diseases, the prevalence of all of which increases with age.

Aging is associated with an altered regulation of the immune system with T-cell-mediated immune responses exhibiting the major changes (1). In vitro, the proliferative response of human and rodent lymphocytes to phytohemagglutinin (PHA) and concanavalin A (Con A) becomes depressed with age. Several groups have shown that antigen and mitogen-stimulated interleukin (IL)-2 production declines with age and contributes to T cell-mediated defects observed with aging while changes in B cell response and IL-1 production are equivocal.

Short-term supplementation with 4.6 g/day of n-3 FA has been shown to decrease the inducible production of IL-1 and tumor necrosis factor (TNF) (2). The effect of lower levels of supplementation with n-3 FA for longer periods of time on IL-1, TNF, other cytokines, and lymphocyte proliferation of healthy subjects has not been studied. Furthermore, the question of age difference in n-3 induced changes has not been addressed. The latter point is especially important in light of the age-associated changes of cell-mediated immune function.

We, therefore, investigated the effect of supplementation with 2.4 g/day of n-3 FA for up to 3 mo on cytokine production and lymphocyte proliferation of young and older females.

MATERIALS AND METHODS

Six healthy young (23-33 yr) and six healthy older (51-68 yr) women were recruited from the Boston area. Each subject's usual diet was supplemented with n-3 FA contained in six capsules of Pro-Mega (Parke Davis, Warner Lambert Co., Morris Plains, NJ) daily for 12 wk. Each subject therefore received 1680 mg of eicosapentaenoic acid (EPA), 720 mg of docosahexaenoic acid (DHA), 600 mg of other FA and 6 IU of vitamin E per day.

Compliance was monitored by measurement of total plasma FA. Blood was collected on two consecutive days. The means of these two determinations were used for further analysis. Samples were collected at baseline and at the end of 1, 2 and 3 mo of supplementation with FO. Heparinized blood (40 ml) was collected for in vitro immunological tests and 6 ml of blood was collected in EDTA for WBC differential, FA and vitamin E analysis. Mitogenic response of lymphocytes to T cell mitogens Con A and PHA was measured as described before (3). Con A stimulated IL-2 production was measured as described by Gillis et al. (4). Con A stimulated IL-6 production was measured by

RIA (5). Endotoxin-stimulated IL-1β and tumor necrosis factor (TNF) production were measured by RIA (6,7). PHA-stimulated PGE$_2$ production was measured by RIA (3).

RESULTS AND DISCUSSION

Compliance was confirmed by a significant increase in plasma EPA (0.64+0.04% before vs. 3.6+0.91% after supplementation, p<0.04 in young women and 0.73+0.05% before supplementation vs. 7.30+0.28% after supplementation, p<0.001 in older women) and DHA (1.81+0.12% before supplementation vs. 2.96+0.44% after supplementation, p<0.06 in young women and 1.76+0.17% before supplementation vs. 4.30+0.36% after supplementation, p<0.001 in older women) and a significant decrease in arachidonic acid (AA)/EPA ratio. These changes were more dramatic in older women than young women so that the AA/EPA ratio decreased 12 fold in older women and only 4 fold in young women. Similarly the decrease in PGE$_2$ production was more dramatic in older women (71% decrease in older women and 31% decrease in young women).

Plasma tocopherol level, total number of WBC and the percentage of mononuclear and polymorphonuclear cells did not change as a result of treatment or age.

IL-1β, TNF, and IL-6 production was not significantly different between young and older women prior to FO supplementation. FO supplementation significantly decreased production of these cytokines in both young and older women. The decrease was more dramatic in older women than young women so that older women had significantly lower production of IL-1β, TNF and IL-6 than young women after 3 mo of FO supplementation (Table 1). Interleukin (IL)-1β and TNF production after 8 wk of supplementation was < 50% of baseline values. Further reductions were observed after 12 wk of supplementation. This demonstrates that substantial reduction in cytokine production can be achieved without the consumption of large quantities of n-3 FA. Although the pre-supplementation production of IL-1β and TNF was not different between young and older women, the n-3 supplementation induced a greater reduction in older women compared to younger women. This was associated with a larger increase in plasma EPA and DHA and a greater decrease in AA/EPA ratio seen in older women compared to young women following n-3 supplementation.

Older women had significantly lower production of IL-2 and mitogenic response to PHA and Con A than young women (p<0.01 for IL-2 and p<0.04 for mitogenic response) (Table 1). FO supplementation resulted in a significant reduction in IL-2 production and mitogenic response of lymphocytes to PHA in older women only. A statistically non-significant reduction was also observed in young women. The reduction by n-3 supplementation in IL-2 production and PHA mitogenesis in older women is of great interest since T cell-mediated functions decrease with aging. The decline in T cell-mediated function has been implicated as a contributory factor in the increased incidence of infectious diseases and tumors in the elderly. In our study a significant reduction in PHA-stimulated mitogenesis was observed only in older adults. This decrease in cytokine production and lymphocyte proliferation may compromise cell-mediated immunity and is supported by the study of Yoshino and Ellis (8) who showed that Sprague-Dawley rats fed FO concentrate had lower delayed type hypersensitivity response than those fed water, oleic acid or safflower oil.

TABLE 1-Effect of n-3 FA supplementation on PBMC cytokine production and lymphocyte proliferation of young and older women

Parameter	Young Baseline[a]	% Change[b]	Older Baseline[a]	% Change[b]
IL-1β (ng/ml)[c]	3.67± 0.63	-48	5.97± 1.20	-90
IL-6 (ng/ml)[d]	0.57± 0.05	-30	0.49± 0.04	-60
TNF (ng/ml)[c]	1.62± 0.23	-58	1.55± 0.30	-70
IL-2 (U/ml)[d]	88.20±27.80	-57	60.40±22.13	-63
Mitogenic response to PHA (CCPm x 10^3)[e]	84.40±15.71	- 7	53.86±5.97	-36

[a] Mean ± SEM, N=6
[b] Represent percent change after 3 mo of supplementation with n-3 FA compared to baseline values.
[c] 5×10^6 PBMC/ml were stimulated with 1 ng/ml LPS for 24 hr; total i.e. cell-associated plus secreted IL-1β and TNF were determined by RIA.
[d] 1×10^6 PBMC/ml were cultured in presence of 10 μg/ml Con A or PHA for 48 hr. Cell free supernatant were used for measurement of IL-2 by bioassay using CTLL cells and measurment of IL-6 by RIA.
[e] 1×10^6 PBMC/ml were cultured in presence or absence of 5 μg/ml PHA for 72 hr in presence of autologous plasma. Lymphocyte proliferation was measured by incorporation of ^{3}H thymidine into DNA after a 4 hr pulse. Data represent corrected counts per minute (CCPM) which is the CPM of stimulated cultures minus CPM of unstimulated cultures.

The decrease in cytokine production and lymphocyte proliferation can not be readily explained by a decrease in PGE_2 production. PGE_2 has been shown to suppress IL-1, IL-2 production and lymphocyte proliferation. The effect of n-3 FA supplementation, therefore, appears to be independent of PGE_2 changes. On the other hand, a reduction in LTB_4 by n-3 FA can suppress IL-1, IL-2 production and the subsequent lymphocyte proliferation since LTB_4 in some but not all studies has been shown to increase IL-1 as well as IL-2 production and lymphocyte proliferation (9). Santoli and Zurier (10) showed that polyunsaturated FA can reduce IL-2 production directly and independently of changes in cyclooxygenase products.

The clinical implications of our findings need to be determined. IL-1β, TNF, and IL-6 have been implicated in the pathogenesis of inflammatory diseases and a reduction in the synthesis of these cytokines by n-3 FA of FO may contribute to the reported beneficial effect of n-3 FA in rheumatoid arthritis (11) and amyloidosis (12). Furthermore, IL-1 is implicated in the pathogenesis of osteoporosis by virtue of its ability to induce bone reabsorption (13). The incidence of both arthritis and osteoporosis increases in older women, therefore, n-3 FA supplementation may prove to be beneficial in retarding the development of these disease states. Conversely, the reduction in older women of IL-2 and IL-6 production may compromise B and T cell proliferation and their differentiation into effector cells. Further clinical trials are needed to define the level of n-3 supplementation which provides an anti-inflammatory effect and minimizes the reduction of cell-mediated immunity.

REFERENCES

1. Siskind, G.W. (1980): In: Biological Mechanism in Aging, edited by R.T. Schimke, pp. 455-467, USDA, NIH.
2. Endres, S., Ghorbani, R., Kelley, V.E., Georgilis, K., Lonnemann, G., Van der Meer, J.W.M., Cannon, J.G., Rogers, T.S., Klempner, M.S., Weber, P.C., Schaefer, E.J., Wolff, S.M., and Dinarello, C.A. (1989): N. Engl. J Med. 320:265-271.
3. Meydani, S.N., Barklund, P., Liu, S., Meydani, M., Miller, R.A., Cannon, J.G., Morrow, F.D., Rocklin, R., and Blumberg, J.B. (1990): Am. J. Clin. Nutr. (In press).
4. Gillis, S., Fern, M.M., Ou, W., and Smith, K.A. (1978): J. Immunol. 120:2027-2032.
5. Brown, B.A. (1984): Hematology: Principles and Procedures, 4th edition. Lea and Febiger, Philadelphia.
6. Endres, S., Ghorbani, R., Lonnemann, G., Van der Meer, J.W.M., and Dinarello, C.A. (1988): Clin. Immunol. Immunopath. 49:424-438.
7. Van der Meer, J.W.M., Endres, S., Lonnemann, G. et al. (1988): J. Leukocyte Biol. 43:216-223.
8. Yoshino, S., and Ellis, E.F. (1987): Int. Arch. Allergy Appl. Immunol. 84:233-240.
9. Rola-Pleszczynski, M. (1985): Immunol. Today 6:302-307.
10. Santoli, D., and Zurier, R.B. (1989): J. Immunol. 143:1303-1309.
11. Leslie, C.A., Gonnermann, W.A., Ullman, M.D., Hayes, K.C., Franz-Blau, C., and Cathcart, E.S. (1985): J. Exp. Med. 162:1336.
12. Cathcart, E.S., Leslie, C.A. Meydani, S.N., and Hayes, K.C. (1987): J. Immunol. 139:1850-1854.
13. Gowen, M., and Mundy, G.R. (1986): J. Immunol. 136:2478-2482.

PAF RECEPTOR MEDIATED PGE$_2$ PRODUCTION IN LPS PRIMED P388D$_1$ MACROPHAGE-LIKE CELLS

Keith B. Glaser, Reto Asmis, and Edward A. Dennis

Department of Chemistry and Center for Molecular Genetics, University of California at San Diego, La Jolla CA 92093 USA

The role of eicosanoids (prostaglandins, thromboxanes, leukotrienes and hydroxyperoxyeicosatetraenoic acids) in the inflammatory response has been well documented. The rate-limiting event in eicosanoid biosynthesis appears to be the availability of arachidonic acid, which is found predominantly esterified in the sn-2 position of membrane phospholipids. The most direct mechanism which would release arachidonic acid is the activation of phospholipase A$_2$ (PLA$_2$) which could directly cleave arachidonic acid from the sn-2 position of membrane phospholipids (7). Since the release of arachidonic acid and the biosynthesis of eicosanoids is an early event in the activation of a primary immunoinflammatory cell, the macrophage, this cell provides an important tool to investigate the mechanisms which control the activation of PLA$_2$ for arachidonic acid release (15).

The macrophage-like P388D$_1$ cell line (13) provides a homogeneous population of cells to serve as a model for the study of the enzymatic mechanisms possibly involved in arachidonic acid release (20). The phospholipases have been characterized in this cell line (19) and several purified and kinetically characterized (14,20,23). The most likely candidate for the phospholipase which releases arachidonic acid is a Ca^{2+}-dependent membrane-associated PLA$_2$; this enzyme has been purified (20), kinetically characterized (14) and evaluated with regard to several inhibitors of phospholipase A$_2$ (15).

Manoalide (8) and manoalogue (18) are potent and irreversible inhibitors of venom PLA$_2$ (10,16,18). The P388D$_1$ PLA$_2$ is dose-dependently inhibited by manoalide and manoalogue; however, this inhibition appears to be

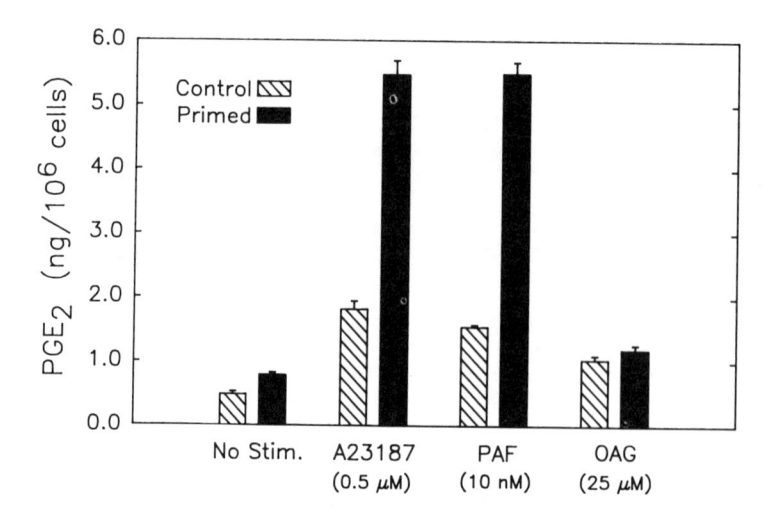

FIG. 1. Effect of LPS Priming on PGE$_2$ Production in Response to Various Stimulants. P388D$_1$ cells were primed with 100 ng/ml LPS RE 595 for 1 h and then stimulated for 4 h with no stimulant, A23187 (0.5 μM), PAF (10 nM) or OAG (25 μM). PGE$_2$ production was measured by specific radioimmonoassay. Reprinted with permission from Glaser et al. (9).

reversible in nature (15). The general effects of manoalide and manoalogue on the P388D$_1$ PLA$_2$ are also observed on prostaglandin E$_2$ (PGE$_2$) production in the intact P388D$_1$ cell (11,15). With the similarities observed between inhibition of the isolated P388D$_1$ PLA$_2$ and PGE$_2$ production in the intact P388D$_1$ cell, we have now investigated the mechanisms involved in the activation of PLA$_2$ for arachidonic acid release. The present study was carried out using a receptor mediated event, platelet-activating factor (PAF) stimulation of PGE$_2$ production (15,21).

Lipopolysaccharide Priming of P388D$_1$ Cells

Bacterial lipopolysaccharides (LPS) are potent immunomodulators and produce profound effects on macrophage function (17). One of these effects is the ability to prime macrophages for enhanced eicosanoid biosynthesis (1,2). P388D$_1$ cells do not respond directly to LPS to produce PGE$_2$ (15), but can be primed by low doses of LPS to produce enhanced levels of PGE$_2$ in response to Ca^{2+} ionophore A23187 and PAF stimulation (9). Normal unprimed cells upon stimulation with Ca^{2+} ionophore A23187 or PAF produce approximately 3-5 fold the constitutive PGE$_2$ levels (15); however, upon priming, these cells produce 10-13 fold constitutive levels of PGE$_2$ (FIG. 1).

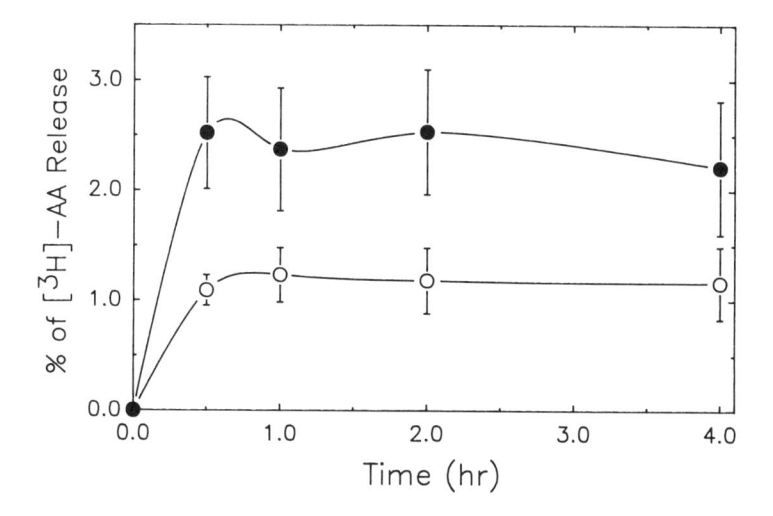

FIG. 2. [³H] Arachidonic Acid Release from Unprimned (○) and LPS Primed (●) Cells in Response to PAF. The % release of [³H] in response to PAF (10 nM) less the constitutive % release of [³H] is shown. The maximum % release was 5% of total incorporated [³H] arachidonic acid in LPS primed cells in response to PAF. P388D$_1$ cells were prelabeled with [³H] arachidonic acid for 18 h prior to LPS priming (100 ng/mg) and PAF stimulation. Reprinted with permission from Glaser et al. (9).

The priming is specific for those stimulants which are able to stimulate PGE$_2$ production in unprimed cells, (9) e.g. priming does not induce the cells to become responsive to OAG (FIG. 1). The LPS priming is also dependent on the concentration of LPS and is independent of the type (i.e. rough or smooth LPS) of LPS which is used to prime the cells (9). Prolonged exposure of P388D$_1$ cells to LPS results in a hypo-responsive state where they no longer respond to the stimulus (9) and this effect is also similar to the hyporesponsiveness observed in RAW 264.7 murine macrophage-like cells (22).

LPS priming of normal murine peritoneal macrophages results in a primed state which is maintained for up to 72 hours before returning to the unprimed state (1). It is of interest that the primed state in P388D$_1$ cells is unstable and deactivates with an apparent half-life of 1.75 h (9). This aspect of LPS priming makes this an attractive model in which both priming and deactivation of priming can be studied in a relatively short period of time.

To study the mechanism of LPS priming we evaluated the enzymes most likely involved in PGE$_2$ production, the Ca$^+$-dependent membrane associated PLA_2 and the cyclooxygenase. Neither of these enzyme activities were enhanced in the primed $P388D_1$ cells (9), suggesting an effect on the mechanisms which transduce the stimulus signal. This was evident when we observed the enhancement of [^{3}H]-arachidonic acid release from prelabelled cells (FIG. 2) (9). As shown in FIG. 2, both the extent and rate of [^{3}H]-arachidonic acid release are enhanced in the primed $P388D_1$ cells stimulated with PAF. Therefore, the LPS priming is controlling the availability of arachidonic acid for eicosanoid biosynthesis and is not necessarily downregulating or preventing the de novo synthesis of enzymes which may be involved in eicosanoid biosynthesis.

Inhibitor Effects on LPS Priming

Various inhibitors were evaluated to elucidate both the mechanism of LPS priming and PAF receptor mediated PGE_2 production in the $P388D_1$ cells. The dual inhibitor of cyclooxygenase and lipoxygenase BW755c at concentrations which inhibit PGE_2 production by greater than 95% had little effect on LPS priming (9). This observation suggests that lipoxygenase and/or cyclooxygenase products are not necessary for the LPS priming event. The phospholipase A_2 inhibitor manoalogue (18) did not block LPS priming but did effectively inhibit primed PAF-stimulated PGE_2 production with a similar IC_{50} as observed for unprimed Ca^{2+} ionophore A23187 stimulated cells. These results suggest that similar enzymes are being inhibited by manoalogue in both unprimed and LPS primed $P388D_1$ cells.

Stimulatory doses of LPS have been shown to increase mRNA for various oncogenes and competence genes and the synthesis of short-lived early proteins (12). It was of interest to determine if LPS priming was blocked by either inhibition of mRNA synthesis by actinomycin D or protein synthesis by cyclohexamide. When present during LPS priming, actinomycin D (3 μM) but not cyclohexamide (10 μM) prevented the generation of the primed state. However, when present during primed PAF-stimulated PGE_2 production, cyclohexamide (10 μM) but not actinomycin D (3 μM) inhibited PGE_2 production (9). These results suggest that LPS is more dependent on mRNA synthesis than protein synthesis during the 1 hr LPS exposure required for generation of the primed state. Primed PAF-stimulated PGE_2 production is dependent on new protein synthesis as cyclohexamide (10 μM) reduced protein biosynthesis, as measured by [^{3}H]-leucine incorporation into TCA precipitable material, by greater than 95% and completely blocked PAF stimulated PGE_2 production. These results suggest that a rapidly turning over protein is involved in receptor mediated arachidonic acid release and subsequent PGE_2 production.

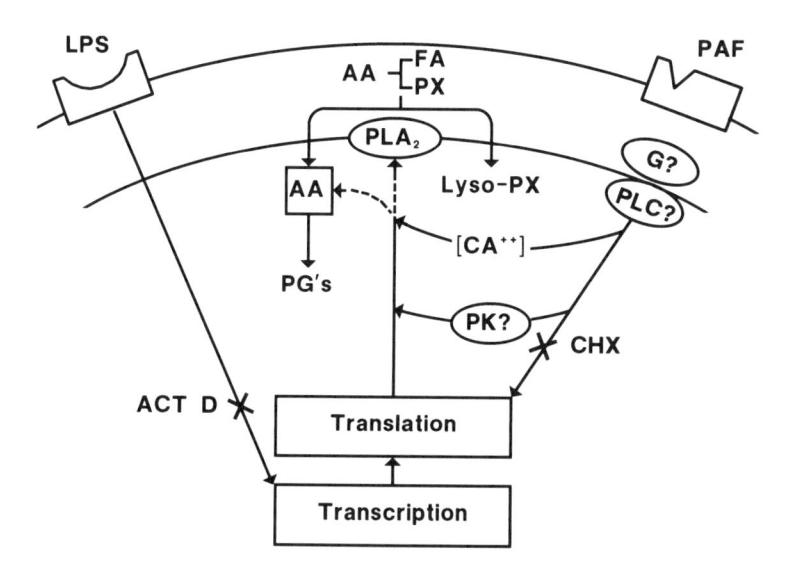

FIG. 3. Possible Stimulus-Response Coupling Pathways in P388D$_1$ Cells. Both LPS priming and PAF-stimulated arachidonic acid (AA) release from membrne phospholipids by phospholipase A$_2$ (PLA$_2$) to form prostaglandins (PG's) is shown. Possible roles for G-proteins (G), phospholipase C (PLC) Ca^{++}, and protein kinases (PK), possibly tyrosine-specific, are indicated as well as inhibition by actinomycin D (ActD) and cyclohexamide (CHX). Reprinted with permission from Glaser et al. (9).

These results are consistent with those reported for normal peritoneal macrophages (3). Various protein kinases, especially protein kinase C, have been implicated in LPS priming but their role is unclear (5,6). Therefore, we investigated the effect of various protein kinase activators/inhibitors on LPS priming and primed PAF stimulation (9). The protein kinase C activator PMA (phorbol myristate acetate) at stimulatory and desensitizing concentrations had little or no effect on LPS priming or on primed PAF stimulation (9). The protein kinase C inhibitor H-7 also had no effect on LPS priming or primed PAF stimulation. Genistein, a selective tyrosine-specific kinase inhibitor (4), partially prevented LPS priming at high doses $\geq$ 10 μM, whereas genistein was a potent inhibitor (IC$_{50}$ = 7 μM) of primed PAF stimulation (9). These results are the first which implicate a tyrosine protein kinase in PAF mediated PGE$_2$ production.

Signal Transduction Mechanisms in P388D$_1$ Cells

The studies reported herein describe a complex regulation of the mechanisms which control arachidonic acid release and the subsequent generation of PGE$_2$ in P388D$_1$ cells (FIG. 3). LPS exposure results in a signal which generated a primed state in P388D$_1$ cells. This priming event appears to involve transcription and ultimately translation of the induced message. The priming event is very sensitive to actinomycin D and less so to cyclohexamide, indicating message accumulation is an important facet of LPS priming. PAF receptor mediated PGE$_2$ production in LPS primed cells is dependent on a rapidly turning over protein induced upon stimulation, sensitive to cyclohexamide. The PAF mediated PGE$_2$ production also appears to involve a protein kinase, possibly activation of a tyrosine protein kinase which is inhibited by genistein.

Based on these results and the effects of manoalogue and those inhibitors involved in characterizing the primed state in P388D$_1$ cells (9), LPS priming appears to lead to a greater activation of a phospholipase A$_2$ in the P388D$_1$ cells which results in greater arachidonate availability and subsequently greater PGE$_2$ production.

Acknowledgements

This work was supported by grants GM 20,501 and HD 27,171 from the National Institutes of Health.

References

1. Aderem, A.A., Cohen, D.S., Wright, S.D., and Cohn, Z.A. (1986): *J. Exp. Med., 164*: 165-179.
2. Aderem, A.A., and Cohn, Z.A. (1988): *J. Exp. Med., 167*: 623-631.
3. Aderem, A.A., Scot, W.A., and Cohn, Z.A. (1986): *J. Exp. Med., 163*: 139-154.
4. Akiyama, T., Ishida, J., Nakagawa, S., Ogawara, H., Watanabe, S., Itoh, N., Shibuya, M., and Fukami, Y. (1987): *J. Biol. Chem., 262*: 5592-5595.
5. Bass, D.A., Gerard, C., Olbrantz, P., Wilson, J., McCall, C.E., and McPhail, L.C. (1987): *J. Biol. Chem., 262*: 6643-6649.
6. Bass, D.A., McPhail, L.C., Schmitt, J.D., Morris-Natschke, S., McCall, C.E., and Wykle, R.L. (1989): *J. Biol. Chem., 264*: 19610-19617.
7. Dennis, E. A. (1987): *Bio/Technology*, 5: 1294-1300.
8. de Silva, E.D., and Scheuer, P.J. (1980): *Tetrahedron Lett., 21*: 1611-1614.
9. Glaser, K. B., Asmis, R., and Dennis, E. A. (1990): *J. Biol. Chem., 265*:

8658-8664.
10. Glaser, K.B., and Jacobs, R.S. (1986): *Biochem. Pharmacol., 35*: 449-453.
11. Glaser, K. B., Lister, M. D., Ulevitch, R. J., and Dennis, E. A., (1990): in *"Phospholipase A$_2$: Role and Function in Inflammation"* (P. Y-K Wong and E. A. Dennis, Edits.) Plenum Press, New York. In press.
12. Hamilton, T.A., and Adams, D.O. (1987): *Immunology Today, 8*: 151-158.
13. Koren, H. S., Handwerger, B. S., and Wunderlich, J. R. (1975): *J. Immunol., 1114*: 894-897.
14. Lister, M. D., Deems, R. A., Watanabe, Y., Ulevitch, R. J, and Dennis, E. A. (1988): *J. Biol. Chem., 263*: 7506-7513.
15. Lister, M. D., Glaser, K. B., Ulevitch, R. J., and Dennis, E. A. (1989): *J. Biol. Chem., 264*: 8520-8528.
16. Lombardo, D., and Dennis, E. A. (1985): *J. Biol. Chem., 260*: 7234-7240.
17. Morrison, D.C., and Ulevitch, R.J. (1978): *Am. J. Path., 93*: 527-617.
18. Reynolds, L. J., Morgan, B. P., Hite, G. A., Mihelich, E. D., and Dennis, E. A. (1988): *J. Am. Chem. Soc., 110*: 5172-5177.
19. Ross, M. I., Deems, R. A., Jesaitis, A. J., Dennis, E. A., and Ulevitch, R. J. (1985): *Arch. Biochem. Biophys., 238*: 247-258.
20. Ulevitch, R. J., Sano, M, Watanabe, Y., Lister, M. D., Deems, R. A., and Dennis, E. A. (1988): *J. Biol. Chem., 263*: 3079-3085.
21. Valone, F. (1988): *J. Immunol., 140*: 2389-2394.
22. Virca, G.D., Kim, S.B., Glaser, K.B., and Ulevitch, R.J. (1989): *J. Biol. Chem., 264*: 21951-21956.
23. Zhang, Y., and Dennis, E. A. (1988): *J. Biol. Chem., 263*: 9965-9972.

ARACHIDONIC ACID RELEASE IN RAT PERITONEAL MACROPHAGES: ROLE OF CALCIUM IONS

S. Nicosia and O. Letari

Institute of Pharmacological Sciences, via Balzaretti 9
20133 Milan, Italy

INTRODUCTION

Macrophages contain an unusually high proportion of arachidonic acid (AA) incorporated into their membrane phospholipids (7), and this fatty acid can be released (and subsequently metabolized to eicosanoids) upon stimulation with a variety of particulate and soluble stimuli (5-7). Thus, these cells constitute a good model for the study of the control of AA release.

It is well known that AA is released from phospholipids by activation of phospholipases (PL), mainly PLA_2, but the molecular mechanisms underlying such activation have not yet been fully clarified. Among the second messengers, calcium ions have been suggested to play a role in this process (4, 8). However, both calcium-dependent and calcium-independent PLA_2 have been described in many cells, and both forms coexist in macrophages (10).

Aim of our work was to elucidate the role of cytosolic calcium ions, $[Ca^{++}]_i$, in the modulation of AA release. To this purpose, we compared the increase in release, elicited by either the calcium ionophore A 23187 or opsonized zymosan (OpZy), with the variations of $[Ca^{++}]_i$, assayed directly with the fluorescent probe Fura2 (1).

METHODOLOGY

Resident peritoneal macrophages were obtained from male rats by peritoneal lavage (2), and purified by adhesion to 12 mm ø round glass coverslips. The adherent macrophages were loaded with Fura2 by incubation with Fura2 acetoxymethyl ester for 45 min at 15°C in Dulbecco's Modified Eagle Medium. After removing excess Fura2, the cells were placed in Hepes-buffered saline (with 1 mM Ca^{++}) for fluorescence monitoring (Perkin Elmer Fluorescence Spectrometer LS 5, 345 nm excitation and 505 nm emission) at 30°C. The fluorescence values, both basal and after stimulation, were converted to $[Ca^{++}]_i$ values by calibration according to Tsien et al. (9) and Grynkiewicz et al. (1).

AA release was assessed in parallel experiments by preincubation of the adherent macrophages with ^{3}H-AA (1 µCi/dish) for 2 hrs, washing to remove unincorporated ^{3}H-AA, and incubation with the indicated stimuli for 15 min at 30°C. The radioactivity (^{3}H-AA plus ^{3}H-metabolites) released in the medium at the end of the incubation was taken as a measure of total ^{3}H-AA release.

RESULTS AND DISCUSSION

In the presence of extracellular calcium ions, the calcium ionophore A 23187 dose-dependently stimulated the release of ^{3}H-AA (assayed as total ^{3}H-products released in the medium) from macrophages that had been preincubated with ^{3}H-AA. As expected, A 23187 was also able to increase the levels of $[Ca^{++}]_i$ significantly (Table 1).

The pattern of response was totally different when a particulate stimulus, i. e. OpZy, was used. In fact, as shown in Table 1, OpZy was able to elicit a dose-dependent increase in ^{3}H-AA release, albeit to a lesser extent than A 23187, but it did not modify $[Ca^{++}]_i$ to any significant extent. Indeed, the increase in fluorescence observed upon addition of OpZy was never higher than the intrinsic autofluorescence of the stimulus itself; in addition, it was demonstrated, by subsequent addition of A 23187, that real increases in $[Ca^{++}]_i$ could be detected even in the presence of the autofluorescent OpZy (data not shown). Thus, the variations in fluorescence elicited by the particulate stimulus cannot be ascribed to variations in $[Ca^{++}]_i$.

These findings gave the first indication that an elevation in the average concentration of cytosolic calcium ions might not be necessary to promote AA release.

In order to investigate in more detail the role of calcium in the control of arachidonate release, a series of experiments was performed in the absence of extracellular calcium. Under these conditions, the basal concentration of cytosolic calcium ions was much reduced (from 230 to approximately 56 nM, Table 1), as expected. The calcium ionophore, at concentrations of 200 nM or higher, was still able to elicit measurable transient increases in $[Ca^{++}]_i$ which should derive from discharge of intracellular stores; however, such increase did not attain statistical significance. Once again, in the absence of extracellular Ca^{++} as in its presence, OpZy did not cause any increase in fluorescence that could be interpreted as an increase in $[Ca^{++}]_i$.

As for the release of ^{3}H-AA, the removal of extracellular calcium greatly blunted the response to A 23187, which elicited a significant increase only at 500 nM. At variance with this result, the effect of OpZy on ^{3}H release was actually augmented (2- to 3-fold, approximately) in the absence of extracellular Ca^{++} with respect to this presence.

Taken together, these results indicate that a genaralized increase in [Ca^{++}]$_i$ is not a necessary trigger for arachidonic acid release. One could hypothesize that OpZy induces AA release through a stimulation of either a calcium-independent PLA$_2$, which has been demostrated to exists in macrophages (10), or a PLA$_2$ that is maximally stimulated at resting calcium levels. Alternatively, OpZy could exert its action through the combined action of a PLC and a digliceride lipase. Indeed, zymosan has been demonstrated to activate a PLC at basal [Ca^{++}]$_i$ ().

At this stage, however, we cannot rule out the possibility that OpZy induced a rapid and transient increase in [Ca^{++}]$_i$, or an increase limited to only a discrete cell site. If this were the case, it is possible that the average [Ca^{++}]$_i$ in the whole cell population would not be significantly affected. Only a study performed on single cells, loaded with Fura2, could reveal whether these transient or localized [Ca^{++}]$_i$ changes do indeed occur.

TABLE I

^{3}H-AA release and citosolic calcium ion levels in rat peritoneal macrophages

Agent	with extracellular Ca^{++}		without extracellular Ca^{++}	
	released dpm	[Ca^{++}]$_i$	released dpm	[Ca^{++}]$_i$
None	2651 ± 242	230 ± 20	2028 ± 373	55.6 ± 9.6
A23187 50 nM	11727 ± 1749*	410 ± 10*	5673 ± 434	52.0 ± 15.4
A23187 200 nM	17144 ± 2059**	1220 ± 20**	3682 ± 509	86.5 ± 26.5
A23187 500 nM	26994 ± 317**	1750 ± 30**	7490 ± 1483*	76.7 ± 24.3
Op Zy 10 g/ml	2429 ± 267	260 ± 70	7087 ± 186**	40.0 ± 12.2
Op Zy 30 g/ml	3015 ± 337	200 ± 50	7419 ± 602**	82.4 ± 28.9
Op Zy 100 g/ml	4018 ± 151*	220 ± 60	9040 ± 307**	63.2 ± 17.9

Extracellular Ca^{++} was 1mM. When extracellular Ca^{++} was removed, EGTA 5 mM was added. Data are means + SE of at least 3 experiment, each performed in duplicate. Op Zy: opsonized zymosan. * p <0.05; ** p <0.01 vs basal

REFERENCES

1. Grynkiewicz G., T. Poenie and R.J. Tsien (1985): J. Biol. Chem. 260: 3440-3450.
2. McCarron R.M., D.K. Goroff, J.E. Luhr, M.A. Murphy and H.B. Herscowitz (1984): Meth. Enzymol. 108: 274-284.
3. Moscat J., C. Herrero, P. Garcia-Barreno and A.M. Municio (1987): Biochem. J. 242: 441-445.
4. Pawlowski N.A., G. Kaplan, A.L. Hamill, Z.A. Cohn and W.A. Scott, (1983): J. Exp. Med. 158: 393-412.
5. Rouzer C.A., W.A. Scott, Z.A. Cohn, P. Blackburn and J.M. Manning (1980): Proc. Natl. Acad. Sci. USA 77: 4928-4932.
6. Scott W.A., N.A. Pawlowski, M. Andreach and Z.A. Cohn (1982): J. Exp. Med. 155: 535-547.
7. Scott W.A., J.M. Zrike, A.L. Hamill, J. Kempe and Z.A. Cohn (1980): J. Exp. Med. 152: 324-335.
8. Tripp C.S., M. Mahoney and P. Needleman (1985): J. Biol. Chem. 260: 5895-5898.
9. Tsien R.Y., T. Pozzan and T.J. Rink (1982): J. Cell Biol. 94: 325-334.
10. Wightman P.D., J.L. Humes, P. Davies and R.J. Bonney (1981) Biochem. J. 195: 427-433.

MODULATION OF MAST CELL EICOSANOID SYNTHESIS BY ATTACHMENT

B.A. Jakschik and L. Xu

Washington University School of Medicine, Department of Pharmacology,
St. Louis, Missouri 63110, U.S.A.

Mouse mast cells (mucosal type) can be readily cultured from bone marrow cells in the presence of IL-3 (WEHI-3b conditioned media). In general, these mast cells grow in suspension. There are also some attached cells present in these cultures which resemble macrophages in their morphological appearance, phagocytose zymosan and do not release detectable amounts of eicosanoids when stimulated with IgE/Ag. However, histological studies of these attached cells showed that they stain metachromatically, identifying them as mast cells. In earlier studies we attempted to culture rodent connective tissue mast cells which were purified from peritoneal cells. Upon culture, some of the mast cells attached and subsequently the cultured mast cells lost their capacity to synthesize eicosanoids when challenged with IgE/Ag. Furthermore, RBL-2H3 cells, a rat mucosal mast cell line, has appreciable amounts of the 5-lipoxygenase protein, but upon stimulation with IgE/Ag they produce relatively little leukotrienes. These cells attach while in culture. Therefore, cultured connective tissue and mucosal mast cells seem to behave in a similar manner. Mast cells are important inflammatory cells which produce potent eicosanoids. It is essential to understand their arachidonic acid metabolism as they change their phenotype. The different phenotypes which seem to emerge with alteration of culture conditions may reflect similar changes occurring in various tissue environments.

Down Regulation of Eicosanoid Formation by Attachment

In order to determine the reason for the lack of eicosanoid synthesis after antigen challenge, experiments were designed to test whether the defect resides at the level of the IgE receptor, phospholipase or the 5-lipoxygenase and cyclooxygenase. Attached mast cells were sensitized with IgE and challenged with antigen alone or with 10 μM arachidonic acid or stimulated with A23187 in the presence or absence of arachidonate. No leukotriene formation was observed with any of the stimuli examined. The lack of leukotriene production with A23187 indicates that there is a block at the phospholipase level. Addition of arachidonate to A23187 stimulated cells did not result in leukotriene release, therefore, 5-lipoxygenase activity was also undetectable. Similar deficits were observed with IgE/Ag challenge. Determination of TXB_2 formation confirmed the lack of phospholipase stimulation. However, appreciable amounts of TXB_2 were observed when arachidonic acid was added to the cells. Therefore, cyclooxygenase activity was intact.

Effect of Attached Mast Cells on Eicosanoid Synthesis by Floating Mast Cells

We also investigated whether the attached mast cells have an effect on eicosanoid production by mast cells in suspension. For these experiments mast cells were grown in the absence of the attached cells and their eicosanoid synthesis compared to that by mast cells cultured in the presence of attached cells. Removal of the mast cells from the attached cells caused a marked increase in eicosanoid production upon challenge with IgE/Ag (Fig. 1) (10). Both leukotriene and thromboxane formation were upregulated to approximately the same extent. Similar results were obtained when mast cells were stimulated with the calcium ionophore A23187. Therefore, the increase in eicosanoid production is not limited to antigen stimulation, but seems to occur with any stimulus which elevates intracellular calcium concentrations.

Careful time course studies showed that a considerable amount of time was needed for the elevation in eicosanoid synthesis to occur. A 2- to 16-fold elevation was observed after overnight culture without the attached cells. In some experiments an increase was already evident by 8 hr (10). This suggested that new protein synthesis might be involved in this process. To further test this possibility, cycloheximide (CHX) or actinomycin D (ACD) was added to the mast cells upon removal from the attached cells, followed by overnight culture. Inhibition of transcription with ACD completely abolished the upregulation of eicosanoid formation. The translational inhibitor CHX had a similar effect (Fig. 1). Therefore, new protein synthesis seems to be necessary for the observed enhancement of eicosanoid production.

Eicosanoid synthesis can be regulated at various levels of phospholipase or 5-lipoxygenase and cyclooxygenase. Experiments were designed to test these possibilities. Therefore, 10,000 x g supernatants of mast cell homogenates were incubated with 100 μM arachidonate, 1.5 mM calcium and 2 mM ATP. HPLC analysis for all the 5-lipoxygenase products formed showed that there was no significant difference in 5-lipoxygenase activity in the two sets of mast cells. Possible changes in cyclooxygenase activity were determined by incubating cells with 30 μM arachidonic acid and measuring TXB_2 formation. Similar to the 5-lipoxygenase, cyclooxygenase activity was not altered (10). Effects on the phospholipase were examined by prelabelling mast cells with [H^3]arachidonic acid and monitoring release of label upon challenge with IgE/Ag or A23187. A substantial enhancement (2 to 3 fold) of the release of [^{3}H]arachidonic acid and/or its products was observed with the mast cells which had been removed from the attached cells. Both stimuli, IgE/Ag and A23187, produced equivalent results. Similar to the effect on the increase on eicosanoid production, the transcriptional inhibitor ACD and the translational inhibitor CHX blocked the upregulation of the phospholipase activity. Therefore, it appears that factors from the attached mast cells suppress their own phospholipase activity as well as that of mast cells in suspension. It is possible that mast cells upon attachment to the plastic tissue cultureware become activated by the charge and then downregulate their eicosanoid production as well as that of the surrounding cells.

The experiments with ACD and CHX show that new protein synthesis is required for the increase in phospholipase activity after the removal of the mast cells from the attached cells. It is not clear whether the new protein synthesis involves production of new enzyme and/or other substances which regulate phospholipase activity. It is also possible that factors from the attached cells may suppress their own cytokinin formation as well as that in

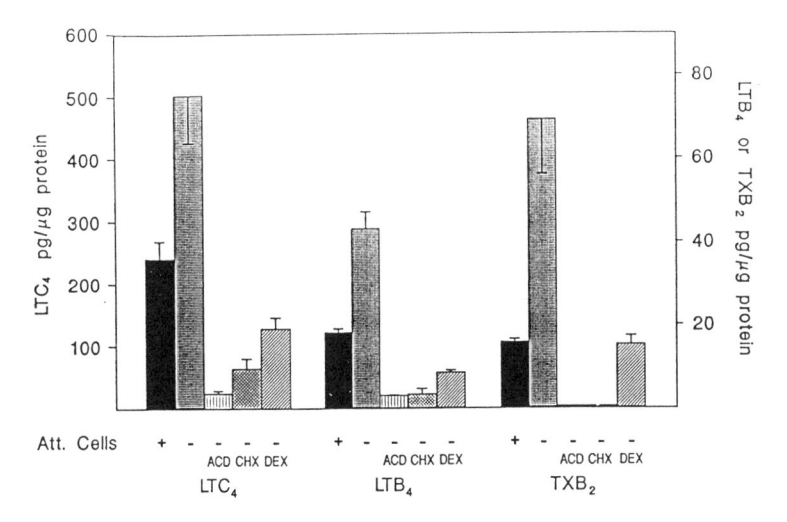

FIGURE 1. UPREGULATION OF MAST CELL EICOSANOID SYNTHESIS UPON REMOVAL FROM ATTACHED CELLS. Floating mast cells were removed from the attached cells (Att. Cells) and incubated overnight in the presence or absence of 1 μM actinomycin D (ACD), 10 μM cycloheximide (CHX) or 40 nM dexamethasone (DEX). The mast cells were sensitized with anti-DNP IgE and challenged with 10 ng/ml DNP-BSA. The supernatants were analyzed for eicosanoids by specific immunoassay. Mean ± SEM, n=3.

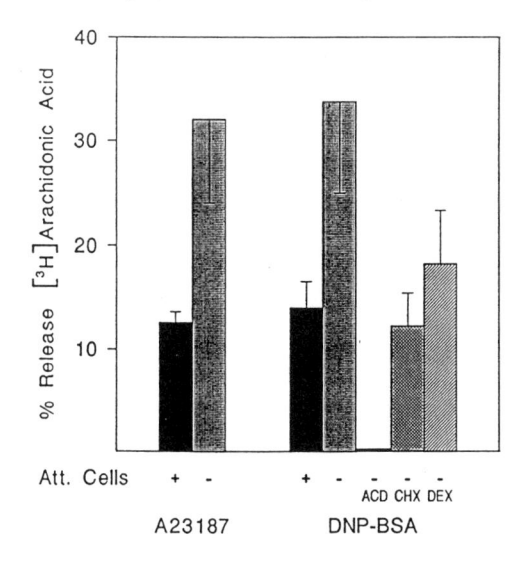

FIGURE 2. EVALUATION OF PHOSPHOLIPASE ACTIVITY. Mast cells were incubated overnight as in Fig. 1 and labeled with [^{3}H]arachidonic acid (10 μCi/ml, spec. activity 76 Ci/mmol) for one hr. The mast cells were stimulated with IgE/Ag as in Fig. 1 or with 1 μM A23187. The supernatants were analyzed for radioactivity.

mast cells in suspension. It has been reported recently that mast cells can synthesize IL-1, 3, 4, 5 and 6, GM-CSF and a TNF-like peptide (1,7,9). These cytokinins from mast cells in turn might be responsible for stimulating the synthesis of new phospholipase or factors activating this enzyme. Cytokinins, such as IL-1 and TNF are known to modulate eicosanoid synthesis (2,6,8). A peptide which activates phospholipase and which is inhibitable by protein synthesis blockers has also been described (3).

The effect of dexamethasone on the upregulation of eicosanoid production and phospholipase activity was tested (Fig 1 and 2). Dexamethasone prevented the increase in eicosanoid synthesis and phospholipase activity. Glucocorticoids generally act by inducing new protein synthesis. Therefore, dexamethasone may cause the formation of a peptide which inhibits phospholipase. This has been reported for other cell types (5). This phospholipase inhibitor is probably not lipocortin. It is thought that glucocorticoids cause the release and synthesis of lipocortins (5). In our experiments no immediate action of dexamethasone on phospholipase activity was observed. Furthermore, the action of lipocortins on phospholipase A_2 has been recently questioned (4).

SUMMARY

The experiments discussed above indicate that a change in phenotype occurs when cultured mast cells attach. This modification in phenotype is associated with a downregulation of their own eicosanoid production and that of cocultured mast cells in suspension. The eicosanoid production of the floating mast cells is markedly elevated after removal from attached cells. This enhancement appears to be due to an upregulation of phospholipase activity. Experiments with actinomycin D and cycloheximide indicate that new protein synthesis is necessary for the increase to occur. This suggests that either new enzyme and/or peptides modulating phospholipase are generated.

ACKNOWLEDGEMENT: This work was supported by NIH grant HL21974.

REFERENCES

1. Burd, P.R., Rogers, H.W., Gordon, J.R., Martin, C.A., Jayaraman, S., Wilson, S.D., Dvorak, A.M., Galli, S.J. & Dorf, M.E. (1989) J. Exp. Med. 170:245-257.
2. Chang, J., Gilman, S.C., & Lewis, A.J. (1986) J. Immun. 136:1283.
3. Clark, M.A., Littlejohn, D., Conway, T.M., Mong, S., Steiner, S., & Crooke, S.T. (1986) J. Biol. Chem. 261:10713-10718.
4. Davidson, F.F., & Dennis, E.A. (1989) Biochem. Pharm. 38:3645-3651.
5. Flower, R.J. (1984) Adv. Inflammation Res. 8:1-34.
6. Mohri, M., Spriggs, D.R. & Kufe, D. (1990) J. Immunol. 144:2678-2682.
7. Plaut, M., Pierce, J.H., Watson, C.J., Hanley-Hyde, J., Nordan, R.P., & Paul, W.E. ((1989) Nature 339:64-67.
8. Raz, A., Wyche, A. & Needleman, P. (1989) Proc. Natl. Acad. Sci. USA 86:1657-1661.
9. Wondnar-Filipowicz, A., Heusser, C.H., & Moroni, C. (1989) Nature 339:150-152.
10. Xu, L., and Jakschik, B.A. (submitted).

A NOVEL MECHANISM OF GLUCOCORTICOSTEROID (GC) ACTION IN SUPPRESSION OF PHOSPHOLIPASE A$_2$ (PLA$_2$) ACTIVITY STIMULATED BY Ca^{2+} IONOPHORE A23187 : INDUCTION OF PROTEIN PHOSPHATASES

[1]U. ZOR, [1]E. HER, [2]P. BRAQUET, [3]E. FERBER and [4]N. REISS

[1]Dept. of Hormone Research, Weizmann Institute of Science, REHOVOT, Israel

[2]Institut Henri Beaufour, 17, avenue Descartes, 92930 LE PLESSIS-ROBINSON, France

[3]Max Planck Institute für Immunobiologie FREIBURG, West Germany

[4]Dept. of Clinical Endocrinology, Hebrew University Hadassa Medical School, JERUSALEM, Israel

SUMMARY

The present article deals with the stimulation of membrane PLA$_2$ induced by activated protein kinase C (PKC), and the effect of a deficiency in cellular PKC activity in reducing in PLA$_2$ activity. The mode of glucocorticoid (GC) inhibition action in regulation of PLA$_2$ activity, by enhancement of protein dephosphorylation in general, and PLA$_2$ in particular, is hypothesized and discussed.

Indirect evidence strongly suggests that activated PKC enzyme is essential for the stimulation of membrane PLA$_2$ activity induced by the Ca^{2+} ionophore A23187 and other agonists. Our hypothesis suggests that membrane-associated PKC directly phosphorylates PLA$_2$ leading to its activation. Dephosphorylation of activated PLA$_2$, possibly by a serine/threonine protein phosphatase reduces PLA$_2$ activity. GC could induce membrane protein phosphatases which mediate their inhibitory action on PLA$_2$ activity. This mode of action of GC is complementary to their effect in reducing in elevated [Ca^{2+}]$_i$, which is essential for full expression of PLA$_2$ activity. Thus, GC exhibits multiple actions which specifically culminate in suppression of PLA$_2$ and other phospholipases (PI-PLC and PLD) and generally in cellular inactivation (relaxation) and reduction of allergic and inflammatory responses.

INTRODUCTION

PLA$_2$ is a key enzyme involved in the release of arachidonic acid (AA) and consequently regulates production of various eicosanoids. Under basal conditions, most of the PLA$_2$ activity is located in the cytosol. Upon stimulation with Ca^{2+}ionophore, diacylglycerol (DG) derivatives, hormones, antigen or ras oncogene protein, this enzyme is translocated to plasma membrane where it meets its phospholipid substrate and becomes activated (6). PLA$_2$ activity is positively regulated by three distinct essential second messengers : a) high Ca^{2+} concentration (2) ; b) phosphorylation by PKC (1) ; c) GTP-binding proteins (4,5).

Using different cell types and various agonists, several groups clearly showed that activated PKC is essential for full expression of PLA$_2$ activity (for review, see ref. 6). Indirect evidence has shown that short term treatment with TPA (or DG derivatives) on their own, sometimes leads to activation of PLA$_2$. More significantly, however, was the potentiation by TPA of AA release, stimulated by Ca^{2+} ionophores and other various agonists. However, PKC activity is essential although not sufficient for PLA$_2$ activity. Indeed, high [Ca^{2+}]$_i$ and/or high levels of GTP-binding proteins are essential as well (5).

Pretreatment with GC such as dexamethasone (DEX) leads to suppression of PLA$_2$ activity induced by antigen, Ca^{2+} ionophore, DG derivative, various hormones and growth factors (6). The GC are potent inhibitors of elevated [Ca^{2+}]$_i$ (2). They also probably interfere with the function of GTP-binding protein (a second messenger in activation of PI-PLC), since they are potent inhibitors of PI-PLC activation induced by antigen (6).

The current idea with regard to the mechanism of GC action in the suppression of allergic and inflammatory responses in general, and PLA$_2$ activity in particular, is initially related to their interaction with a nuclear steroid receptor, leading to induction of a family of proteins termed lipocortins (LCs). Indeed, GC have a delay effect (several hours), which is dependent on controlled cellular protein synthesis machinery and which is cycloheximide sensitive (2).

The defined mechanism by which LCs inhibit PLA$_2$ activity and the inflammatory response is a controversial issue. The "classical" current idea is that LCs (which are Ca^{2+} and phospholipid-binding proteins) bind to membrane phospholipid (PL) substrates and therefore mask them from interacting with PLA$_2$. This attractive view however, has some limitations ; this effect is not specific in nature, since albumin has similar binding properties to PL, as LCs (6). In addition, LCs mainly (if not exclusively) bind to acidic phospholipids (PS, PI) but not to PC and only to a very low extent to PE. These latter two PLs are the main membrane substrates for PLA$_2$. Moreover, in several cell types, GC suppresses PLA$_2$ activity without either enhancing mRNA to LCs or LC formation (1). In some cell types, GC even stimulates the release of AA (while decreasing certain PGs such as PGD$_2$), rather than the usual inhibition of AA that is usually noted (6). These discrepancies lead us to hypothesize that GC and their mediators LCs may have different (and possible various) mode of action on inhibition of PLA$_2$ activity, rather than the current "substrate depletion" theory.

GC are known inducers of alkaline phosphatase and possible other protein phosphatases as well (3). In the liver, GC induce protein phosphatase(s) which dephosphorylate both glycogen synthetase and phosphorylase (3), leading to enhanced glycogen synthesis and accumulation. GC may induce membrane protein phosphatases which dephosphorylate activated PLA$_2$ (in its phosphorylated state) and therefore reduce its activity. In addition, GC could induce plasma membrane Na$^+$/K$^+$ ATPase which could reduce ATP concentration in the plasma membrane below the Km needed for PKC activity. Thus, the "native" LC which are responsible for inhibition of PLA$_2$ activity could belong to a protein phosphatase family. This hypothesis is testable and under current investigation. Preliminary results with regard to this possible action of GC are presented and discussed in this article.

RESULTS

Ca^{2+} ionophore A23187 on its own is almost inactive in stimulating ^{3}H-AA release in NIH 3T3 cells (50 % above basal release, data not presented), in contrast to its potent action (10 fold increase) in RBL cells. This stimulation was partially (50 %) inhibited by pretreatment with DEX. On the contrary, TPA on its own was active in inducing ^{3}H-AA release (300 % above basal level) from 3T3 cells but was devoid of direct effect on RBL cells. Combined treatment with both agonists led to higher release of ^{3}H-AA in both cell types (data not presented). Incubation of the cells with DEX prevented the stimulation induced by combined treatment with Ca^{2+} ionophore and TPA in 3T3 fibroblasts, while having little inhibitory action in RBL cells (Fig. 1). Thus, TPA overcame the inhibitory action of DEX on Ca^{2+} ionophore induced ^{3}H-AA release in RBL cells. Staurosporine (St), an efficient inhibitor of PKC activity, was active in inhibiting ^{3}H-AA release from

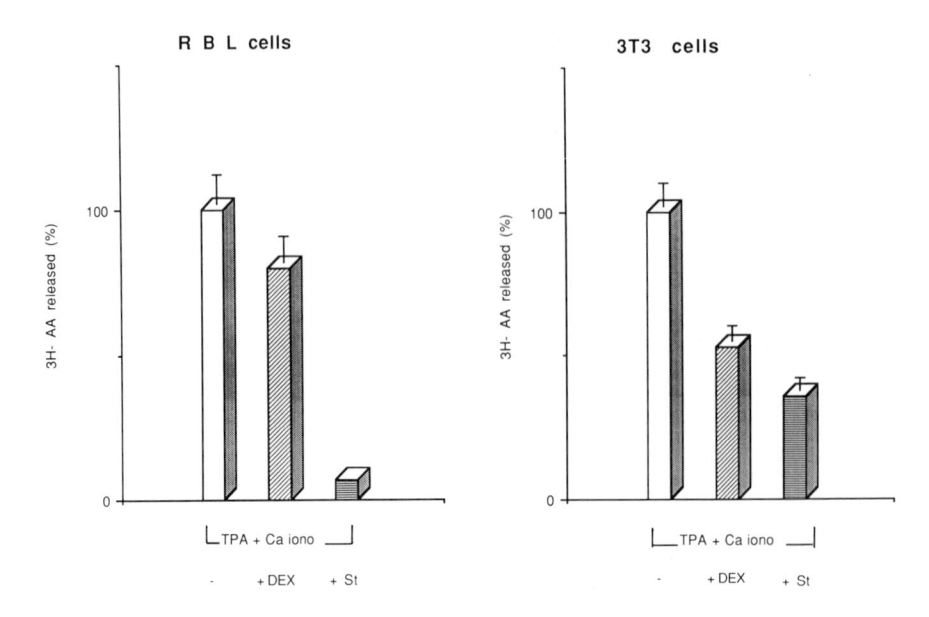

Figure 1. - Stimulation of ^{3}H-AA release from RBL and NIH 3T3 cells by combined short term treatment with TPA and Ca2+ionophore (Ca iono) : inhibition by dexamethasone (DEX) and staurosporine (St).
Ca^{2+} ionophore 3 µM, TPA 100 ng/ml added for 30 min. DEX (10^{-7}M) was administered for 16 hr. St (0.3 µM) was added 5 min before addition of the stimulants.

both cell types (Fig. 1), suggesting that the effect of Ca^{2+} ionophore and/or TPA on ^{3}H-AA release is mediated fully or partly by activation of PKC.
^{32}P incorporation to 3T3 cell proteins was examined with or without treatment with DEX (Fig. 2). The results demonstated that even the basal phosphorylation of certain proteins was reduced by DEX (an average of 50% seen in several different experiments). DEX retreatment of the cells also reduced protein phosphorylation induced by the Ca^{2+} ionophore, TPA or their combination (data not shown). DEX reduced the specific activity (cpm ^{32}P/µg protein) of various phosphorylated proteins. Similar results were obtained using RBL cells.

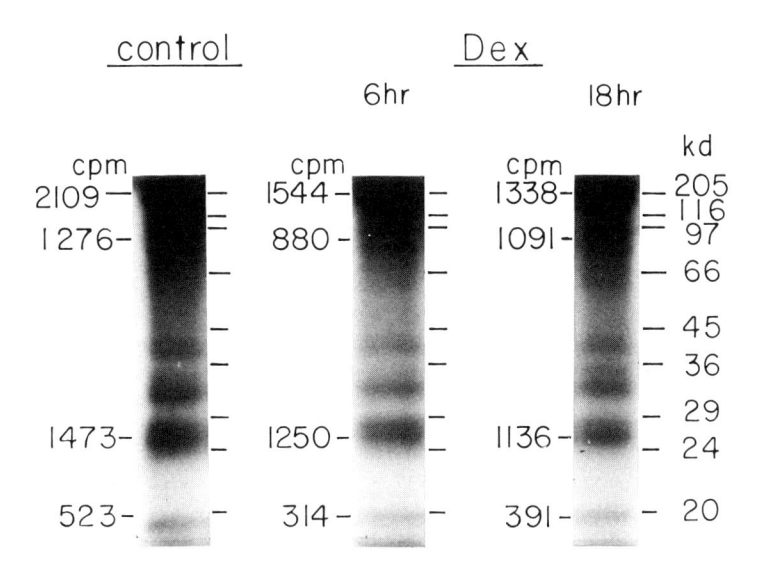

Figure 2. - Autoradiograph of polyacrylamide gels of NIH-3T3 cells labelled with [^{32}P] orthophosphate : reduction in the extent of protein phosporylation was induced by treatment with DEX (10^{-7} M) for 6 or 18 hr. Similar results were obtained by using RBL cells. For other details, see ref. 6.

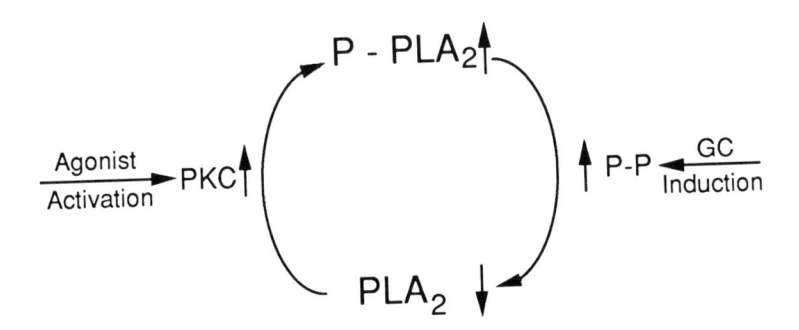

Figure 3. - Hypothetical model of activation and inactivation of PLA$_2$ by induction of phosphorylation (by PKC and possibly by TPK) and dephosphorylation (by protein phosphatases), respectively. P-PLA$_2$, phosphorylated (activated) PLA$_2$; P-P protein phosphatase; ↑ increasing ; ↓ decreasing.

DISCUSSION

Indirect evidence strongly suggests that PKC enzyme activity is essential and intimately involved in the regulation of PLA_2 activity (6). Such an involvment of PKC in the regulation of other key enzymes such as glycogen synthetase and EGF receptor tyrosine kinase has already been reported. This evidence is based on the ability of short term treatment of the cells with TPA to potentiate (and in some cases to stimulate) Ca^{2+} ionophore-induced AA release and PG production. The inability of Ca^{2+} ionophore to release AA in PKC-depleted cells or staurosporine-treated ones, supports this hypothesis. Although some groups have suggested that TPA or DG derivatives have this pharmacological effect, which may not be related directly to activation of PKC (6), many others support the ided that the effect of TPA (or DG) is mediated mainly via PKC activation (6).

The substrate for PKC phosphorylation with regard to PLA_2 activation has not yet been defined. It has been suggested that phosphorylation of LC may enhance their degradation or render them inactive, leading to increased PLA_2 activity. However, it is probably that PKC directly phosphorylates and therefore activates PLA_2, similarly to the well known stimulatory effect of membrane EGF receptor containing tyrosine protein kinase (TPK stimulated by EGF) on PI-PLC activity. Moreover, recently it has been shown that TPK activity is also essential for PLA_2 activation induced by EGF (1). It would be extremely attractive to determine whether purified PKC (and PTK) could directly phosphorylate PLA_2 and increase its activity. This possibility is currently under investigation.

Baird's group recently showed (5) that exogenous PLA_2 (derived from Naja or pancreatic origin) could be incorporated into the membrane of intact RBL cells. This invasive PLA_2 activity was even stimulated by administration of antigen and/or GTPγS. These data suggest that, at least, in RBL cells, exogenous PLA_2 could be coupled to membrane IgE receptors and be linked to GTP - binding protein. Obviously, the inhibitory action of DEX is currently being examined in this promising and elegant system.

Although this area of research is still in a preliminary stage, there is enough scientific basis and available practical techniques to challenge the idea that regulation of PLA_2 activity is controlled (at last partly) by phosphorylation-dephosphory-lation. The inhibitory action of DEX (and other GC) is partially related to induction of protein phosphatases, therefore, leading to protein dephophorylation (inactivation). In 1994, in the next PG Conference in Florence, we and possibly other groups, may have more data and could challenge this important issue which may give us a clue to the mechanism of GC inhibitory activity in allergy and inflammation.

REFERENCES

1. -Goldberg, H.J., Viegas, M.M., Margolis, B.J., Schlessinger, J. and Skorecki, K.L. (1990) Biochem. J. 267, 461-465.
2. -Her, E., Weissmann, B.A. and Zor, U. (1990): Biochim. Biophys. Acta, 1051:203-206.
3. -Hers, H.G., De Wulf, H. and Stalmans, W. (1970). FEBS Lett. 12: 73-81.
4. -Murayama, T., Kajiyama, Y. and Nomura, Y. (1990) J. Biol. Chem. 265: 4290-4295.
5. -Narasimha, V., Howka, D. and Baird, B. (1990) J. Biol. Chem. 264: 1459-1464.
6. -Zor, U., Her, E., Harrel, T., Fischer, G., Naor, Z., Braquet, P., Ferber., E. and Reiss, N. Biochim. Biophys. Acta (submitted).

PURIFICATION OF A MULTIMERIC PHOSPHOLIPASE A_2 FROM RABBIT RENAL CORTEX

Aubrey R. Morrison and Carl Irwin

Departments of Medicine and Pharmacology
660 South Euclid Avenue
Washington University School of Medicine
St. Louis, Missouri USA

Phospholipase A_2 (phosphatide 2-acylhydrolase) is a widely distributed enzyme involved in numerus biological functions. Some of these include phospholipid digestion as part of the digestive process (for pancreatic phospholipase A_2), toxic effects for the enzymes present in numerous snake or insect venoms, antibacterial defense as in the polymorphonuclear neutrophil, membrane phospholipid turnover, and regulation of arachidonic acid release and of eicosanoid biosynthesis. These different functions have been ascribed to the soluble or membranous enzymes so far identified in many tissues (6, 7). Over the past two decades, phospholipase A_2 (PLA_2) enzyme activities have been purified and characterized from various tissues, cultured cells and exudates from several organisms. These isolated activities have been reported to vary in molecular weight, pH optima, Ca^{2+} requirements and solubility. From these observations it would appear that mammalia contain several distinct forms of PLA_2 each having its own unique properties and roles.

Experimental evidence obtained in $HgCl_2$ induced renal failure (2) and toxic injury to $LLC-PK_1$ cells in culture (5) have suggested that there is selective turnover early in the injury of phosphatidyl ethanolamine. Because of evidence in the literature suggesting specificity for the substrate by phospholipases (1, 4, 3), we sought to determine if there was a phosphatidyl ethanolamine specific or selective phospholipase A_2 in rabbit kidney cortex.

Methods

New Zealand white rabbits 2-3 kg were utilized in our studies. The kidneys were removed, cortex isolated and homogenized in 4 vols of 10 mM. Tris pH 7.5, 2 mM EDTA, 10 μM leupeptin, 10 μM pepstatin A, 3 mg/L soybean trypsin inhibitor, 0.25 ml DFP and 0.02% sodium azide. The homogenate was centrifuged at 15,000 x g for 15 min and the low speed supernatant (LSS) centrifuged for 60 min at 100,000 x g in a Beckman L2 ultracentrifuge. The high speed supernatant was then subjected to sequential chromatography starting with hydrophobic interactin chromatography on a Biogel TSK-phenyl-5PW column, ion exchange chromatography on TSK-DEAE-5PW, chromatofocusing on MONO-P, ion exchange on MONO-Q and gel filtration on Biosil TSK 250. Protein electrophoresis was carried out on 12% acrylamide gels and protein bands detected by silver staining. PLA_2 activity was assayed using 1-palmitoyl-2-[1-^{14}C] arachidonyl phosphatidyl ethanolamine (55 mCi/mmol).

Results

Table 1 gives the distribution of activity in the various subcellular components and indicates the major activity against PE resided in the HSS accounting for 81% of the activity.

Table 1. Distribution of PLA_2 Acting Against PE

	Activity cpm AA Release/10 µl/min	Total Volume	Total Activity cpm/10 min	% Activity
LSS	7095	83	58.9 x 10^6	100
HSS	6042	79	47.9 x 10^6	81
HSP	2366	16.5	3.9 x 10^6	6.6
0.5 M NaCl wash of HSP	2111	13.5	2.8 x 10^6	4.8
Resuspended HSP	1069	16.5	1.7 x 10^6	2.9

From hydrophobic interaction chromatography, the peak of activity eluted towards the end of the $(NH_4)SO_4$ gradient. This activity was resolved into two peaks by DEAE chromatography. The later eluting peak had activity against both PE and PC and was not evaluated further here. The peak eluting at lower ionic strength had activity against PE and none against PC. This peak was chromatofocused on MONO-P and appeared to give two under resolved peaks of activity. The activity was pooled and run on MONO-Q ion exchange chromatography where in the absence of 20% glycerol, the activity elutes as one peak but with 20% glycerol in mobile phase, there appears an additional peak eluting earlier. Both peaks of activity when run on gel filtration gave apparent Mr of 85 kD. SDS-PAGE demonstrated that peak A, the earlier eluting peak from the MONO-Q, had major protein bands at 88 kD and 44 kD. While the later eluting peak B gave protein bands at 44 kD and 23 kD. Kinetic analysis suggested that both peaks had a Km of 30 µM againse PE substrate, but the Vmax of peak A was 286 nmol/mg protein/min while for peak B was 25 nmol/mg protein/min.

Discussion

The present study demonstrated an unusual phospholipase A_2 which is purified from the high speed supernatant of rabbit renal cortex. The enzyme appears to be labile as it is purified towards homogeneity and in the presence of 20% glycerol demonstrates high catalytic activity and by gel electrophoresis suggests a MW of 88 kD. In the absence of glycerol to "stabilize" the enzyme, it appears to break down into its monomeric form giving proteins of 44 and 23 kD by SDS PAGE. The enzyme is purified about 1500 fold or greater (Table 2) and appears to be a tetramer with a monomeric subunit of 23 kD. It appears to have higher activity when in its tetrameric form when compared with its monomeric or dimeric form. Our enzyme displays an obligatory requirement for Ca^{2+} and appears to exert selectivity for PE >> PI >> PC with arachidonate in the Sn-2 position.

Table 2. Purification Table

Step	Volume ml	Protein Conc. mg/ml	Enzyme Activity nmoles/ml/min	Total Activity nmoles/min	Specific Activity nmoles/mg/min	Fold Purification
LSS (homogenate 10,000 x g spin)	120	14.3	1.21	145	0.09	1
HSS	110	7.25	1.28	141	0.18	2.1
HIC	65	1.14	1.48	95	1.30	15.3
DEAE-5PW	35	0.09	1.50	52	16.7	196
Mono P	3	0.08	2.23	6.7	27.5	323
Mono QA	1.5	0.01	1.32	2.0	132.0	1553
Mono QB	2	0.02	0.71	1.4	35.4	416

References

1. Gassama-Diagne, A., Fauvel, J., and Chap, H. (1988): *J. Biol. Chem.* 264:9470-9475.

2. Morrison, A.R. and Pascoe, N. (1986): *Kidney Int.* 29:496-501.

3. Ono, T., Tojo, H., Kuramitsu, S., Kagamiyama, H., and Okamoto, M. (1988): *J. Biol. Chem.* 263:5732-5738.

4. Tojo, H., Onot, H., Kuramitsu, S., Kagamiyama, H., and Okamoto, M. (1988): *J. Biol. Chem.* 263:5724-5731.

5. Troyer, D.A., Kreisberg, J.L., and VenKatachalam, M. (1986) *Kidney Int.* 29:530-538

6. van den Bosch, M. (1980): *Biochim. Biophys. Acta*, 604:191-246.

7. Waite, M. (1987): In: *Phospholipases*, pp. 111-133, Plenum Publishing Corp., New York.

ACTIVATION OF GROUP II PHOSPHOLIPASE A_2 GENE VIA TWO DISTINCT MECHANISMS IN RAT VASCULAR SMOOTH MUSCLE CELLS

H. Arita, T. Nakano, O. Ohara and H. Teraoka

Shionogi Research Laboratories, Shionogi & Co., Ltd., Fukushima-ku, Osaka 553, Japan

Phospholipase A_2 (PLA_2) is an enzyme which releases fatty acids esterified at the $\underline{sn}$-2 position of phospholipids. From the pathological view point, the secretory type of the enzyme is supposed to be an important mediator of inflammation diseases (1). Two types of mammalian secretory PLA_2 have been well characterized so far. Group I PLA_2 is mainly produced in the pancreas while group II PLA_2 (PLA_2-II) of high level is often found in some inflammatory regions (2-4). PLA_2-II also causes inflammatory responses when it is injected into animal. Thus, PLA_2-II has been thought to participate in promoting inflammatory processes. However, until recently it was impossible to examine the regulation of PLA_2 production. The cloning in recent years of cDNA for PLA_2-II from human and rat has made it possible to investigate the regulation of the expression of PLA_2-II at the gene level (5). In this study using cultured rat vascular smooth muscle cells (VSMCs), we investigated the mechanisms which up-regulated the expression of PLA_2-II gene in the cells, as well as the effects of glucocorticoid, a potent antiinflammatory agents, on the expression of PLA_2-II.

METHODS

Rat VSMCs were isolated by enzymatic digestion (6) of media of thoracic aorta from male Sprague-Dawley rats, and cultured in Dulbecco's modified Eagle's medium containing 20% fetal calf serum. Confluent VSMCs were incubated with inhibitors and/or stimuli for 24 h. At the end of incubation, the supernatant was removed for use in the PLA_2 assay and immunoblotting, and RNA was extracted from the cells for use in RNA blotting. PLA_2 activity was measured by the hydrolysis of [^{3}H]oleic acid-labeled E. coli phospholipids.

RESULTS

Activation of PLA_2 Gene Expression

As illustrated in Table I, two potent inflammatory mediators, interleukin 1 (IL-1) and tumor necrosis factor (TNF), as well as lipopolysacharide (LPS) increased PLA_2 release from VSMCs. The agents which increase intracellular cAMP levels, such as forskolin (FK), isobutylmethylxanthine (IBMX) and dubutyryl cAMP, also stimulated the release. On the other hand, dibutyryl cGMP and phorbol myristate acetate (PMA) had no effects on the secretion of PLA_2. These findings suggested that cAMP participated in the elevation of the PLA_2 release activated by the inflammatory factors, however neither TNF, IL-1 nor LPS has been shown to elevate cAMP levels in VSMCs (7). Immunoblotting study using anti rat PLA_2-II IgG revealed that the PLA_2 released from the VSMCs was PLA_2-II (7). Actinomycin D, an inhibitor of transcription, prohibited the PLA_2 release, suggesting that de novo RNA synthesis was necessary for enhancing the release of PLA_2-II (Table I). Indeed, RNA blotting study showed the increase of PLA_2-II mRNA concomitantly with the increased PLA_2 release (7). From these results, we concluded that the level of rat PLA_2-II mRNA is controlled at least by two distinct mechanisms, one involves cAMP and the other is mediated by TNF, IL-1 and LPS (Fig. 1).

Table I. Release of PLA_2 activity from VSMCs

Addition	Phospholipase activity
Control	1.0
IL-1 (10 U/ml)	12.6
TNF (1000 U/ml)	37.3
LPS (100 ng/ml)	33.4
FK (10 uM)	17.3
IBMX (0.5 mM)	7.5
dbcAMP (1 mM)	14.9
dbcGMP (1 mM)	1.6
PMA (100 nM)	1.2
Act.D (1 uM) + FK	0.8
Act. D (1 uM) + TNF	1.1

Effect of Glucocorticoid on PLA_2-II synthesis

Inhibition of PLA_2 by glucocorticoids had been accounted for by the induction of PLA_2 inhibitory proteins known as lipocortins. However, some recent reports have described results negative to the theory. Then, we investigated the effect of glucocorticoid on PLA_2-II synthesis in VSMCs in order to further characterize the antiinflammatory action of glucocorticoid (8). Both FK-induced and TNF-induced PLA_2-II release responses were almost completely blocked by 10 nM and 100 nM dexamethasone, respectively, as assayed by protein blotting and PLA_2 activity assays. Dexamethasone-mediated inhibition of PLA_2-II release appeared to be mediated by the glucocorticoid receptor. Dexamethasone at concentrations > 10 nM inhibited FK-induced elevation of the PLA_2-II mRNA level but not the TNF-induced one. These results suggest that the mechanism mediating FK-induced mRNA accumulation is sensitive to glucocorticoid but the mechanism mediating TNF-induced one is not. Inhibition of the PLA_2-II release induced by TNF may be explained by the blocking of post-transcriptional synthesis of the PLA_2 (Fig. 1). The inhibitory effect of glucocorticoid on PLA_2-II synthesis may provide one possible explanation of the glucocorticoid-mediated PLA_2 suppression.

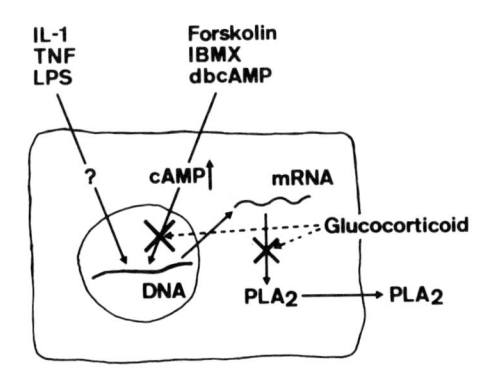

Fig. 1. Regulation of PLA_2-II expression in VSMCs

DISCUSSION

This study using cultured rat VSMCs suggests that PLA_2-II plays an important role in the pathogenesis of vascular inflammatory processes such as atherosclerosis and vasculitis. In vascular system, production of the PLA_2-II may be specific to VSMCs, because cultured rat endothelial cells did not respond to TNF or forskolin to release the PLA_2 (unpublished result). This finding also indicates that some tissue-specific factors may be involved in the expression of the gene. With these considerations in mind, it would be very important to clarify the regulation mechanism of the PLA_2-II gene in detail on the molecular basis and to clarify the physiological role of the PLA_2-II in the progression of inflammatory diseases.

REFERENCES

1. Vadas, P., and Pruzanski, W. (1986): Laboratory Inv., 55: 391-404.
2. Forst, S., Weiss, J., Elsbach, P., Maranganore, J. M., Reardon, I., and Heinrikson, R. L. (1986): Biochemistry, 25: 8381-8385.
3. Chan, H. W., Kudo, I., Tomita, M., and Inoue, K. (1987): J. Biochem. (Tokyo), 102: 147-154.
4. Hara, S., Kudo, I., Matsuta, K., Miyamoto, T., and Inoue, K. (1988): J. Biochem. (Tokyo), 104: 326-328.
5. Ishizaki, J., Ohara, O., Nakamura, E., Tamaki, M., Ono, T., Kanda, A., Yoshida, N., Teraoka, H., Tojo, H., and Okamoto, M. (1989): Biochem. Biophys. Res. Commun., 162: 1030-1036.
6. Chamley-Campbell, J., Campbell, G. R., and Ross, R. (1979): Physiol. Rev., 59: 1-61.
7. Nakano, T., Ohara, O., Teraoka, H., and Arita, H. (1990): FEBS Lett., 261: 171-174.
8. Nakano, T., Ohara, O., Teraoka, H., and Arita, H. (1990): J. Biol. Chem., in press.

THE EICOSANOID LIPID PRECURSORS DIACYL-GLYCEROL AND PHOSPHATIDIC ACID ARE FORMED BY PHOSPHOLIPASE D IN NEUTROPHILS

M. Motasim Billah, Stephen Eckel, Theodore J. Mullmann, Jin-Keon Pai, Marvin I. Siegel and Robert W. Egan

Schering-Plough Research, Department of Allergy and Immunology, New Jersey USA 07003

The importance of phospholipase D (PLD) has gone virtually unnoticed until recently, because the phospholipase C (PLC) could account for diglyceride (DG) and, when coupled to a diglyceride kinase (DGK), could also form phosphatidic acid (PA) and because there were no reagents to categorically recognize PLD in the presence of other lipid metabolizing enzymes. Nevertheless, with PLD and a phosphatidate phosphohydrolase (PPH), one can also make PA then DG. The concomitant products, choline and phosphocholine, can also be exchanged, so that these cannot differentiate the pathways either. However, the tools to distinguish these pathways now exist and have been very revealing. By labeling cellular PC with ^{32}P and ^{3}H (6) or by utilizing the PLD-catalyzed transphosphatidylation reaction of PC with ethanol to give PEt (5), we can and have defined the PLD reaction both qualitatively and quantitatively.

We radiolabel the cells with 1-0-alkyl lysoPC rather than diacyl lysoPC to avoid scrambling the label into a variety of lipids, but this has not turned out to be a problem (4). The lysoPC is incorporated and acylated endogenously into membrane PC, the desired substrate. We have labeled the PC in the sn-1 fatty acid with tritium, in the phosphate with ^{32}P or in both.

PLD would make PA directly and the ratio of ^{32}P to ^{3}H would remain the same as in the PC (1,4,6). Because everything is normalized to the starting PC, the ratio in PA would be 1.

On the other hand, were the PA to arise from PLC and DGK, the ^{32}P would be removed and replaced with cold phosphate from unlabeled ATP and the ratio would be 0. For example, a $^{32}P/^{3}H$ ratio of 0.5 indicates an equal contribution from each pathway.

To indicate the relative importance of PLD, the $^{32}P/^{3}H$ ratios in neutrophils or differentiated HL-60 cells with various stimulators have been measured. For example, at shorter times, in the HL-60 cell, PLD contributes 85 and 100% of the PA with fMLP and PMA, respectively. At longer times, the PLC pathway could be contributing up to 50% of the PA with fMLP. The bottom line is that with labeled alkylPC, and we also know with acylPC, PLD is the dominant pathway for PA formation in these cells. Bear in mind that this analysis applies only to the labeled PC and that metabolism of other lipids is transparent.

TABLE 1
MASS, SPECIFIC ACTIVITY AND $^{32}P/^{3}H$ RATIO OF PC, PA AND PEt IN HUMAN NEUTROPHILS

Washed human neutrophils were double-labeled in alkyl-PC by incubation with [^{3}H]alkyl-lysoPC and alkyl-[^{32}P]-lysoPC. Triplicate samples containing these double-labeled cells (5 x 10^{7} cells) and 1.5 mM $CaCl_2$ were incubated with 5 μM cytochalasin B for 5 min before adding buffer or 100 nM fMLP for 30 s in the absence or the presence of 0.5% ethanol. PC, PA and PEt containing ^{3}H and ^{32}P were separated by TLC and analyzed for mass and radioactivity.

Parameters	Vehicle PC	fMLP PA	fMLP + EtOH PA	fMLP + EtOH PEt
Mass (nmol/10^7 cells)	30.0 ± 0.6	1.07 ± 0.01	0.71 ± 0.03	0.37 ± 0.04
^{3}H (dpm/nmol)x10^{-3}	22.6 ± 0.2	20.8 ± 1.4	26.8 ± 2.6	20.0 ± 0.4
^{32}P (dpm/nmol)x10^{-3}	16.8 ± 0.7	18.0 ± 0.1	19.6 ± 1.1	15.0 ± 0.4
$^{32}P/^{3}H$ ratio (normalized)	1.0	1.2	1.0	1.0

We determine the mass of PA colorimitrically following PCA digestion of the PA that was separated by TLC from the other lipids following Bligh & Dyer extraction of the incubations (2). Because the neutrophils are labeled with ^{3}H and ^{32}P, we could also determine the radioactivity in the PA and, from mass and radioactivity, we established the specific activity (Table 1). First, note that about 3% of the total PC is converted into PA following stimulation with 100 nM fMLP and 5 µM cytochalasin B. The specific activity of the PC prior to stimulation was 23 x 10^3 dpm/nmol for ^{3}H and 17 x 10^3 dpm/nmol for ^{32}P. Then, note that the specific activities in the PA formed in the presence or absence of 0.5% ethanol are virtually identical, 21 and 27 with ^{3}H or 18 and 20 with ^{32}P. Were other lipids contributing to the PA, the specific activity would decrease because the other lipids are not labeled with either radioisotope. These mass measurements, therefore, indicate that PLD is responsible for virtually all the PA mass and, as expected, the ^{32}P/^{3}H ratios remains at a normalized value of about 1 for the radiolabeled PA.

It has been demonstrated that propranolol inhibits the PPH (3,7), and we have used this tool along with DG mass measurements to investigate the pathways for DG formation. At concentrations much higher than those required for β-blocking, propranolol inhibits the conversion of PA to DG by the PPH. Using ^{3}H PC labeled neutrophils, 200 µM propranolol inhibits labeled DG formation completely (2). This is not the result of inhibiting the PLD because phosphatidyl ethanol formation is completely unchanged at this concentration. As expected, there is an increase in PA when the PPH is inhibited.

DG mass was measured by converting it to PA with an E.coli diglyceride kinase in the presence of [^{32}P]ATP then separating the resultant PA by TLC, counting and determining the mass from the known specific activity of the ATP (2). Figure 1 shows the effect of propranolol on the DG levels in fMLP/CB stimulated neutrophils (2). Propranolol was added 5 min prior to stimulation with 100 nM fMLP and the reaction was terminated by extraction 3 min later. Note in the open circles that without fMLP there are about 100 pmole/10^7 cells of DG that are unaffected by propranolol. On the other hand, propranolol inhibits stimulated DG formation in a dose dependent fashion, with virtually complete inhibition at 200 µM. Therefore, the preponderance of the mass as well as the labeled DG arises from the PLD/PPH pathway. In these and in other experiments, higher concentrations of propranolol never reduced the DG level below the baseline suggesting that the maintenance levels were sustained by PLC.

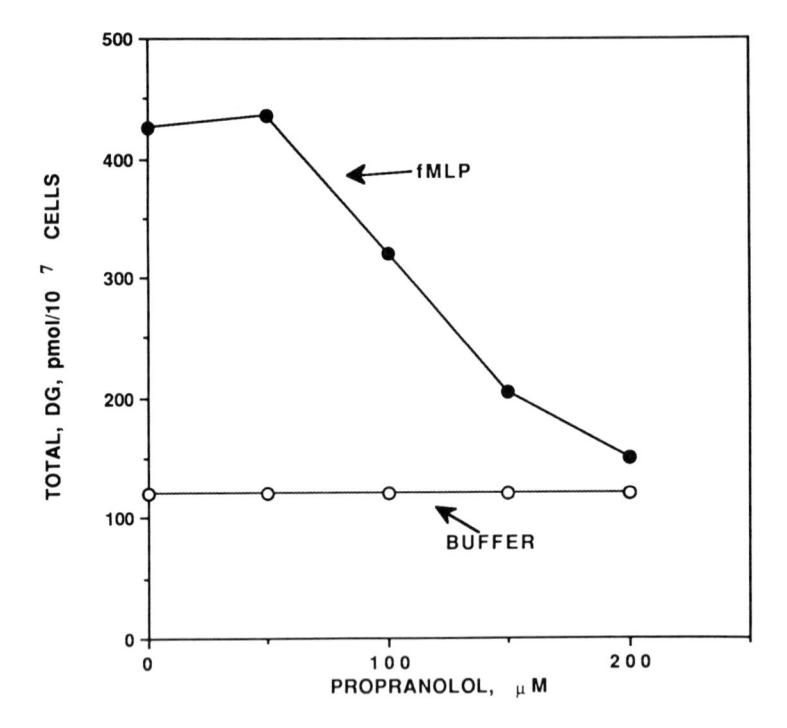

FIG. 1. Effect of propranolol on total DG mass formation by fMLP-stimulated neutrophils: Duplicate samples containing 5 x 10^6 neutrophils, 1.5 mM $CaCl_2$ and 5 µM cytochalasin B were incubated with various concentrations of propranolol for 5 min before adding either buffer (○) or 100 nM fMLP (●) for an additional 3 min. DG mass was determined by enzymatic conversion to [^{32}P]PA.

In summary, PLD is involved in the activation of neutrophils and is ubiquitous to many other cells where it is receptor linked through a G-protein and requires extracellular Ca^{2+}. In the neutrophil, it prefers PC as substrate. As measured by radioactive PC turnover to PA and PEt, PLD is turned on rapidly and maintains a sustained activity. PLD is responsible for virtually all the PA mass formed in neutrophils and, in conjunction with PPH, is also responsible for the increases in the mass of DG during neutrophil stimulation. Thus, the class of PLD enzymes is integral to many aspects of cell activation.

ACKNOWLEDGMENT

The authors thank Lisa Ramirez for typing the manuscript.

REFERENCES

1. Billah, M.M., Pai, J.-K., Mullmann, T.J., Egan, R.W., and Siegel, M.I. (1989): *J. Biol. Chem.*, 264:9069-9076.
2. Billah, M.M., Eckel, S., Mullmann, T.J., Egan, R.W., and Siegel, M.I. (1989): *J. Biol. Chem.*, 264:17069-17077.
3. Koul, O., and Houser, G. (1987): *Arch. Biochem. Biophys.*, 253:453-461.
4. Mullmann, T.J., Siegel, M.I., Egan, R.W., and Billah, M.M. (1990): *J. Immunol.*, 144:1901-1908.
5. Pai, J.-K., Siegel, M.I., Egan, R.W., and Billah, M.M. (1988): *Biochem. Biophys. Res. Commun.*, 150:355-364.
6. Pai, J.-K., Siegel, M.I., Egan, R.W., and Billah, M.M. (1988): *J. Biol. Chem.*, 263:12472-12477.
7. Pappu, A.S., and Hauser, G. (1983): *Neurochem. Res.*, 8:1565-1575.

PHOSPHOLIPASE D IN THE PANCREATIC ISLET: EVIDENCE SUGGESTING THE INVOLVEMENT OF PHOSPHATIDIC ACID IN SIGNAL TRANSDUCTION

S. Metz[*], M. Dunlop[+]

From the Medical & Research Services, Denver VA Medical Center[*] (111H), 1055 Clermont Street, Denver, CO 80220, USA

(and) the Department of Medicine[+]
Royal Melbourne Hospital, Clinical Sciences Bldg., the University of Melbourne, Parkville 3050, Victoria, Australia

A role for phosphatidic acid (PA) in ion fluxes, accumulation of cyclic nucleotides, inositol phospholipid turnover and growth has been proposed for many cells. In pancreatic islet cells, PA can be derived via the phosphorylation of diglyceride, or de novo from products of glucose's metabolism (3); however, the most direct route would be via the activation of a phospholipase of the D type (PLD). Since a PLD had not previously been identified in peptide-secreting endocrine cells, we investigated the presence and effects of PLD in pancreatic islet cells.

DISPERSED NEONATAL ISLET CELLS VS. INTACT ADULT RAT ISLETS

Although results with these two models are qualitatively similar, certain important quantitative differences exist. For example, stimulatory effects of exogenous arachidonic acid (13) or PA (4) on insulin release can be demonstrated with facility in the former, whereas special conditions are required to deliver arachidonate to the ß cell-rich interior of intact islets (9,10). The same appears to be true for PA. This is probably due in part to the limited solubility and permeation of these hydrophobic moieties (9).

In addition, the metabolism of choline differs somewhat in the two models. We have observed that in the former, an overnight (18-20 hr) labelling period in the presence of [^{14}C-Me]choline yields a distribution of cellular water-soluble choline metabolites as follows: free choline, 2-9%; phosphorylcholine, 18-31%; glycero-phosphorylcholine (GPC), 55-73% (betaine and CDP-choline make only minor contributions); in intact adult islets, these figures are 5-10%, 53-86%, and 7-31%, respectively. In addition, in the former model, exposure to the phorbol ester TPA (2 μM) increases the total release of free [^{14}C]choline (cells plus medium) to 300% of basal (5) in the presence of a 25 μM choline chase. In contrast, while a significant increase is elicited in intact adult islets, it is of the order of only $\leq$ 25% of basal, even in the presence of 1 mM unlabelled choline, and most of this increase is found in the medium. These quantitative differences in cellular choline and phosphorylcholine content might reflect a greater activity of choline kinase and/or a greater difficulty in achieving an adequate "chase" in intact islets and possibly may explain the failure of Turk et al. to see increments in cellular choline after glucose stimulation of intact adult islets (17). The marked accumulation of GPC in the neonatal cells (5) may reflect greater phospholipase A activity and/or impaired clearance of GPC, since, in preliminary studies, we have been unable to convincingly demonstrate de novo synthesis of GPC, as proposed by Infante (8).

PHOSPHOLIPASE D ACTIVATION IN ISLET CELLS

Despite quantitative differences in the two models, PLD is activated in both systems by TPA, ionomycin or sodium fluoride (NaF), as indicated by release of free choline and a concomitant accumulation of PA (5). In addition, in the presence of alcohols (methanol, ethanol, propanol or butanol) or glycerol, a phosphatidyl group (principally from phosphatidylcholine) is transferred to the alcohol (rather than to water - i.e., hydrolysis), yielding phosphatidyl-alcohols (11) in a process called "transphosphatidylation". The accumulation of these unnatural phospholipids provides a sensitive, unambiguous and specific marker for PLD activation and confirms the activation by TPA, ionomycin or NaF (11). It is unlikely that phosphatidylethanol derives via a base exchange-like mechanism or via the de novo synthesis of phospholipid, since it was accompanied by release of choline, was not reduced by 35µg/ml dioctanoylglycerol (to dilute labelled endogenous diglyceride stores used for phospholipid synthesis) or by 1mM 5'-deoxy-5-isobutylthio-adenosine (an inhibitor of the CDP-choline pathway in islets; 7). Furthermore, the effect of ethanol was not reduced by the endogenous bases choline (250µM) and myo-inositol (35µg/ml).

In the case of TPA, PLD is selectively activated; in the case of ionomycin or NaF, PLD activation is accompanied by additional evidence of activation of a phospholipase C (probably directed against inositol lipids) and a considerable accumulation of diglyceride (5). Provision of ethanol reduces the PA formation induced by TPA presumably by fostering transphosphatidylation; the PA induced by NaF or ionomycin is refractory to inhibition (11), presumably because this pool of PA arose via the phosphorylation of diglyceride. However, two caveats should be kept in mind in extrapolating these findings to other situations: First, ethanol can activate PA phosphohydrolase in some cells (16), thereby directly accelerating the removal of PA. Second, ethanol can interfere with Ca^{++} (and other ion) channels (6); since phosphatidylinositol-directed phospholipase C is Ca^{++}-activated in some tissues (probably including the islet), ethanol theoretically could impede diglyceride formation, with a secondary decline in PA. However, ethanol also has some other effects to potentiate phospholipase C activation (15) and these may more than offset any effects due to alterations in ion fluxes.

EFFECTS OF OTHER AGONISTS ON ISLET PLD

In contrast to some other tissues, in preliminary studies of adult rat islets, 250 µM Na_2ATP or 1 mM carbachol did not increase phosphatidylethanol formation detectably, although phospholipase C was probably activated. In preliminary studies of neonatal islet cells, the physiologic carbohydrate dl-glyceraldehyde (15-20 mM) did increase phosphatidylethanol by two-fold whereas the amino acid secretagogue ketoisocaproic acid (KIC) was inactive in this respect. These findings are of interest since they indicate not only that some physiologic secretagogues are active, but also that PLD activation is not merely secondary to insulin release (since KIC does stimulate secretion). In addition, it is worth noting that the former agonist lowers intracellular pH in islet cells whereas the latter may elevate it (1); since the pH optimum of many PLDs is acidic, a role of pH in the physiologic regulation of PLD is suggested. In adult islets, we have thus far not seen elevations of phosphatidylethanol induced by glucose or glyceraldehyde. However, the provision of 1.5% ethanol as acceptor may have impeded Ca^{++} mobilization (see <u>above and following</u>) and thereby blocked the signal for PLD activation; future studies, therefore, may have to use acceptors (e.g., glycerol) other than ethanol.

ENDOGENOUS PA PROMOTES INSULIN RELEASE

In adult islets, treatment with bacterial PLD selectively augmented the formation of <u>endogenous</u> PA in [^{14}C] myristate- or [^{14}C] arachidonate-labelled islets and, in close parallel (r = 0.98-0.99), promoted non-toxic insulin release (12). This secretion did not require the presence of Ca^{++}_o. It was blocked by Co^{++} or dantrolene in the absence of any inhibition of PA formation, suggesting that these pharmacologic probes may antagonize the cellular effects of PA. These observations support our previous observations (4) that <u>exogenous</u> PA augments insulin release from dispersed neonatal islet cells. However, it remains to be determined whether increments in PA due to <u>de novo</u> synthesis or derived from the phosphorylation of DG are also insulinotropic, since the fatty acid composition of PA from the three sources is likely to be different (17).

Some evidence suggests that the molecular species of PA may indeed modify its insulinotropic potency. Whereas neonatal islet cells respond briskly to exogenous PA, they seem to respond sluggishly to endogenous PA (augmented via the provision of exogenous PLD) as compared to adult islets. While this could be due to a deficiency in paracrine augmentation (glucagon-containing α cells are absent) in this dispersed cell preparation, it is intriguing to note that the neonatal preparation seemed (in preliminary studies) to generate a greater percentage of a second species of PA having an R_F slightly greater than that of the diacyl-PA standard and which is tentatively identified as an alkyl-linked PA species. Thus, this second, minor PA species may be relatively inactive (or even inhibitory) with regard to secretion.

If the hypothesis is correct that PA, generated via PLD activation, promotes physiologic insulin release, then provision of ethanol should impede such secretion (by promoting phosphatidylethanol at the expense of PA). This could contribute to the known inhibitory effects of ethanol on secretion (14), especially since PA, which is pro-secretory, would be replaced by phosphatidylethanol which, in addition, may directly impair the membrane fusion process (2) critical to exocytosis. Indeed in preliminary studies, we observed that ethanol does reduce glucose-induced insulin release. However, it also inhibited (by 73%) the insulin release induced by depolarizing concentrations of K^+ (control, at glucose 3.3 mM = 135 $\pm$ 18 μU/10 islets/30 min; 50 mM K^+ = 562 $\pm$ 33; 50 mM K^+ and 2.5% ethanol = 278 $\pm$ 20; x $\pm$ SEM; p < .001) even though 50 mM K^+ does <u>not</u> activate islet PLD (5). These findings again suggest the presence of confounding, direct effects of ethanol on ion fluxes (see <u>above</u>) and again reinforce the need to study alternate phosphatidyl acceptors.

POSSIBLE ROLE OF PLD IN THE "TOXIC" EFFECTS OF CHRONIC HYPERGLYCEMIA AND ALCOHOLISM

One hypothesis for the complications of hyperglycemia in diabetes is that glucose (having unrestricted access to insulin-independent tissues) is converted by aldose reductase to sorbitol, which in turn accumulates to levels which are detrimental to cell function. However islet (and other) cells can "transphosphatidylate" using glycerol as acceptor; we would speculate that they could do the same using sorbitol, leading to the accumulation of a unique phospholipid (phosphatidylsorbitol) which might be responsible for some of the observed cell dysfunction. Our recent studies showed that endogenous phosphatidylethanol is relatively slowly removed from membranes of intact islets <u>in situ</u> (40-50%/hr). Thus, this lipid might build-up in the membranes of alcoholics, just as membranes of diabetics might have increased phosphatidylsorbitol levels. This latter event would be fostered not only because glucose would generate the phosphatidyl acceptor (sorbitol) but also because glucose metabolism yields diglyceride (3,17), which may (like TPA; see above) activate PLD.

ACKNOWLEDGMENTS

This work was supported by the Veterans Administration, the National Health and Medical Research Council of Australia, and the National Institutes of Health (DK 37312).

REFERENCES

1. Best, L., Yates, A.P., Gordon, C., Tomlinson, S. (1988): Biochem. Pharmacol., 37:4611-4615.
2. Bondeson, J., Sundler, R. (1987): Biochim. Biophys. Acta, 899:258-264.
3. Dunlop, M.E., Larkins, R.G. (1985): Biochem. Biophys. Res. Commun., 132:467-473.
4. Dunlop, M.E., Larkins, R.G., (1989): Diabetes, 38:1187-1192.
5. Dunlop, M., Metz, S.A. (1989): Biochem. Biophys. Res. Commun., 163:922-928.
6. Gandhi, C.R., Ross, D.H. (1989): Experientia, 45:407-413.
7. Hoffman, J.M., Laychock, S.G. (1988): Diabetes, 37:1489-1498.
8. Infante, J.P. (1984): FEBS Lett., 170:1-14.
9. Metz, S. (1988): Prostagland. Leukotri. Essent. Fatty Acids - Reviews, 32:187-202.
10. Metz, S.A., Draznin, B., Sussman, K.E., Leitner, J.W. (1987): Biochem. Biophys. Res. Commun., 142:251-258.
11. Metz, S., Dunlop, M. (1990): Abstracts of the 72nd Annual Meeting of the Endocrine Society, in press.
12. Metz, S., Dunlop, M. (1990): Diabetes (Suppl 1), 39:57a.
13. Metz, S., VanRollins, M., Strife, R., Fujimoto, W., Robertson, R.P. (1983): J. Clin. Invest., 71:1191-1205.
14. Patel, D.G., Singh, S.P. (1979): Metabolism, 28:85-89.
15. Rubin, R., Hoek, J.B. (1988): Biochem. J., 254:147-153.
16. Savolainen, M.J., Hassinen, I.E. (1978): Biochem. J., 176:885-892.
17. Wolf, B.A., Easom, R.A., Hughes, J.H., McDaniel, M.L., Turk, J., (1989): Biochemistry, 28:4291-4301.

EFFECT OF DEXAMETHASONE AND PHORBOL MYRISTATE ACETATE ON LIPOCORTIN 1, 2 AND 5 mRNA AND PROTEIN SYNTHESIS

E. Solito, G. Raugei, M. Melli and L. Parente

Sclavo Research Centre, Laboratory of Pharmacology and Molecular Biology, Via Fiorentina, 53100, Siena, Italy

Lipocortins (LCT) are a family of Ca^{2+} and phospholipid-binding proteins which have been implicated in the anti-phospholipase and anti-inflammatory action of glucocorticoids (for review see ref. 6). However, conflicting results have been reported on the ability of steroid drugs in inducing the synthesis of lipocortins. Stimulation of the synthesis of the protein by glucocorticoids has been observed in macrophages (2), neutrophils (8), renomedullary interstitial cells (4), thymocytes (5, 14), Swiss 3T3 fibroblasts (13). Negative results have been reported in human skin fibroblasts (3), lymphocytes (3), alveolar macrophages (3), endothelial cells (9), U-937 cells (1,10). Recent studies have also shown that differentiation of U-937 (10) and HL-60 (15) cells is associated with increased synthesis of LCTs. In order to obtain further information on the regulation of expression of LCTs, we have investigated the effect of phorbol 12-myristate 13-acetate diester (PMA) and dexamethasone on LCT 1,2 and 5 mRNA and protein synthesis in U-937 cells and rat peritoneal macrophages.

METHODS

Cell cultures

U-937 cells were cultured in RPMI 1640 (Gibco,U.K.) containing 2mM glutamine, 50 µg/ml gentamycin and 10% foetal calf serum. To induce differentiation, cells were plated at 10^7 per well (6x35 mm) in the presence of 1 nM PMA for 24 or 48 hours. Peritoneal cells were collected from male Wistar rats and macrophages purified by 2 hours adherence in RPMI with 20% FCS. Dexamethasone (1 µM) was incubated with the cells for 2 hours.

Ex vivo experiments

Peritoneal cells were collected from adrenalectomized (ADX) or sham-operated (SHO) rats 2 hours after saline (2 ml/kg i.p.) or dexamethasone (0.5 mg/kg i.p.) administration.

Northern and Western blot analysis

Northern and Western blots were performed according to Pepinsky et al.(11). Hybridization probes for LCT 1, 2 and 5, encompassing the entire coding region, were isolated from a cDNA library utilizing either the polymerase chain reaction method (LCT 1 and 5) or the oligonucleotide plaque screening (LCT 2). The cDNA library was obtained from human placenta mRNA utilizing λgt11 fage vector. The anti-LCT antibodies (rabbit polyclonal antisera 1/1000) were kindly provided by Dr.J.L. Browning, Biogen, Cambridge, MA.

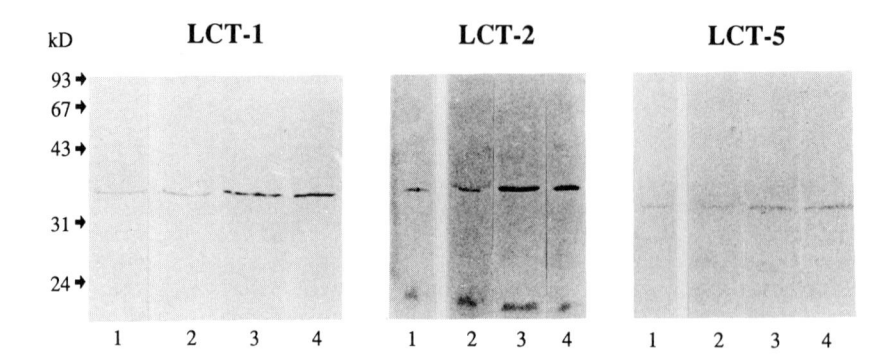

FIG. 1. Western blot analysis of lipocortin (LCT) 1, 2 and 5 in U-937 cells. Lane 1, control cells. Cells were incubated with dexamethasone (1 μM for 2 hr, lane 2) or with PMA (1nM for 24 hr, lane 3, and 48 hr, lane 4).

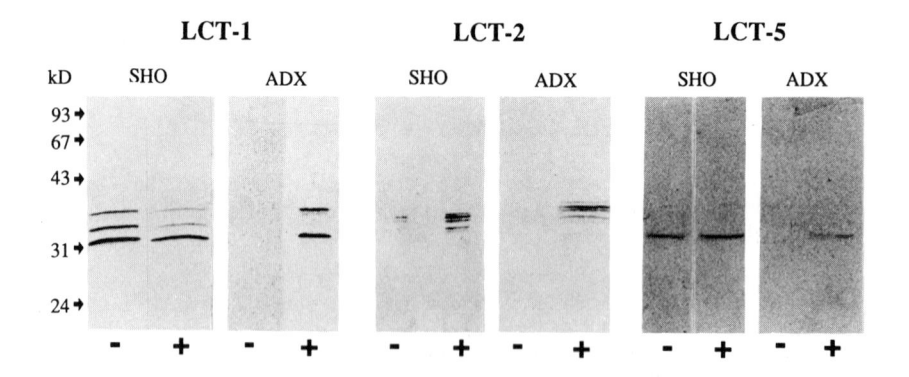

FIG.2. Western blot analysis of lipocortin (LCT) 1, 2 and 5 in peritoneal cells collected from sham-operated (SHO) and adrenalectomized (ADX) rats treated 2 hr before with 2 ml/kg i.p. saline (-) or 0.5 mg/kg i.p. dexamethasone (+).

RESULTS AND DISCUSSION

Northern blot analysis revealed constitutive expression of mRNA for the three LCTs in both U-937 and peritoneal macrophages. The steady-state amount of LCT 2 mRNA was higher than that of LCT 1 and 5. The addition of dexamethasone (1 μM for 2 hr) to the incubation medium of U-937 cells did not alter the amount of LCT mRNAs (not shown). Addition of PMA (1 nM) for 24 or 48 hr also did not modify the quantity of LCT mRNAs. We have observed a similar lack of effect by glucocorticoids and 1 nM PMA on LCT mRNA amounts in different cell lines: HL-60, human skin fibroblasts, HeLa, THP-1 (not shown). Preliminary results have shown increase of mRNA in U-937 cells incubated for 24 hr with 10 nM PMA. Western blot analysis revealed that LCT 1, 2 and 5 are constitutively synthetized in U-937 cells (Fig.1, lane 1) and in peritoneal macrophages (not shown). In agreement with Northern blot results the amount of LCT 2 was higher than that of LCT 1 and 5 . Fig.1 also shows that in U-937 cells the amount of the three LCTs was not modified by dexamethasone (lane 2) whereas it was increased by 1 nM PMA incubated for 24 and 48 hr (lanes 3 and 4). These results indicate that under our experimental conditions dexamethasone does not affect the amount of LCT 1, 2 and 5 mRNAs and proteins. The increase caused by PMA supports a role of these proteins in cell differentiation as previously suggested (10,15).

In the *ex vivo* experiments constitutive expression of LCT mRNAs was observed in peritoneal cells collected from both ADX and SHO rats. Also in these cells the amount of LCT 2 mRNA appeared to be higher than that of LCT 1 and 5. The administration of dexamethasone did not change the mRNAs (not shown). Constitutive expression of the three proteins was observed in peritoneal cells collected from control SHO animals (Fig.2). In these cells the amount of LCT 2, but not of LCT 1 and 5, was increased by the *in vivo* administration of dexamethasone. On the other hand, the three proteins were not detected in peritoneal cells collected from control ADX rats. A marked increase of the synthesis of the three LCTs was observed in cells from ADX rats after the *in vivo* administration of the glucocorticoid (Fig.2). These data confirm the inefficacy of steroid drugs in the induction of LCT mRNAs and suggest that glucocorticoids regulate *in vivo* LCT synthesis at a post-transcriptional level. It is noteworthy that in previous experiments an increased synthesis of LCT 1 by fluocinolone was observed only in the presence of serum, suggesting the existence of a serum factor acting synergistically with glucocorticoids (13). Finally the undetectable amount of LCTs in cells from ADX rats may provide the physiological explanation of the increased severity of the inflammatory process observed in ADX animals which may be ascribed to a de-regulated phospholipase A_2 activation (7,12).

REFERENCES

1. Bienkowski, M.J., Petro,M.A., and Robinson, L.J. (1989): *J.Biol.Chem.*, 264:6536-6544
2. Blackwell, G.J., Carnuccio, R., Di Rosa, M., Flower, R.J., Parente, L., and Persico, P. (1980): *Nature*, 287:147-149
3. Bronnegard, M., Andersson, O., Edwall, D., Lund, J., Norstedt, G., and Carlstedt-Duke, J. (1988): *Mol.Endocrinol.*, 2:732-739
4. Cloix, J.F., Colard, O., Rothhut, B., and Russo-Marie, F. (1983): *Br.J.Pharmacol.*,79:313-321

5. Errasfa, M., Rothhut, B., and Russo-Marie, F. (1989): *Biochem.Biophys.Res.Comm.*, 159:53-60
6. Flower, R.J. (1988): *Br.J.Pharmacol.* 94:987-1015
7. Flower, R.J., Parente, L., Persico, P., and Salmon, J.A. (1986): *Br.J.Pharmacol.*, 87:57-62
8. Hirata, F., Schiffmann, E., Venkatasubramanian, K., Salomon, D., and Axelrod, J. (1980): *Proc.Natl.Acad.Sci.USA*, 77:2533-2536
9. Hullin, F., Raynal, P., Ragab-Thomas, J.M.F., Fauvel, J., and Chap, H. (1989): *J.Biol.Chem.*, 264:3506-3513
10. Isacke, C.M., Lindberg, R.A., and Hunter, T. (1989): *Mol.Cell.Biol.*, 9:232-240
11. Pepinsky, R.B., Tizard, R., Mattaliano, R.J., Sinclair, L.K., Miller, G.T., Browning, J.L., Chow, E.P., Burne, C., Huang, K.S., Pratt, D., Wachter, L., Hession, C., Frey, A.Z., and Wallner, B.P. (1988): *J.Biol.Chem.*, 263:10799-10811
12. Perretti, M., Becherucci, C., Scapigliati, G., and Parente, L. (1989): *Br.J.Pharmacol.*, 98:1137-1142.
13. Philipps, C., Rose-John, S., Rincke, G., Furstenberger, G., and Marks, F. (1989): *Biochem.Biophys.Res.Comm.*, 159:155-162
14. Piltch, A., Sun, L., Fava, R.A., and Hayashi, J. (1989): *Biochem.J.*, 261:395-400
15. William, F., Mroczkowski, B., Cohen, S., and Kraft, A.S. (1988): *J. Cell.Physiol.*, 137:402-410

A CRITICAL APPROACH TO EICOSANOID ASSAY

Elisabeth Granström and *Hans Kindahl

Department of Reproductive Endocrinology,
Karolinska Hospital, S-104 01 Stockholm, Sweden, and
*Department of Obstetrics and Gynaecology,
Swedish University of Agricultural Sciences,
S-750 07 Uppsala, Sweden.

Quantification of eicosanoids has now been done for over 20 years, with considerable variation in approach as well as success. With increasing knowledge of the biochemistry of this family of compounds, we have become aware of a number of problems that complicate the assay methods and/or the interpretation of data. In addition to "pure" assay problems there are also metabolic and chemical phenomena that may interfere with the results.

METABOLIC PROBLEMS

One of the first complications to be recognized was the artifactual production of the primary prostaglandins and thromboxanes during collection and processing of the samples (reviews, 6,15). This is generally interpreted as due to mechanical stimulation of cells with high capacity for eicosanoid biosynthesis, and should thus only occur with blood, tissue or other cell-rich samples. The phenomenon should not complicate the analysis of e.g. urine or cell culture media. This undesired contribution of the analyzed prostanoid can be reduced but probably not completely suppressed by the prior addition of a cyclooxygenase inhibitor to the sample tube.
Recently, the picture has become more complex by the discovery of Morrow et al. (11) that a large number of prostaglandin F isomers can be formed by radical catalyzed reactions, independent of the cyclooxygenase. They are formed in vitro as well as in vivo in fairly large amounts, and they are also excreted into the urine (12). This discovery may cast some doubt on previously published PGF data from any biological material.
Another well-known metabolic problem is the rapid uptake and degradation of the eicosanoids, once they have reached the blood stream (15). Thus, the plasma levels of the primary prostaglandins and thromboxanes usually do not exceed the low picogram range. This particular assay problem can however usually be solved by monitoring a more long-lived metabolite instead, which may accumulate to considerably higher levels in the circulation (4,5,15).
Metabolic interconversion of many compounds in this field adds to the uncertainty in interpretation of data. If a rise in a cer-

tain PGF metabolite, for example, has been detected in some biological system, it does not necessarily mean that an overproduction of PGF has taken place. The formation of PGF compounds, both α and β, from prostaglandins of the E type has long been known. PGF_α is also formed non-enzymatically from the endoperoxides, PGG and PGH. High levels of a circulating PG metabolite, 15-keto-13, 14-dihydro-$PGF_{2\alpha}$, have been found in a number of conditions which may or may not be associated with overproduction of mainly $PGF_{2\alpha}$: luteolysis, pregnancy and parturition, asthma, anaphylaxis, medullary carcinoma of the thyroid, cold urticaria, etc. (6). One disease known to involve overproduction of PGD_2 rather than $PGF_{2\alpha}$, viz. systemic mastocytosis (14), also displays increased levels of mainly PGF metabolites, although in this case most compounds have the 9α,11β-configuration (10). These are however easily confused with the corresponding 9α,11α compounds (1).

Even prostacyclin, PGI_2, can be metabolized into a PGF_α metabolite, although an unusual one, pentanor-$PGF_{1\alpha}$ (6).

A fourth metabolic problem concerns variations in metabolism, which may cause greater problems than has so far been recognized. The probably best known case of variable metabolism was found in the catabolism of PGD_2 in normal subjects compared with mastocytosis patients (10,14). The major break-down product was 2,3-dinor-PGF_2 in the disease, whereas normals formed larger amounts of 9α, 11β-dihydroxy-15-keto-2,3,18,19-tetranorprost-5-ene-1,20-dioic acid.

In our own research, we have occasionally encountered other metabolic variations, which are difficult to explain. In a series of experiments aimed at monitoring the profile of circulating prostaglandin metabolites (4,5), the tritium-labeled compound was given by i.v. injection and blood samples were collected from the contralateral side. Analysis was done with two-dimensional TLC and autoradiography (3). When $PGF_{2\alpha}$ was given, the results were the expected ones, regardless of species: a very rapid disappearance of the parent compound and corresponding appearance of metabolites (4,5). Surprisingly, when PGE_2 was injected, the most prominent compound in blood co-chromatographed with reference $PGF_{2\alpha}$, even 15-20 min after the PGE_2 injection. Very little 15-ketodihydro-$PGF_{2\alpha}$ seemed to be formed under these circumstances (Fig. 1).

An even more puzzling finding is illustrated in Fig. 2, which shows the profile of circulating products of tritium-labeled $PGF_{2\alpha}$ in a human subject, 20 min after an injection was given which was a technical failure: instead of going i.v., the compound was deposited perivascularly in the forearm. This failure could be deduced from several facts: first, no radioactivity was detected in the samples collected from the contralateral arm until about 20 min later, and then only very small amounts which soon decreased. Second, excretion of products into urine showed a pronounced lag period. This happened a total of three times in a series of similar experiments, and every time the metabolic profile in blood displayed the same pattern (Fig. 2): one major product only, co-chromatographing with reference $PGF_{2\alpha}$, and very small amounts of

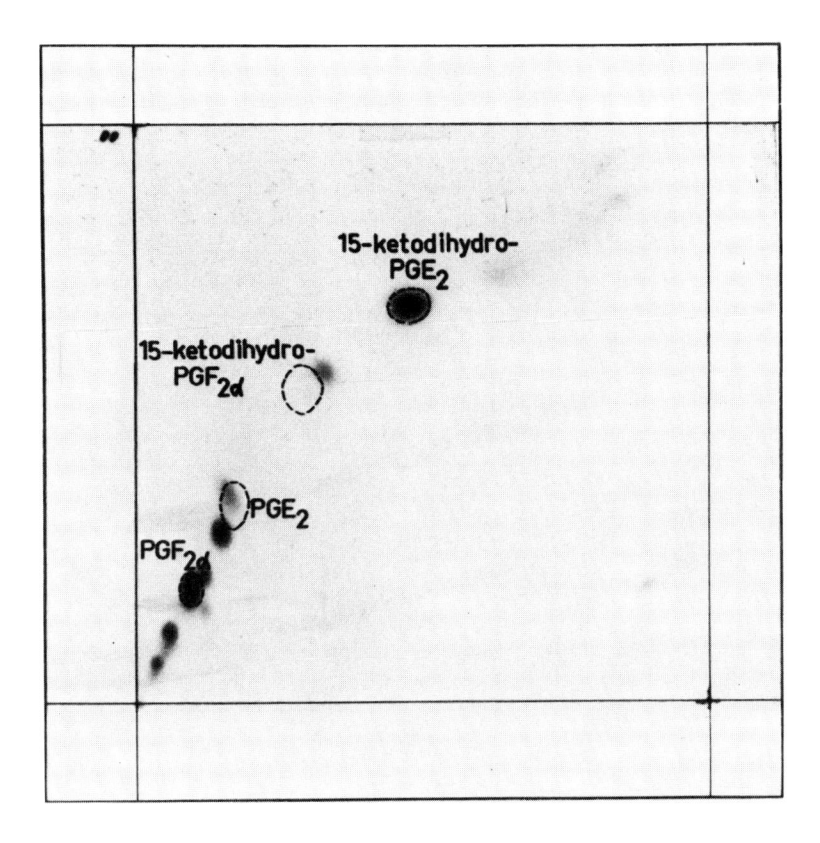

Fig. 1. Two-dimensional TLC of circulating ^{3}H-labeled metabolites of PGE$_2$ in a rabbit. The compound was given by i.v. bolus injection in the ear vein, and the above sample was taken from the opposite ear 15 min after the injection. For extraction and analysis of the sample, see (4).

the expected metabolites (cf. 5). Why PGF$_{2\alpha}$ should survive undegraded in these circumstances (Figs 1 and 2) is unclear. An alternative explanation is that it was dihydro-PGF$_{2\alpha}$, which would not separate well from PGF$_{2\alpha}$ in the employed chromatographic systems. However, dihydro-PGF$_{2\alpha}$ is usually a minor metabolite in blood, and we would then only be facing a different metabolic problem: why should this compound be formed in particularly large amounts in these conditions and not in others?

CHEMICAL PROBLEMS

Many chemical problems add difficulties to analytical experiments. For example, several of the eicosanoids are chemically un-

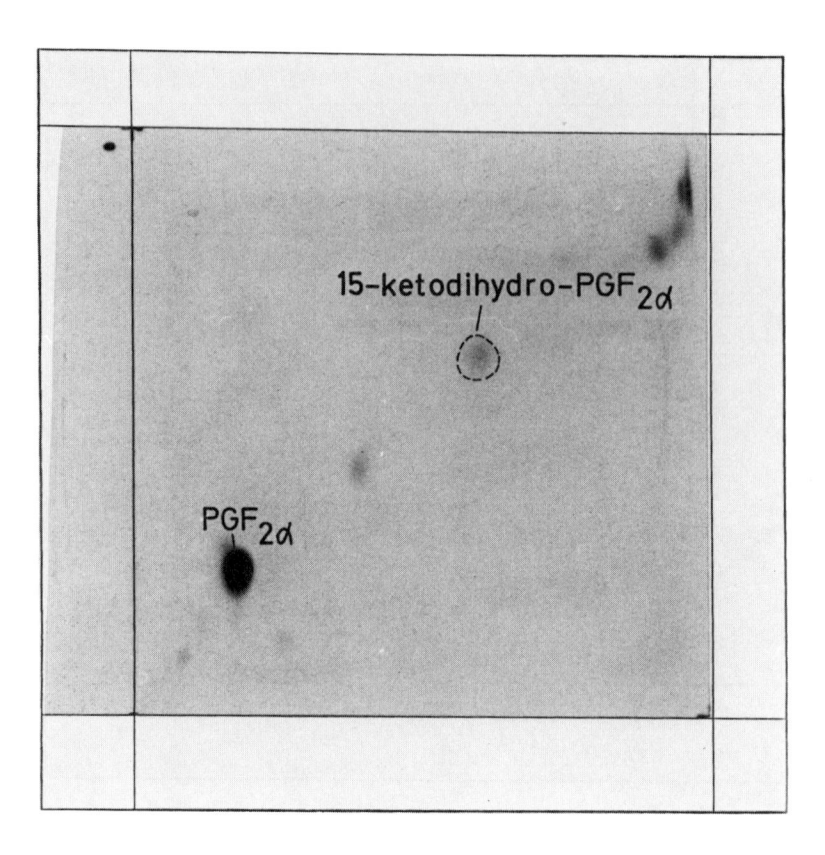

Fig. 2. Two-dimensional TLC of circulating ^{3}H-labeled metabolites of PGF$_{2\alpha}$ in a human: the compound was accidentally deposited perivascularly in one forearm, instead of given i.v. The above sample was taken 20 min after the injection from the opposite arm. For extraction and analysis, see (5).

stable and decompose more or less rapidly into a mixture of degradation products (16). Characteristically, this decomposition may proceed at different rates, varying with for example the concentration of the compound, the presence of albumin, etc. (2,16).

A number of the eicosanoids may also exist in several different forms in equilibrium - an equilibrium that may require rather long incubation times to reach, as is for example the case with some lactones and their corresponding open forms (7).

A different kind of difficulty may arise from the use of isotope labeled compounds. Some labeled atoms may be lost during metabolism or otherwise, without the scientist's being aware of it. Metabolic isotope effects may further distort the picture.

ASSAY PROBLEMS

Only a few of the numerous assay problems will be dealt with here, namely some reasons for non-specificity of GC/MS as well as immunoassays. Two specific questions will be discussed. How should one interpret, first, a **measured** high level or increase of an eicosanoid; and second, a measured **real** high level or increase of an eicosanoid?

A few years ago, we studied the roles of $PGF_{2\alpha}$ in the reproductive cycle and pregnancy in the bovine. $PGF_{2\alpha}$ is a well-known endogenous luteolytic substance in this species, and its biosynthesis is normally completely suppressed during early pregnancy (8). Our interest then turned to animals who repeatedly aborted during early pregnancy. Since $PGF_{2\alpha}$ is also a potent abortifacient, we were specifically looking for an overproduction of the compound in the animals. In the first part of the study, the non-pregnant animals' cycles were monitored.

All animals displayed what seemed to be a dramatic increase in their $PGF_{2\alpha}$ production, measured as 15-ketodihydro-$PGF_{2\alpha}$ in peripheral blood. This "increase" however occurred on the same date in all animals, regardless of the stage of their cycle. This date we changed our regular sample tubes (heparinized Vacutainer tubes) to another brand, also containing heparin.

In vitro tests soon revealed that the inhibition of the antibody binding of the labeled ligand, which had initially been interpreted as due to prostaglandin, was caused by a water-soluble factor from the new brand of tubes. Various chromatographic systems, together with glucuronic acid assay (9), indicated that this strongly interfering substance was heparin. The reason why this particular heparin disturbs the antigen-antibody reaction so strongly, whereas Vacutainer heparin does not, is not known at present. However, heparin is not one, well-defined compound, but a rather large group of related substances, which differ in molecular weight and structure of the disaccharide repeat unit as well as the degree of sulfation (9). It is also known that the numerous effects that heparin displays in the body can vary, in a rather unpredictable way, with variations in this structure (13).

The heparin obtained from 10 of the new brand of tubes was injected i.v. to two sheep, one of which had been pretreated with Flunixin, a cyclooxygenase inhibitor, in a dose large enough to completely suppress its endogenous PG biosynthesis. Blood samples were taken repeatedly before and after the injection during a total of 6 hrs, and the plasma was analyzed using our regular 15-ketodihydro-$PGF_{2\alpha}$ RIA. The results are shown in Fig. 3.

The animal treated with only heparin displayed a pronounced peak in "measured 15-ketodihydro-$PGF_{2\alpha}$". That this is not due to a real PG release, elicited by heparin, can however be seen from the similar pattern in the Flunixin treated animal. The half-life of the measured substance was estimated at 20-40 min, which suggests heparin.

It is worth noting that a biological experiment, analyzed with

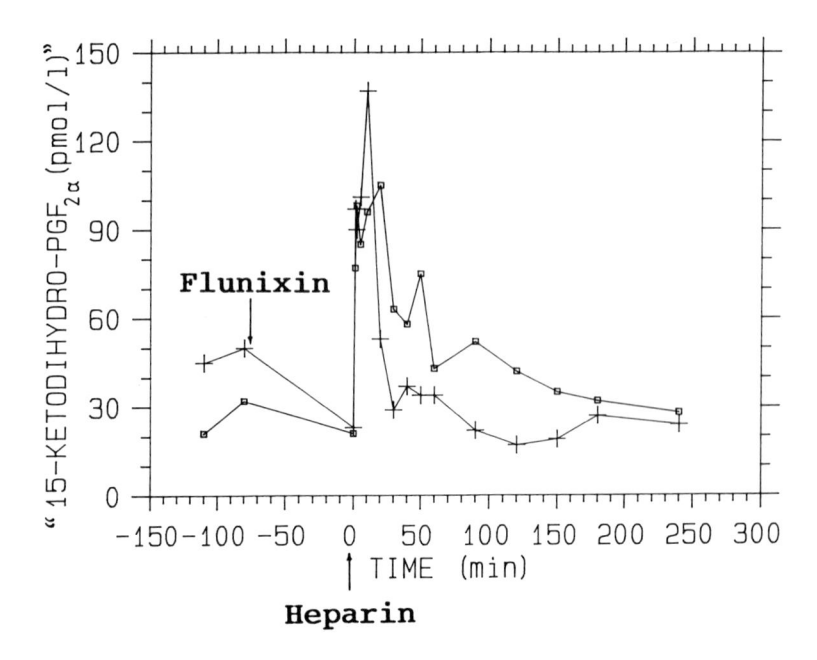

Fig. 3. Heparin extracted from a batch of commercially available plastic tubes given by i.v. injection to two sheep. Each animal received the amount obtained from 10 tubes. One animal (+---+) was pretreated with Flunixin.

a highly specific antibody, can give results like those seen in Fig. 3 and yet have nothing to do with prostaglandins. Many scientists run their experiments in heparinized biological systems and may be unaware of this risk.

How should one then interpret a measured **real** increase or high level of an eicosanoid? By real increase is meant one that is verifiable with mass spectrometry; that it is possible to suppress by the use of a specific inhibitor, and so on.

A very common type of study is to administer a drug or some other compound to a biological system to find out whether it can trigger the arachidonic acid cascade, and whether its biological effects can perhaps be explained by one or more of the formed eicosanoids.

A rather typical such substance is endotoxin: lipopolysaccharides from the cell wall of Gram-negative bacteria. It is well known that endotoxin can activate the arachidonic acid cascade, and no doubt some of the many biological effects of endotoxins can be explained by this. For example, it causes luteolysis in many species, and abortion if the animal is pregnant, and these events are known to be accompanied by large increases in inter alia $PGF_{2\alpha}$.

It is however less well known that endotoxins are ubiquitous contaminants in the environment. They can be found in food, dust, distilled water, chemicals, and even drugs and medical devices, such as surgical gloves (review, 17).

In a study where the enzyme superoxide dismutase (SOD) was given to an animal model, results regarding body temperature, peripheral blood cell profile, and prostaglandin release differed greatly when SOD from different sources was used (17). Quantitative assays for endotoxin showed that two of the employed SOD preparations were heavily contaminated, and that the results were far better explained as endotoxin effects. An endotoxin-free SOD preparation gave virtually no changes in the monitored parameters.

To return to non-specificity of assay methods, it is now becoming clear that also GC/MS methods can be quite non-specific, in contrast to what was earlier thought. One reason is that the most common type of quantitative GC/MS is the NICI type, with monitoring of only one major ion. If isomers of the monitored compound are present, they may give misleading information (cf. 1,10). Interestingly, it is likely that immunoassays in such circumstances may be more specific, since antibodies usually discriminate quite well between stereoisomers.

Because of the rapid expansion of this area, with frequent disconveries of new enantiomers and diastereomers, it is likely that much more emphasis will have to be put on the separation methods before the GC/MS step.

ACKNOWLEDGMENTS

This study was supported by grants from the Swedish Medical Research Council (proj. no. 03X-5915), the Swedish Council for Forestry and Agricultural Research and Pharmacia Leo AB.

REFERENCES

1. Barrow, S.E., Heavey, D.J., Ennis, M., Chappell, C.G., Blair, I.A., and Dollery, C.T. (1984): Prostaglandins, **28**:743-754.

2. Fitzpatrick, F.A. and Wynalda, M.A. (1983): J. Biol. Chem., **258**:11713-11718.

3. Granström, E. (1982): Methods Enzymol., **86**:493-511.

4. Granström, E. and Kindahl, H. (1982): Biochim. Biophys. Acta, **713**:555-569.

5. Granström, E., Kindahl, H., and Swahn, M.-L. (1982): Biochim. Biophys. Acta, **713**:46-60.

6. Granström, E. and Kumlin, M. (1987): In: Prostaglandins and Related Substances, A Practical Approach, edited by C. Benedetto, R.G. McDonald-Gibson, S. Nigam, and T.F. Slater. pp. 5-27. IRL Press, Oxford.

7. Granström, E., Kumlin, M., and Kindahl, H. (1987). Ibid., pp. 167-195.

8. Kindahl, H., Edqvist, L.-E., Bane, A., and Granström, E. (1976): Acta Endocrin. (Kbh), **82**:134-149.

9. Lindahl, U. and Höök, M. (1978): Annu. Rev. Biochem., **47**: 385-417.

10. Liston, T.E. and Roberts, L.J.II (1985): J. Biol. Chem., **260**: 13172-13180.

11. Morrow, J.D., Harris, T.M., and Roberts, L.J.II (1990): Anal. Biochem., **184**:1-11.

12. Morrow, J.D., Hill, K.E., Burk, R.F., Nammour, T.M., Badr, K.F., and Roberts, L.J.II (1990): 7th International Conference on Prostaglandins and Related Compounds, Florence (Italy), May 28-June 1, Abstract, p. 12.

13. Naggi, A., Torri, G., Casu, B., Pangrazzi, J., Abbadini, M., Zametta, M., Donati, M.B., Lansen, J., and Maffrand, J.P. (1987): Biochem. Pharmacol., **36**:1895-1900.

14. Roberts, L.J.II and Sweetman, B.J. (1985): Prostaglandins, **30**: 383-400.

15. Samuelsson, B., Granström, E., Gréen, K., Hamberg, M., and Hammarström, S. (1975): Annu. Rev. Biochem., **44**:669-695.

16. Stehle, R.G. (1982): Methods Enzymol., **86**:436-458.

17. Yagoda, C.R., Bylund-Fellenius, A.C., Adner, N. and Kindahl, H. (1990): Acta Vet. Scand. (in press).

DEVELOPMENT OF SCINTILLATION PROXIMITY ASSAYS FOR PROSTAGLANDINS AND RELATED COMPOUNDS

P.M.Baxendale, R.C.Martin, K.T.Hughes, D.Y.Lee and N.M.Waters

Amersham International plc, Cardiff Laboratories, Whitchurch, Cardiff, CF4 7YT. United Kingdom

During the past ten years significant advances have been made in our understanding of the actions of arachidonic acid and its metabolites, the prostaglandins, thromboxanes and leukotrienes. Many of these advances have only been made possible by the development of suitable measurement techniques.

Since prostaglandins occur in biological fluids at low concentrations, highly sensitive techniques are required for their accurate determination. Numerous methods have been used including gas chromatography/mass spectrometry (GC/MS) and bioassay, but the most applicable and widely used technique is radioimmunoassay (RIA).

RIA techniques are both sensitive and specific, however traditional methodology suffers a number of limitations: There is a need to separate the antibody bound from the unbound ligand which usually requires centrifugation and hence is difficult to automate. In addition the process may decrease assay precision and contribute to the non-specific binding. Secondly, there is a need to use a liquid scintillation cocktail for tritium detection which is both expensive and hazardous. Scintillation proximity assay (SPA) is a novel technique applicable to radioligand-binding assays which eliminates the need for a separation step and addition of liquid scintillant.

PRINCIPLE OF SCINTILLATION PROXIMITY RADIOIMMUNOASSAYS

In an aqueous environment weak ß emitters, notably ^{3}H and ^{125}I (Auger electrons) need to be close to scintillant molecules in order to produce light, otherwise the energy is dissipated and lost in the solvent (2). This concept has been used to develop homogeneous assays which overcome many of the limitations of present RIA systems.

In common with conventional radioimmunoassays, scintillation proximity assays are based on the competition between unlabelled ligand and a fixed quantity of radiolabelled ligand for a limited number of binding sites on a specific antibody. Antibody bound ligand is then reacted with the scintillation proximity assay reagent which contains a second antibody or protein A bound to fluomicrospheres. Fluomicrospheres are support bodies in the form of beads that are impregnated with a material capable of fluorescence when excited by radioactive energy. Any radiolabelled ligand that is bound to the primary antibody will be immobilized on the fluomicrosphere and the fluorescer integrated in the beads is placed in close enough proximity to allow the radiation energy emitted to activate the fluorescer and emit light energy (3,5,7). The level of light emitted, which is an indicator of the extent of antibody-radioligand binding, may be measured in a liquid scintillation counter (LSC).

Ligand molecules that are not bound to the antibody are located too far away to enable any radiation energy emitted to reach the fluomicrosphere. Consequently no separation of the bound from unbound fraction is necessary. In addition, the requirement to add liquid scintillant to tritium based assays is eliminated.

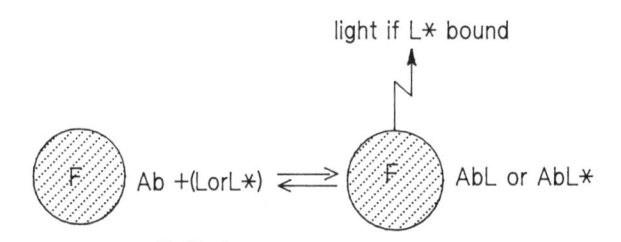

Fig. 1., Diagramatic representation of the principle of scintillation proximity assay. F, fluomicrosphere with second antibody or protein A; Ab, primary antibody; L*, radiolabelled ligand; L, unlabelled ligand.

METHODS

Scintillation proximity assays have been developed for the important arachidonic acid metabolites: thromboxane B_2 (TxB_2), 6-keto-prostaglandin $F_{1\alpha}$ (6-keto-$PGF_{1\alpha}$), prostaglandin E_2 (PGE_2), prostaglandin D_2, prostaglandin $F_{2\alpha}$, leukotriene C_4 and leukotriene B_4. The assay protocol common to all is summarized in Table 1.

TABLE 1. SPA Assay Protocol

1. Pipette standard or unknown into polypropylene mini-scintillation vial (100µl).
2. Add tracer - either ^{3}H or ^{125}I (100µl).
3. Add antiserum (100µl).
4. Add SPA reagent (100µl).
5. Cap tubes, incubate with shaking between 15-20 hours at 15-30°C.
6. Count in an LSC

Note: Samples for PGE$_2$ determination require methyl oximation according to the procedure of Kelly (6) prior to assay.

Assays were developed by simple substitution of the charcoal or second antibody separation reagent in heterogeneous assay kits (Amersham International plc, UK) for the respective second antibody or protein A coupled SPA reagent (1).

As an alternative to performing assays in mini-scintillation vials, assays can be carried out in T trays and microtitre plates applicable to the Pharmacia-Wallac Betaplate and Micro-Beta instruments.

RESULTS AND DISCUSSION

Sensitivity

Sensitivities, determined at the 95% confidence level for SPA assays (TxB$_2$, 1.0pg; 6-keto-PGF$_{1\alpha}$, 3.0pg; PGE2, 1.0pg) were similar to heterogeneous assays (1.0;pg; 6.0pg; 0.8pg respectively). In addition curve shapes were superimposable over the major part of the range.

Precision

It is well accepted that the separation procedure has a considerable effect on RIA assay precision (4). Improved precision of SPA assays support this observation. Fig. 2A. compares precision profiles for SPA and a heterogeneous TxB$_2$ assay using charcoal separation. Data were obtained after counting all assay tubes from 10 curves to accumulate 10,000 cpm (1% counting error). The profile differences therefore result solely from errors associated with the technical operation of the assays.

The counting efficiency of the solid SPA scintillant in some old LSCs is 36% lower than using a liquid cocktail, for example Optiphase MP, available from Pharmacia. Consequently the counting error of SPA assays will be higher when counting for the same time. Nevertheless, the overall precision of the TxB$_2$ assay (Fig.2B) is still superior over the important range of the curve after 2 minute counting.

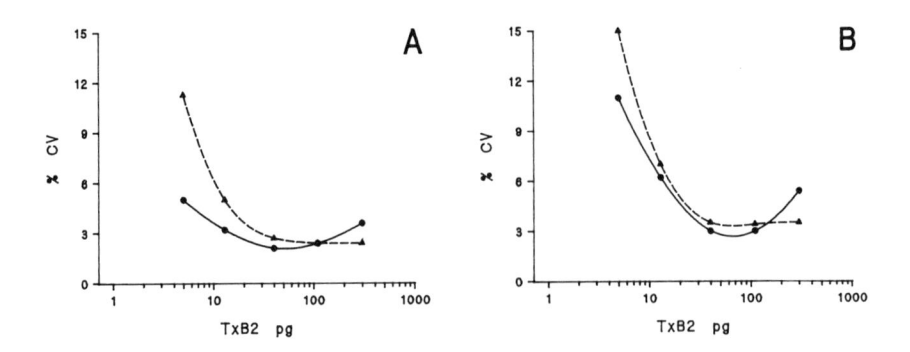

FIG. 2., Comparison of TxB$_2$ precision profiles of SPA (circles) and heterogeneous (triangles) assays.
A - count until 10,000cpm. B - count for 2 minutes.

Convenience

Scintillation proximity assay technology greatly simplifies the ease of performing RIAs. Only 4 pipetting steps are required, thus reducing 'hands on' and total assay time. The assay is carried out in one tube and the addition of liquid scintillant is not required. Assays are readily amenable to automation, a feature that has been difficult to achieve in traditional assays. The technique is also compatible with the new generation multi-head LSCs, thereby providing a simple means of increasing assay throughput.

REFERENCES

1. Baxendale, P.M. Marenghi, A.S., and Jessop, R.A. (1989): Proc.Int.Physiol.Sci., XVII: 390.
2. Bertoglio-Matte, J.H. (1986): US Patent Number 4568649.
3. Bosworth, N. and Towers, P. (1989): Nature, 341:167-168.
4. Chard, T. (1982): An Introduction to Radioimmunoassay and Related Techniques, Elsevier, Amsterdam/New York.
5. Hart, H.E. and Greenwald, E.B. (1979): Mol.Immunol., 16: 265-267.
6. Kelly, R.,W., Graham, B.J.M. and O'Sullivan, M.J. (1989): Prostag.Leuk. and Essential Fatty Acids, 37: 187-191.
7. Udenfriend, S., Gerber, L.D., Brink, L. and Spector, S. (1985): Proc.Natl.Acad.Sci., U.S.A., 82: 8672-8676.

IMMUNOQUANTITATION OF THROMBOXANE SYNTHASE IN HUMAN TISSUES

R. Nüsing and V. Ullrich

Faculty of Biology, University of Konstanz,
P.O.Box 5560, D-7750 Konstanz, FRG

Thromboxane (Tx) A_2 is an unstable cyclooxygenase product of arachidonic acid with potent proaggregatory effects on platelets and strong vasoconstriction properties (1). TxA_2 is not only responsible for clot formation but is also released in certain types of shock and may contribute to the altered circulatory pattern under these conditions (6). Tx-synthase, the microsomal enzyme responsible for Tx biosynthesis, was purified by us from human platelets and its proteinchemical (4) and catalytic (5) properties have been well investigated.
We have recently raised and characterized polyclonal and monoclonal antibodies directed to purified human platelet Tx-synthase (8). We now describe a sensitive and convenient enzyme-linked immunoassay of the sandwich-type to determine the Tx-synthase content in different human cells and tissues.

Methods

Thromboxane synthase was purified from human platelets as described by us recently (4). Tx-synthase activity was measured by the addition of PGH_2 to the microsomal fraction. Biosynthesized TxB_2 was assayed by radioimmunoassay.
Microsomes of isolated or cultured cells and of human tissues were prepared as described in (9). For immunoenzymometry 1400 µg of microsomal protein were solubilized by addition of 1/10 V of 10% Triton X-100 solution. After standing for 30 min on ice, the mixture was centrifuged at 160000 g for 15 min and the supernatant solution was used as the solubilized enzyme. Polyclonal antibodies raised in rabbits against purified Tx-synthase were precipitated by a 40% saturated ammoniumsulphate solution and further purified by DEAE chromatography. The purified antibodies were diluted in 50 mM $NaHCO_3$ pH 8.3 and coated in microtiter plates for 1 h at room temperature. The ELISA was further performed as described in (8).

Results

The use of an ELISA to quantitate a particular antigen requires the binding of the antigen to be independent of the protein concentration. We used polyclonal antibodies to avoid the problem of competition for binding to microtiter wells by other proteins of solubilized microsomes. The antiserum directed to purified Tx-synthase was generated in rabbits and partially purified by ammoniumsulphate precipitation and DEAE-chromatography. The polyclonal antibodies reacted selectively and were used for trapping of Tx-synthase out of crude enzyme preparations.

Our immunoenzymometric assay of Tx-synthase was applied to various human cells and tissues. Since the enzyme is known to be a membrane-bound enzyme, a microsomal fraction was prepared from each cell suspension or tissue and the enzyme was solubilized with the non-ionic detergent Triton X-100 and the insoluble fraction separated by high-speed centrifugation. Quantitation of Tx-synthase by the sandwich-ELISA was performed by diluting microsomal protein in a suitable concentration range for each assay and employing 4 assay points in duplicate per sample. From parallelism between the absorbance curves of diluting series of samples and standard we assume that Tx-synthase from all cells and tissues tested had the same antigenicity as that of the platelet enzyme as a standard.

Table 1 Thromboxane synthase content in different human cells

	Enzyme Content ng/mg	Specific Activity nmol TxB$_2$/min/mg	Molecular Activity[a] 1/min
Platelets	2187	23.7	628
Monocytes	1548	10.1	380
Granulocytes	n.d.	< 0.05	/
Fibroblasts	64	0.49	439
HL-60 Cells	87	0.59	395
U-937 Cells	277	2.12	441

[a] Molecular activity is expressed in term of mol TXB$_2$ × min^{-1} × mol enzyme^{-1}

The quantity of Tx-synthase in different human cells is indicated in Table 1. It demonstrates large differences in the distribution of this enzyme. As assumed, the highest content of 2187 ng Tx-synthase/mg microsomal protein was found in platelets but also a similar high concentration was found in human blood monocytes, which were prepared essentially free of platelets. Human lung fibroblasts of the IMRI-90 line and promyelocytic cells such as HL-60 and U-937 apparently have a low content in Tx-synthase of 64, 87 and 277 ng enzyme/mg protein, respectively. Interestingly, no enzyme could be detected in purified human granulocytes which is at variance with other reports (2). Table 2 indicates that Tx-synthase is present in all tissues tested but to significantly different extents. High amounts were found in lung and liver, whereas the enzyme was low in spleen, kidney, brain, lymph nodes and gall bladder.

Table 2 Thromboxane synthase content in different human tissues.

Tissue	Enzyme Content ng/mg	Specific Activity nmol TxB$_2$/min/mg	Molecular Activity[a] 1/min
Liver	324	3.73	667
Bile duct	15	0.38	1500
Heart	25	0.30	698
Adrenal	103	1.07	606
Lung	765	5.46	416
Kidney	80	0.68	488
Colon	242	1.56	378
Gall bladder	31	0.47	893
Brain	50	0.64	740
Spleen	64	0.69	623
Lymph node	51	0.72	827

[a] Molecular activity expressed in term of mol TXB$_2$ x min^{-1} x mol enzyme^{-1}

Given the specific content of Tx-synthase in a tissue and the molecular mass of 58 800 (4), one can calculate the molecular activity by measuring the specific activity in the preparation (Tab.1,2).

Discussion

In earlier immunohistochemical studies employing the same antibodies we could qualitatively demonstrate the presence of the enzyme in cells of the mononuclear phagocytotic system (7). Our present results corroborate these data and allow to

conclude on the maximum capacity of a tissue to produce TxA₂. The unresolved question whether granulocytes possess the ability to produce TxA₂ must now be answered in terms of lack of their biosynthetic capacity. In contrast, monocytes contained almost as much enzyme as platelets which supports the significance of these cells in mediating TxA₂-effects in tissues. Histiocytes and macrophages are present in all tissues and therefore explain the positive ELISA response in all tissues and organs. The levels, however, vary greatly. The inconsistencies in the molecular activities between different tissues unlikely reflect errors in the ELISA or in the activity measurements but are rather due to a varying degree of enzyme inactivation. The tissues were obtained from three to four donors 4-8 h post mortem and the microsomal fractions pooled because of their small quantities. Whereas the immunological properties remain, a partial inactivation of Tx-synthase activity during preparation can not be excluded.
The availability of the presented ELISA for determination of Tx-synthase will provide a valuable tool for probing the function of the enzyme in various physiological and pathophysiological states.

References

1. Ellis, E.F., Oek, O., Roberts, L.J., Payne, N.A., Sweetman, B.J., Nies, A.S., Oates, J.A. (1976): *Science*, 193:1135-1137.
2. Goldstein, J.M., Mahnsten, C.L., Kindahl, H., Kaplan, H.B., Radmark, O., Samuelsson, B., Weissmann, G. (1978): *J. Exp. Med.*, 148:787-792.
3. Hammarström, S., Falardeau, P. (1977): *Proc. Natl. Acad. Sci.*, 74:3691-3695.
4. Haurand, M., Ullrich, V. (1985): *J. Biol. Chem.*, 260:15059-15067.
5. Hecker, M., Ullrich, V. (1989): *J. Biol. Chem.*, 264:141-150.
6. Lefer, A.M. (1989): *Adv. Prostagland. Thromboxane Leukotriene Res.*, 19:321-326.
7. Nüsing, R., Lesch, P., Ullrich, V. (1990): *Eicosanoids*, 3:53-58.
8. Nüsing, R., Wernet, M.P., Ullrich, V. (1989): *Blood*, accepted.
9. Ullrich, V., Haurand, M. (1983): *Adv. Prostagland. Thromboxane Leukotriene Res.*, 11:105-110.

REVERSE PHASE HPLC PROFILING OF ARACHIDONIC ACID METABOLITES IN BLOOD STIMULATED EX VIVO

A. Odeimat, P.E. Poubelle and P. Borgeat

Unité de Recherche *Inflammation et Immunologie-Rhumatologie*
Centre de Recherche du CHUL
2705, boul. Laurier, Québec, Canada, G1V 4G2

INTRODUCTION

Stimulation of whole blood with the ionophore A23187 or zymosan leads to formation of lipoxygenase products (3-7). The measurement of arachidonic acid metabolites generated in blood ex vivo makes the assessment of the in vivo effects of drugs on arachidonic acid metabolism in various blood cells possible. We describe here a simple procedure which enables the simultaneous assay of several products of the arachidonic acid cascade in blood; we also point out experimental conditions that have a major impact on the formation of eicosanoids in blood ex vivo.

MATERIALS AND METHODS

Ionophore A23187, zymosan and prostaglandin (PG) B_1 were purchased from Sigma (St. Louis, MO). Leukotrienes (LTs) were given by Dr. R. Young (Merck Frosst, Montreal). A 23187 was used in solution in dimethylsulfoxide; zymosan was washed in phosphate buffered saline and sonicated before use. Nineteen-hydroxy-PGB_1 (19-OH-PGB_1) was prepared as described for 19-OH-PGB_2 (1).

Venous blood was obtained from healthy donors who had been fasting for 15 hr, and collected in heparinized tubes. One ml blood aliquots were dispensed in plastic tubes and incubated at 37°C in the presence of A23187 or zymosan. Incubations were terminated by cooling the blood samples in a ice-water bath. The samples were centrifuged (400 x g, 15 min, 4°C) and the plasma collected. One hundred µl plasma samples were denatured with 400 µl of methanol/acetonitrile (1/1, V/V) containing 10 ng each of PGB_1 and 19-OH-PGB_1, as internal standards. After standing 2 hr or more at -20°C, the denatured samples were centrifuged (400 x g, 15 min, 4°C) and the supernatants were analyzed by RP-HPLC as described previously (2) using on-line extraction procedures and UV detection at 229 and 280 nm.

RESULTS AND DISCUSSION

Stimulation of blood with zymosan led to selective induction of 5-lipoxygenase product synthesis and formation of LTB_4 and 5-OH-eicosatetraenoic acid (5-HETE) as major products (data not shown). A23187 was a more potent activator of the synthesis of the 5-lipoxygenase products, and in addition to LTB_4 and 5-HETE, 20-OH-LTB_4, 20-COOH-LTB_4 and LTE_4 were formed in detectable amounts (Fig. 1). A23187 stimulation also led to the formation of the 12-lipoxygenase and cyclooxygenase products, 12-HETE and 12-OH-heptadecatrienoic acid (HHTrE), respectively, presumably from platelets. The stimulatory effect of A23187 and zymosan were maximal at 30 μM and 2 mg/ml respectively. Time course studies indicated that the products analyzed reached near maximal concentrations in blood in about 30 min.

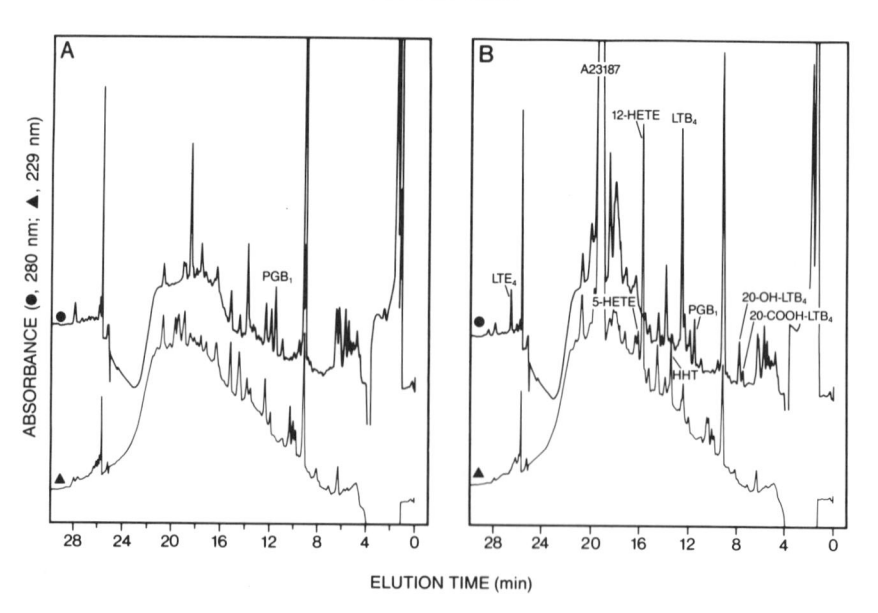

FIG. 1. HPLC chromatograms of 100 μl plasma samples (denatured) from unstimulated (A) and A23187-stimulated blood. Blood samples were incubated 30 min at 37°C with or without 30 μM A23187. Attenuation settings were 0.01 and 0.04 absorbance units (full scale) at 280 and 229 nm respectively.

The use of EDTA or citrate as anticoagulants prevented the synthesis of 5-lipoxygenase products, but not of 12-HETE and HHTrE. Interestingly, preincubation of the blood at either 4°, 20° or 37°C led to a rapid and marked decrease of the stimulatory effect of A23187 on 5-lipoxygenase product synthesis, with a 75% reduction of LTB$_4$ and 5-HETE formation after a 90 min preincubation period. Preincubation (up to 90 min) had no significant effect on the stimulatory action of zymosan (data not shown).

The role of platelets in the generation of LTs in blood ex vivo was also investigated. Blood samples were centrifuged (150 x g, 15 min, 20°C), the platelet-rich plasma (PRP) was collected taking care of not removing the white cell layer (buffy coat), the platelets were removed from the PRP by centrifugation (600 x g, 15 min, 20°C) and the plasma was added back to the red cell pellet; this procedure was performed 3 times and allowed reduction of the platelet count

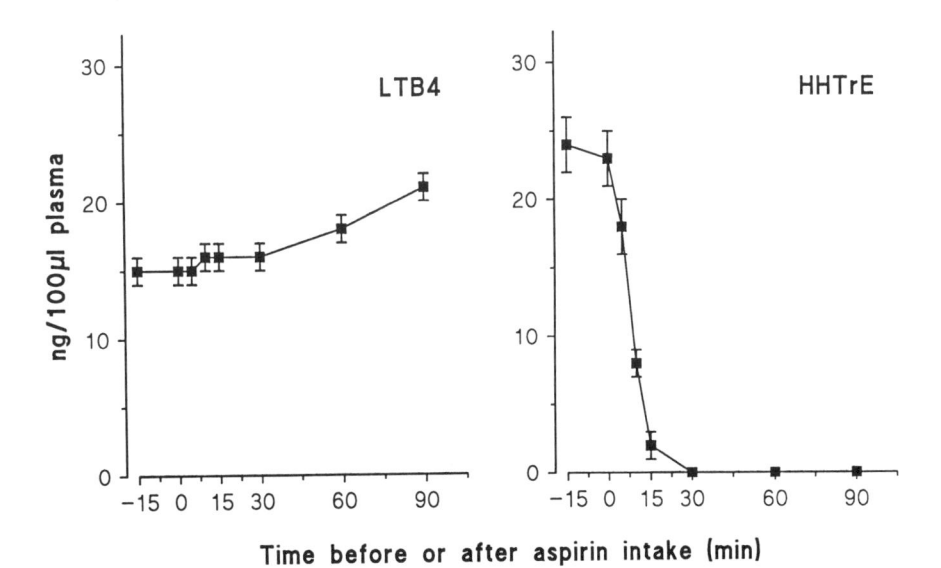

FIG. 2. Effect of acetyl salicylic acid (ASA, aspirin) intake on LTB$_4$ and HHTrE synthesis in A23187-treated blood. Three healthy volunteers received a single oral dose of 600 mg ASA. Blood samples were obtained 15 min before and at various times after ASA intake, up to 90 min. Blood samples were stimulated with 30 µM A23187 for 30 min immediately after blood collection, and plasma samples were analyzed by RP-HPLC. The data show rapid and complete inhibition of the synthesis of the cyclooxygenase product HHTrE while the synthesis of the 5-lipoxygenase product LTB$_4$ was not inhibited (the elevation of LTB$_4$ synthesis was not significant); 12-HETE and other 5-lipoxygenase products were not inhibited (data not shown). The results are the mean ± S.E.M. of the values obtained for the 3 subjects. Incubations were performed in triplicate at all time points.

by more than 80%. As expected, synthesis of the platelet products 12-HETE and HHTrE was not detectable upon stimulation of the platelet-depleted blood samples with A23187; interestingly LTB$_4$ and 5-HETE synthesis were decreased by more than 70% indicating that platelets contributed to synthesis of 5-lipoxygenase products by neutrophils (and monocytes) in A23187-stimulated blood, possibly by providing arachidonic acid. Accordingly, LTB$_4$ and 5-HETE synthesis were not altered in platelet-depleted blood stimulated with zymosan, a phagocyte-specific stimulus (data not shown).

In summary, RP-HPLC can be used for the profiling of various eicosanoids in plasma (obtained from blood stimulated ex vivo) following a simple deproteinization procedure. Measurement of compounds derived from the 5- and 12-lipoxygenases as well as of HHTrE from the cyclooxygenase, enables the assessment of the in vivo effects of drugs on the different pathways of the arachidonic acid cascade in blood cells (ex vivo) (Fig. 2). Our study also pointed out that the time elapsed between blood collection and stimulation dramatically alters A23187-induced LT synthesis in whole blood. Finally, our study supports the concept that transcellular metabolism occurs in whole blood stimulated ex vivo (4), and indicates a crucial role for platelets in A23187-activated blood; these data also question the validity of expressing LT synthesis on the basis of neutrophil counts.

REFERENCES

1. Borgeat, P. and Picard S. (1988): Anal. Biochem., 171: 283-289.
2. Borgeat, P., Picard, S., Vallerand, P., Bourgoin, S., Odeimat, A., Sirois, P., and Poubelle, P.E. In: *Methods in Enzymology*, edited by R.C. Murphy, and F. Fitzpatrick, Academic Press, Boca Raton, FL. In press.
3. Carey, F., and Forder, R.A. (1986): Prostaglandins Leukotrienes Med., 22: 57-70.
4. Fradin, A., Zirrolli, J.A., Maclouf, J., Vausbinder, L., Henson, P.M., and Murphy, R.C. (1989): J. Immunol., 143: 3680-3685.
5. Gresele, P., Arnout, J., Coene, M.C., Deckmyn, H., and Vermuylen, J. (1986): Biochem. Biophys. Res. Commun., 137: 334-342.
6. Kikawa, Y., Nakai, A., Shigematsu, Y., and Sudo, M. (1989): J. Chromatogr., 491: 193-199.
7. Sweeney, F.J., Eskra, J.D., and Carty, T.J. (1987): Prostaglandins Leukotrienes Med., 28: 73-93.

A STABLE ISOTOPE DILUTION MASS SPECTROMETRIC ASSAY FOR THE MAJOR URINARY METABOLITE OF PGD$_2$

Jason D. Morrow, Chandra Prakash, Tanya A. Duckworth, William E. Zackert, Ian A. Blair, John A. Oates, L.J. Roberts II

Division of Clinical Pharmacology,
Departments of Pharmacology and Medicine,
Vanderbilt University,
Nashville, TN 37232-6602

Prostaglandin D$_2$ is the principal cyclooxygenase product produced by mast cells (7). Overproduction of PGD$_2$ occurs in patients with systemic mastocytosis and PGD$_2$ has been shown to be the principal mediator of episodes of flushing and vasodilatory hypotension experienced by these patients (8). Therefore, a means for assessing endogenous production of PGD$_2$ in humans to explore its role in disorders of mastocyte activation and other human diseases is of considerable clinical importance. Toward the eventual goal of developing a mass spectrometric assay for a urinary metabolite of PGD$_2$ for this purpose, we previously carried out studies examining the metabolic fate of PGD$_2$ in humans.

These studies revealed that PGD$_2$ is initially transformed by 11-ketoreductase stereospecifically to 9α,11β-PGF$_2$. 9α,11β-PGF$_2$ then undergoes further metabolic degradation to yield the 15-keto, dihydro, tetranor dicarboxylic acid metabolite which we identified as the major urinary metabolite of PGD$_2$ in humans and termed PGD-M (Figure 1, Compound I) (2).

PGD-M is an interesting compound in that it was isolated from urine and identified in a tricyclic form. In the presence of acid, the compound initially forms a hemiketal ring (Figure 1, Compound II) followed by additional cyclization to form a γ-lactone (Figure 1, Compound III). The assay method that was developed for quantification of this metabolite takes advantage of the ability of this compound to cyclize and uncyclize allowing for the formation of a novel ester derivative and a powerful purification-extraction step. Procedures involved in performing the assay as well as potential uses of the assay in assessing the role of PGD$_2$ in human disease are summarized.

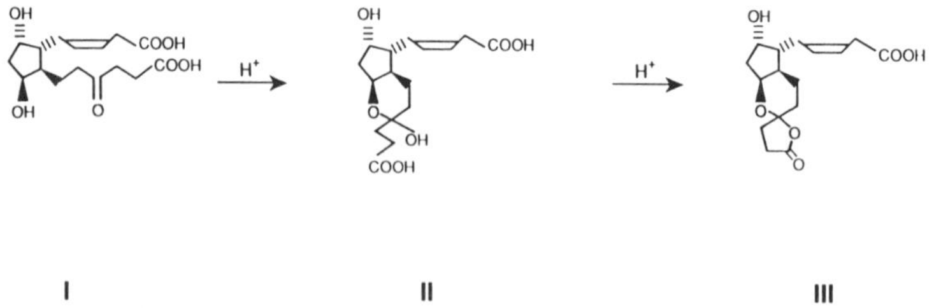

FIG. 1: Cyclized and uncyclized forms of the major urinary metabolite of PGD$_2$

METHODS TO ASSAY PGD-M

Preparation of the Standard

Quantification of PGD-M is accomplished using combined gas chromatography (GC) negative ion chemical ionization (NICI)/mass spectrometry (MS) employing stable isotope dilution techniques. To provide sufficient material for the internal standard used in the assay, we chemically synthesized PGD-M as previously reported (6). Subsequently, the metabolite was converted to an [$^{18}O_4$]-labelled derivative for use as an internal standard. This was accomplished by the method of Murphy et al. involving successive steps of methylation and alkaline hydrolysis in the presence of ^{18}O-water (4). After this was carried out, the unlabelled blank of the internal standard was found to be only 1 part of 10,000 and remained unaltered when the standard was subjected to the assay procedure subsequently developed.

Sample Purification and Analysis

To 1 ml of urine is added several nanograms of the [$^{18}O_4$]-labelled internal standard. The urine is then acidified to pH 3 and allowed to stand at room temperature for 30 min. This quantitatively results in cyclization of the molecule to compound III (in Figure 1), which is the tricyclic hemiketal γ-lactone. Following cyclization of the metabolite, it is solid phase extracted using a C-18 Sep-pak (Waters Associates, Milford, MA) and subsequently eluted through a silica Sep-pak. The upper side chain carboxyl is then converted to a methyl ester with diazomethane. However, the lower side chain carboxyl is not methylated by this treatment because of the lactone ring. Following this, treatment with methoxyamine·HCl results in ring opening and the formation of a methoxime derivative of the C-15 keto group. At this point, the upper side chain carboxyl is esterified whereas the lower side chain contains a free carboxyl group. However, other potentially interfering carboxylic acids present, that are incapable of undergoing cyclization, have been methylated by the previous treatment with diazomethane. Therefore, considerable purification can be accomplished by extracting the urine at pH 7 with ethyl acetate to remove these compounds. Because of the free carboxyl group on the lower side chain of the metabolite, it will not extract into the ethyl acetate at neutral pH and remains in the aqueous phase. The aqueous phase is then acidified to pH 3 and the metabolite extracted into ethyl acetate. After the ethyl acetate is evaporated, the lower carboxyl is converted to a pentafluorobenzyl ester and subjected to further purification by TLC. After the metabolite is eluted from the TLC plate, it is converted to a trimethylsilyl ether derivative and analyzed by GC NICI/MS.

GC is carried out using a 15 meter DB1701 fused silica capillary column (J & W Scientific, Folsom CA). The major ion generated by endogenous PGD-M is m/z 514 which represents the carboxylate anion of the compound formed as a result of loss of the pentafluorobenzyl moiety. The corresponding ion generated by the [$^{18}O_4$]-internal standard is m/z 522. Quantification of endogenous PGD-M in a sample is determined by comparing the ratio of m/z 514 to m/z 522.

We have found this assay to be highly sensitive and specific. Lower limits of sensitivity of the assay are in the range of 50 pg. The assay was found to be highly accurate in that it was determined to have a precision of ± 7% and an accuracy of 96%. Normal levels in 9 healthy males and 9 healthy females were found to be 1.08 ± 0.72 ng/mg creatinine (mean ± 2 S.D.). No differences in the levels were found between males and females.

APPLICABILITY OF THE ASSAY TO HUMAN DISEASES

The usefulness of the assay to assess the role of PGD_2 in human disease was explored in several situations in which the release of increased quantities of PGD_2 has been shown to occur. First, patients with systemic mastocytosis overproduce histamine in addition to PGD_2 (8). We have found a good correlation (r = .78) between increased urinary excretion of the histamine metabolite N^τ-methylhistamine and PGD-M in patients with mastocytosis. Increased excretion of N^τ-methylhistamine has been shown to be a very reliable indicator of systemic involvement in patients with mastocytosis. The finding of a good correlation between the levels of the urinary excretion of PGD-M and N^τ-methylhistamine suggests that measuring PGD-M can also be a clinically useful predictor of systemic involvement in patients with proliferative mast cell disease.

Second, treatment of hypercholesterolemia with the hypolipidemic agent niacin is very poorly tolerated because it causes intense flushing (1).

Recently we reported the discovery that oral ingestion of niacin evokes the release of markedly increased quantities of PGD$_2$ assessed by quantification of its metabolite 9α,11ß-PGF$_2$ in plasma (3). Ingestion of niacin in normal volunteers was found to be accompanied by 25-48-fold increases in the excretion of the PGD$_2$ urinary metabolite.

Finally, we had previously demonstrated that antigen challenge in patients with allergic asthma results in increased quantities of PGD$_2$ in bronchoalveolar lavage fluid (5). Antigen challenge in these patients has also been found to be accompanied by striking increases up to 8-fold above normal in the urinary excretion of PGD-M.

SUMMARY

1. A sensitive and specific negative ion chemical ionization mass spectrometric assay for the major urinary metabolite of PGD$_2$ has been developed employing a chemically synthesized [$^{18}0_4$]-labelled internal standard.
2. The finding that increased urinary excretion of this metabolite occurs in a number of clinical situations suggests that the assay may prove to be a valuable tool to explore the role of PGD$_2$ in the pathophysiology of human disease.

ACKNOWLEDGEMENTS

This work was supported by NIH Grant GM 15431.

REFERENCES

1. Hotz, W. (1983): Adv. Lipid. Res., 20:195-217.
2. Liston, T.E., and Roberts, L.J. (1985): J. Biol. Chem., 260:13172-13180.
3. Morrow, J.D., Parsons, W.G., and Roberts, L.J. (1989): Prostaglandins, 38:263-274.
4. Murphy, R.C., Clay, K.L. (1982): Meth. Enzymol., 86:547-551.
5. Murray, J.J., Tonnel, A.B., Brash, A.R., Roberts, L.J., Gosset, P., Workman, R., Capron, A., Oates, J.A. (1986): N. Engl. J. Med., 315:800-804.
6. Prakash, C., Saleh, S., Roberts, L.J., Blair, I.A. (1988): J. Chem. Soc. Perkin Trans I., 2821-2826.
7. Roberts, L.J., Lewis, R.A., Oates, J.A., Austen, K.F. (1979): Biochem. Biophys. Acta., 575:189-192.
8. Roberts, L.J., Sweetman, B.J., Lewis, R.A., Austen, K.F., Oates, J.A. (1980): N. Engl. J. Med., 303:1400-1404.

MEASUREMENT OF LEUKOTRIENES BY ENZYME IMMUNOASSAYS USING ACETYLCHOLINESTERASE AS LABEL

Catherine Antoine [1,2], Jacques Maclouf [2] and Philippe Pradelles [1]

1 Section de Pharmacologie et d'Immunologie, Département de Biologie, Commissariat à l'Energie Atomique, CEN/Saclay, 91191 Gif/Yvette Cédex, France and 2 U 150 INSERM, Hôpital Lariboisière, 6 rue Guy Patin, 75475 Paris, France.

Leukotrienes (LTs) represent a class of biologically active lipids that derive from the oxidative metabolism of arachidonic acid (1). Clarification of their function in allergic, inflammatory disorders or cardiovascular diseases require accurate and reliable quantitative methods. Radioimmunoassays have turned out to be the most convenient method to measure all LTs (2). However, the obtention of antisera against the various LTs with sensitivities adapted to biological problems has remained difficult because of the limitations in availability of synthetic material necessary to generate antibodies In addition, the current radioactive tracers are limited to specific activities of approximately 3.7-8.8 TBq/mmol for tritium allowing current sensitivities (IC 50) of 0.3 pmol (3) and lack of corresponding ^{125}I-LT tracers prevents the improvement of some applications. Further, increasing costs of disposal of radioactivity has become a serious problem for the extensive use of radiolabeled ligands such as in RIAs techniques.

We have previously used successfully acetylcholinesterase from Electrophorus electricus as a label for most eicosanoids providing enzyme immunoassays with sensitivities equal to or superior to those achieved with ^{125}I radioactive tracers (4,5). We have undertaken similar approach for LTs B_4, C_4 and E_4. However, because of the specific problems raised by these molecules, we have combined a dual strategy to prepare the protein-LT conjugates necessary for the generation of antibodies and corresponding enzyme tracers. In this work, we will describe the procedures followed for the development of such assays and their application.

METHODS:

In brief, we have added an amino group to LTB_4 using ethylene diamine so that we could use a similar approach for all LTs (3). We have then coupled the LTs to bovine serum albumin using glutaraldehyde and the immunizations were performed as described earlier (6). Succinimidyl 4-(N-maleimidomethyl) cyclohexane-1-carboxylate was selected to attach the LTs to the acetylcholinesterase and the tracers were purified similarly to other eicosanoids conjugates (4). The procedure used for all enzyme immunoassays was similar to that described previously (4,5). Briefly, standards or samples (50 µl) were added to each well of a 96-well microtiter plate (Nunc 96F with certificate) which was previously coated with mouse monoclonal anti-rabbit IgG antibody. Tracers and specific antisera were then added (50 µl each) at appropriate dilutions. After incubation at 4 or 22 °C, 18-48 hours, the plates were washed using an automatic washer (Flow equipment). Each well was then filled with 200 µl of the Ellman's reagent as the enzymatic substrate and chromogen (acetylthiocholine and 5-5'-dithiobis (2-nitrobenzoic acid)). After shaking 1 hour in the dark at room temperature, the absorbance of a yellow colored product in each well was measured at 414 nm using a spectrophotometer (Flow laboratories). Results were expressed in terms of B/Bo x 100 where B and Bo represent the absorbance of LT label measured on the bound fraction in the presence or in the absence of LTs competitors, respectively. Fitting of the standard curves and calculations were done with a microcomputer (Apple IIe) using a linear log-logit transformation (7).

RESULTS AND DISCUSSION:

TABLE I: Binding parameters of some anti-LTs antisera [a]

Antiserum	Dilution (final)	Sensitivity (IC_{50}) (pg)
LTC_4	1/120,000	5
LTE_4	1/90,000	6.5
LTB_4	1/150,000	3

[a] Incubation was performed overnight at 22 °C.

Table I presents the sensitivity and titer of the various antisera obtained following the above mentioned protocols. As can be seen, the titers are high for all systems and the sensitivity allowed a detection in the low picogram range. It should be noted that sensitivities depended on the temperature of incubation and for all systems, incubation at 4 °C resulted in a gain of factor 5-10 as compared to room temperature, depending on the system. However, lowering of the temperature also resulted in an increased cross reactivity of the different antisera vis à vis the heterologous systems. The technique, was validated by performing analysis of neutrophil supernatant after their stimulation in plasma, Sep-Pak extraction and HPLC purification. As can be seen in figure 1, stimulated neutrophils generated LTB_4 and a small amount of LTC_4; however, the amount of either compound was greater than that measured in plasma alone. It is noteworthy that in spite of a solid phase extraction and HPLC, analysis of the plasma samples alone exhibited a significant degree of immunoreactivity as already observed in a similar study (3). Great care should be taken to interpret correctly such data and a threshold of specificity should be established i.e. significant increase above backround such as that shown in the presence of activated neutrophils.

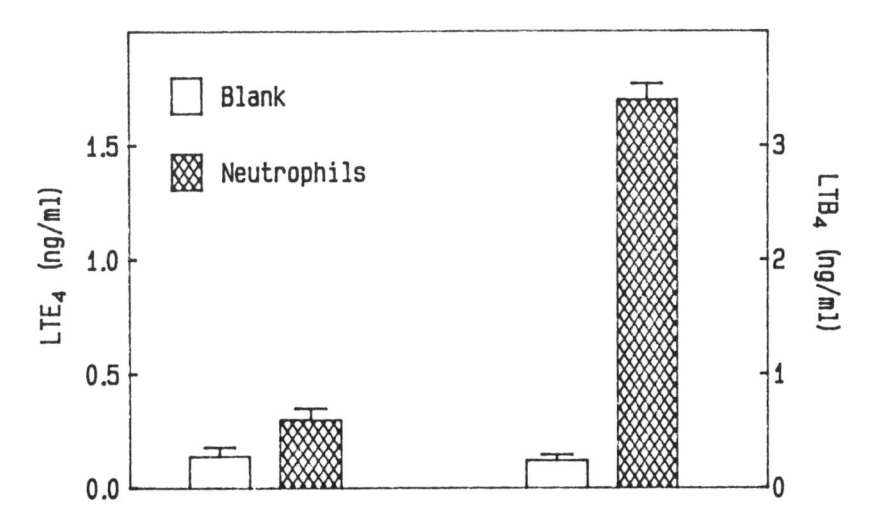

Figure 1: Analysis of neutrophils incubates suspended in plasma after 10 min. stimulation by 20 µM ionophore A23187 (5 x 10^6 neutrophils/ml).

In conclusion, we have succeeded to develop a common approach for the preparation of the different LTs-albumin conjugates necessary for the obtention of specific antibodies as well for that of the corresponding enzymatic tracers. From previous experience, the success of these assays is the result of several parameters. The use of selected coupling reagents allowed us to obtain an optimization in the attachment of the LTs to the immunogen with a minimization of the undesirable recognition of the coupling moiety on the enzymatic label by the antibodies. Thus, enzyme immunoassays using acetyl cholinesterase as a label have now been successfully applied to all eicosanoids with the same simplicity of use (i.e. competitive assay, semi-automation) and advantages inherent to the enzyme (elevated turnover rate resulting in a high sensitivity, stability of the enzyme conjugates).

REFERENCES:

1. Samuelsson, B., Dahlen, S. E., Lindgren, J. A., Rouzer, C. A., Serhan, C. N. (1984): Science. 237:1171-1176.

2. Zweering, H. R., Limjuco, G. A., Hayes, E. C. (1987): In Radioimmunoassay in Basic and Clinical Pharmacology. Edited by Patrono, C. and Peskar, B. A. pp 481-501. Springer-Verlag, Berlin-Heidelberg.

3. Rockach, J., Hayes, E. C., Girard, Y., Lombardo, D. L., Maycok, A. L., Rosenthal, A.L., Young, R.N., Zamboni, R., Zweering, H. J. (1984): Prostaglandins Leukotrienes Med. 13:21-25.

4. Pradelles, P., Grassi, J., Maclouf, J. (1985): Anal. Chem. 57:1170-1173.

5. Maclouf, J., Grassi, J., Pradelles, P. (1987): In Prostaglandin and Lipid Metabolism in Radiation Injury. Edited by Walden and Hughe. pp 355-364. Plenum Press, New York.

6. Vaïtukaitis, J. L. (1981): Methods. Enzymol. 73:46-52.

7. Rodbard, D., Bridson, W., Rayford, P. L. (1969): J. Lab. Clin. Med. 74:770-776.

8. Heavey, D.J., Soberman, R.J., Lewis, R.A., Spur, B. and Austen, K.F. (1987): Prostaglandins 33:693-708.

A NOVEL METHOD FOR THE ANALYSIS OF PAF AND ALKYL-ETHER PHOSPHOLIPIDS BY MASS SPECTROMETRY

Michael Balazy, Jacques Cluzel and Nicolas G. Bazan

LSU Eye Center and Neuroscience Center
Louisiana State University Medical Center School of Medicine
2020 Gravier Street, Suite B
New Orleans, Louisiana 70112, U.S.A.

The structural characterization of platelet-activating factor (PAF) as 1-O-alkyl-2-acetyl-sn-glycero-3-phosphatidylcholine rapidly led to the recognition of the role of ether phospholipids in the mediation of many pathological conditions (3). The biosynthesis of PAF involves the acylation of its immediate, inactive precursor, lyso-PAF, which is also its initial metabolite. The formation of lyso-PAF from phospholipid precursors may occur through the stimulation of calcium-dependent phospholipase A_2. One of these precursors, 1-O-alkyl-2-arachidonoyl-GPC, (AA-GPC) is unique because it may form lyso-PAF and free arachidonic acid upon enzymatic hydrolysis and therefore may serve as a common precursor for both PAF and eicosanoids (prostaglandins, leukotrienes). These mediators have been observed in several cells and tissues under conditions of phospholipase stimulation. Leukocytes have been shown to produce prostaglandin E_2, leukotriene B_4 and PAF (5). The release of free polyunsaturated fatty acids and formation of prostaglandins, leukotriene C_4, and PAF in electroconvulsive shock and in cerebral and retinal ischemia have been observed by us (2) and others. However, testing of the PAF-eicosanoids relationship is difficult to conduct due to the limitations of current analytical techniques employed to study phospholipid molecular species. We have sought methods to convert these phospholipids in a single step to derivatives amenable to GC/MS and ancillary techniques.

We report here a direct derivatization of PAF, lyso-PAF and AA-GPC with pentafluorobenzoyl chloride (PFBCl) at elevated temperatures. The hexane-extractable products were structurally characterized by chromatographic and spectroscopic techniques and showed adequate GC/MS properties. The quantitation of PAF and lyso-PAF is illustrated here in ionophore-stimulated leukocytes by isotope-dilution technique using newly synthesized deuterium-labeled phospholipid analogs with deuterium placed in the 1-O-hexadecyl chain.

MATERIALS AND METHODS

Standards Tritium-labeled phospholipids were from New England Nuclear; 1-*O*-[16,16,16-^{2}H$_3$]-hexadecyl-2-acetyl-GPC (PAF-D$_3$) was a generous gift from Dr. R. Zipkin (Biomol). *Lyso*-PAF-D$_3$ was prepared by enzymatic hydrolysis of PAF-D$_3$; *AA*-GPC-D$_3$ was prepared by acylation of *lyso*-PAF-D$_3$ with arachidonoyl anhydride and *N,N*-dimethyl-4-aminopyridine.

Instrumentation Mass spectrometry was conducted on an HP-5988A GC/MS system additionally equipped with a particle-beam (PB) LC/MS unit. Sample analysis was performed in negative chemical ionization (NCI) mode using methane as a reagent gas at a source pressure of 1 torr. A fused capillary column (5m x 0.25 mm, SP-2330, Supelco) was temperature-programmed from 100 °C to 300 °C at a rate of 25 °C/min.

Cell preparation and phospholipid quantitation Leukocytes were isolated from rabbit venous blood by density gradient centrifugation on plasma-Percoll and resuspended in Krebs Ringer phosphate buffer at 2x10^7 cells/ml. Cells were stimulated at 37 °C by addition of calcium ionophore A23187 to 2 µM final concentration. In control cells an equal volume of DMSO was added. The cell suspensions were extracted by Bligh and Dyer procedure along with added internal standards. The concentrated extracts were chromatographed on an LK5 plate in chloroform/methanol/ glacial acetic acid/water (50/25/8/4). The silica was scraped at R$_f$: 0.13, 0.29 and 0.77 to extract *lyso*-PAF, PAF and *AA*-GPC, respectively. Phospholipids were reacted with PFBCl for 4 h at 150 °C (*AA*-GPC overnight at 120 °C in chloroform), and derivatives were purified by TLC (hexane/ethyl acetate, 3/1, R$_f$: 0.67) prior to GC/MS analysis. Using selected ion monitoring, the abundance ratio of ions (see Figure 2) corresponding to endogenous and deuterated phospholipid was measured and its amount was calculated from the standard curve.

RESULTS AND DISCUSSION

As can be seen in Figure 1 the reaction of tritium-labeled alkyl-ether phospholipids with PFBCl at elevated temperature followed by hexane extraction resulted in a time-dependent accumulation of radiolabeled products in the hexane extract. PAF and *lyso*-PAF were converted with 95 and 50% yield, respectively, after reacting for 4 h at 150 °C. *AA*-GPC was converted with 90% yield after reacting for 18 h at 120 °C in PFBCl/chloroform. Each extract was analyzed by GC/MS and by HPLC with an on-line UV and mass-spectrometric detection using the novel technique of PB-LC/MS. In separate experiments fractions were collected to determine the distribution of radioactivity by scintillation counting. Milligram amounts of derivatives were also prepared to record NMR spectra. The data from these experiments, combined, indicate that the phospholipids were converted into single derivatives containing a pentafluorobenzoyl group which substituted the original phosphatidylcholine group. Additionally, *lyso*-PAF formed a new derivative containing chlorine in place of a hydroxyl group (1).

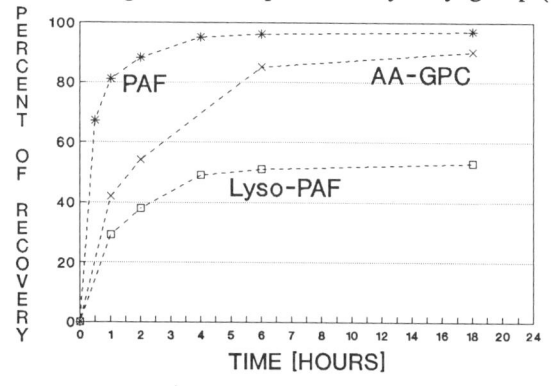

Figure 1. Conversion of tritiated ether phospholipids into hexane-extractable products following the reaction with PFBCl: PAF and *lyso*-PAF at 150 °C, *AA*-GPC at 120 °C (in PFBCl/chloroform).

Figure 2. Structures of PAF, *AA*-GPC and *lyso*-PAF (C_{16}) PFB derivatives. Corresponding ions in NCI/MS are indicated for native and deuterium-labeled compound.

The PFB derivatives of PAF and *lyso*-PAF can be detected at 1 pg injected onto the GC column with signal-to-noise greater than 3. Approximately 20 pg of these phospholipids can be derivatized and detected by NCI-GC/MS. The standard curves were found to be linear in the picogram and nanogram range. The application of the direct derivatization for the analysis of PAF and lyso-PAF in rabbit leukocytes stimulated with calcium ionophore is shown in Figure 3. We are currently studying the changes in cellular concentrations of AA-GPC following stimulation with calcium ionophore.

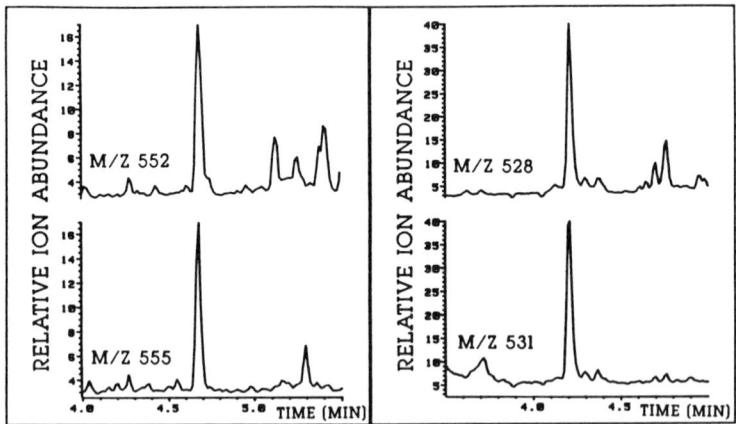

Figure 3. Electron-capture GC/MS analysis of PAF (left) and lyso-PAF as PFB-derivatives in rabbit leukocytes challenged with 2 µM ionophore A23187 for 10 min. The concentration of PAF and lyso-PAF was 34.4 pmol/10^6 cells and 15.4 pmol/10^6 cells, respectively.

CONCLUSIONS

Direct derivatization of PAF and related phospholipids with PFBCl at elevated temperatures produces in one step derivatives suitable for NCI-GC/MS analysis. The amount of isomerization or side products was insignificant. The reaction is nearly quantitative for PAF and AA-GPC. Novel internal standards showed excellent isotopic composition and stability during extraction and GC/MS analysis. The described method can be conveniently applied to analyze simultaneously different phosphatidylcholines in biological samples. This approach could potentially eliminate the use of phospholipase C in PAF assays, which has been reported to affect adversely the mass spectrometric analysis (4). *NIH EY05121.*

REFERENCES

1. Balazy, M., Braquet, P., Bazan, N.G. *in preparation.*
2. Bazan, N.G. (1989): In: *Extracellular and Intracellular Messengers in the Vertebrate Retina*, edited by D. Redburn & H. P. Morales. pp. 269-300, Alan R. Liss, N.Y.
3. Braquet, P., Touqui, L., Shen, T.Y., and Vargaftig, B.B. (1987): *Pharm. Rev.,* **39**: 97-145.
4. Haroldsen, P.E., Clay, K.L., and Murphy, R.C. (1987): *J. Lipid Res.,* **28**: 42-49.
5. O'Flaherty, J.T., and Wykle, R.L. (1983): *Clin. Rev. Allergy.,* **1**: 353-367.

DETERMINATION OF PLATELET-ACTIVATING FACTOR IN BIOLOGICAL SAMPLES BY HIGH RESOLUTION MASS SPECTROMETRY.

F. Magni,
*F. Berti
L. De Angelis, G. Rossoni, G. Galli

Istituto Scientifico San Raffaele ,V.Olgettina 60, 20132, Milan, Italy.
Institute of Pharmacological Sciences, School of Pharmacy, University of Milan, V.Balzaretti 9, 20133 Milan, Italy.
*Department of Medical Pharmacology, Chemoterapy and Toxicology, School of Medicine, University of Milan, V.Vanvitelli 32, 20133 Milan, Italy.

INTRODUCTION

Platelet activating factor (PAF; 1-O-alkyl-2-acetyl-sn-glycero-3-phosphocholine) is a phospholipid derived product generated in response to a variety of stimuli from various cells and tissues which has been shown to play an important role in immunological and inflammatory reactions (4). In view of the relevant biological activities of this lipidic mediator, it is of primary importance to be able to accurately determine its concentration in different biological samples. Recently, PAF analyses have been carried out by fast-atom-bombardament (FAB) (5,10) and gas chromatography-mass spectrometry (GC-MS) (7) because the previously described bioassay was not accurate and specific enough due to the variable bioactivity associated with the O-alkyl chain lenght (9) and to the contribution to biological activity of compounds structurally unrelated to PAF. Higher sensitivity of detection (10^{-12}-10^{-14}g) was improved further by GC-negative ion chemical ionization mass spectrometry (GC-NICI) (8). However, several purification steps were necessary for this kind of analysis to be specific enough, due to the presence of interfering compounds in the biological matrix. Results reported here show that by GC-NICI with high resolution PAF can be specifically evaluated in rather crude extracts.

EXPERIMENTAL

GC-MS was carried out using a VG-70SEQ instrument with a DB-1 fused silica capillary column (15mx0.22mm ID). Temperature was programmed from 60°C to 280°C at 25°C/min after 1 min holding at the initial temperature. Helium flow-rate was 1ml/min. The mass spectrometer operated in NICI using ammonia ($6x10^{-5}$ Torr) as the reagent gas. Analyses were performed in selected-ion-recording (SIR), monitoring the molecular anions at 552.2874 and 555.3063 and 580.3187 for the derivatives of hexadecyl-PAF, [$^2H_3$]-PAF and octadecyl-PAF, respectively, at 10000 resolution. The amount of hexadecyl-PAF in biological samples was calculated from a calibration curve with each point (range for hexadecyl-PAF 250pg-40ng) processed as the biological samples.

To each sample 1-0-hexadecyl-2-[$^2H_3$]-acetyl-sn-glycerophosphocholine (10 ng) was added as internal standard (5). Extraction was then carried out according to the Bligh and Dyer procedure (3). The dried organic phase was applied to a silicic acid column (0.5 g) in 1 ml of chloroform : methanol (50:50;v:v). The column was washed with 10 ml of the same solvent mixture and PAF and the internal standard were eluted with 10 ml of methanol:28% aqueous ammonia (98:2;v:v). Hydrolysis of the purified extract was performed with phospholipase C for 60 min at 37°C (8). The hydrolized mixture was extracted (3) and evaporated to dryness. The residue was dissolved in 20µl of anhydrous toluene, added with 10 µl of pentafluorobenzoyl chloride and heated at 90°C for 60 min. These derivatization conditions were preliminarly assessed by using a mixture of tritiated PAF and hexadecyl- and octadecyl-PAF heated at different temperatures (60°C, 90°C and 120°C) for 15, 30, 60 min. The derivatized products were then separated from the unreacted material by TLC using diethyl ether: ethyl acetate (75:25;v:v) as the elution mixture , and the peak area was measured by radio-chromatoscanning to estimate the percentage of the reacted meterial. After evaporating solvent and excess of reagent, the derivatized mixture was dissolved in 20 µl of hexane for the GC-MS analysis.

Male albino rabbit hearts were rapidly removed and mounted in a warm glass chamber (2). Briefly, the hearts were retrogradely perfused with Krebs-Henseleit solution, containing 0.2% of bovine serum albumin gassed with carbogen. The perfusion rate was adjusted to obtain a coronary perfusion pressure of 40-50 mmHg with a flow rate of 20 ml/min. The hearts were paced at the frequency of 180 beats/min with rectangular impulses (duration 1 ms, voltage 10% above threshold). The perfused buffer was collected for 10 min intervals.

RESULTS AND DISCUSSION

In the present study we describe a simplified method to determine the ability of tissues to sinthesize and release PAF. Under the analytical conditions described here, at high resolution (10000 RP), we were able to obtain reproducible results with a single chromatographic purification. PAF was quantitatively extracted from the buffer perfused through isolated rabbit hearts (% recovery 95±1.5,

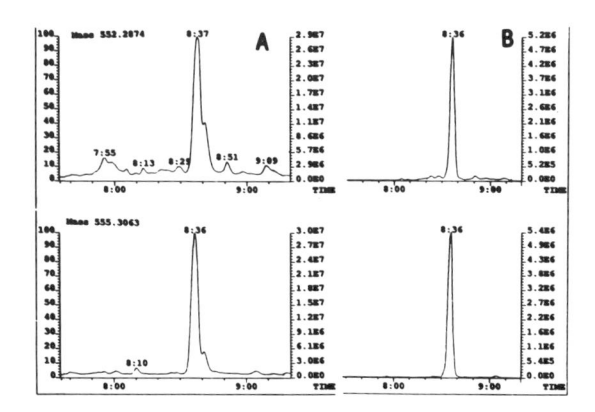

FIG. 1. GC-NICI of hexadecyl-PAF (upper trace) and [^{2}H$_3$]-PAF (lower trace) at resolution 1000 RP (A) and 10000 RP (B).

mean±S.D.,n=5) and purification was carried out on silicic acid (% recovery 82±7.8). Time and temperature for optimal derivatization were determined and on the basis of the results, heating at 90°C for 1hr were the selected reaction conditions.

When this work was completed other authors reported PAF evaluation in plasma (11) and urine (1) after single step purification. Analysis was then carried out by GC-NICI on the the pentafluorobenzoyl derivative at 1000 RP. At this resolution our samples presented an interfering peak which did not allow the accurate quantification of PAF (Fig.1A). At higher resolution (10000 RP) the interference was eliminated (Fig.1B) and still 10 pg of the hexadecyl-PAF derivative gave rise to a clear signal. PAF measurement was linear in the 250 pg to 40 ng range (r=0.997) with a intra-assay coefficient of variation of 7.1% (at 250 pg).

The basal release of PAF from isolated rabbit hearts was found by the described method to be 5.4±1.2 ng/min (n=11) when determined during perfusion at the normal flow rate of 20 ml/min. The release became 19.7±2 ng/min in the 10 min of reperfusion at the same rate following a 40 min ischemic period obtained by reducing the flow to 0.2 ml/min. The described method appears therefore to be useful in studies on the physiological role of PAF and on its pharmacological modulation.

REFERENCES

1. Benfenati, E., Macconi, D., Noris, M., Icardi, G., Bettazzoli, L., De Bellis, G., Gavinelli, M., Rotondo, S., and Remuzzi ,G. (1989): J. Lipid Res., 30:1977-1981.
2. Berti, F., Rossoni, G., Magni, F., Caruso, D., Omini, C., Puglisi, L., and Galli, G. (1988): J. Cardiovasc. Pharmacol., 12:438-444.
3. Bligh, E.G., and Dyer, W.J. (1959): Can. J. Biochem. Physiol., 37:911-919.
4. Braquet, P., Touqui, L., Shen, T.Y., and Vargaftig, B.B.(1987): Pharmacological Reviews, 39:97-145.
5. Clay, K.L., Stene, D.O., and Murphy, R.C. (1984): Biomed. Mass Spectrom., 11:47-49.
6. Demopoulus, C.A., Pickard, R.N., and Hanahan, J. (1979): J.Biol.Chem., 254:9355-9358.
7. Oda, M., Satouchi, K., Yasunaga, K., and Saito, K. (1985): J. Immunol., 134:1090-1093.
8. Ramesha, C.S., and Pickett, W.C. (1986): Biomed. Mass Spectrom., 13:107-111.
9. Satouchi, K., Pickard, R.N., and Hanahan, D.J. (1981): Arch. Biochem. Biophys., 211:683-688.
10. Verenne, P., Das, B.C., and Tence, M. (1985): Biomed. Mass Spectrom., 12:6-10.
11. Yamada, K., Asano, O., Yoshimura, T., and Katayama, K, (1988): J. Chromatogr., 433:243-247.

CHARACTERIZATION OF THROMBOXANE A$_2$/PROSTAGLANDIN H$_2$ RECEPTORS OF VARIOUS TISSUES USING A NEW RADIOIODINATED THROMBOXANE A$_2$/PROSTAGLANDIN H$_2$ MIMETIC, I-BOP

Thomas A. Morinelli, Masao Naka, Atsushi Masuda, John E. Oatis, Jr., Anselm K. Okwu, *Dale E. Mais, *David L. Saussy,Jr. and Perry V. Halushka

Departments of Cell and Molecular Pharmacology and Experimental Therapeutics and Medicine, Medical University of South Carolina, Charleston, South Carolina, 29425 and *Lilly Research Laboratories, Lilly Corporate Center, Indianapolis, IN 46285

INTRODUCTION

The presence of thromboxane A$_2$/ prostaglandin H$_2$ (TXA$_2$/PGH$_2$) receptors on platelets, blood vessels and other tissues was originally established using pharmacologic approaches (4). In recent years radiolabeled ligands are being used to more extensively characterize these and other receptors (4). Both ^{3}H and ^{125}I-labelled ligands have been used. The latter having the advantage of a much greater specific activity (29 Ci/mMole versus ~2000Ci/mMole).

[^{125}I]-PTA-OH, a TXA$_2$/PGH$_2$ receptor antagonist, has a high affinity for canine and human platelet receptors, but not for vascular tissue (8). In an attempt to develop high affinity ^{125}I-labelled ligands for TXA$_2$/PGH$_2$ receptors in vascular and other tissues, I-BOP([1S-(1α,2β(5Z), 3α1E,3R*)4α)]-7-[3-(3-hydroxy-4-(4'-iodophenoxy)-1-butenyl)-7-oxabicyclo-[2.2.1]heptan-2-yl]-5-heptenoic acid) was synthesized. I-BOP has an EC$_{50}$ value for inducing platelet shape change of 210 pM, for inducing platelet aggregation, 11 nM and for inducing increases in intracellular free calcium in platelets of 4 nM (15). Thus, I-BOP appears to have a high enough affinity for use as a radiolabeled ligand in platelets and vascular tissue. The binding characteristics of [^{125}I]-BOP as well as its activation of functional responses in platelets and vascular tissues are presented.

MATERIALS AND METHODS

I-BOP and [^{125}I]-BOP (Figure 1) were synthesized in our laboratory as previously described (15).

Washed platelets were prepared from whole blood that was drawn into indomethacin (10 μM) and EDTA (5 mM) (final concentrations) as previously described (9). Platelet functional studies were performed as described previously (15).

Rat aortic and human saphenous vein smooth muscle cells were cultured from explants of tissue as described previously (11,16).

Radioligand binding experiments using [^{125}I]-BOP

Binding assays using isolated rat platelets and suspensions of cultured rat aortic smooth muscle cells were performed with [^{125}I]-BOP as previously described (11). Briefly, platelets (1 x 10^7) or smooth muscle cells (5 x 10^5) in their respective buffers, were incubated with [^{125}I]-BOP (~20,000 cpm, 40 pM) and increasing concentrations of ^{127}I-BOP in a final volume of 0.2 ml in the platelet studies and 0.4 ml in the smooth muscle studies. After an incubation period of thirty minutes at 30°C, the reaction was stopped by the addition of 4 ml of ice cold buffer followed by filtration, under vacuum through Whatman GF/C glass fiber filters (Whatman, Inc., Clifton, N.J.). The filters were then washed with three additional 4ml volumes of ice cold buffer and then counted for bound radioactivity.

Binding assays using human platelets and suspensions of vascular smooth muscle cells were performed in a similar manner as described in detail previously (15,16).

Binding assays in which crude homogenates of guinea pig lung used conditions as previously described (18).

In all cases, non-specific binding was defined as the amount of radioactivity bound in the presence of the TXA$_2$/PGH$_2$ receptor antagonists L657925 (10 μM)(3) or SQ29548 (10).

RESULTS

I-BOP caused a concentration-dependent shape change of isolated human platelets that was inhibited by the TXA$_2$/PGH$_2$ receptor antagonist SQ29548. I-BOP also produced a concentration-dependent increase in intracellular free calcium and platelet aggregation.

In both cases, these responses were inhibited by the TXA$_2$/PGH$_2$

receptor antagonist L657925. In the three functional responses of human platelets tested, I-BOP has proven to be more potent than the most commonly used TXA_2/PGH_2 receptor agonist U46619. In fact, I-BOP has proven to be more potent than either of the naturally occurring prostanoids TXA_2 or PGH_2 in causing platelet aggregation (Table 1).

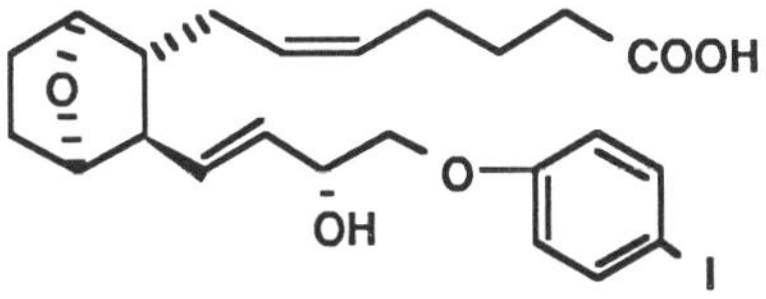

FIG. 1. Structure of I-BOP

TABLE 1.   Summary of platelet functional responses
EC_{50} (nM)

	I-BOP	U46619	PGH_2	TXA_2
Shape change	0.21#	40*	---	---
Ca^{++} transients	4.2#	14	---	---
Aggregation	11#	121#	45+	163+

* (14); #(15): +(12)

In suspensions of cultured rat aortic smooth muscle cells, I-BOP was shown to produce increases in intracellular free calcium, as measured by Fura-2 fluorescence. The EC_{50} value of I-BOP in these studies was reported to be 20 nM (11). Isolated rings of canine saphenous veins were stimulated to contract in a concentration-dependent manner with the addition of I-BOP (Figure 2). The EC_{50} value in this system was 0.038 nM (15).

Equilibrium binding studies indicated that I-BOP bound specifically and in a saturable mannner in human (15) and rat platelets (10) and vascular smooth muscle cells (11,16), as well as preparations of guinea pig lung membrane homogenates (18). The binding was of relatively high specificity and affinity (Table 2).

In competition binding experiments using a series of TXA_2/PGH_2 receptor agonists and antagonists, I-BOP was displaced by the competing ligands with rank order potencies that indicated that I-BOP was interacting with the respective TXA_2/PGH_2 receptors of rat and human platelets and vascular smooth muscle (15,16,11).

In addition to the equilibrium binding assays mentioned above, I-BOP has been used to characterize the TXA_2/PGH_2 receptor in both crude homogenates as well as detergent solubilized membranes of human platelets.

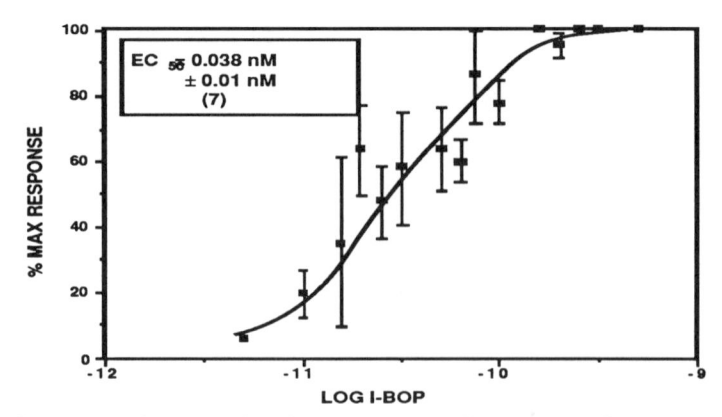

FIG. 2. I-BOP stimulated contraction of canine saphenous vein. Saphenous veins were prepared as described (9) and stimulated by various concentrations of I-BOP. A cumulative concentration response curve is shown from average values from 7 different segments of saphenous vein.

TABLE 2. Summary of I-BOP equilibrium binding data

	Human Platelet[#]	Smooth Muscle[+]	Rat* Platelet	Smooth Muscle	Guinea pig lung membranes[@]
K_d (nM)	2.2	2.6	0.2	0.3	0.087
B_{max} (sites/cell)	1700	33,540	771	10,872	82 fmoles/mg
%Specific binding	90	48	90	60	>90

[#](15); [+](16). *(11). [@](18)

In crude homogenates of platelet membranes I-BOP was found to show a K_d of 0.4 nM with a B_{max} of 1.8 pmoles/mg. In CHAPS solubilized human platelet membranes I-BOP also showed specific and saturable binding; K_d = 2.5 nM, B_{max} = 1.3 pmoles/mg (Figure 3).

I-BOP has also been used to examine the influence of pH on the platelet TXA_2/PGH_2 receptor. The optimum pH at which I-BOP was found to bind to human platelets was 6.0. In washed human platelets the affinity as well as the number of TXA_2/PGH_2 receptors for I-BOP was found to significantly increase at pH 6.0 vs. 7.4. In fact, at the lower pH, I-BOP was found to interact with two classes of TXA_2/PGH_2 receptors. One class of higher affinity revealed a K_d

of 0.23 nM with 1104 sites/platelet and a second class of lower affinity receptors, K_d = 3.9 nM and 5316 sites/platelet (13).

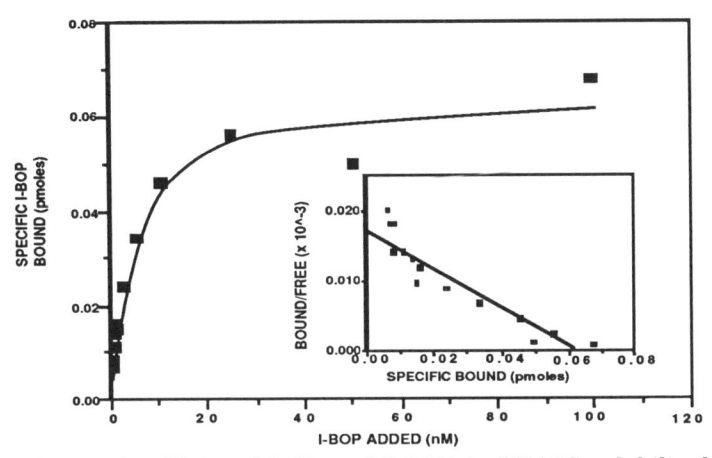

FIG. 3. Equilibrium binding of I-BOP to CHAPS solubilized human platelets. Binding conditions were; 180,000 cpm (~0.4 nM) of [^{125}I]-BOP was incubated with 40 µg of solubilized receptor, along with increasing concentrations of I-BOP (0.1-100 nM) in a final volume of 0.2 ml in 5mM CHAPS buffer at pH 6.5. The incubation and washing conditions were as described. Data were analysed using LIGAND (17). K_d = 2.9 nM; B_{max} = 1.3 pmoles/mg.

DISCUSSION

I-BOP is the first ^{125}I-labeled agonist for the TXA$_2$/PGH$_2$ receptor. I-BOP produced a concentration-dependent increase in platelet shape change, increase in intracellular free calcium and aggregation of washed human platelets. All of these functional responses caused by I-BOP were inhibited by known antagonists of the TXA$_2$/PGH$_2$ receptor, indicating that I-BOP produces its effects through interaction with the platelet TXA$_2$/PGH$_2$ receptor. Additionally, I-BOP has proven to be more potent than either TXA$_2$ or PGH$_2$ in causing aggregation of washed human platelets.

In equilibrium binding studies, I-BOP has been shown to be a highly specific ligand for the TXA$_2$/PGH$_2$ receptor in washed platelets, crude and solubilized platelet membranes and also in crude lung membranes. In each of the tissues and cell types tested, competition binding studies using analogs of either TXA$_2$ or PGH$_2$ indicated that I-BOP bound to the respective TXA$_2$/PGH$_2$

receptor in a specific manner. The rank order potency for the analogs to displace [125I]-BOP from its receptor was comparable to the published pharmacological potencies for the same compounds to either inhibit or induce TXA_2/PGH_2 mimetic activation of the cells under investigation.

Of particular significance is the fact that [125I]-BOP was stereoselectively displaced from its receptor by the stereoisomeric pair of TXA_2/PGH_2 receptor antagonists L657925 and L657926 (3) in human platelets (15) and vascular smooth muscle cells (16) and in rat platelets and vascular smooth muscle cells (11).

Previous studies examining the TXA_2/PGH_2 receptor of various cells and/or tissues with radioligands have employed the antagonists [125I]-PTA-OH (8) and [3H]-SQ29548 (5) or the agonists [3H]-U44069 (1) or [3H]-U46619 (6,7,14). The studies using the tritiated agonists have found similar values for platelet receptor density as we have reported in the studies with I-BOP. The affinity of the agonists for the receptor, however, were much lower in those studies, ranging from 20 nM (7) to 131 nM (6). I-BOP represents a significant advance over the previously employed radiolabelled agonists.

I-BOP has an additional advantage because of its high specific activity. The specific activity of [125I]-BOP should be that of the theoretical activity of 125I; ~2000 Ci/mmol. Because of this, I-BOP can be used to detect smaller amounts of receptor than the tritiated ligands. This is of particular advantage in studies designed to characterize and subsequently purify the TXA_2/PGH_2 receptor from various tissues where small amounts may be present.

Using I-BOP, preliminary studies have shown the existence of TXA_2/PGH_2 receptors in rat glomerular and aortic membrane homogenates, in equine mononuclear cells (unpublished observations) and rabbit aortic membranes (19).

In summary, I-BOP should prove to be a valuable ligand that can be used for the characterization of TXA_2/PGH_2 receptors in cells and tissues from various sources.

REFERENCES

1. Armstrong, R.A., Jones, R.L. and Wilson, N.H. (1983): *Br. J. Pharmacol.* 79:953-964.
2. Dorn, G. W. III (1989): *J. Clin. Invest.* 84:1883-1891.
3. Gillard, J.W., Morton, H.E., Fortin, R., Yoakim, C., Girard, Y., Lord, A., Ethier, D., Leveille, C., Letts, G., Evans, J. and Jones T.R. (1989): in *Prostaglandins in Clinical Research; Cardiovascular system*, editors K. Schror and H. Sinzinger Alan R. Liss, Inc, New York. 579-583.
4. Halushka, P.V., Mais, D.E., Mayeux, P.R. and Morinelli, T.A.

(1989): *Annu. Rev. Pharm. Tox.* 29:213-239.
5. Hedberg, A., Hall, S.E., Ogletree, M.L., Harris, D.N. and Liu, E.C.K. (1988): *Jour. Pharm. Exper. Therap.* 245:786-792.
6. Johnson, G.J., Dunlop, P.C., Leis,L.A. and From, A.H.L. (1988): *Circ. Res.* 62:494-505.
7. Liel, N., Mais, D.E. and Halushka, P.V. (1987): *Prostaglandins* 33:789-797.
8. Mais, D.E., Kochel, P.J., Saussy, D.L.Jr. and Halushka, P.V. (1985): *Mol. Pharmacol.* 28:163-169.
9. Mais, D.E., DeHoll, D., Sightler, H. and Halushka, P.V. (1988): *Eur. J. Pharmacol.* 148: 309-315.
10. Mais,D.E., Yoakim, D., Guindon, Y., Gillard, J., Rokach, J. and Halushka, P.V. (1989): *Bioch. Biophys. Acta.* 1012:184-190.
11. Masuda, A., Mais, D.E., Oatis, J.E.Jr. and Halushka, P.V. (1990):(submitted)
12. Mayeux,P.R., Morton, H.E., Gillard, J., Lord,A., Morinelli, T.A., Boehm, A., Mais, D.E. and Halushka, P.V. (1988):*Biochem. Biophy. Res. Comm.* 157:733-739.
13. Mayeux, P.R., Morinelli, T.A., Williams, T.C., Hazard,E.S., Mais,D.E., Oatis, J.E.Jr., Baron,D.A. and Halushka, P.V. (1990): *Jour. Biol. Chem.* (in press).
14. Morinelli, T.A., Niewiarowski, S., Daniel, J.L. and Smith, J.B. (1987): *Am. J. Physiol.* 253:H1035-H1043.
15. Morinelli, T.A., Oatis, J.E.Jr., Okwu,A.K., Mais,D.E., Mayeux,P.R., Masuda,A., Knapp, D.R. and Halushka, P.V. (1989): *Jour. Pharm. Exper. Therap.* 251:557-562.
16. Morinelli, T.A., Mais, D.E., Oatis, J.E.Jr., Crumbley,A.J. III and Halushka, P.V. (1990): *Life Sciences*, 46:1765-1772.
17. Munson, P.J. and Rodbard, D. (1980): *Anal. Biochem.* 107:220-239.
18. Saussy, D.L.Jr., Mais, D.E., Magee, D.E., Dube, G.P., Brune, K.A., Kurtz, W.L. and Williams, C.M. (1990): *FASEB Jour.* 4:A324.
19. Sessa,W.C., Halushka, P.V., Okwu,A. and Nasjletti (1990): Circ.Res. (in press).

PURIFICATION AND CHARACTERIZATION OF THE HUMAN PLATELET TXA$_2$/PGH$_2$ RECEPTOR

Shuh Narumiya, Fumitaka Ushikubi, Masatoshi Nakajima, Masakazu Hirata and *Minoru Okuma

Departments of Pharmacology and *Internal Medicine, Kyoto University Faculty of Medicine, Sakyo-ku, Kyoto 606, Japan

Thromboxane (TX) A$_2$, a major arachidonate metabolite in platelets, is a potent stimulator of platelet aggregation and constrictor of vascular and respiratory smooth muscles. However, its mechanism of action has not been fully elucidated. Pharmacological studies using stable structural analogues of TXA$_2$ have suggested the presence of a receptor for this very unstable compound (2, 10, 11, 19), and radioligand binding experiments using radiolabeled derivatives of these analogues have revealed the existence of a class of binding sites in platelets which appears to represent this putative TXA$_2$ receptor (1, 9, 18, 20). The specificity of this binding also suggested that the PG endoperoxide, PGH$_2$, shares this same receptor with TXA$_2$. Halushka and his collaborators reported solubilization of this putative TXA$_2$/PGH$_2$ receptor from platelet membranes and partially characterized it by gel permeation and density gradient centrifugation (5, 6). However, isolation and further characterization of the receptor have not been reported so far, probably because the solubilized receptor quickly loses the binding affinity to the above ligands (5). Recently a series of compounds having a bicycloheptane ring and a sulfonamide linkage have been developed as new TXA$_2$ receptor antagonists (14, 17). Based on these compounds we have developed new ligands for the TXA$_2$ receptor which bind to the solubilized receptor without significant loss of the binding affinities (21). Using these ligands, we have purified the TXA$_2$/PGH$_2$ receptor from the membranes of human blood platelets (22).

DEVELOPMENT OF NEW LIGANDS AND LIGAND-AFFINITY GEL

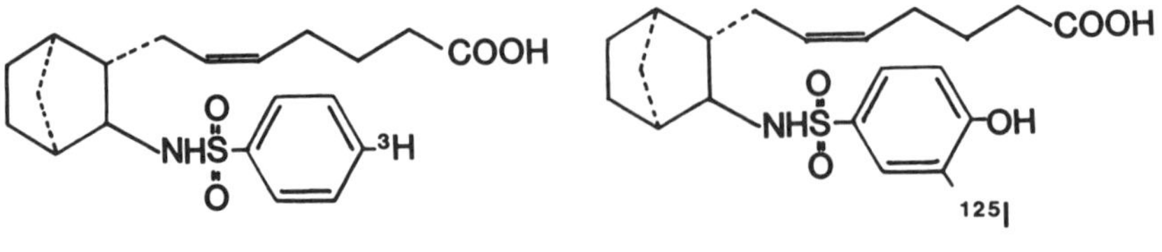

Figure 1. Structures of [^{3}H]S-145 and [^{125}I]I-S-145-OH

The structures of the ligands we developed, [^{3}H]S-145 and [^{125}I]I-S-145-OH, are shown in Fig. 1. These radioligands bound to washed human platelets as well as the solubilized TXA$_2$ receptor in a time dependent manner, and in either of the two preparations, specific binding displaceable by 500-fold excess of unlabelled ligand was more than 90% of the total binding. The specific binding appeared to be reversible, because similar extent of the binding was displaced by the addition of excess amount of an unlabelled ligand after the binding equilibrium had been reached, although the dissociation of the ligand from washed platelets was much slower than that from the solubilized receptor. The binding of these ligands occurred in a saturable manner. The Scatchard analyses of the [^{3}H]S-145 and [^{125}I]I-S-145-OH bindings to washed human platelets and the solubilized receptor showed a straight line in each preparation, suggesting a single class of binding sites for these ligands. The Kd and Bmax of [^{3}H]S-145 binding to washed platelets were 3.64 ± 0.48 nM and 196 ± 28 fmol/10^8 platelets, respectively, (mean ± S.D. of four experiments) and those of [^{125}I]I-S-145-OH binding were 5.72 ± 1.38 nM and 196 ± 22 fmol/10^8 platelets, respectively (mean ± S.D. of four experiments). The Kd and Bmax of [^{3}H]S-145 binding to the solubilized receptor were 8.22 ± 2.13 nM and 1.70 ± 0.39 pmol/mg of solubilized protein, respectively, (mean ± S.D. of six experiments), and those of [^{125}I]I-S-145-OH were 4.09 ± 0.60 nM and 1.68 ± 0.14 pmol/mg of solubilized protein, respectively, (mean ± S.D. of six experiments). Affinity of [^{3}H]S-145 binding to the solubilized receptor was also determined by the association and dissociation rate constants, and this fits well with the value from the Scatchard analysis. Thus, the two ligands showed no loss of binding affinity on solublization of TXA$_2$ receptor from platelet membranes. This character is more clearly shown by comparing them with the affinities of other TXA$_2$/PGH$_2$ analogues to these receptor preparations. The comparison was carried out by examining displacement of specific [^{3}H]S-145 binding with these analogues in washed platelets, platelet membranes and solubilized receptor. Table 1 summarizes Ki values of these analogues calculated from IC$_{50}$ values of the binding. Consistent with the above findings, both S-145 and I-S-145-OH showed relatively constant IC$_{50}$ values to all three preparations., and they showed the highest affinity to the receptor among the analogues. On the other hand, other analogues such as SQ-29548, STA$_2$, ONO-11120 and U-46619 showed lower affinities than S-145 and I-S-145-OH in washed platelets, and their affinities to the receptor further decreased on membrane preparation and receptor solubilization.

Another advantage of S-145 and I-S-145-OH as ligands of the TXA$_2$ receptor is that modification of their α-carboxyl group has no effect on its binding affinity to the receptor. This property was made use of in preparation of affinity gel for purification of TXA$_2$ receptor in which S-145 was immobilized by conjugating its α-carboxylic group with the amino group of Affigel 102 (Fig. 2) (22).

Table 1. Affinities of Various TXA$_2$/PGH$_2$ Analogues to Various Receptor Preparations (from ref. 21)

Analogues	Washed Platelets	Platelet Membranes	Solubilized Receptor
		(Ki, nM)	
S-145	4.4	4.6	12.2
I-S-145-OH	10.9	2.4	8.1
SQ-29548	24.7	125	204
STA2	36.1	75.5	206
ONO-11120	222	1,360	1,690
U-46619	603	2,580	9,030

*Values for some componds are higher than those previously reported (18, 20). This appeared due to aged platelet preparation we used in this study.

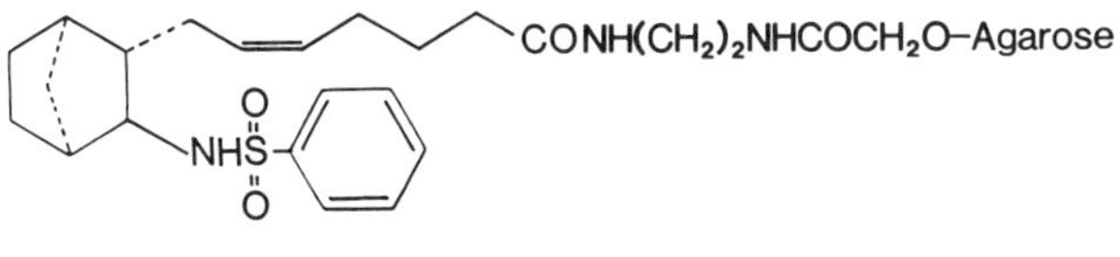

Fig. 2. Chemical structure of S-145 Affinity Gel

RECEPTOR ISOLATION

Human platelet membranes were solubilized with 10 mM CHAPS in the presence of 20%(w/v) glycerol by vortexing at room temperature for 2 min. The solubilized extract was obtained as a supernatant of centrifugation at 200,000 x g for 60 min. About 30% of the binding activity was solubilized by these procedures. The TXA$_2$ receptor was purified from the extract by a series of column chromatographies described below. Asolectin was added to some of the buffers, because it not only restored the ligand binding activity of the solubilized receptor but also improved recovery of the activity from the columns. The solubilized extract was mixed first with S-145 Affigel described above, and the mixture was gently agitated overnight. The activity bound to the gel in a time-dependent manner, and more than 70% of it was adsorbed in 8 h. The suspension was then transferred to a glass column. After the column was washed, the activity was eluted with the buffer containing 0.1 mM S-145. The elution of the activity from the Affigel column required a large volume of the elution buffer containing the cold ligand and caused dilution of the binding activity. We, therefore, connected a WGA-Agarose column in sequence to the Affigel column, and recycled the eluate through the two columns. The activity eluted from the Affigel column was thus successively adsorbed to a WGA-Agarose column. The activity collected on a WGA-Agarose column was then eluted with N-acetyl-D-glucosamine. This combined-affinity chromatography purified the receptor about 1,600-fold with 22% recovery. This Affigel-WGA fraction was next applied to a column of Red Agarose. After the column was washed, elution was performed with a linear gradient between 0 and 0.7 M KCl. The activity was eluted as a broad peak between 0.2 and 0.5M KCl. The active fractions were pooled (the Red Agarose fraction), concentrated and applied to a TSKgel G-3000SW column. Gel permeation was performed in the presence of 0.5 M KCl at a flow rate of 0.3 ml/min. The peak fractions were concentrated and injected again onto a TSKgel G-3000SW column. The activity was eluted as a symmetrical peak which overlapped exactly with an ultraviolet absorption peak. The active fractions were pooled as the final receptor preparation.

A representative purification of the TXA$_2$ receptor from the membranes of human platelets is shown in Table 1. About 8,700-fold purification was achieved from the solubilized extract with a recovery of 6%.

Table 2. Purification of the TXA$_2$ receptor from human blood platelets (from ref. 22)

Fraction	Protein	[3H]S-145 total amount	Binding specific activity	Purification	Recovery
	mg	pmol	pmol/mg	-fold	%
Solubilized extract	2,886	6,395	2.22	1	100
Affigel-WGA	0.399	1,425	3,570	1,620	22
Red-Agarose	0.197	996	5,060	2,300	16
1st TSKGel	0.052	657	12,600	5,730	10
2nd TSKGel	0.020	384	19,200	8,730	6

PROPERTIES OF THE PURIFIED RECEPTOR

Samples from each purification step were analyzed by SDS-polyacrylamide gel electrophoresis (Fig. 3). The final preparation (the 2nd TSKgel fraction) showed a broad protein band (lane 6), the molecular weight of which was estimated to be 57,000. This protein band was broader than those of the marker proteins, and this is probably due to the glycoprotein nature of this protein as evidenced by its behavior on the WGA-Agarose column. Such broadness of protein bands was also noted for α-adrenergic receptor and muscarinic receptor, and suggested to be caused by microheterogeneity in the carbohydrate residues (7).

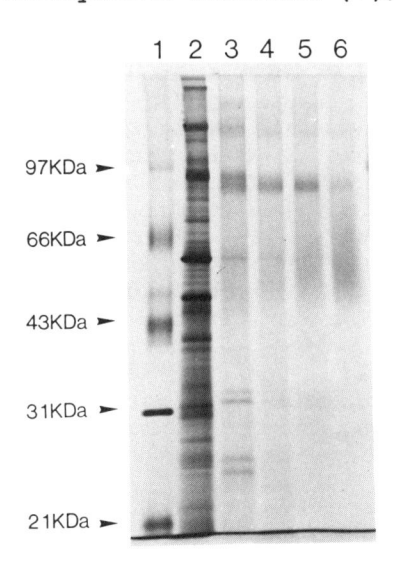

Fig. 3. SDS-polyacrylamide gel electrophoresis of the various receptor preparations. Lane 1, molecular weight markers; Lane 2, the solubilized extract; lane 3, the Affigel-WGA fraction; lane 4, the Red Agarose fraction; lane 5, the 1st TSKgel fraction; lane 6, the 2nd TSKgel fraction. An arrow indicates an Mr 57,000 protein band. (from ref. 22)

The purified receptor showed a time-dependent and reversible [^{3}H]S-145 binding as in intact platelets. Scatchard analysis of the binding yielded a single straight line, suggesting a single class of binding sites. The Kd and Bmax values were estimated to be 29.8 nM and 19.2 nmol/mg protein, respectively. Assuming that the molecular weight of this receptor protein is 57,000, the theoretical Bmax value is 17.5 nmol/mg protein. This suggests that the 57 KDa protein purified here binds one ligand per molecule. The specificity of [^{3}H]S-145 binding was examined by competition of the binding with various compounds. The binding was specifically displaced by various TXA_2/PGH_2 analogues such as S-145 and ONO-3708 (both antagonists) and STA_2 and U-46619 (both agonists) in a concentration dependent manner to the level of the nonspecific binding. The Ki values calculated from the IC_{50} values were 21, 110, 870, and 19,900 nM for S-145, ONO-3708, STA_2 and U-46619, respectively. These values were in good agreement with those observed for the solubilized receptor as described above. On the other hand, the binding was not effectively competed by other PGs such as TXB_2, PGD_2, PGE_1 and $PGF_{2\alpha}$. Thus, the specificity of the binding to the final preparation correlated well with that found in intact platelets and the crude membranes.

THE TXA_2 RECEPTOR IN ERYTHROLEUKEMIA CELLS

The above results clearly demonstrated that we purified the platelet TXA_2 receptor to apparent homogeneity and can make use of it for amino acid sequencing analysis. In order to carry out cDNA cloning based on such analysis, we examined the expression of the TXA_2 receptor in several lines of cultured leukemia cells (16). We found specific binding of [^{125}I]I-S-145-OH in two lines of human erythroleukemia cells, HEL and K-562, but not in other leukemia cells such as HL-60 and L1210 cells. The binding in HEL and K-562 cells consisted of the high and low affinity bindings; the Kd of the high affinity binding were 2.4 and 2.8 nM and those of the low affinity 58 and 18 nM for HEL and K-562, respectively. The specificity of the high affinity binding was similar to that found in human platelets. Furthermore, the addition of 12-O-tetradecanoyl-phorbol-13-acetate to the culture of HEL and K-562 cells induced both classes of the bindings in concentration and time-dependent manners. These findings suggest that these cells can serve as a mRNA source for cloning of this receptor.

PERSPECTIVE AND SUMMARY

Here we report development of new TXA$_2$ receptor ligands, purification using these ligands of the platelet TXA$_2$/PGH$_2$ receptor and identification of the similar, if not identical, receptor in human erythroleukemia cells. Based on these studies, cDNA cloning of the TXA$_2$/PGH$_2$ receptor is currently carried out. This will clarify the structure of the TXA$_2$/PGH$_2$ receptor in near future. It will also contribute to identify molecular heterogeneity of receptor subtypes found in platelets and smooth muscles (12,13). With these knowledges it will also become clear how the TXA$_2$ receptor transduces signals in these tissues. Several groups (3, 4, 8, 15) have suggested that the TXA$_2$ receptor couples with a GTP-binding protein which is distinct from Gs and Gi/Go. Identity of this putative GTP-binding protein will be revealed by reconstitution experiment using the purified receptor and cadidate GTP-binding proteins.

In conclusion, we have purified the platelet TXA$_2$ receptor. This work should facilitate understanding the mechanism of PG actions in more details at the molecular level.

Acknowledgements

The authors are grateful to Japanese Red Cross Society for their supply of outdated platelets for research purpose. We are also grateful to the Shionogi Research Laboratories and ONO Pharmaceutical Co. for their generous supply of various compounds. This work was supported in part by Grants in aid for Scientific Research from the Ministry of Education, Science and Culture of Japan (No. 02240207, 02220210, 02262213, 01480147), a Research Grant for Cardiovascular Diseases (1A-1) from the Ministry of Health and Welfare of Japan and by grants from the Japan Intractable Diseases Research Foundation and the Ono Medical Research Foundation.

References

1. Armstrong, R.A., Jones, R.L., and Wilson, N.H. (1983) Br. J. Pharmacol., 79, 953-964
2. Armstrong, R.A., Jones, R.L., Peesapati, V., Will, S.G., and Wilson, N.H. (1985) Br. J. Pharmacol., 84, 595-607
3. Avdonin, P.V., Svitina-Ulitina, I.V., Leytin, V.L., and Tkachuk, V.A. (1985) Thromb. Res., 40, 101-112
4. Brass, L.F., Shaller, C. C., and Belmonte, E. J. (1987) J. Clin. Invet., 79, 1269-1275
5. Burch, R.M., Mais, D.E., Saussy, D.L., Jr., and

Halushka, P.V. (1985) Proc. Natl. Acad. Sci. USA, 82, 7434-7438
6. Burch, R.M., Mais, D.E., Pepkowitz, S.H., and Halushka, P.V. (1985) Biochem. Biophys. Res. Commun., 132, 961-968
7. Haga, K., and Haga, T. (1985) J. Biol. Chem., 260, 7927-7935
8. Houslay, M.D., Bojanic, D., and Wilson, A. (1986) Biochem. J., 234, 737-740
9. Hung, S.C., Ghali, N.I., Venton, D.L., and Le Breton, G.C. (1983) Biochim. Biophys. Acta, 728, 171-178
10. Jones, R.L., Peesapati, V., and Wilson, N.H. (1982) Br. J. Pharmacol., 76, 423-438
11. Le Breton, G.C., Venton, D.L., Enke, S.E., and Halushka, P.V. (1979) Proc. Natl. Acad. Sci. USA, 76, 4097-4101
12. Lefer, A.M., Smith, E.F.III., Araki, H., Smith, J.B., Aharony, D., Claremon, D.A., Magolda, R.L., and Nicolaou, K.C. (1980) Proc. Natl. Acad. Sci. USA, 77, 1706-1710
13. Mais, D.E., Saussy, D. L., Jr., Chaikhouni, A., Kochel, P.J., Knapp, D.R., Hamanaka, N., and Halushka, P.V. (1985) J. Pharmacol. Exp. Ther., 233, 418-424
14. Naka, M., Hamanaka, N., Sugioka, M., Iwamura, H., Sakata, M., Kira, H., Okegawa, T., and Kawasaki, A. (1989) in Biosignalling in Cardiac and Vascular Systems (ed. M. Fujiwara, S. Narumiya and S. Miwa), pp. 422-425, Pergamon Press, Oxford.
15. Nakahata, N., Matsuoka, I., Ono, T., and Nakanishi, H. (1989) Eur. J. Pharmacol., 162, 407-417
16. Nakajima, M., Yamamoto, M., Ushikubi, F., Okuma, M., Fujiwara, M., and Narumiya, S. (1989) Biochem. Biophys. Res. Commun., 158, 958-965
17. Narisada, M., Ohtani, M., Watanabe, F., Uchida, K., Arita, H., Doteuchi, M., Hanasaki, K., Kakushi, H., Otani, K., anad Hara, S. (1988) J. Med. Chem., 31, 1847-1854
18. Narumiya, S., Okuma, M., and Ushikubi, F. (1986) Br. J. Pharmacol., 88, 323-331
19. Nicolaou, K.C., Magolda, R.L., Smith, J Aharony, D., Smith, E.F., and Lefer, A.M. (1979) Proc. Natl. Acad. Sci. USA, 76, 2566-2570
20. Saussy, D.L., Mais, D.E., Burch, R.M., and Halushka, P.V. (1986) J. Biol. Chem., 261, 3025-3029
21. Ushikubi, F., Nakajima, M., Yamamoto, M., Ohtsu, K., Kimura, Y., Okuma, M., Uchino, H., Fujiwara, M., and Narumiya, S. (1989) Eicosanoids, 2, 21-27
22. Ushikubi, F., Nakajima, M., Hirata, M., Okuma M, Fujiwara, M. and Narumiya, S. (1989) J. Biol. Chem., 264, 16496-16501

Advances in Prostaglandin, Thromboxane, and Leukotriene Research, Vol. 21,
edited by B. Sameulsson et al.
Raven Press, Ltd., New York © 1990.

Binding of a Radioiodinated Agonist to Thromboxane A_2/ Prostaglandin H_2 (TXA_2/PGH_2) Receptors in Guinea Pig Lung Membranes

Dale E. Mais, David L. Saussy, Jr., David E. Magee
and Carl M. Williams
Lilly Research Laboratories
Lilly Corporate Center
Indianapolis, IN 46285

Introduction

The arachidonic acid metabolites prostaglandin H_2 (PGH_2) and thromboxane A_2 (TXA_2) are potent stimulators of airway mouth muscle contraction and may mediate some of the pulmonary effects of leukotrienes (1-2). Presumably these actions are mediated via specific TXA_2/PGH_2 receptors. TXA_2/PGH_2 receptors from platelets and vascular smooth muscle have been characterized using both pharmacologic and radioligand binding studies (3), however, the TXA_2/PGH_2 receptor from the lung has not been as well characterized. Previous studies indicate that the lung TXA_2/PGH_2 receptor may play an important role in the bronchoconstrictor response to allergen challenge and its chemical mediators such as LTD_4. Thus it is important to further characterize the lung TXA_2/PGH_2 receptor in order to facilitate investigations into the role of TXA_2 in airway disease.

Recently, the synthesis of a new radioiodinated TXA_2 mimetic IBOP, shown in Figure 1, and its binding to TXA_2/PGH_2 receptors in washed human platelets was described (4). IBOP was found to bind with high affinity and high specific binding. In this paper we describe the characterization of $[^{125}I]BOP$ binding to membranes prepared from guinea pig lung.

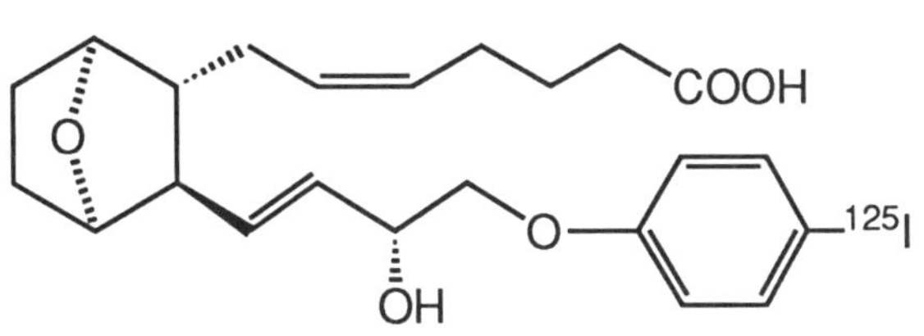

Figure 1. Structure of $^{125}IBOP$

Methods

Guinea pig lung membranes were prepared by differential centrifugation of homogenates of lungs perfused with EGTA-saline. Radioligand binding assays were performed in silanized glass tubes at 30°C. Incubations (222 µl final vol.) typically contained 50 ug of protein in a 25mM MOPS, 100mM NaCl, 5mM $MgCl_2$ at a pH of 6.5 (assay buffer) and containing ~100,000 cpm of ^{125}IBOP (0.1 nM) and displacing ligands or vehicle as appropriate. The reaction was terminated by addition of 4 ml ice cold buffer (25 mM Tris, pH 7.4), followed immediately by rapid vacuum filtration through Whatman GF/C glass fiber filters. Non displaceable binding was determined in the presence of 10 uM SQ29548 and was generally <10% of total binding.

Results and Discussion

Binding of ^{125}IBOP to guinea pig lung membranes was linear with protein concentration over a range of 7.8 to 62.5 mg per tube (data not shown). Scatchard analysis of the binding data are shown in figure 2. Analysis of the data using the nonlinear curve fitting program LUNDON-1 yielded a best fit of the data by a one site model with a Kd value of 87 ± 12 pM and a B_{max} of 82 ± 8 fmoles per mg protein (n = 3).

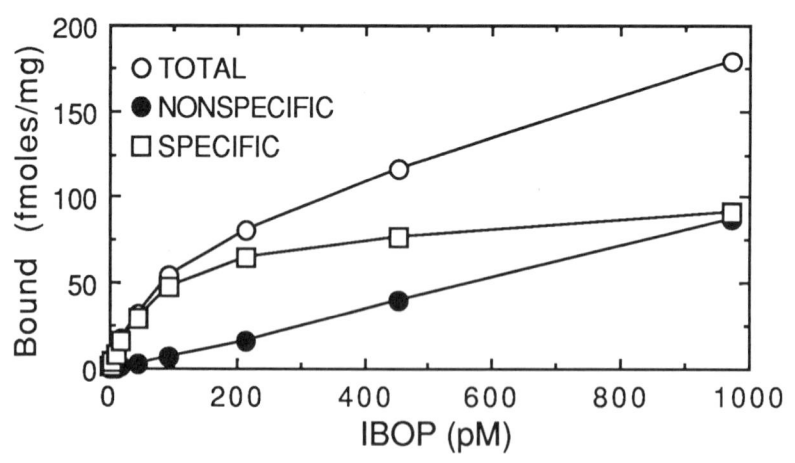

Figure 2. Saturation of ^{125}IBOP binding to guinea pig lung membranes.

Pretreatment of membranes with 10mM dithiothreitol or N-ethylmaleimide for 30 min resulted in a 30-36% inhibition of displaceable binding. However, neither GTP nor the nonhydrolysable GTP analogs GTP-gamma-S and GPPNHP had any effect on displaceable binding in concentrations from 1nM to 300uM.

A number of structurally dissimilar compounds that act as mimetics or antagonists at the TXA_2/PGH_2 receptor in other tissues were found to compete for $^{125}IBOP$ binding in lung membrane. A summary of these results is shown in Table 1. In addition, we examined the ability of a variety of prostanoids to compete with $^{125}IBOP$ binding since it has been proposed that the TXA_2/PGH_2 receptor mediates the contractile responses to PGD_2, PGE_2 and PGF_{2a} and the PGD_2 metabolite 9a,11b-PGF_2 in guinea pig lung parenchyma and trachea (5-8). A summary of IC_{50} values for these prostanoids and TXB_2 is presented in Table 1.

Table 1. Inhibition of $^{125}IBOP$ binding to guinea pig lung membranes by TXA2/PGH2 analogs and prostanoids.

COMPOUND	IC_{50}
SQ29548	30 ± 2 nM
BM13505	184 ± 22 nM
IPTAOH	384 ± 35 nM
IBOP	320 ± 30 pM
SQ26655	1.12 ± 0.06 nM
U46619	6.2 ± 0.3 nM
PGD_2	687 ± 108 nM
9a,11b-PGF_2	779 ± 129 nM
PGF_{2a}	1.39 ± 0.09 µM
PGE_2	4 ± 0.67 µM
TXB_2	> 10 µM

In summary, these studies represent the first characterization of lung TXA_2/PGH_2 receptors using a radioligand assay and demonstrate the utility of $^{125}IBOP$ to conduct such studies. The preparation of lung membranes with a binding site for both TXA_2/PGH_2 agonists and antagonists provides the opportunity for further analysis of these receptors in the lung.

Acknowledgements
David Magee was supported by a Charles Dana Scholarship from DePauw University. The authors wish to thank Ms. Sherry Pike for her secretarial assistance.

References
1. Svensson JK, Strandberg T, Tuvemo R and Hamberg M. Prostaglandins 1977; 14:425-436
2. Coleman, RA. Humphrey PPA, Kennedy I, Levy GP and Lumley P Br J Pharmacol 1981; 73:773-778
3. Halushka PV, Mais DE, Mayeux PR and Morinelli TA Annu Rev Phamacol Toxicol 1989; 29:213-239
4. Morinelli TA, Oatis , Jr. JE, Okwu AK, Mais DE, Mayeux PR, Masuda A, Knapp DR and Halushka PV J Pharmacol Exp Ther 1989; 251:557-562
5. McKennif M, Rodger IW, Norman P and Gardiner PJ Eur J Pharmacol 1988; 153:149-159
6. Coleman RA and Kennedy I Prostaglandins 1985; 29:363-375
7. Beasley CRW, Robinson C, Featherstone RL, Varley JG, Hardy CC, Church MK and Holgate ST J Clin Invest 1987; 79:987-983
8. Featherstone RL, Robinson C, Holgate ST and Church MK Br J Pharmacol 1988; 94:336P

ON THE MECHANISM OF THE PROLONGED ACTION IN MAN OF GR32191, A THROMBOXANE RECEPTOR ANTAGONIST.

J.M. Ritter, H.S. Doktor, N. Benjamin, S.E. Barrow
& P. Stewart-Long[a]

Department of Clinical Pharmacology, UMDS, Guy's Hospital, LONDON, SE1 9RT, and [a]Clinical Research Division Glaxo Group Research Limited, Greenford Road, GREENFORD, Middlesex UB6 0HE

SUMMARY

Twenty four healthy men were treated with GR32191, a thromboxane receptor antagonist with a long duration of action, in a double blind placebo-controlled crossover study. Platelet aggregation in response to a thromboxane (TX) mimetic (U46619) was studied turbidometrically using platelet rich plasma (PRP) prepared 12 h after dosing (80 mg po) and 1.5 h after a second dose (40 mg po). To determine whether the long lasting inhibition caused by GR32191 is associated with persistent inhibitory activity in plasma (from residual drug or from an active metabolite), platelet poor plasma (PPP) from treated subjects was mixed with PRP from placebo treated controls. 12 h after dosing this caused 40-80% inhibition, consistent with the plasma concentration of GR32191. Inhibition of U46619 in PRP from GR32191 treated subjects mixed with PPP from controls was even greater (essentially 100%). We conclude that the prolonged activity of GR32191 is due in part to a reduction in available thromboxane receptors and in part to its persistence in plasma for longer than had previously been appreciated.

INTRODUCTION

GR32191 is a potent and specific thromboxane receptor antagonist (5,6). Following administration to man (0.25 mg/kg by mouth) its biological activity persists for >12 h (13). This could be explained by permanent blockade or loss of thromboxane receptors, and there have been two recent reports of such irreversible inactivation (1,12). We have studied the action of GR32191 on platelet aggregation *ex vivo*, with particular reference to the additional possibility of persistent biological activity in plasma attributable either to the drug itself or to an active metabolite. This was investigated by means of mixing experiments in which PRP from placebo-treated subjects acted as a bioassay to detect residual activity in PPP from subjects previously treated with GR32191. In addition, serum TXB_2 was determined as a measure of thrombin-stimulated platelet thromboxane synthesis.

METHODS

Twenty four healthy non-smoking men (18-40 years) consented to participate in the study. The trial was performed according to a double-blind crossover design, each subject being randomly allocated to receive placebo on one occasion and GR32191 on another, two weeks or more apart. A balanced block randomisation permitted subjects to be studied blindly in pairs, such that one member was treated with active drug and one with placebo on each occasion. Venous blood (5 ml) was obtained using a 19 gauge needle for preparation of serum (8) for TXB_2 determination. Subjects received GR32191 (80 mg po) or matched placebo at 8.00 pm. At 8.00 am the following morning venous blood (25 ml) was obtained as before. One portion was used to prepare serum for TXB_2 determination, one portion was heparinised for preparation of plasma for GR32191 determination by HPLC (9), and the remainder was anticoagulated with trisodium citrate (0.31% w/v final concentration) for preparation of PPP and PRP. The platelet count in PRP was adjusted using PPP from the same subject to 400,000/µl. Aggregation was studied at 37 °C in a four channel PAP-4 aggregometer.

Aggregation was measured in PRP diluted 1:1 with PPP 1 min before addition of U46619, according to a code prepared by the Biometrics Department, Glaxo Group Research. Aggregation was recorded as % change in light transmission 4 min after agonist; 100% was taken as the transmission of PPP. After blood sampling, subjects received a second dose of the same medication as 12 h previously: either GR32191 (40 mg) or placebo. Blood was sampled 1.5 h following this, and PRP and PPP prepared and studied as before.

Data are presented as means ± s.e.m.. Differences between aggregation to U46619 in mixtures of PPP with PRP were evaluated using a non-parametric analysis of variance (Friedman's method). TXB_2 measurements before and after active treatment or placebo were compared by paired t-test (2-tailed). Differences were considered significant when $P < 0.05$.

RESULTS

The effect of GR32191 on platelet aggregation caused by U46619 is shown in Figure 1.

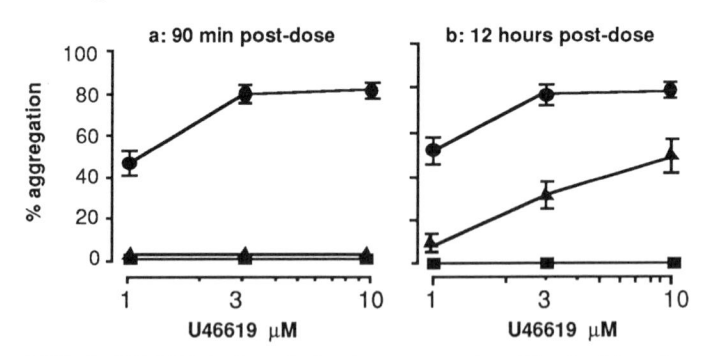

FIG. 1. U46619-induced platelet aggregation 90 min (a) and 12 h (b) after GR32191 or placebo. GR32191 active (■), placebo (●), mix (▲). For details of mixing experiment, see text.

U46619 (1, 3 and 10 µM) caused dose dependent aggregation in PRP from placebo treated controls. Treatment with GR32191 90 min before blood sampling abolished the effect of U46619 on PRP and admixture of PPP from GR32191-treated subjects abolished aggregation to U46619 in PRP from placebo treated subjects (Figure 1a). Twelve hours after dosing (Figure 1b),

PPP from GR32191-treated subjects inhibited aggregation to U46619 of platelets from placebo treated controls by 40-80%, significantly (P < 0.001) less than the inhibition in PRP from GR32191 treated subjects. Mean plasma concentrations of GR32191 were 36.6 ± 2.7 nM at 12 h and 431.9 ± 23.6 nM at 90 min. Serum TXB_2 concentrations are shown in table 1.

TABLE 1: Effect of GR32191 on serum TXB_2 concentration (ng ml^{-1})

Placebo		GR32191	
Baseline	12 h	Baseline	12 h
240.8 ± 21.8	234.1 ± 20.8	268.3 ± 21.4	204.1 ± 13.8*

(*differs from baseline and placebo day, each P < 0.02)

Serum TXB_2 was significantly inhibited by prior ingestion of GR32191 by approximately 20%.

DISCUSSION

These observations confirm that GR32191 causes prolonged inhibition of responses of platelets to U46619 (13). The mixing experiment reported here is relevant to the mechanism of this protracted activity, by showing that plasma from treated subjects contains persistent biological activity 12 h after dosing. This could be explained either by residual plasma GR32191 or by an active metabolite. The pA_2 of GR32191 measured at concentrations of around 30 nM in acute experiments on human platelets *in vitro* is reported to be 8.3 (7). The dose ratio in the mixing experiment 12 h after dosing was approximately 10 with a mean concentration of GR32191 of 36.6 nM, corresponding to an estimated pA_2 of 8.4. The surprisingly close agreement between these estimates argues strongly against prolonged biological activity being due to an active metabolite, and indicates that in addition to the reduction in thromboxane receptors observed by others (1,12), prolonged activity of GR32191 after oral dosing in man is also due to its persistence in plasma for longer than had previously been appreciated.

The findings also bear on the question of the role of TXA_2 in platelet activation. Since activated platelets produce TXA_2, which is itself a potent stimulus to aggregation, TXA_2 may act as a positive feedback amplifying an initial stimulus. Such reinforcement would be interrupted by a TX receptor antagonist. This could account for the highly significant reduction in TXB_2 in serum from clotted blood from subjects treated with GR32191 as compared with the same subjects treated with placebo. When blood is allowed to clot *ex vivo* thrombin is formed and stimulates platelet TXA_2 synthesis (11). TXA_2 could reinforce this action of thrombin and GR32191 would antagonise this, explaining the observed reduction of serum TXB_2 concentration. By contrast to the reduction in serum TXB_2 described here, we have previously reported that urinary TXB_2 and 2,3-dinor TXB_2 excretion are not affected by GR32191 (9). These breakdown products reflect basal TXA_2 biosynthesis. This therefore argues against involvement of TXA_2 in reinforcing platelet activation under basal conditions in healthy non-smoking young men. Platelet activation in healthy subjects may occur as platelets are activated intermittently at spatially discrete sites within the circulation, without concomitant platelet-platelet interaction (aggregation). The situation is quite different in pathological states such as unstable angina in which thrombosis occurs on a ruptured atheromatous plaque and TX production is increased (4,10). Thromboxane biosynthesis is also increased in apparently healthy cigarette smokers (2,3,7). It will therefore be of great interest to determine whether a TX receptor antagonist such as GR32191 will inhibit TX synthesis in such circumstances.

ACKNOWLEDGEMENT

This work was supported by Glaxo plc. Ella Trasankowska (Glaxo) performed the HPLC analysis of GR32191. We thank Paul Morrison (director: Guy's Drug Research Unit) for invaluable discussions.

REFERENCES

1. Armstrong, R.A., Lumley, P., and Humphrey, P.P.A. (1990): *Br. J. Pharmac.*, 99: 113P.

2. Barrow, S.E., Ward, P.S., Sleightholm, M.A., Ritter, J.M., and Dollery, C.T. (1989): *Biochim. Biophys. Acta*, 993: 121-127.

3. Fischer, S., Bernutz, C., Meier, H., and Weber, P. (1986): *Biochim. Biophys. Acta*, 876: 194-199.

4. Fitzgerald, D.J., Roy, L., Catella, F., and FitzGerald, G.A. (1986): *N. Engl. J. Med.*, 315: 983-989.

5. Lumley, P., Collington, E.W., Hallett, P., Hornby, E.J., Humphrey, P.P.A., Wallace, C.J., Jack, D., and Brittain, R.T. (1987): *Thromb. Haemostas.*, 58: 261.

6. Lumley, P., White, B.P., and Humphrey, P.P.A. (1989). *Br. J. Pharmac.*, 97: 783-794.

7. Nowak, J., Murray, J.J., Oates, J.A., and FitzGerald, G.A, (1987): *Circulation*, 76: 6-14.

8. Patrono, C., Ciabbatoni, G., Pinca, E., Pugliesi, F., Castrucci, G., de salvo, A., Satta, M.A., and Peskar, B.A. (1980): *Thromb. Res.*, 17: 317-327.

9. Ritter, J.M., Benjamin, N., Doktor, H.S., Barrow, S.E., Mant, T.G.K., Schey, S. and Stewart-Long P. (1990): *Br. J. Clin. Pharmac.*, 29: 431-436.

10. Sherman, C.T., Litvack, F., and Grundfest, W. (1986): *N. Engl. J. Med.*, 315: 913-919.

11. Shuman, M.A., and Levine, S.P. (1980): *J. Clin. Invest.*, 65: 307-313.

12. Takahara, K., Murray, R., FitzGerald, G.A., and Fitzgerald, D.J. (1990): *J. Biol. Chem.*, 265: 6836-6844.

13. Thomas M., Lumley, P., Ballard, P., and O'Brien, J.R. (1987): *Thromb. Haemostas.*, 58: 181.

Advances in Prostaglandin, Thromboxane, and Leukotriene Research, Vol. 21,
edited by B. Sameulsson et al.
Raven Press, Ltd., New York © 1990.

EFFECT OF BAY U 3405, A NEW THROMBOXANE ANTAGONIST, ON ARACHIDONIC ACID INDUCED THROMBOEMBOLISM

F. Seuter, E. Perzborn and V.B. Fiedler

Institute of Pharmacology, BAYER AG,
Aprather Weg 18 a, 5600 Wuppertal 1, FRG

Thromboxane A_2 (TXA_2) induces platelet aggregation, vasoconstriction and bronchoconstriction (6,8). TXA_2 antagonists may be useful for the treatment of ischaemia, thromboembolic and respiratory diseases.

BAY U 3405, an enantiomerically pure compound (7), potently inhibits platelet aggregation in vitro and ex vivo (10,11), vasoconstriction (5), bronchoconstriction (3,4) and coronary artery thrombosis (2).

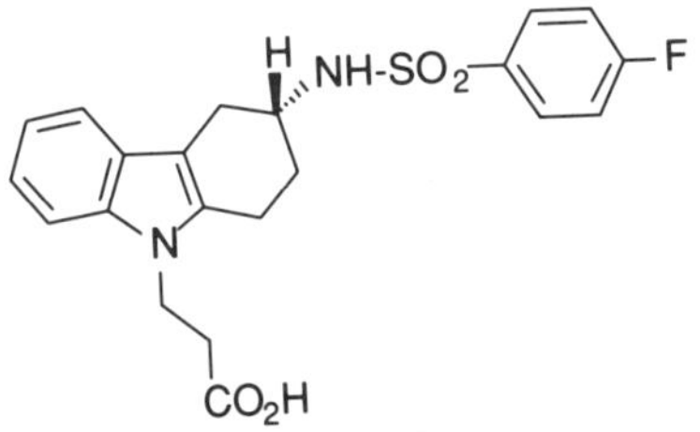

Fig. 1. BAY U 3405, (3R)-3-(4-Fluorophenylsulfonamido)-1,2,3,4-tetrahydro-9-carbazolepropanoic acid

The purpose of this study was to investigate the effect of BAY U 3405 on sudden death provoked by arachidonic acid (AA), an experimental model introduced by Silver et al. in 1974 (12). Sudden death most likely is caused by embolized platelet aggregates, direct TXA_2 mediated cardiovascular effects and bronchoconstriction.

MATERIALS AND METHODS

All experiments were carried out in urethane (1 g/kg i.m. and again after 30 min 0.5 g/kg i.v. into a marginal ear vein) anesthetized male CHBB:HM rabbits (Thomae, Biberach/FRG) weighing about 2 kg. The animals were fed a standard diet for 1-2 weeks and then fasted for 16 h before the experiments.

Arachidonic acid (Sigma^R A 6382, 99 % pure, MW 304.5) was dissolved in an equimolar sodium hydroxide solution, and was further diluted with physiologic saline up to 2.5 mmol/l. 1.5 mg/kg sodium arachidonate solution was injected into a marginal ear vein over 30 s causing respiratory distress, seizures and death of more than 90 % in the control group within a few minutes.

An equimolar solution of sodium hydroxyde was used to prepare a solution of the sodium salt from the acid form of BAY U 3405. The drug was administered orally to conscious animals using a rubber stomach tube, 1 h before injection of the challenging agent. Results were statistically analyzed by the chi-square method.

RESULTS

Following AA injection 97 % of the animals died in the vehicle treated group. Pretreatment with oral doses of 1,3 and 10 mg/kg BAY U 3405 resulted in a dose-dependent protection of the animals from eicosanoid induced sudden death (Fig. 2).

The survival rate was 100 % after 10 mg/kg, 58 % at 3 mg/kg and 10 % at 1 mg/kg. The effects achieved are statistically significant at both 3 and 10 mg/kg p.o. compared to control.

20 min after administration of 10 mg/kg p.o. BAY U 3405 40 % of the animals survived, reaching 100 % after 60 min (Fig. 3). This effect persisted for up to 16 h, but declining to base-line at 24 h. 3 mg/kg p.o. was less effective (Fig. 3).

SUMMARY AND CONCLUSIONS

The model of AA-induced sudden death employed in these investigations seems to be appropriate for studying the efficacy of TXA_2-antagonists. The actions of TXA_2 on platelets, respiratory and vascular tissue are considered as key events resulting in the death of the animals (1,9).

The results obtained in this study, using BAY U

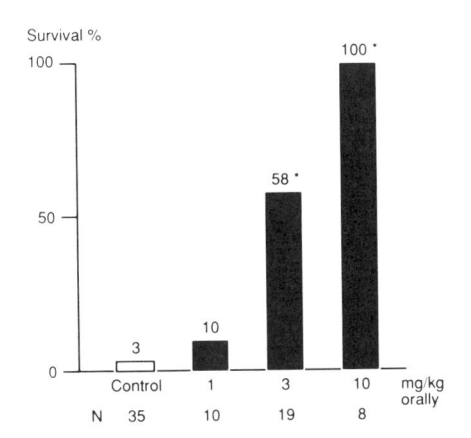

FIG. 2. Effect of BAY U 3405 on AA induced sudden death in rabbits. BAY U 3405 was administered 1 h before AA injection.
* Significantly different by chi-square test ($p < 0.01$).

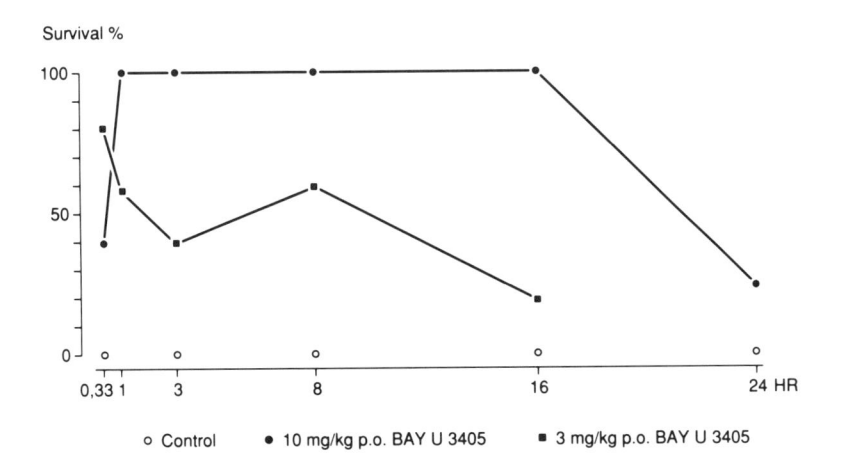

FIG. 3. Duration of action of BAY U 3405 on AA induced sudden death in rabbits.

3405 as a selective TXA_2 receptor antagonist (5), clearly show that TXA_2 mediated processes are effectively abolished by this type of drug.

Since TXA$_2$ is implicated in the pathophysiology of many diseases (6,8), potent TXA$_2$ antagonists appear to be useful for treatment of these disorders. BAY U 3405 seems to fulfil these requirements. The threshold dose is 1 to 3 mg/kg p.o.. In addition, there is a rapid onset and long duration of action at 10 mg/kg p.o. under the experimental conditions used.

REFERENCES

1. Darius, H., and Lefer, A.M. (1985): Thromb.Res., 40:663-675.
2. Fiedler, V.B., Perzborn, E., Seuter, F., Rosentreter, U., and Böshagen, H. (1989): Arzneim.-Forsch., 39:1527-1530.
3. Francis, H.P., Greenham, S., Patel, U., Thompson, A.M., and Gardiner, P.J. (1990): Br.J.Pharmacol., 99 (Proc.Suppl.):60P.
4. McKenniff, M.G., Norman, P., and Gardiner, P.J. (1990): Br.J.Pharmacol., 99 (Proc.Suppl):59P.
5. Perzborn, E., Seuter, F., Fiedler, V.B., Rosentreter, U., and Boeshagen, H. (1989): Arzneim.-Forsch., 39:1527-1530.
6. Peterson, M.B. (1989): In: Prostaglandins in Clinical Practice, edited by W.D. Watkins, M.B. Peterson, and J. R. Fletcher. pp. 21-44. Raven Press, New York.
7. Rosentreter, U., Böshagen, H., Seuter, F., Perzborn, E., and Fiedler, V.B. (1989): Arzneim.-Forsch., 39:1519-1521.
8. Said, S.I., and Mojarad, M. In: Prostaglandins in Clinical Practice, edited by W.D. Watkins, M.B. Peterson, and J. R. Fletcher. pp. 45-58. Raven Press, New York.
9. Seuter, F., and Busse, W.-D. (1979): In: Arachidonic acid metabolism in inflammation and thrombosis, edited by K. Brune, and M. Baggiolini. pp. 175-183. AAS4. Birkhaeuser, Basel.
10. Seuter, F., Perzborn, E., Fiedler, V.B., Rosentreter, U., and Boeshagen, H. (1989a): Thromb. Haemostas., 62:345.
11. Seuter, F., Perzborn, E., Fiedler, V.B., Rosentreter, U., and Boeshagen, H. (1989b): Arzneim.-Forsch., 39:1525-1527.
12. Silver, M.J., Hoch, W., Kocsic, J.J., Ingerman, C.M., and Smith, J.B. (1974): Science, 183:-1085-1087.

Advances in Prostaglandin, Thromboxane, and Leukotriene Research, Vol. 21,
edited by B. Sameulsson et al.
Raven Press, Ltd., New York © 1990.

RATIONAL DESIGN OF THROMBOXANE A2 ANTAGONISTS

N. Hamanaka, T. Seko, T. Miyazaki and A. Kawasaki

Minase Research Institute, Ono Pharmaceutical Co., Ltd.,
Shimamoto, Mishima, Osaka 618, Japan

Thromboxane A2 (TXA2) is well known to play a very important role in cardiovascular system and it is proposed to be an origin of some kinds of diseases, *e.g.*, angina and thrombosis. Therefore, TXA2 antagonist is of great importance in order to develop a therapeutic agent for these diseases.

We have been working on the development of novel and significant drugs which antagonize the actions of both TXA2 and PGH2. In the course of this investigation, the compounds **1** (ONO-NT-026) (1, 4) and **2** (ONO-NT-126) have been found to show the potent antagonistic activities (platelet aggregation and smooth muscle contraction) (2). The absolute configurations of the ring systems of the compounds **1** and **2** are opposite to each other. This result can be interpreted only by the conformational similarity of these compounds. Here we describe a clear function of chirality for TXA2 antagonist using the spectroscopic method and the computer aided molecular dynamics. Based on these findings, the rational design of new antagonists is now possible.

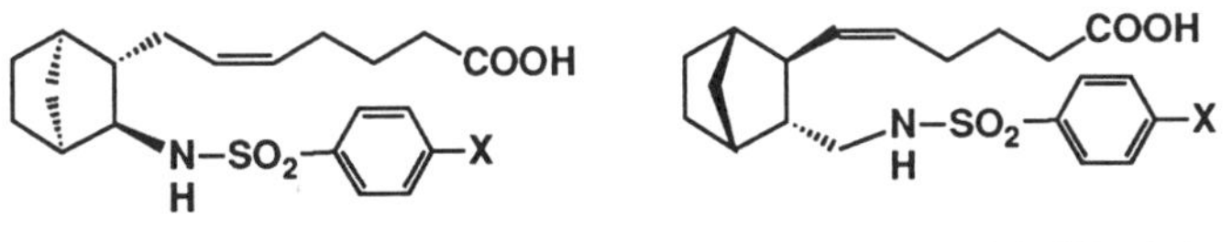

1 X=CH3 (ONO-NT-026)
X=H (S-145)

2 X=CH3 (ONO-NT-125)
3 X=Br (ONO-NT-126)

Fig. 1

In order to confirm the conformational similarity between **1** and **2**, a careful NMR analysis was carried out. Selective proton-proton one dimensional NOE and two dimensional NOE experiments on **1** showed the following results. Irradiation of the olefinic protons (C5-H and C6-H are not separated at 500 MHz) resulted in observation of a weak NOE with the aromatic protons and of clear NOE with C12-H and C9-H. This revealed that **1** is an equilibrium mixture of two conformers, **1a** and **1b**. A Newman projection formula seen from C8 to C7 is shown in Fig. 2.

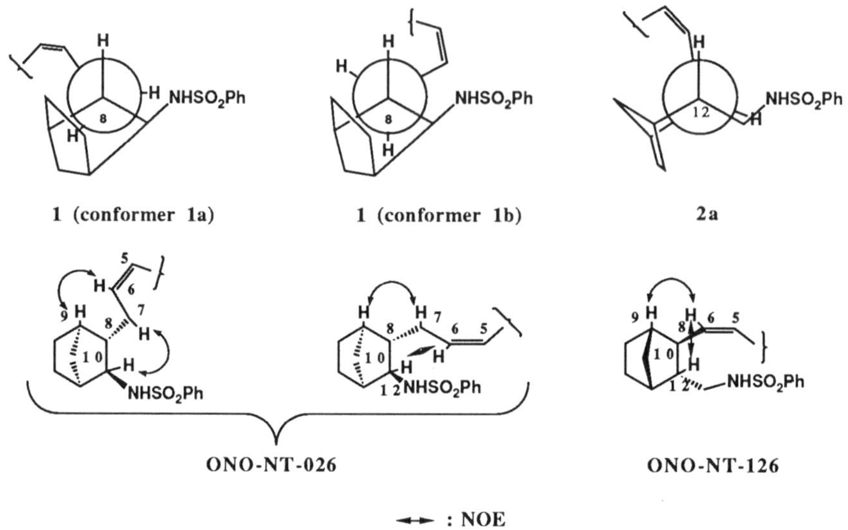

Fig. 2

The same NMR experiments on **2** showed that the olefinic C6-H does not have only a weak NOE with C9-H but also a clear NOE with C10 endo-H and C12-H. Thus, the conformation **2a** should be relatively fixed. A Newman projection formula seen from C12 through C8 is also shown in Fig. 2, and it is in good agreement with that of **1a**. It seems that the difference in biological activities between **1** and **2** must be the result of the difference in fixation of the active conformation.

For further information on the conformation of **1** and **2**, the possible conformers were calculated by molecular dynamics. Since there are no generally accepted parameters at present for the sulfonylamide function, CHARMm (3) was utilized in the molecular dynamics. A rough approximation was enough for our primary aim, and in order to eliminate the effects of the minor conformational mobility, C1-C3 moiety was excluded from the calculation. The results are shown in Fig. **3** where only a few conformers were selected from a group of similar ones. As expected from the previous results of NMR analysis, the sulfonyl amide moiety in both **1** and **2** can rotate freely, and therefore its position in a molecule could not be determined. However, the relationship between the double bond and ring system was completely identifiable as that shown in the NMR analysis. Thus, there are two preferred conformers for **1** and one for **2**. The energy difference in the conformers **1a** and **1b** was approximately 0.3-0.7 kcal/mol, which is the same as that of **2a**. We therefore concluded that the bioactive general conformer is **3**.

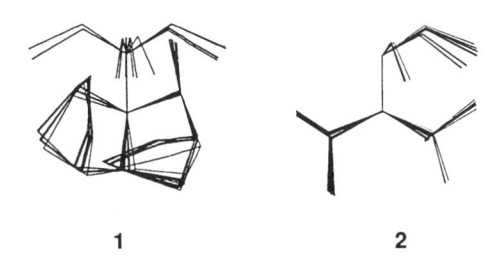

1   2

Computer generated conformers

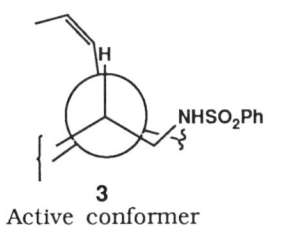

3
Active conformer

Fig. 3

To construct the active comformer by the another structre, we used the cyclopentane ring. In Fig. **4** the structurs of four optical isomers of cyclopentane derivatives and their antaginistic activities are shown. Among these, the compound **4** showed the potent antagonistic activity. Two Newman projection formula of the compound **4** seen from C4 to C3, **4a** and from C2 to C3, **4b**, are shown in Fig. 5. The structure **4a** did match the conformer **1a**. The others could not take the active conformer energetically.

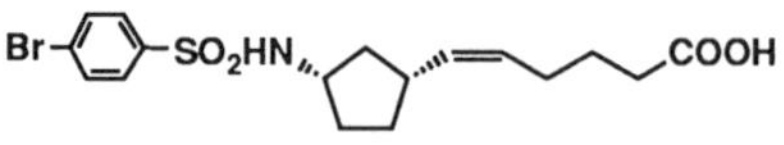

4 0.03 μM

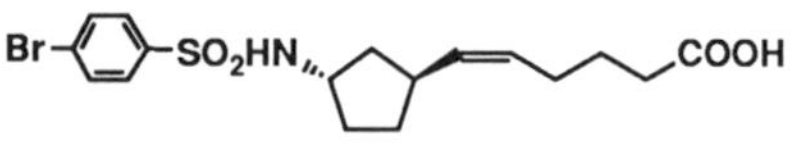

5 0.66 μM

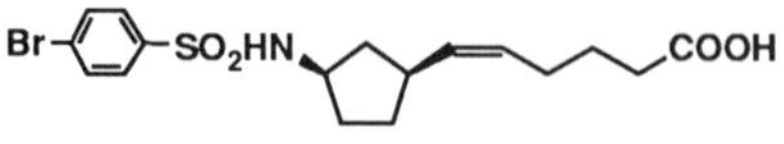

6 0.51 μM

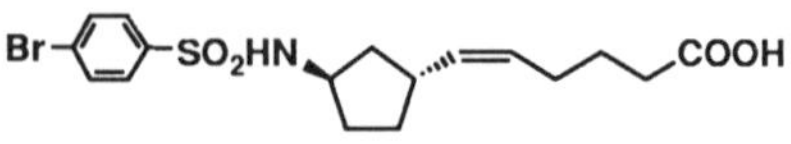

7 0.13 μM

Inhibition of human platelet aggregation induced by STA$_2$ (IC$_{50}$)

Fig. 4

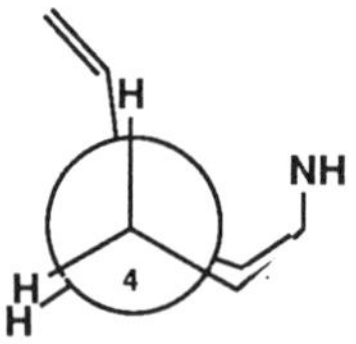

4a (C4 to C3)

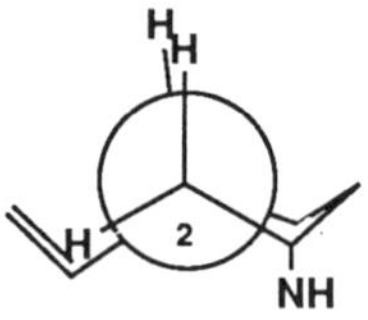

4b (C2 to C3)

Fig. 5

References

1. Furuta, K., Hayashi, S., Miwa, Y., Yamamoto, H. (1987): Tetrahedron Lett., 28: 5841.
2. Hamanaka, N., Seko, T., Miyazaki, T., Naka, M., Furuta, K., Yamamoto, H. (1989): Tetrahedron Lett., 30: 2399.
3. Pettitt, B. M., Karplus, M. (1985): J. Am. Chem. Soc., 107: 1166.
4. Similar compound was reported by Shionogi company: Narisada, M., Ohtani, M., Watanabe, F., Uchida, K., Arita, H., Doteuchi, M., Hanasaki, K., Kakushi, H., Ohtani, K. (1988): J. Med. Chem., 31: 1847.

PHORBOL ESTER-INDUCED EXPRESSION OF THE COMMON, LOW-AFFINITY BINDING SITE FOR PRIMARY PROSTANOIDS IN VASCULAR SMOOTH MUSCLE CELLS

K. Hanasaki, M. Kishi, and H. Arita

Shionogi Research Laboratories, Shionogi & Co.,Ltd., Fukushima-ku, Osaka 553, Japan

Biochemical charcterization of prostaglandin (PG) receptors has been carried out using radioligand-binding assays and regulation mechanisms for the receptor functions have been reported in several cell types (1,5). However, the mechanisms on the gene expression of the PG receptors have not yet been clarified.

We have previously shown the presence of two specific binding sites for thromboxane A2 (TXA2) agonists in cultured rat vascular smooth muscle cells (VSMC), as depicted in Fig. 1 (2). One is a high-affinity binding site corresponding to the "TXA2 receptor", which mediates the TXA2-induced contraction of vascular smooth muscles. The other is a common, low-affinity binding site for primary prostanoids, called the "primary PG site", which is recognized by TXA2 agonists as well as primary PGs, such as PGE1, PGD2 and PGF2α, but not by TXA2 antagonists (3).

The first objective of the present paper is to evaluate the structural requirements for recognition of the primary PG site. Next, we examined the differences in the modulation by protein kinase C (PKC) activators between the TXA2 receptor and the primary PG site, since PKC has been reported to regulate the binding characteristics in some receptor systems (7).

METHODS

VSMC were prepared from explants of the thoracic aorta of Sprague-Dawley rats by the method of Ross (6). The cells were cultivated in Dulbecco's modified Eagle's medium supplemented with 20% fetal bovine serum (GIBCO) and antibiotics in a humidified atmosphere of 95% air and 5% CO2. For binding assay, confluent VSMC were washed twice with phosphate buffered saline, then harvested in 0.125% trypsin solution containing 0.01% EDTA and finally suspended with Hanks' medium (pH 7.6) containing 0.1% BSA. The binding study was performed by incubating VSMC (1.5 x 10^6 cells) with each [3H]-labeled radioligand in 0.5 ml at 24°C. Specific binding is defined as the differences between binding in the presence and absence of 10 uM of the respective unlabeled ligand. The TXA2 receptor was evaluated using [3H]SQ29,548, one of the selective TXA2 antagonists, as a radioligand. The primary PG site was characterized using [3H]PGF2α and [3H]PGE1.

RESULTS AND DISCUSSION

In order to determine the binding specificity of the primary PG site, a number of structurally modified analogs of PGF2α were examined for their abilities to displace the specific bindings of [3H]PGF2α (1.8 nM) and [3H]PGE1 (4.3 nM). Among various PGF2α analogs, 9α-11β-PGF2 showed a similar displacement potency (IC_{50} = ca. 100 nM) with primary PGs as well as TXA2 agonists, demonstrating a loose recognition for substituents on the cyclopentane ring of PGs. In contrast, PGF2α analogs with modification in the 15-hydroxy group and 13,14-dihydro-PGF2α blocked the bindings with much lower potency ($IC_{50} > 3$ μM), indicating that the primary PG site

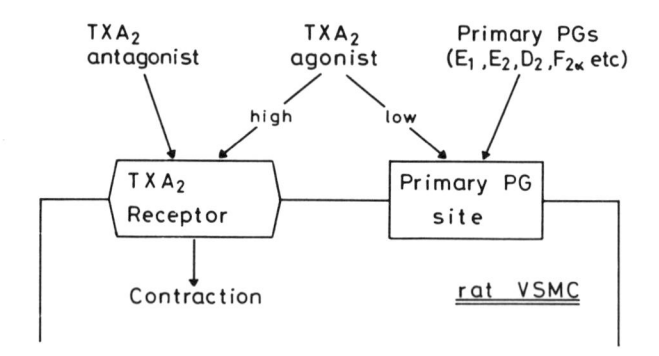

FIG. 1. Two specific binding sites for TXA2 agonists in rat cultured vascular smooth muscle cells.

strictly recognize the allyl alchol moiety of the ω-side chain of PGs. This view is further supported by the lower inhibition activities of the TXA2 antagonists which definitely modified in the ω-side chain. However, 12(S)-hydroxy-5,8,10-heptadecatrienoic acid, which contains the ω-side chain structures of PGs, could not suppress the [3H]PGF2α binding at up to 3 µM, demonstrating an essential recognition of the ring structures of PGs.

Next, the effect of phorbol myristate acetate (PMA), a known PKC activator (4), on the binding activities for the TXA2 receptor and primary PG site was examined. After 4-h treatment of VSMC with 100 nM PMA, significant increases were observed in the binding activities of [3H]PGF2α and [3H]PGE1, and both activities reached the maximum level after 12-h treatment. The maximum magnitude of the increment was about 8-fold the binding level in the control VSMC. In contrast, the [3H]SQ29,548 binding activity for the TXA2 receptor did not significantly change even after 34-h treatment with PMA. As

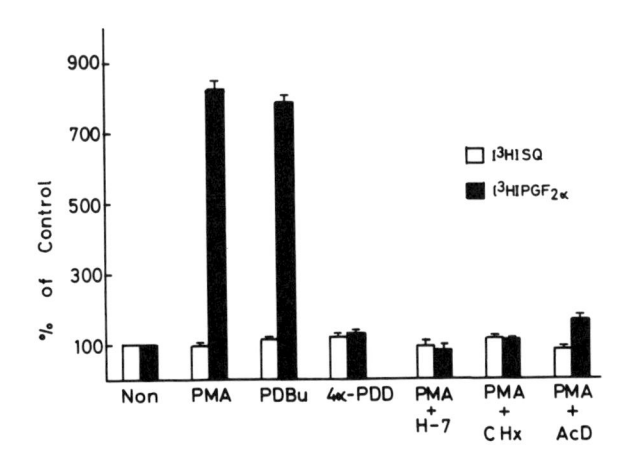

FIG. 2. Effects of various agents on the binding activity for the primary PG site in VSMC. Rat VSMC were pretreated with 1 µM of PMA, PDBu, 4α-PDD, PMA plus 50 µM H-7, PMA plus 10 µg/ml CHx or PMA plus 2.5 µg/ml AcD for 24 h. After washing, specific binding activities for the VSMC were examined by incubating them with 1.8 nM [3H]PGF2α (■) or 5.6 nM [3H]SQ29548 (□) at 24°C for 120 min. The control value was defined as the specific binding for the nontreated VSMC.

shown in Fig. 2, phorbol dibutylate (PDBu), another PKC-activating phorbol ester, was also effective for enhancing the [3H]PGF2α binding. However, 4α-phorbol didecanoate (4α-PDD), which does not stimulate PKC, had no effect at 1 μM. Furthermore, PKC inhibitor, H-7, completely blocked the PMA effects, suggesting that PMA-induced up-regulation of the primary PG site depends on PKC-mediated mechanism. The PMA-induced increment of [3H]PGF2α binding was also effectively suppressed by pretreatment with cycloheximide (CHx) and actinomycin D (AcD), indicating the requirement of protein synthesis as well as transcription. However, the binding activity of [3H]SQ29,548 was unaltered by pretreatment with these agents. Scatchard analyses revealed that treatment with PMA caused an approximately 8-fold increase in the binding density of the primary PG site without significant changes in the binding affinity.

In conclusion, our work has provided the first evidence of an expression mechanism of a primary PG site through a pathway involving PKC. Angiotensin II, which is known to activate PKC through receptor binding, also possessed the increment effects on the primary PG site. Thus, the expression of the primary PG site might be heterologously regulated by the physiological agonists which can activate PKC. Since the 15-hydroxy group and the 13,14-double bond in the ω-side chain is known as an essential structure for physiological activities of PGs, the primary PG site might represent the site necessary for the induction of some functional activities.

REFERENCES

1. Hanasaki, K., Mizuno, Y., Ikeda, M., Shimonishi, M., Yoshimura, S., Tomita, K., and Ichikawa, A. (1987) Biochim. Biophys. Acta 927: 261-268.
2. Hanasaki, K., and Arita, H. (1989) Biochim. Biophys. Acta 1013: 28-35.
3. Hanasaki, K., Kishi, M., and Arita, H. (1990) J. Biol. Chem. 265: 4871-4875.
4. Nishizuka, Y. (1986) Science 233: 305-312.
5. Robertson, R. P. (1986) Prostaglandins 31: 395-411.
6. Ross, R. (1971) J. Cell. Biol. 50: 172-186.
7. White, S. S., and Ojeda, S. R. (1981) Endocrinology 108: 347-349.

Ca²⁺ TRANSIENTS EVOKED BY PROSTANOIDS IN SWISS 3T3 CELLS SUGGEST AN FP-RECEPTOR MEDIATED RESPONSE

D.F. WOODWARD, C.E. FAIRBAIRN, D.D. GOODRUM,
A. H-P. KRAUSS, T.L. RALSTON, and L.S. WILLIAMS

Allergan Pharmaceuticals, Department of Biochemistry
2525 Dupont Drive, Irvine, CA 92715, U.S.A.

The FP-receptor is described by the working classification for prostanoid receptors as specific for $PGF_{2\alpha}$ and is currently characterized according to the rank order of potency for natural prostanoids and fluprostenol in $PGF_{2\alpha}$-sensitive preparations (1,2). The studies described herein further characterize the pharmacology of the putative FP-receptor by using the Ca²⁺ transient in Swiss 3T3 cells as a convenient $PGF_{2\alpha}$-sensitive system.

MATERIALS AND METHODS

PGD_2, PGE_2, $PGF_{2\alpha}$, U-46619, and 11-deoxy PGE_1 (Cayman Chemical, Ann Arbor, MI) and BW 245C (Burroughs Wellcome, Beckenham, UK) were dissolved in Na_2CO_3 and neutralized. PGI_2 (Cayman Chemical) was dissolved in TRIS and Daltroban (Boehringer-Mannheim, West Germany) was dissolved in Na_2CO_3 to pH 8.5. fluprostenol (Cooper, Berkhampsted, UK) and sulprostone (Berlex, Cedar Knolls, NJ) were dissolved in saline. PDGF (Sigma) was dissolved in 1N CH_3COOH.

Measurement of intracellular [Ca²⁺] was achieved by incorporating the Ca²⁺-sensitive fluorescent probe Fura-2AM into Swiss 3T3 cells in suspension as previously described (6). Fluorescence was measured in a Perkin-Elmer LS-5 spectrophotometer at excitation and emission wavelengths of 340 and 492 nM, respectively. Each experimental determination employed 10⁶ cells suspended in Schmuells buffer. For studies in Ca²⁺-free Schmuells buffer, each cuvette also contained 0.4 mM EGTA. Calibration of the Fura 2 signal was as previously described for Quin 2 (5) and Fura 2 (6). Briefly the cells were lysed with digitonin (10 µl x 100 mg/ml in DMSO). EGTA (100 mM) and sufficient 10N NaOH to adjust the pH to 8.5 were then successively added to obtain minimum fluorescence.

RESULTS AND DISCUSSION

The effects of fluprostenol and the natural prostanoids PGD_2, PGE_2, $PGF_{2\alpha}$, and PGI_2 on $[Ca^{2+}]$ of Swiss 3T3 cells suspended in Schmuells medium containing 1.4 mM $CaCl_2$ are depicted in fig. 1. All, except PGI_2, caused a dose-dependent Ca^{2+} transient with the following rank order of potency: fluprostenol $\geq$ $PGF_{2\alpha}$ > PGD_2 > PGE_2 > PGI_2. The effects of relatively selective prostanoid receptor subtype agonists on $[Ca^{2+}]$ in Swiss 3T3 cells were similarly examined (fig. 2). Representative prostanoid receptor agonists were as follows: BW 245C, DP-agonist; sulprostone, EP_1/EP_3 agonist; 11-deoxy PGE_1; EP_2-agonist; U-46619, TP-agonist (1-4). BW 245C and 11-deoxy PGE_1 were essentially inactive over a 10^{-7} - 10^{-4}M concentration range. U-46619 and sulprostone exhibited relatively weak activity compared to fluprostenol. Since U-46619 is a potent TxA_2-mimetic, the effect of the TxA_2-antagonist Daltroban (BM 13505) on U-46619 induced Ca^{2+} transients was examined, but found ineffective.

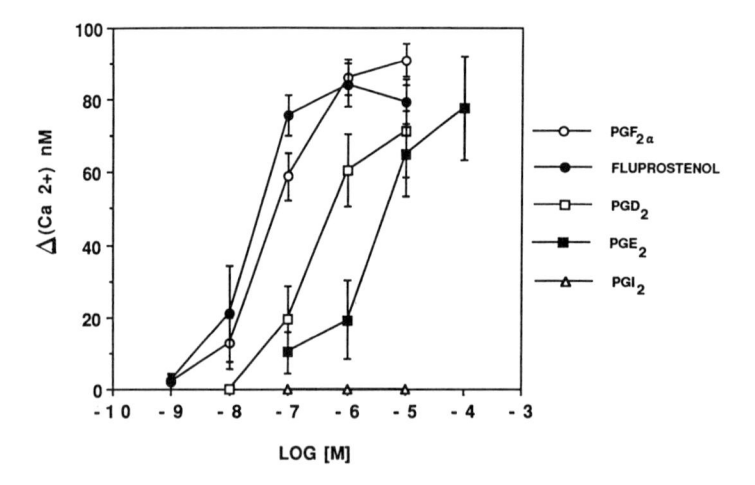

FIG. 1 Effect of fluprostenol and natural prostanoids on intracellular $[Ca^{2+}]$ in Swiss 3T3 cells.
Values are mean $\pm$ SEM; n=4.

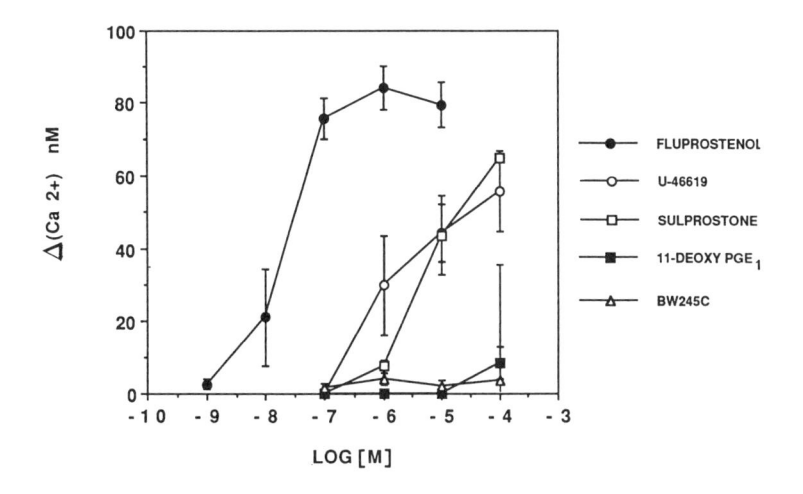

FIG. 2 Effect of prostanoid analogues on intracellular [Ca^{2+}] in Swiss 3T3 cells. Values are mean ± SEM; n = 4.

Studies in Ca^{2+}-free medium demonstrated that the increase in cytosolic [Ca^2] evoked by fluprostenol, PGF$_{2\alpha}$, PGD$_2$, and PGE$_2$ was mainly of intracellular origin. Sequential addition provided indirect evidence pertaining to the number of possible receptor subtypes involved in prostanoid induced Ca^{2+} transients (6). In these studies, cells were pretreated with a maximally effective dose of each prostanoid and the [Ca^{2+}] was allowed to re-equilibrate to a new basal level. Subsequently, a cumulative dose-response experiment was performed in the presence of the prostanoid originally added. Cells pretreated with a maximally effective dose of fluprostenol were refractory to subsequent addition of PGF$_{2\alpha}$, PGD$_2$, or PGE$_2$. Likewise, dose-response curves to fluprostenol could not be obtained after a maximal dose of PGF$_{2\alpha}$, PGD$_2$, or PGE$_2$. In contrast, the Ca^{2+} transient to PDGF was inaffected by prostanoid pretreatment (fig. 3 gives representative examples).

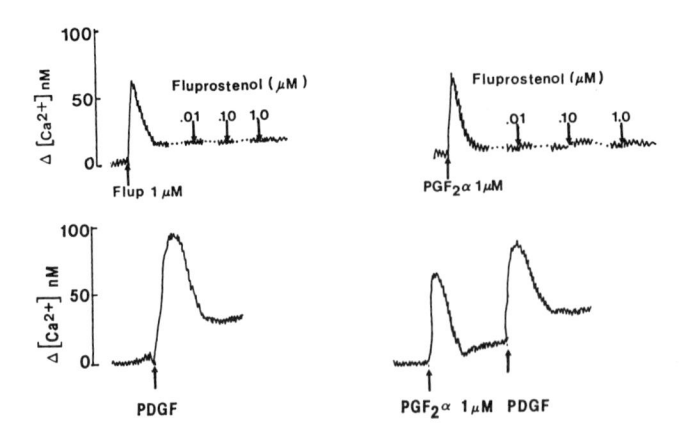

FIG. 3 Successive additions of prostanoids and PDGF (approximately 10 ng/ml) on intracellular $[Ca^{2+}]$ in Swiss 3T3 cells. For graded doses of prostanoids, additions are at 5 minute intervals.

These Ca^{2+} second messenger studies suggest that prostanoids stimulate Ca^{2+} release from the same intracellular pool and provide indirect evidence for the singular involvement of the FP-receptor as follows: a) rank order of potency (1,2); b) successive addition studies (6); c) PGD_2 and U-46619 effects are independent of DP- and TP-receptor stimulation.

REFERENCES

1. Coleman, R.A., Humphrey, P.P.A., and Kennedy, I. (1982) Trends in Autonom. Pharmacol. 3:35-49.

2. Coleman, R.A., Humphrey, P.P.A., and Kennedy, I., and Lumley, P. (1984) T.I.P.S. 5:303-305.

3. Dong, Y.J., and Jones, R.L. (1982) Br. J. Pharmacol. 76:149-155.

4. Narumiya, S. and Toda, N. (1985) Br. J. Pharmacol 85:367-375.

5. Tsien, R.Y., Pozzan, T., and Rink, T.J. (1982) J. Cell Biol. 94:325-334.

6. Yamaguchi, D.T., Hahn, T.J., Becker, T.G., Kleeman, C.R., and Muallem, S. (1988) J. Biol. Chem. 263:10745-10753.

SIGNAL TRANSDUCTION COUPLED TO PROSTAGLANDIN D_2

Seiji Ito, Manabu Negishi, Kazushige Sugama, Emiko Okuda-Ashitaka, and Osamu Hayaishi

Department of Cell Biology, Osaka Bioscience Institute, 6-2-4 Furuedai, Suita 565, Japan

Prostaglandin D_2 (PGD_2) produces a broad range of biological effects such as sleep induction, bronchoconstriction, vasoconstriction, and inhibition of platelet aggregation (2). Pharmacological analyses have indicated the presence of two groups of PGD_2-sensitive tissues and cells based on the difference in the order of potency of PGD_2 and its analogues (6). The action of PGD_2 is believed to be mediated by PGD_2 receptors on the plasma membrane. Most cells have at least two major signaling systems for transducing information mediated by receptors on the membrane. One system depends on the generation of cyclic AMP (cAMP), while the other system induces rapid turnover of inositol phospholipids as well as Ca^{2+} mobilization. In human platelets, PGD_2 is well known to inhibit aggregation by increasing intracellular cAMP. We (3) also recently reported that a fibroblastic cell line EBTr specifically responds to PGD_2 by elevating cAMP level and that ZK110841 (8) and AH6809 (4) serve as an agonist and an antagonist of PGD_2 for cAMP formation in EBTr cells, respectively. Here we report that PGD_2 can stimulate phosphoinositide metabolism through a receptor different from that coupled to the adenylate cyclase system.

RESULTS

PGD_2-induced Ca^{2+} Mobilization in Swiss 3T3 cells

It was reported that PGE_1 caused a rapid increase in cAMP level and also elevated cytoplasmic free Ca^{2+} concentration ($[Ca^{2+}]i$) in Swiss 3T3 cells (9). We examined whether these two responses to PGE_1 were mediated by the same receptor or not. PGE_1 induced a time- and dose-dependent increase in cAMP levels in the cells. Iloprost, a stable analogue of PGI_2, was one order more potent than PGE_1, and PGE_2 did not increase cAMP level in Swiss 3T3 cells, indicating that cAMP formation is mediated by PGI_2/PGE_1 receptor.

Next we observed rapid changes in $[Ca^{2+}]i$ in individual cells by PGs with a digital imaging fluorescence microscope. The resting [Ca^{2+}]i in fura-2-loaded cells was calculated to be 142 ± 3.3 nM. PGE$_1$ did not increase [Ca^{2+}]i at all and PGE$_2$ slightly increased it at 1 µM. Unexpectedly, when PGD$_2$ was challenged to the cells, it elicited a rapid and dose-dependent increase in [Ca^{2+}]i in most cells in a field, which returned to the basal level within 2 min. In contrast to cAMP formation in human platelets, ZK110841 and BW245C, another PGD$_2$ mimetic, showed no or a very weak effect on [Ca^{2+}]i in Swiss 3T3 cells. As reported previously, PGF$_{2\alpha}$ also elevated [Ca^{2+}]i. Although PGD$_2$ was 0.5-1 order less potent than PGF$_{2\alpha}$, a peak [Ca^{2+}]i obtained with PGD$_2$ was almost equivalent to that with PGF$_{2\alpha}$ at higher concentrations. PGD$_2$- or PGF$_{2\alpha}$-induced [Ca^{2+}]i change was also observed in a Ca^{2+}-free medium containing 0.5 mM EGTA, suggesting that Ca^{2+} was released from intracellular stores via inositol trisphosphate (IP$_3$).

Phosphoinositide Metabolism Stimulated by PGD$_2$

We next examined whether PGD$_2$ could stimulate phosphoinositide metabolism in Swiss 3T3 cells. [^{3}H]Inositol-labeled chromaffin cells were treated with 1 µM PGD$_2$ in the presence of 10 mM LiCl. PGD$_2$ induced rapid rises in IP$_3$ and inositol bisphosphate (IP$_2$) followed by a slower accumulation of inositol monophosphate. [^{3}H]IP$_3$ and [^{3}H]IP$_2$ levels were 250-300% of the control at 30 sec and continued to increase up to 10 min in a biphasic fashon.

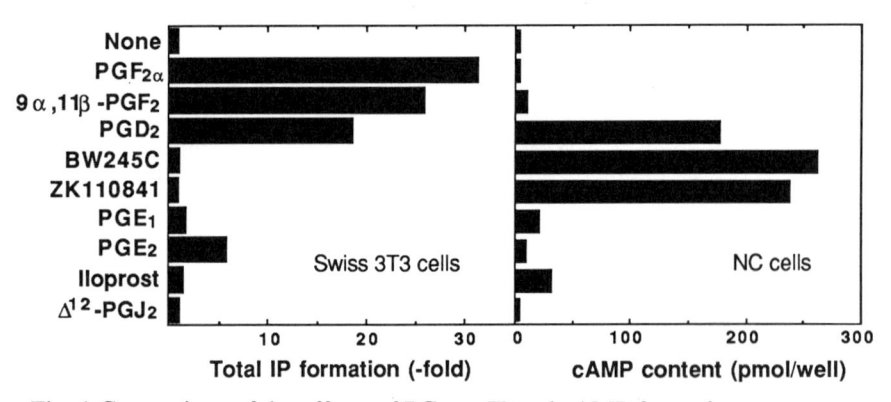

Fig. 1 Comparison of the effects of PGs on IP and cAMP formation.

Figure 1 shows the effect of various PGs on IP formation in Swiss 3T3 cells during 10-min incubation. PGF$_{2\alpha}$, 9α,11β-PGF$_2$ and PGD$_2$ were most potent in IP formation in this order and the total IP level increased 18-30-fold over the control at 10 min. Being consistent with the effect on [Ca^{2+}]i, BW245C, ZK110841, and Δ^{12}-PGJ$_2$, a dehydrate of PGD$_2$, showed no effect on IP formation. These results suggest that IP formation in Swiss 3T3 cells may be mediated by PGF$_{2\alpha}$/PGD$_2$ receptor.

Previously we (7) reported that nonchromaffin (NC) cells prepared from bovine adrenal medulla specifically responded to PGD$_2$ by elevating cAMP levels. In NC cells, BW245C and ZK110841 increased cAMP level, equipotent to or more than PGD_2 (Fig. 1), but $PGF_{2\alpha}$ and $9\alpha,11\beta$-PGF_2 showed negligible effect. While AH6809 antagonized the elevation of cAMP levels in NC cells by PGD_2, it did not affect IP formation in Swiss 3T3 cells by PGD_2 or $PGF_{2\alpha}$. These results demonstrate that PGD_2 may couple to phosphoinositide metabolism and the adenylate cyclase system through different receptors.

DISCUSSION

Narumiya and Toda (6) reported that PGD_2-sensitive tissues and cells can be classified into two groups. Human platelets, mast cells and rabbit stomach strip belong to one receptor group coupled to the activation of adenylate cyclase. The other group consists of guinea-pig trachea and dog cerebral artery. They suggested that PGD_2 may act on the receptors of $PGF_{2\alpha}$ and/or thromboxane to elicit contraction in these tissues. In agreement with pharmacological studies, the present study clearly demonstrate that PGD_2 is coupled to two signal transduction systems. As summarized in Table 1, one is coupled to adenylate cyclase through PGD_2-specific receptor and the other may be coupled to phosphoinositide metabolism through $PGF_{2\alpha}/PGD_2$ receptor. In fact, PGD_2 is a potent competitor for binding of [^{3}H]$PGF_{2\alpha}$ to the $PGF_{2\alpha}$ receptor on ovine luteal cells (1). Previously, Miwa et al. (5) demonstrated that $PGF_{2\alpha}$, $9\alpha,11\beta$-PGF_2, and PGD_2 increased [Ca^{2+}]i in mouse neuroblastma X rat glioma hybrid NG108-15 cells. Here we first demonstrate that PGD_2 stimulates phosphoinositide metabolism and that this effect of PGD_2 can be discriminated from that coupled to the adenylate cyclase system by using BW245C, ZK110841, and AH6809.

Table 1. Signal transduction coupled to PGD_2.

Signal transduction	Receptor	Cells
1. Activation of adenylate cyclase	PGD_2 receptor	platelets
		mast cells
		EBTr cells
		NC cells
2. Phosphoinositide metabolism/ Ca^{2+} mobilization	$PGF_{2\alpha}/PGD_2$ receptor	Swiss 3T3 cells
		NG108-15 cells

$PGF_{2\alpha}$ and PGD_2 are bronchoconstrictors which are released under allergic conditions such as asthma. Inhalation of these PGs produces bronchoconstriction in asthmatic subjects. In the literature, PGD_2 is more potent than $PGF_{2\alpha}$ in both asthmatic and normal men, whilst the potency is reverse in human isolated bronchus. Furthermore, PGD_2 is a major product of antigen-stimulated pulmonary tissue and human lung mast cells as well as rat brain homogenates. These results taken together suggest that PGD_2 may couple to phosphoinositide metabolism through $PGF_{2\alpha}/PGD_2$ receptor in tissues under pathophysiological conditions.

ACKNOWLEDGEMENTS

This work was supported by grants-in-aid for scientific research from the Ministry of Education, Science, and Culture of Japan and by a grant from Ono Medical Research Foundation. Authentic PGs, ZK110841, BW245C, and AH6809 were kindly provided by Ono Pharmaceuticals (Osaka, Japan), Schering (Berlin, F. R. G.), Wellcome (Beckenham, U. K.) and Glaxo (Hertfordshire, U. K.), respectively.

REFERENCES

1. Balapure, A.K., Rexroad, C.E., Kawada, K., Watt, D.S., and Fitz, T.A. (1989): *Biochem. Pharmacol.*, 38: 2375-2381.
2. Ito, S., Narumiya, S., and Hayaishi, O. (1989): *Prostaglandins Leukotrienes and Essential Fatty Acids*, 37: 219-234.
3. Ito, S., Okuda, E., Sugama, K., Negishi, M., and Hayaishi, O. (1990): *Br. J. Pharmacol.*, 99: 13-14.
4. Keery, R.J. and Lumley, P. (1988): *Br. J. Pharmacol.*, 94: 745-754.
5. Miwa, N., Sugino, H., Ueno, R., and Hayaishi, O. (1988): *J. Neurochem.*, 50: 1418-1424.
6. Narumiya, S. and Toda, N. (1985): *Br. J. Pharmacol.*, 85: 367-375.
7. Sugama, K., Tanaka, T., Yokohama, H., Negishi, M., Hayashi, H., Ito, S., and Hayaishi, O. (1989): *Biochim. Biophys. Acta*, 1011: 75-80.
8. Thierauch, K.-H., Stürzebecher, C.-ST., Schillinger, E., Rehwinkel, H., Radüchel, B., Skuballa, W., and Vorbrüggen, H. (1988): *Prostaglandins*, 35: 855-868.
9. Yamashita, T., Tsuda, T., Hamamori, Y., and Takai, Y. (1986): *J. Biol. Chem.*, 261: 16878-16882.

CHARACTERISATION OF PGE₂ RECEPTORS MEDIATING INCREASED VASCULAR PERMEABILITY IN INFLAMMATION

R.A. Armstrong, J.S. Matthews, R.L. Jones and N.H. Wilson

Department of Pharmacology, University of Edinburgh
1 George Square, Edinburgh, EH8 9JZ, U.K.

PGE$_2$ has little effect on vascular permeability when injected alone into rabbit skin, but potentiates the local exudation produced by other inflammatory mediators. This has been attributed to its vasodilator activity (5). However, there are potential difficulties with using PGE$_2$ as an agonist since it is known to act on (at least) three receptor subtypes, designated EP$_1$, EP$_2$ and EP$_3$ (3,4). We have investigated the ability of more selective PGE analogues to potentiate bradykinin (BK)-induced plasma exudation in rabbit skin (leakage of ^{125}I albumin (6)).

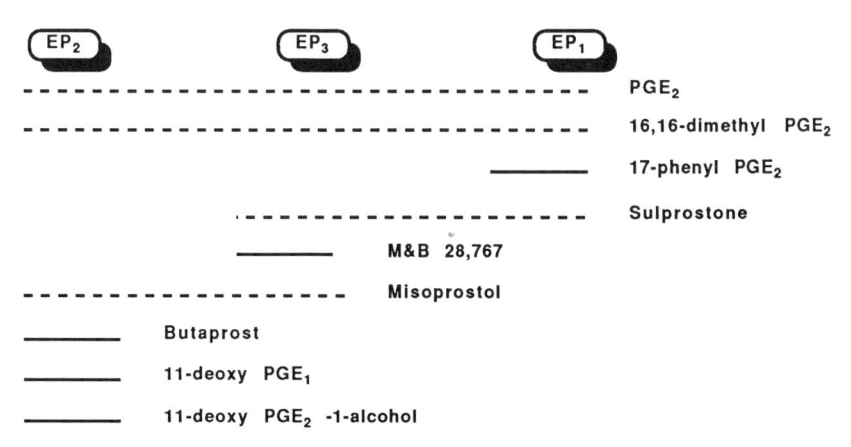

EP$_2$	EP$_3$	EP$_1$	
--------------------------------	----	PGE$_2$
--------------------------------	----	16,16-dimethyl PGE$_2$
		———	17-phenyl PGE$_2$
	--------------------	Sulprostone
	———	M&B 28,767
-------------------		Misoprostol
———			Butaprost
———			11-deoxy PGE$_1$
———			11-deoxy PGE$_2$ -1-alcohol

FIG. 1 Specificity of action of the PGE analogues used in this study.

EP$_1$ receptors mediate contraction of the guinea-pig ileum, fundus and trachea *in vitro*; the action of PGE$_2$ is antagonised by SC 19220 and AH 6809 (2). EP$_2$ receptors mediate relaxation of cat trachea, guinea-pig trachea and rabbit jugular vein *in vitro*, and dog hind limb arterial vessels *in vivo*;. EP₃ actions are characterised *in vitro* by contraction of the chick ileum, inhibition of transmitter release in the guinea-pig vas deferens and inhibition of secretion in the rat isolated gastric mucosa. No antagonists are available for EP₂ or EP₃ receptors.

PLASMA EXUDATION BY EP₂ AGONISTS

We set up the rabbit skin model in the expectation that we would readily characterise the prostanoid receptor mediating the potentiation of exudation as an EP₂ receptor, since vasodilatation is the archetypal EP₂ effect. However, the initial results were surprising in that the potent EP₂ agonists butaprost (1000 ng), 11-deoxy PGE₁ (5000 ng) and 11-deoxy PGE₂-1-alcohol (5000 ng) were poor potentiating agents, achieving +69%, +98% and +38% of the BK control respectively. Only misoprostol (1000 ng) could achieve the maximal potentiation seen with PGE₂ (+265% at 1000 ng) (FIG. 2). Furthermore, whereas PGE₂ at only 1 ng gave a potentiation of +108%, the EP₂ agonists showed little activity below concentrations of 100-1000 ng. The weak effects were not due to a partial agonist action, since pre-treatment with 11-deoxy PGE₂-1-alcohol (5000 ng intradermally) did not antagonise potentiation by PGE₂ or misoprostol, but produced additive effects (n=4).

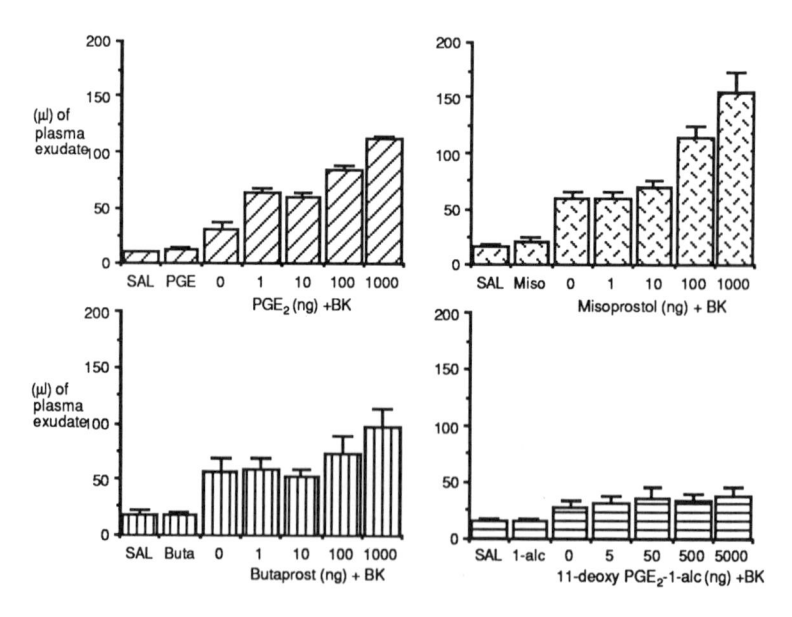

FIG 2. The ability of PGE₂, misoprostol, butaprost and 11-deoxy PGE₂-1-alcohol to potentiate plasma exudation in rabbit skin induced by intradermal bradykinin (500ng). SAL and Drug columns represent injections of saline and drug at the highest concentration tested, but in the absence of BK. Values are the mean ± s.e.m of at least 4 experiments.

PLASMA EXUDATION BY EP₃ AGONISTS

EP₃ activity was examined using sulprostone and M&B 28,767, whose true activity could be assessed only after its thromboxane (TP) agonist activity had been blocked by the TP receptor antagonist GR 32191 (2 mg/kg i.v.). M&B 28,767 (1 ng) significantly increased plasma exudation to +78% (FIG. 3) (as compared to +20% in the absence of GR 32191). Unfortunately TP receptor block is difficult to achieve in the rabbit, and a dose-ratio of only 15 was achieved against U 46619-induced pulmonary hypertension. While higher concentrations of M&B 28,767 may overcome the TP block, neither M&B 28,767 nor sulprostone showed further potentiation with higher concentrations (100-1000 ng) and both are devoid of EP₂ activity.

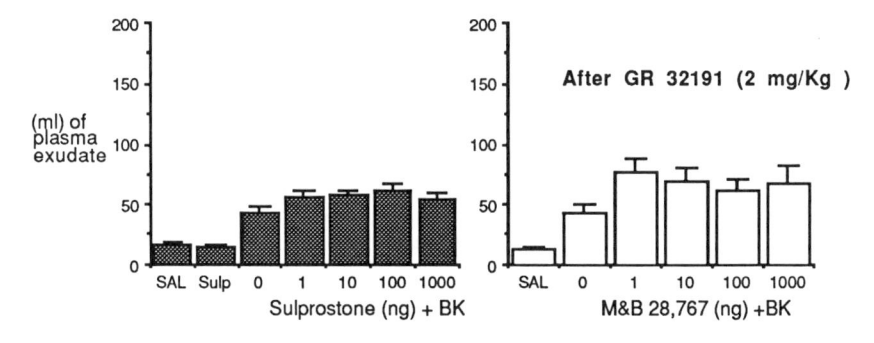

FIG. 3. The ability of sulprostone and M&B 28,767 (after GR 32191) to potentiate plasma exudation. Conditions as in FIG. 2.

DILATATION IN THE SKIN

FIG. 4 shows dilatation in the skin, measured by a ^{133}Xe clearance technique (6).

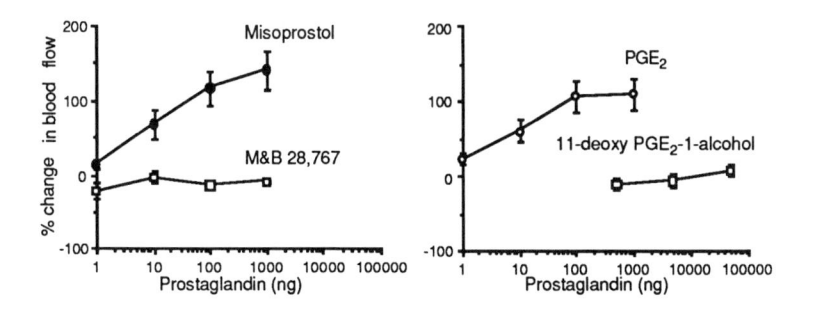

FIG. 4. The ability of PGE₂, misoprostol, M&B 28,767 (in the presence of 2mg/kg GR 32191) and 11-deoxy PGE₂-1-alcohol to increase blood flow in rabbit skin. Drugs were mixed with ^{133}Xe (5-10 µCi per injection) and injected intradermally. Values are the mean ± s.e.m. of at least 4 experiments.

PGE$_2$ and misoprostol are potent dilators, although at 1 ng PGE$_2$ produces little dilatation. M&B 28,767(even after TP receptor block) and sulprostone (1000 ng, n=4) did not dilate. The EP$_2$ agonist 11-deoxy PGE$_2$-1-alcohol which did not potentiate BK-exudation did not induce dilatation, and butaprost which was slightly more effective, induced some dilatation (50% at 1000 ng,n=3)

CONCLUSIONS

Potentiation of BK-induced exudation by PGE$_2$ may have two components. Neither is mediated by an EP$_1$ receptor as 17-phenyl PGE$_2$ does not potentiate BK in concentrations up to 1000 ng (n=4). The high potency (1-10 ng) component may be mediated by an EP$_3$ receptor and appears to be unrelated to dilatation. One possibility is that dilatation induced by BK is potentiating an EP$_3$ receptor-mediated, leukocyte-dependant mechanism, as has been shown with LTB$_4$(1). The lower potency (100-1000 ng) component may be mediated by an EP$_2$ receptor and does correlate with dilatation. However, the low potency of butaprost and the inactivity of 11-deoxy PGE$_2$-1-alcohol suggests that the receptor differs from the conventional EP$_2$ subtype.

ACKNOWLEDGMENTS

This work was supported by The Wellcome Trust. We thank the following pharmaceutical houses for generous gifts of compounds: Schering AG, Berlin; Rhone-Poulenc, U.K.; Searle, U.S.A.; Glaxo, U.K. and Bayer, U.K.

REFERENCES

1. Bray, M. A., Cunningham, F. M., Ford-Hutchinson, A.W., and Smith, M.J.H (1981) : *Br. J. Pharmac* 72 : 483-486
2. Coleman, R. A., Kennedy, I., and Sheldrick, R. L. G. (1985): *Br. J. Pharmac. Proc. Suppl.* 85 : 273P.
3. Coleman, R. A., Kennedy, I., Sheldrick, R. L. G., and Tolowinska, I.Y. (1987):*Br. J. Pharmac. Proc. Suppl.* 91 : 407P.
4. Lawrence, R. A., Jones, R.L., and Wilson, N. H. (1989): *Br. J. Pharmac.Proc. Suppl.* 98 : 796P.
5. Wedmore, C. V. and Williams, T. J. (1981) : *Nature* 289 : 646-650.
6. Williams, T.J. (1979) : *Br. J. Pharmac.* 65 : 517-524.

Advances in Prostaglandin, Thromboxane, and Leukotriene Research, Vol. 21,
edited by B. Sameulsson et al.
Raven Press, Ltd., New York © 1990.

GR63799X – A NOVEL PROSTANOID WITH SELECTIVITY FOR EP_3 RECEPTORS

K.T. Bunce, N.M. Clayton, R.A. Coleman,
E.W. Collington, H. Finch, J.M. Humphray, P.P.A. Humphrey,
J.J. Reeves, R.L.G. Sheldrick and R. Stables

Glaxo Group Research Ltd., Ware, Hertfordshire, SG12 0DP, U.K.

INTRODUCTION

A number of prostanoids have been developed as gastric antisecretory/cytoprotective agents for use in the treatment of peptic ulcers in man. Two such compounds are enprostil and misoprostol, which while undoubtedly effective, can cause various side–effects, including diarrhoea and uterine stimulation (Collins, 1986). It has recently been suggested that the gastric protective effects of these compounds result from their prostanoid EP_3–receptor agonist activity, both enprostil and misoprostol being potent EP_3–receptor agonists (Reeves et al., 1988). It is possible that the side–effects of these compounds arise at least in part from their actions at other prostanoid receptors. We now report some preliminary results obtained with a novel, potent, selective EP_3–receptor agonist, GR63799X (Figure 1).

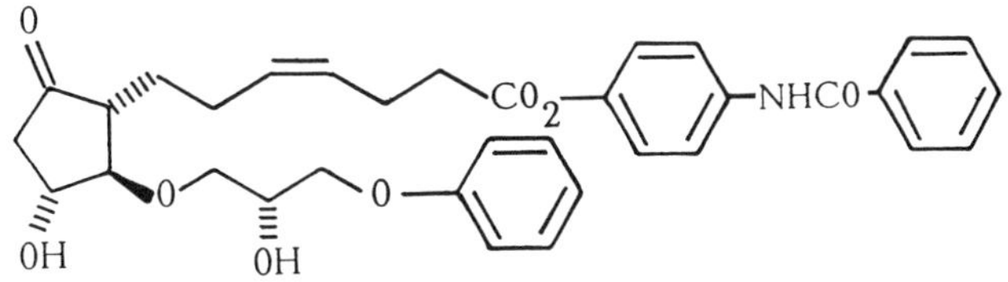

Figure 1. Structure of GR63799X

METHODS

in vitro preparations

The smooth muscle preparations used, guinea–pig fundic strip (GPF), cat trachea (CT), guinea–pig vas deferens (GPVD), dog iris sphincter (DI) and rat aorta (RA) were all prepared as described by Coleman (1987). The rat isolated gastric mucosa preparation (RGM) was set up as described by Reeves and Stables (1985).

in vivo preparations

Gastric mucosal lesions were induced in the rat by the intragastric administration of ethanol as described by Robert et al (1979). Diarrhoeogenic activity was assessed by the appearance of perianal staining in groups of 6 rats examined at 0.5h intervals after drug administration. In order to measure gastric non-parietal secretion, cats were anaesthetized with chloralose (80mgkg^{-1} i.v.) and treated with indomethacin (3.6mgkg^{-1} i.v.). A polythene cannula was inserted per os, into the stomach just below the cardiac sphincter, and a second cannula inserted throught the duodenal wall and into the stomach via the pylorus. The secretion of fluid and electrolytes was measured at 30 min intervals. Drugs were administered close arterially to the stomach by retrograde infusion into the hepatic artery. In order to measure uterine activity, the uterus was connected to a strain gauge by a thread, via an incision in the flank.

RESULTS

Receptor selectivity

GR63799X was compared for agonist activity with PGE$_2$ and the two gastric antisecretory PGE analogues, enprostil and misoprostol, on a range of prostanoid-receptor containing preparations. The results are summarized in Table 1. GR63799X was a potent agonist on the EP$_3$-receptor containing preparations, GPVD and RGM, where it was between 11 and 50-times more potent than PGE$_2$, however it was substantially less potent on all of the other preparations. Enprostil had a similar profile, except for its relatively high potency at FP-receptors, but misoprostol was both less potent and less selective, being a potent agonist on the EP$_2$-receptor containing preparation, CT. Mean concentration-effect curves to GR63799X, enprostil and misoprostol on RGM are illustrated in Fig. 2.

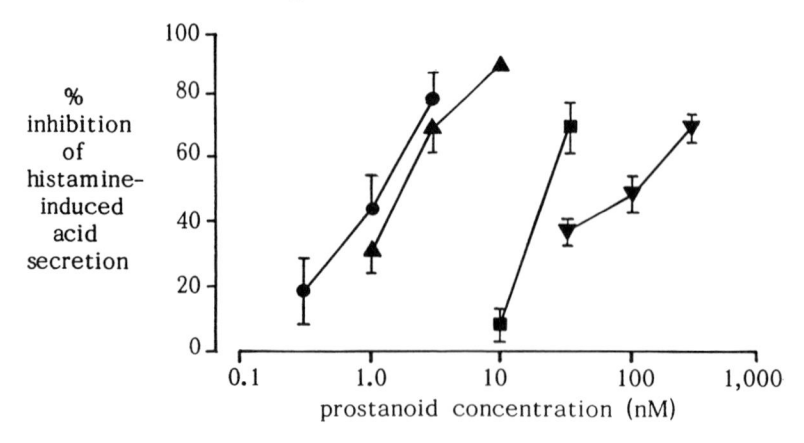

Figure 2   Rat isolated gastric mucosa. Concentration-effect curves for GR63799X (▲), enprostil (●), misoprostol (■) and PGE$_2$ (▼).

Table 1 Receptor selectivity. Equipotent concentration values for PGE_2, GR63799X, enprostil and misoprostol on a range of prostanoid-receptor containing preparations

Agonist	Equipotent Concentration (standard agonist = 1)					
	GPF (EP_1)	CT (EP_2)	GPVD (EP_3)	RGM (EP_3)	DI[1] (FP)	RA[2] (TP)
PGE_2	1	1	1	1	515 (179-1483)	180 (130-240)
GR63799X	4.4 (2.4-7.8)	>1000	0.09 (0.05-0.15)	0.02	232 (93-578)	46 (31-67)
Enprostil	1.8 (1.1-2.9)	850-1580	0.08 (0.03-0.22)	0.02	4.4 (1.8-11)	14 (9-22)
Misoprostol	43 (20-92)	3.7 (1.4-9.4)	1.0 (0.5-2.0)	0.24	>6500 (1400-31,000)	256 (130-504)

Values geometric means (95% C.L.) where n > 4, or range where n=2
1. Standard agonist = $PGF_{2\alpha}$ 2. Standard agonist = U-46619

Gastric protection

The three compounds were compared for their ability to inhibit ethanol-induced gastric lesions in rats. When administered by the oral route, in the dose range 0.1-10μgkg^{-1}, all three compounds caused dose-related inhibition of lesion formation. Furthermore, all three compounds were of similar potency, with ED_{50} values of 0.66 (95% confidence limits = 0.36-1.06, n=20) μgkg^{-1}, 0.36 (0.19-0.63, n=20) μgkg^{-1} and 0.31 (0.08-1.20; n=15) μgkg^{-1} for GR63799X, enprostil and misoprostol respectively.

Diarrhoea

The compounds were evaluated for diarrhoeogenic activity after oral administration to conscious rats. All three compounds induced dose-related diarrhoea at doses higher than those required to protect against ethanol-induced lesions. Enprostil was the most potent, ED_{50} = 47 (n=24) μgkg^{-1}, whereas misoprostol was less potent, ED_{50} = 450 (n=24) μgkg^{-1}, and GR63799X had the lowest diarrhoeogenic potential, ED_{50} = 1300 (n=32) μgkg^{-1}.

Uterine stimulation

The compounds were tested for in vivo uterine stimulant activity in anaesthetized cats, after intragastric instillation. In these experiments, gastric non-parietal secretion was used as an index of gastric protection. All three compounds caused dose-related stimulation of non-parietal secretion in the dose-range $1.2-59\mu gkg^{-1}$, whereas, while misoprostol also caused uterine stimulation at $38\mu gkg^{-1}$, GR63799X and enprostil had no uterine effects at doses up to $590\mu gkg^{-1}$. A gastric/uterine selectivity factor was determined for each compound by dividing the dose causing significant uterine stimulation by that causing significant stimulation of non-parietal secretion. The resulting factors were >125, >170 and 2 for GR63799X, enprostil and misoprostol respectively.

DISCUSSION AND CONCLUSIONS

The novel prostanoid, GR63799X, resembles enprostil and misoprostol in that it is a potent agonist at prostanoid EP_3-receptors, it is an effective inhibitor of gastric acid secretion in isolated preparations of rat gastric mucosa, and it inhibits ethanol-induced lesion formation in conscious rats. However, in vitro it is more selective in its EP_3-receptor agonist activity than misoprostol, and in vivo, it appears to have a much lower diarrhoeogenic potential than enprostil, and a much lower myometrial stimulant potential than misoprostol. This profile suggests that GR63799X should be as potent as enprostil and misoprostol as a gastric mucosal protectant and inhibitor of acid secretion, but should be less prone to cause the side-effects of diarrhoea and uterine stimulation associated with these prostanoids.

REFERENCES

Coleman, R.A. (1987). In: Benedetto, C. et al. (eds) Prostaglandins and related substances, a practical approach. IRL Press, Oxford, 267-303.

Collins, P.W. (1986). J. Med. Chem., 29, 437-443.

Reeves, J.J., Bunce, K.T., Sheldrick, R.L.G. and Stables, R. (1988). Br. J. Pharmacol., 95, 805P.

Reeves, J.J. and Stables, R. (1985). Br. J. Pharmacol., 86 677-684.

Robert, A., Nezamis, J.E., Lancaster, C. and Hanchar, A. (1979). Gastroenterology, 77, 433-443.

MODULATION OF PLATELET ACTIVATION BY PROSTAGLANDIN E$_2$ MIMICS

K.-H. Thierauch and G. Prior

Biochemical Pharmacology, Research Laboratories of Schering AG, Berlin, Muellerstr. 170-178, 1000 Berlin 65, FRG

Prostaglandin E$_2$ at high concentrations inhibits platelet aggregation. At lower concentrations it augments ADP-induced platelet aggregation albeit it is not aggregating platelets by itself. The latter property is also exhibited by the PGE$_2$-analogue sulprostone (5). There are PGE$_2$-receptors described on the platelet surface (3). Are the effects mediated by two different signal transduction pathways?

Utilizing sulprostone, iloprost and ZK 110841, a PGD$_2$-analogue (9,10 and this vol.), we shall demonstrate in assays which measure cAMP content and cyctosolic free calcium concentrations that in human platelets PGE$_2$ activity is the result of two discernible effects possibly via PGI$_2$- and PGE$_2$-receptors.

METHODS

Intracellular free calcium concentration was estimated in FURA II-AM loaded platelet suspensions (3 M) that were gel filtered over Sepharose 2B Cl according to Erne et al.(4). cAMP-levels in platelet rich plasma (PRP) or gel filtered platelet suspensions (GFP) were done as described previously (10).

RESULTS

Fura II-loaded gelfiltered human platelet suspensions will increase fluorescence and therefore intracellular free calcium when U 46619 is added (IC$_{50}$=30nM). 1µM PGE$_2$ shifts the curve rightward and decreases the maximal effect by about 40 %. Sulprostone increases maximal fluorescence obtained with U 46619 (Fig. 1). The U 46619- or thrombin-induced increase in fluorescence can be blocked by PGD$_2$- and PGI$_2$-analogues. The inhibitory curve is then shifted rightward in the presence of low concentrations of PGE$_2$ or sulprostone (Fig 2).

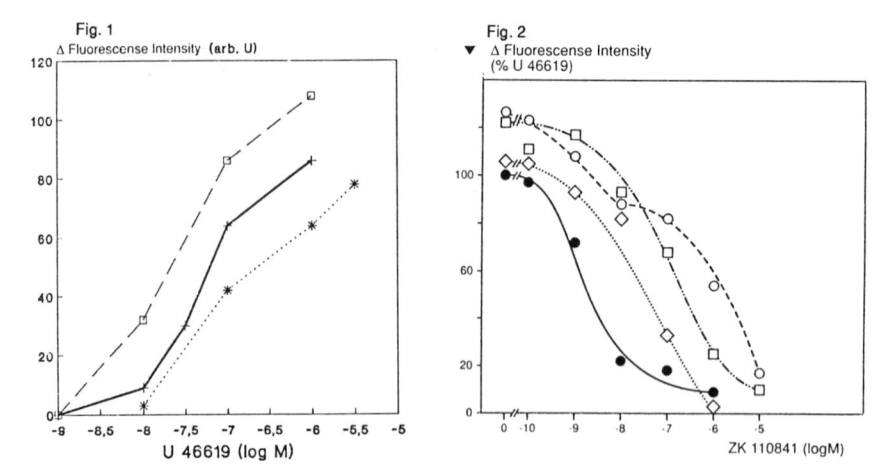

Figure 1: Platelet stimulation with U 46619 in the presence of PGE_2 or sulprostone. FURA II loaded platelets were preincubated with PGE_2 or sulprostone for 5 min before U 46619 was added and fluorescence increase determined. —+— control ····*···· PGE-2 1µM —☐— sulprostone 1µM

Figure 2: Inhibition of U 46619 induced platelet stimulation by ZK 110841 in the presence of sulprostone. Platelet suspensions were treated with sulprostone and ZK 110841 for 30 sec. before 1µM U 46619 was added. ●—● Control; ◇·····◇ + 10^{-8} M Sulprostone; ☐---☐ + 10^{-7} M Sulprostone; ○- -○ + 10^{-6} M Sulprostone

Basal cAMP concentrations of human PRP are not affected by sulprostone, they are increased by PGE_2 (at 10µM < 2 fold), ZK 110841 (at 10µM 10 fold) and iloprost (at 10 nM 20 fold). Sulprostone attenuates the iloprost (Fig. 3) or ZK 110 841 induced cAMP elevation in platelets.

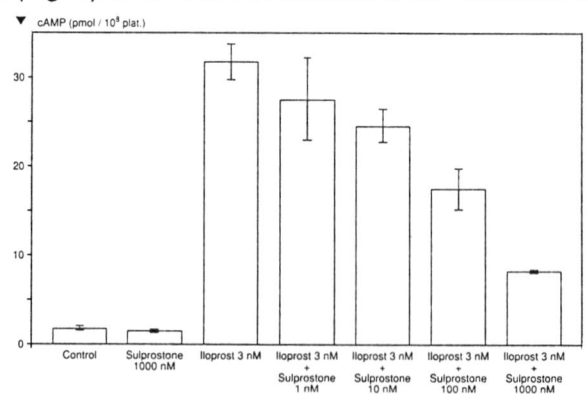

Figure 3: cAMP-levels in PRP. PRP was incubated with the prostaglandin analogues for 30 sec at 37°C before the reaction was stopped by addition of 2 vol. ethanol.

Fig. 4 shows the time curve of cAMP-content in gel filtered platelets after stimulation with PGE$_1$ and ZK 110 841 at equivalent concentrations (10 x IC$_{50}$ of 1 μM U 46619 stimulated platelet aggregation). cAMP levels reach a maximum within a minute and then decline rapidly after PGE$_1$ stimulation. They remain elevated after ZK 110841 treatment for more than 20 min. If sulprostone or PGE$_2$ (not shown) are present the increase induced by iloprost (Fig. 5) or ZK 110841 (not shown) is blunted giving a time curve as that obtained with PGE$_1$.

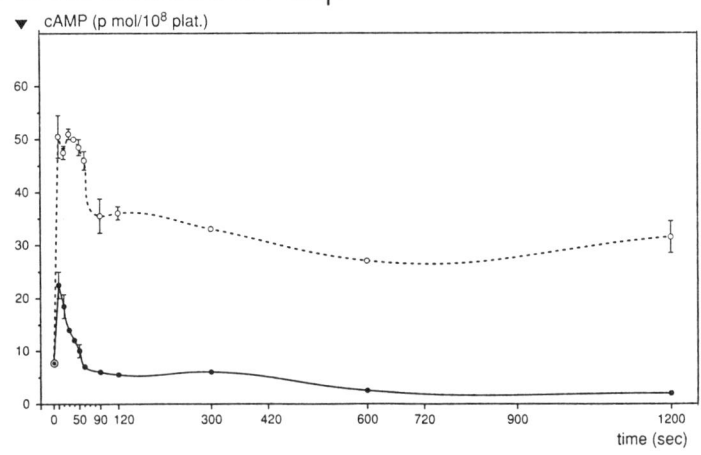

Figure 4: Time courses of cAMP content in GFP after addition of PGE1 or ZK 110841. •——• PGE$_1$ 100 nM   o----o ZK 110 841 100 nM

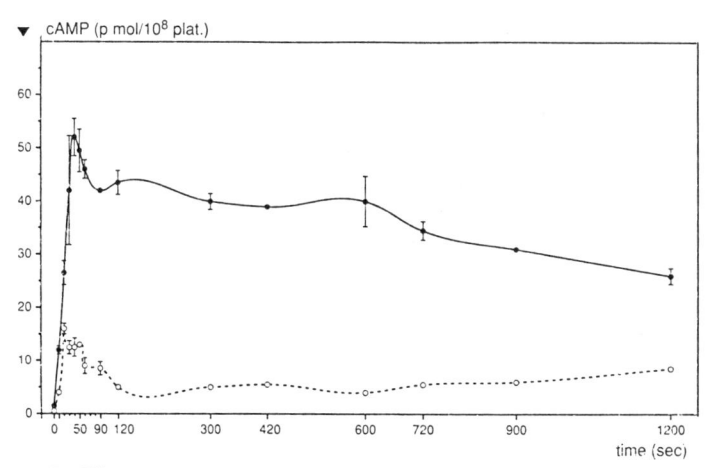

Figure 5: Time course of cAMP-content in GFP after addition of iloprost or iloprost plus sulprostone. •——• Iloprost 3 nM   o----o Iloprost 3 nM + Sulprostone 1 μM

The PGE/D-Antagonist AH 6809 (6) at 1 μM does not reverse the shape of the time curve of PGE$_1$ towards one comparable with PGD$_2$ or

Phorbolmyristateacetate (PMA) does not reduce but rather increases cAMP-content after stimulation with iloprost.

DISCUSSION

Inhibitory effects of PGE_2 on platelet antiaggregatory action of PGE_1 has been observed earlier (8,2). Bonne et al (1). showed that PGE_2 reduces fluoride elevated cAMP production in platelet membranes.

The modulation of cAMP-content in platelets by PGE_2-mimics is not a result of protein kinase C (PMA-effect) nor one that involves stimulation of calcium influx (no effect on [Cai]). It might occur via the inhibitory G-protein as it affects cAMP stimulation heterologously.

In platelet membrane preparations PGE_1 induces the same maximal rate of cAMP-synthesis as does PGI_2 (7) or its analog iloprost. Why does the PGE-like modulation not occur in membrane vesicles? If the binding sites described by Eggerman (3) (high affinity 6/cell; low affinity 60/cell) are mediating the effect, then uneven receptor distribution might be one reason.

ADP attenuates increase in platelet cAMP content (unpublished observation). It is present in adenylate cyclase assays and therefore might prevent prostacyclin stimulated cAMP-synthesis from obtaining theoretically maximal rates. So the observed stimulation is already attenuated.

Thirdly one could postulate a soluble factor which is lost during membrane preparation that transmits the inhibitory effect and couples the inhibitory signal with the stimulatory one.

REFERENCES

1. Bonnè, C. et al. 1981: Thromb. Res. 21, 13-22
2. Menter D.G. et al.1984: Cancer Res. 44, 450-456
3. Eggerman et al. 1986: J. Pharm. Exp. Therap. 236, 586-573
4. Erne, P. et al. 1984: J Rec. Res. 4, 1-6
5. Losert et al. 1978: In: Internat. Sulprostone Sympos. edi. by K. Friebel, A. Schneider, H. Würfel, pp. 47-59, Berlin
6. Keery R.J an Lumley P. 1988: Br. J. Pharmacol. 94, 745-754
7. Gorman R.R. et al. 1977:Prostaglandins 13,377-388
8. Shio, H. and Ramwell, P.W. 1972: Nature (New Biol.) 236, 45-46
9. Thierauch K.-H. et al. 1989: In: Prostaglandins in Clin.Res.: Cardiovas. Sys., edi. by K. Schroer and H. Sinzinger, pp579-601, New York
10. Thierauch K.-H. et al. 1988: Prostaglandins 35, 855-868

BIOSYNTHESIS AND FUNCTION OF LEUKOTRINE B4

IMMUNOCHEMICAL STUDY OF LEUKOTRIENE A4 HYDROLASE AND IDENTIFICATION OF PUTATIVE LEUKOTRIENE B4 RECEPTOR

Takao Shimizu, Nobuya Ohishi*, Ichiro Miki
Motonao Nakamura, and Yousuke Seyama

Department of Physiological Chemistry and Nutrition,
and * Department of 3rd Internal Medicine
Faculty of Medicine, University of Tokyo, Tokyo 113, Japan

Leukotriene (LT) A4 hydrolase catalyzes enzymic hydration of LTA4 to LTB4 (5(S),12(R)-dihydroxy-6,14-cis-8,10-trans-eicosatetraenoic acid), a potent chemotactic and immunoregulatory compound (9, 16, 21-25, 27). The enzyme was originally described in blood cells (leukocytes and erythrocytes) and has been purified to homogeneity from these sources (4, 20, 11). We obtained the evidence, however, that the enzyme activity is ubiquitously distributed in various organs and tissues of mammals (10, 26), and the higher specific activities than those of leukocytes were observed in some organs, including small intestine, lung and so on. The enzyme was then purified from human lung (17, 19), guinea pig lung (1) and liver (8). It was still unclear which kind of cells in these organs carry the enzyme protein, and what the biological roles in these cells are. It is of importance to elucidate fully the mechanism and regulation of LTB4 biosynthesis and its versatile functions. Described herein, (1). immunological quantitation of the enzyme in various tissues, and identification of cell types possessing an enzyme protein. (2). solubilization and partial characterization of LTB4 receptor (binding protein) from spleen.

IMMUNOLOGICAL STUDIES OF LTA4 HYDROLASE

Preparation and Characterization of the Anti-LTA4 Hydrolase Antibody.

The cDNA encoding human LTA4 hydrolase was cloned (6, 14), and the enzyme protein was expressed in *Escherichia coli* (15). The purified enzyme (340 μg) was emulsified with Freund's complete adjuvant, and administered to New Zealand white rabbits by multiple subcutaneous injections. The titer of antisera was determined by enzyme-linked immunosorbent assay (ELISA), using a Clone-SelectorTM. Antisera were combined, and purified by ammonium sulfate fractionation, Mono Q column chromatography, and immunoaffinity column chromatography. The procedure of coupling LTA4 hydrolase to Sepharose 4B is described in Ohishi et al. (18). The IgG fraction was applied to an affinity column, and the adsorbed antibody, which specifically recognized LTA4 hydrolase, was eluted with 0.1 M glycine-HCl buffer, pH 2.5. A typical elution profile is illustrated in FIG. 1.

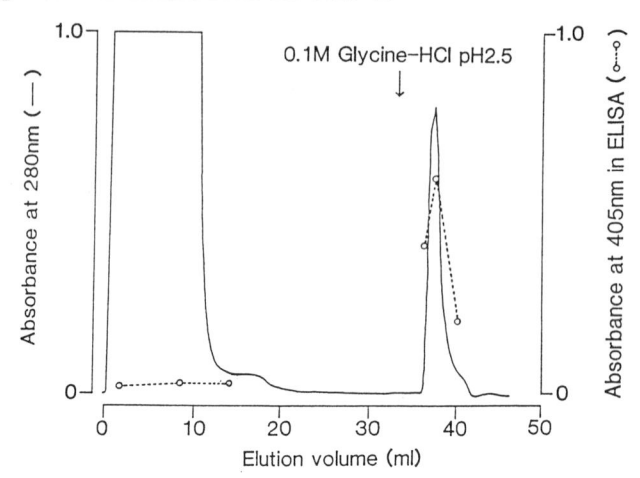

FIG. 1. Affinity Column Chromatography Coupled with Recombinant LTA4 Hydrolase (18).

Immunological Quantitation of LTA4 Hydrolase.

Cytosolic fractions from various tissues of the guinea pig were obtained after animals were perfused with EDTA-containing saline. The native LTA4 hydrolase was purified from guinea pig small intestine, essentially by the method as described previously (1). The purified enzyme (standard) and cytosols with certain amounts of the purified enzyme (sample) were subjected to SDS-polyacrylamide gel electrophoresis and transferred to a nitrocellulose membrane. The membrane fraction containing 60-80 KDa protein was cut out, and incubated for 15 min with the peroxidase reaction mixture. The reaction was quenched by addition of NaN3, and the absorbance at 405 nm was measured. It was plotted against the amount of exogenously-added purified enzyme. These two curves (standard and sample) could be considered as linear (r > 0.95). From the calibration curve in FIG. 2, the enzyme amount (B) was determined. Table 1 summarizes the simultaneous determinations of the LTA4 hydrolase activity and protein content in the cytosolic fraction from each tissue. The enzyme activity was high in small intestine, leukocytes, lung, and colon with values much the same as in our previous report (10). The protein content was also high in small intestine, spleen, lung, adrenal gland, and leukocytes in this order. The calculated enzyme activity (enzyme activity/enzyme amount) ranged mostly between 300 and 550, which accords well with values obtained from the purified enzyme (1, 17, 20). The relatively low values (170 and 240) obtained in liver and adrenal gland suggests the presence of inhibitory substance(s) or suicide-inactivated enzyme, or both. Since chalcone oxide, a potent epoxide hydrolase inhibitor (12), did not affect the enzyme activity, the low value could not be explained by the presence of cytosolic epoxide hydrolase, which also utilizes LTA4.

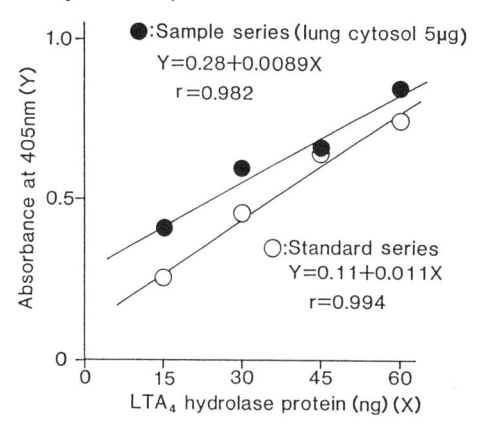

$0.11 + 0.011[A(X+B)] = 0.28 + 0.0089X$

$A = 0.81$
$B = 19 ng/5 \mu g$ lung cytosol

FIG. 2. Determination of LTA4 hydrolase protein content in the guinea pig lung cytosol (18).

TABLE 1. Distribution of LTA4 hydrolase in guinea pig tissues.

Tissues	LTA4 hydrolase activity	LTA4 hydrolase protein amount	Calculated enzyme activity
	nmol/min mg cytosol	μg/mg cytosol	nmol/min mg enzyme
Small intestine	2.5	6.5	390
Lung	1.3	3.8	340
Colon	1.3	2.6	500
Spleen	1.1	3.9	280
Aorta	0.9	1.6	550
Adrenal gland	0.9	3.6	240 *
Heart	0.7	2.0	370
Kidney	0.7	1.8	410
Stomach	0.7	2.2	310
Liver	0.4	2.5	170 *
Leukocytes	1.4	3.6	390

Data from (18). * Relatively lower values were observed as compared with the purified enzyme (500-600).

Immunocytochemical Localization of LTA4 Hydrolase

The organs from guinea pig were excised, cut into small blocks and fixed in 4% (w/v) paraformaldehyde in 0.1 M sodium phosphate buffer, pH 7.4 for 15 h. Tissue blocks were placed in OCT compound, frozen in dry ice/acetone and then sliced into 6-μm sections in a cryostat (18).

As summarized in Table 2, the enzyme protein is present in various parenchymal cells of each tissue. The results provide the first direct evidence that LTA4 hydrolase protein exists in cells other than leukocytes. Control experiments using preimmune serum or antibody which was previously adsorbed with either the purified enzyme or the recombinant enzyme showed negative stainings, suggesting that these stainings were specific to LTA4 hydrolase. Whether or not the enzyme is present in vascular endothelial cells has been controversial (3, 6), our present results indicate the presence of the enzyme protein in guinea pig aorta and small artery. Possible explanations for this discrepancy can be done by species difference or the presence of endogenous inhibitor(s).

The presence of LTA4 hydrolase protein raised the possibility that LTB4 may possess some biological activities in these cells. LTA4 should be supplied either by enzymic production in the same cells, or by the intercellular transfer from neighboring cells. Alternatively, LTA4 hydrolase might be a multi-functional enzyme which has different enzyme activity toward other substrates.

Table 2. Identification of cells with LTA4 hydrolase immunoreactivity.

Tissues	Positive Cells
Ileum	Epithelial cells (enterocytes), Auerbach's plexus, Meisner's plexus, Endothelial cells of arteriol, Infiltrating leukocytes
Stomach	Parietal cells
Colon	Epithelial cells
Trachea	Ciliated pseudostratified columnar epithelial cells
Lung	Bronchial smooth muscle, Bronchial epithelial cells Endothelial cells of pulmonary artery, Alveolar macrophage
Aorta	Smooth muscle cells in the media, Endothelial cells
Spleen	Macrophages

CHARACTERIZATION OF LTB4 RECEPTOR-GTP BINDING PROTEIN

Distribution of LTB4 Binding Activity in Various Tissues of Mammals.

As described above, LTA4 hydrolase is ubiquitously distributed in various tissues and organs. The cellular localization of LTB4 receptor must be elucidated to understand the biological significance of the compound. By using a radiolabeled LTB4, the binding experiments were carried out (13). Detailed procedures were described elsewhere (13). The LTB4 binding activity was high in porcine leukocytes and spleen. The species difference was prominent, since rat spleen had negligible amount of the binding and bovine spleen had weak binding capacity (13).
As to the guinea pig, the specific binding was high in peritoneal leukocytes, spleen, lung, brain, colon, and intestine in this order. The results were essentially in good agreement to those obtained by Cheng et al. (2).

Purification and Characterization of LTB4 Receptor.

The membrane fraction was obtained as described from porcine spleen (13). The LTB4 binding activity was solubilized with the buffer containing 1% (w/v) CHAPS, 10 mM $MgCl_2$, and 20% (w/v) glycerol. The solubilized preparation was applied to a Superose 6 gel-filtration column. The binding activity eluted at a retention volume corresponding to an Mr. about 650 KDa. Divalent cations such as Mg^{2+}, Mn^{2+}, and Ca^2 were stimulatory for the LTB4 binding, whereas NaCl, KCl, LiCl at higher concentration (0.5 - 1 M) were all inhibitory. By scatchard analysis, a single entity of the binding site was observed with Kd and Bmax values of 0.26 nM and 120 fmol/mg protein, respectively. As GTPγS decreased the affinity of LTB4 to this fraction (see below), the receptor is solubilized and parially purified in a complex form with GTP-binding protein(s).

Effect of GTPγS and IAP-Treatment on LTB4 Binding.

As shown in FIG. 3, the receptor was specific to LTB4, Ki values for 20-hydroxy-LTB4, and 20-carboxy-LTB4, both inactive metabolites of LTB4 were significantly low (1. 7 and 1,000 nM, respectively) as compared with LTB4 (0.33 nM) (FIG. 3).
Addition of 10 μM GTPγS strongly inhibited LTB4 binding. The Kd value of the high affinity site increased from 0.26 to 1.6 nM. Furthermore, a low affinity site with a Kd value of 390 nM appeared. LTB4 binding was slightly inhibited by IAP (islet-activating protein)-treatment. The inhibitory effect of GTPγS was significantly enhanced by IAP-treatment; at 10^{-8} M concentration of GTPγS, the inhibition of LTB4 binding was 68% or 29%, either with or without IAP-treatment. The maximal inhibitory effect on LTB4 binding by high concentration of GTPγS was same in IAP-

treated or nontreated sample. ADP-ribosylation study using 32P-labeled NAD showed a single band with an Mr. about 40KDa (unpublished data).

We have shown that the solubilized LTB4 receptor is coupled to GTP-binding protein(s) in porcine spleen. The LTB4 receptors in guinea pig tissues (lung, small intestine, and leukocytes) are also coupled to GTP-binding protein(s) (unpublished data). Although several groups have reported that biological activities of LTB4 were blocked by IAP-treatment of cells (7, 28), direct evidence for the coupling of an IAP-sensitive G-protein and LTB4 receptor has not yet been available. As demonstrated above, IAP-treatment of the solubilized receptor decreased only partially the LTB4 binding, but it significantly enhanced the inhibitory effect of GTPγ on LTB4 binding. These results can be interpreted either by that the solubilized LTB4 receptor is coupled to two GTP-binding proteins (IAP-sensitive and insensitive) or that the ADP-ribosylation of α-subunit partially decreases the affinity of GTP-binding protein to the receptor.

Further studies are ongoing including purification, characterization of functional receptor and GTP-binding protein to elucidate the signal transduction mechanism of LTB4 in the various tissues. This work was supported in part by a Grant-in-Aid from the Ministry of Education, Science and Culture of Japan.

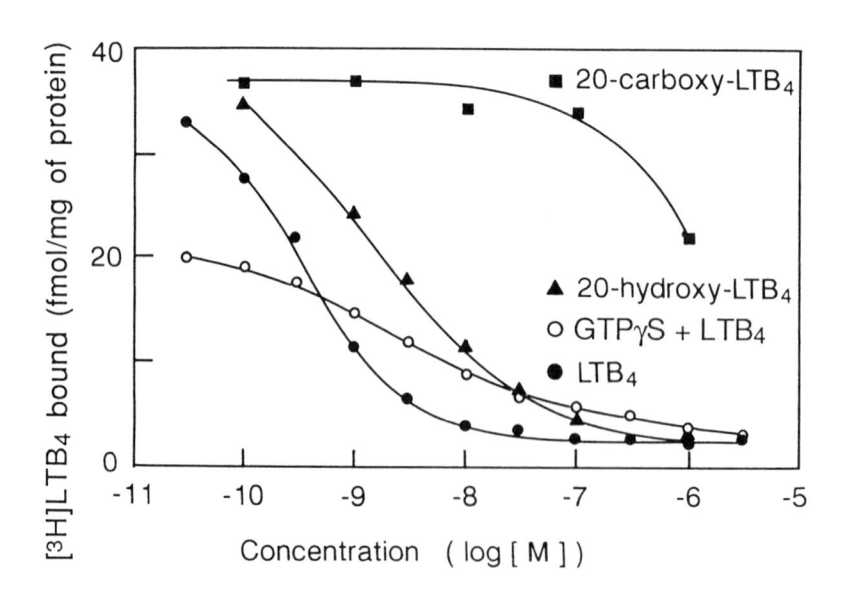

FIG. 3. Inhibition of [3H]LTB4 binding to porcine spleen receptor by GTPγS, LTB4 and its ω-oxidized metabolites (13).

REFERENCES

1. Bito, H., Ohishi, N., Miki, I., Minami, M., Tanabe, T., Shimizu, T., and Seyama, Y: (1989) *J. Biochem.* 105: 261-264

2. Cheng, J. B., Cheng, E. I-P., Kohi, F., and Townley, R. G: (1986) *J. Pharmacol. Exp. Ther.* 236: 126-132

3. Claesson, H.-E., and Haeggström, J: (1988) *Eur. J. Biochem.* 173: 93-100

4. Evans, J. F., Dupuis, P., and Ford-Hutchinson, A. W: (1985) *Biochim. Biophys. Acta* 840: 43-50

5. Feinmark, S. J., and Cannon, P. J: (1986) *J. Biol. Chem.* 261: 16466-16472

6. Funk, C., Rådmark, O., Fu, J-Y., Matsumoto, T., Jornvall, H., Shimizu, T. and Samuelsson, B: (1987) *Proc. Natl. Acad. Sci. U. S. A.* 84: 6677-6681

7. Goldman, D. W., Chang, F.-H., Gifford, L. A., Goetzl, E. J., and Bourne, H. R: (1985) *J. Exp. Med.* 162: 145-156

8. Haeggström, J., Bergman, T., Jörnvall, H., and Rådmark, O: (1989) *Eur. J. Biochem.* 174: 717-724

9. Hammarström, S: (1983) *Annu. Rev. Biochem.* 52: 355-377

10. Izumi, T., Shimizu, T., Seyama, Y., Ohishi, N., and Takaku, F: (1986) *Biochem. Biophys. Res. Commun.* 135: 139-145

11. McGee, J., and Fitzpatrick, F: (1985) *J. Biol. Chem.* 260: 12832-12837

12. Miki, I., Shimizu, T., Seyama, Y., Kitamura, S., Yamaguchi, K., Sano, H., Ueno, H., Hiratsuka, A., and Watabe, T: (1989) *J. Biol. Chem.* 264: 5799-5805

13. Miki, I., Watanabe, T., Nakamura, M., Seyama, Y., Ui, M., Sato, F., and Shimizu, T: (1990) *Biochem. Biophys. Res. Commun.* 166: 342-348

14. Minami, M., Ohno, S., Kawasaki, H., Radmark, O., Samuelsson, B., Jornvall, H., Shimizu, T., Seyama, Y., and Suzuki, K: (1987) *J. Biol. Chem.* 262: 10200-10205

15. Minami, M., Minami, Y., Emori, Y., Kawasaki, H., Ohno, S., Suzuki, K., Ohishi, N., Shimizu, T., and Seyama, Y: (1988) *FEBS Lett.* 229: 279-282

16. Needleman, P., Turk, J., Jakschik, B. A., Morrison, A. R., and Lefkowith, J. B: (1986) *Annu. Rev. Biochem.* 55: 69-102

17. Ohishi, N., Izumi, T., Kitamura, S., Minami, M., Seyama, Y., Ohkawa, S., Terao, S., Yotsumoto, H., Takaku, F., and Shimizu, T: (1987) *J. Biol. Chem.* 262: 10200-10205

18. Ohishi, N., Minami, M., Kobayashi, J., Seyama, Y., Hata, J., Yotsumoto, H., Takaku, F., and Shimizu, T: (1990) *J. Biol. Chem.* 265: 7520-7525

19. Ohishi, N., Izumi, T., Seyama, Y., and Shimizu, T: (1990) *Methods Enzymol.* 187: 289-296

20. Rådmark, O., Shimizu, T., Jörnvall, H., and Samuelsson, B: (1984) *J. Biol. Chem.* 259, 12339-12345

21. Rola-Pleszczynski, M: (1989) *J. Lipid Res.* 1: 149-159

22. Samuelsson, B., Dahlén, S-É., Lindgren, J-Å., Rouzer, C. A., and Serhan, C: (1987) *Science* 237: 1171-1176

23. Samuelsson, B., and Funk, C. D: (1989) *J. Biol. Chem.* 264: 19469-19472

24. Shimizu, T: (1988) *Int. J. Biochem.* 20: 661-666

25. Shimizu, T., and Wolfe, L. S: (1990) *J. Neurochem.* 55: 1-15

26. Shimizu, T., Izumi, T., Honda, Z., Seyama, Y., Kurachi, Y., and Sugimoto, T: (1990) *Advances Prostaglandin, Thromboxane, Leukotriene Res.* 20: in press

27. Yamaoka, K. A., Claesson, H-E., and Rosen, A: (1989) *J. Immunol.* 143: 1996-2000

28. Winkler, J. D., Sarau, H. M., Foley, J. J., Mong, S., and Crooke, S. T: (1988) *J. Pharmacol. Exp. Ther.* 246: 204-210

PHOTOAFFINITY LABELING OF LEUKOTRIENE BINDING SITES IN HEPATOCYTES AND HEPATOMA CELLS

M. Müller, E. Falk*, R. Sandbrink, U. Berger, I. Leier, G. Jedlitschky, M. Huber, G. Kurz*, and D. Keppler

Deutsches Krebsforschungszentrum, Division of Tumor Biochemistry, D-6900 Heidelberg, and *Universität Freiburg, Institut für Organische Chemie und Biochemie, D-7800 Freiburg, Federal Republic of Germany

INTRODUCTION

The liver is the major organ which eliminates the cysteinyl leukotrienes, LTC_4, LTD_4, and LTE_4, from the blood circulation (3) by a temperature- and energy-dependent uptake system at the sinusoidal membrane of hepatocytes (4). Hepatocellular uptake is followed by partial intracellular metabolism and by excretion of cysteinyl leukotrienes and their degradation products into bile (3). Understanding of the biological actions and of the hepatobiliary elimination of leukotrienes at the molecular level requires further characterization of leukotriene receptors, of leukotriene-metabolizing enzymes, and of the respective transport systems.

Photoaffinity labeling has been successfully applied to identify binding polypeptides such as receptors and transport systems interacting with various compounds of physiological or pharmacological interest. Since photoaffinity labeling can be performed not only with purified polypeptides and subcellular fractions but also with intact cells, it can reveal binding sites functioning under physiological conditions.

DIRECT PHOTOAFFINITY LABELING WITH LEUKOTRIENES

Photoaffinity labeling is usually performed with a photolabile derivative of the compound of interest. We have described a novel approach, the direct photoaffinity labeling of leukotriene binding sites in the deep-frozen state using the radioactively labeled leukotriene itself as the photolabile ligand (2). The cysteinyl leukotrienes, e.g. LTE_4, have an absorbance maximum at 280 nm and shoulders at 270 and 292 nm. Leukotrienes are converted in irreversible reactions to molecular species of high reactivity by irradiation with high energy UV-light (300 nm) near to the absorption maximum. After 15 s of photolysis LTE_4 is decomposed by more than 50 % to a compound characterized by a UV maximum at 243 nm (Fig. 1), likely to contain a conjugated diene structure.

Cryofixation eliminates unspecific labeling taking place in solution by photoisomers and photodegradation products of leukotrienes (2). In the frozen state the highly reactive intermediates are fixed in the binding sites and react under formation of covalent bonds between the respective binding site and the radioactive ligand.

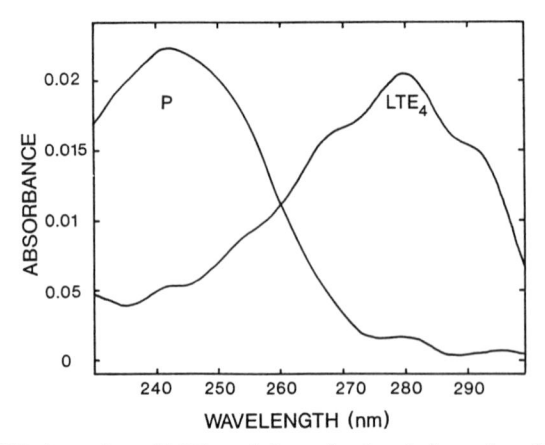

FIG. 1. UV absorption of LTE_4 and the main photolysis product (P) after irradiation of 13 nmol LTE_4 for 15 s at 300 nm (16 x 21 W lamps) in solution at 30 °C. Photolysis products were analyzed by RP-HPLC (65 % aqueous methanol, 0.1 % acetic acid, 1 mM EDTA; pH was adjusted to 5.6 with ammonium hydroxide) with continuous photodiode array recording of the absorbance. Retention times were 22 min for the photolysis product P and 32.8 min for LTE_4.

IDENTIFICATION OF LEUKOTRIENE BINDING SITES

In the intact liver hepatocytes exhibit morphological and functional polarity. LTE_4 is taken up into the hepatocyte through the sinusoidal membrane and is excreted after partial metabolic transformation through the bile canalicular membrane. Freshly isolated hepatocytes have retained a relatively intact intracellular compartmentation. Therefore, direct photoaffinity labeling studies were performed after cryofixation of freshly isolated rat hepatocytes incubated with $[^3H_2]LTC_4$ and $[^3H_2]LTE_4$. SDS-PAGE of the total membrane fraction after photoaffinity labeling in the frozen state indicated a dominant labeling of a polypeptide with an apparent M_r of 48 000 (Fig. 2 A + B). This polypeptide is assumed to be the one predominantly labeled in the subfraction enriched with sinusoidal membranes (2). The polypeptides with apparent M_rs of 68 000, 33 000, and 16 000, which were labeled in the crude particulate fraction of hepatocytes must be localized in intracellular compartments (Fig. 2).

Many labeled polypeptides were found in the soluble fraction. This indicates that the cysteinyl leukotrienes interact after their uptake into intact cells with a number of different polypeptides. The detailed functions of these polypeptides is not known at present. Among these polypeptides, those with apparent M_rs in the range of 27 000 - 25 000 were identified as subunits of glutathione transferases by immunoprecipitation (2). Since photoaffinity labeling was performed with intact hepatocytes after cryofixation, labeling of glutathione transferases suggests a possible function of these proteins in the intracellular transport of cysteinyl leukotrienes.

Whether the plasma membrane polypeptide with the apparent M_r of 48 000 is involved in uptake of cysteinyl leukotrienes or whether it has a different function cannot be decided since photoaffinity labeling only reveals ligand binding and not the function of a polypeptide. The identity of this leukotriene-binding polypeptide with the polypeptides of similar M_rs, which are labeled in rat hepatocytes by photolabile derivatives of bile salts and other amphipathic compounds, and are expected to be part of an uptake system of broad specificity (1), can only be established after purification of the proteins.

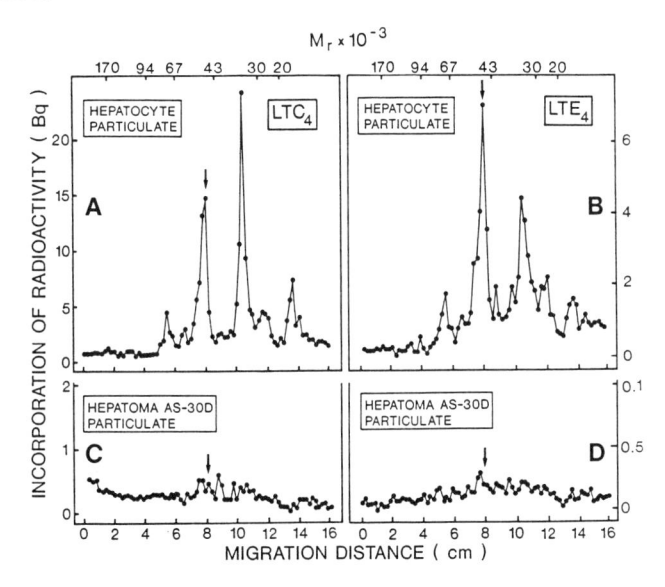

FIG. 2. Distribution of radioactivity after SDS-PAGE of the particulate fraction of labeled hepatocytes and hepatoma cells. Freshly isolated rat hepatocytes (A + B) and AS-30D hepatoma cells (C + D) (0.5 mg protein each) were incubated with 74 kBq [^{3}H$_2$]LTC$_4$ (300 nM) or 74 kBq [^{3}H$_2$]LTE$_4$ (300 nM) at 37 °C for 2 min. After shock-freezing and irradiation of the sample at 300 nm for 5 minutes in the frozen state the particulate fraction was separated and subjected to SDS/PAGE (7 - 20 % acrylamide gradient gel). Arrows indicate the position of M_r 48 000. For further experimental conditions see (2).

Evidence for a function of this leukotriene-binding protein as part of an uptake system for these eicosanoids was obtained from labeling studies with AS-30D ascites hepatoma cells which are deficient in cysteinyl leukotriene uptake (5). Photoaffinity labeling with cysteinyl leukotrienes showed no labeling of polypeptides with an apparent M_r of 48 000 (Fig. 2 C + D). Corresponding results were obtained when we used isolated intact human hepatocytes (Fig. 3 A) and the human hepatoma cell lines PLC (Fig. 3 B) and Hep G2 (Fig. 3 C). The polypeptide with the apparent M_r of 48 000 which was labeled in the plasma membrane of human hepatocytes was not labeled in the dedifferentiated hepatoma cells. For Hep G2 hepatoma cells (Fig. 3 C) the soluble fraction is shown in addition and no significant labeling was detected. This is consistent with the deficient uptake of cysteinyl leukotrienes by hepatoma cells.

SUMMARY

The method of direct photoaffinity labeling in the frozen state using the leukotrienes as suitable photolabile compounds may serve to identify and characterize polypeptides which interact with these eicosanoids during their hepatobiliary transport and metabolism. Furthermore, it will be a helpful technique to evaluate changes in the cell-specific protein pattern during neoplastic dedifferentiation of hepatocytes.

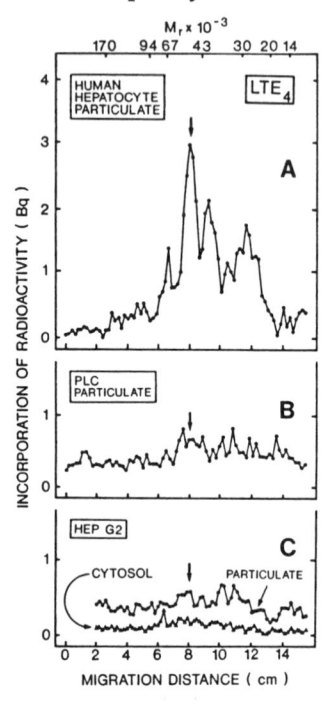

FIG. 3. Distribution of radioactivity after SDS-PAGE of the particulate fraction of labeled human hepatocytes and hepatoma cells. Intact isolated human hepatocytes (A), cultivated hepatoma cells PLC (B), and Hep G2 (C) were incubated with 74 kBq [^{3}H$_2$]LTE$_4$ (300 nM) at 37 °C for 2 min.

REFERENCES

1. Buscher, H.-P., Fricker, G., Gerok, W., Kramer, W., Kurz, G., Müller, M., and Schneider, S. (1986): In: *Receptor-mediated uptake in the liver*. edited by H. Greten, E. Windler, and U. Beisiegel. pp. 189-199. Springer-Verlag, Berlin.
2. Falk, E., Müller, M., Huber, M., Keppler, D., and Kurz, G. (1989): *Eur. J. Biochem.*, 186: 741-747.
3. Huber, M., and Keppler, D. (1990): In: *Progress in Liver Diseases*, vol. 9, edited by H. Popper and F. Schaffner. pp.117-141, W.B.Saunders, Philadelphia.
4. Uehara, N., Ormstadt, K., Örning, L., and Hammarström, S. (1983): *Biochim. Biophys. Acta*, 732: 69-74.
5. Weckbecker, G., and Keppler, D. (1986): *Eur. J. Biochem.*, 154: 559-562.

MECHANISMS OF LEUKOTRIENE B_4-SPECIFIC CHEMOTACTIC DEACTIVATION OF HUMAN POLYMORPHONUCLEAR LEUKOCYTES

J.M. Boggs and E.J. Goetzl

Departments of Medicine and Microbiology-Immunology,
University of California Medical Center,
San Francisco, California 94143-0724

Human polymorphonuclear leukocytes (PMNLs) bear cell-surface receptors for leukotriene B_4, which consist of a high-affinity subset (Kd = 0.4 nM) that mediates chemotaxis and increased adherence to surfaces and a low-affinity subset (Kd = 61 nM) that directs lysosomal degranulation and superoxide anion generation (1-3). Exposure of PMNLs to LTB_4 at 37°C rapidly results in concurrent suppression of high-affinity receptors and chemotactic responses to LTB_4, termed chemotactic deactivation. Deactivation has no effects on the low-affinity subset of LTB_4 receptors or on responses to peptide chemotactic factors (Table 1). Rabbit anti-idiotypic IgG antibodies (a-Id) were developed to the combining site of a mouse monoclonal anti-LTB_4 antibody, which bind to the 60-80 kD membrane protein of LTB_4 receptors in Western blots and block selectively both binding of [^{3}H]LTB_4 to high-affinity receptors and chemotactic responses to LTB_4 (4). The a-Id were used to quantify the diminished expression of LTB_4 receptor antigen in parallel with reduced binding of [^{3}H]LTB_4 in order to elucidate the mechanisms of LTB_4-induced chemotactic deactivation.

TABLE 1. *Previously defined characteristics of human PMNL chemotactic deactivation by LTB_4*

1. Stimulus-specific at low concentrations of LTB_4

2. Selective decrease in chemotactic function

3. Loss of only high-affinity binding of [^{3}H]LTB_4

4. Rapid and rapidly reversible at 37°C

METHODS

Samples of PMNL purified from human blood and isolated PMNL membranes were preincubated for 1-20 min at 37°C without (control) or with LTB_4, cooled to 4°C, and studied for binding of a-Id and $[^3H]LTB_4$. Replicate 100 µL aliquots of suspensions of 1-2×10^7 control and deactivated PMNLs/ml and of 75-100 µg of PMNL membrane protein in 100 µl of buffer were added to 12 x 75 mm polypropylene tubes containing 50 µl of 0.3 nM $[^3H]LTB_4$ and 100 µl of 1,000 nM nonradioactive LTB_4 (nonspecific binding) or buffer alone (total binding). After incubation at 4 °C for 45 min, the bound and free $[^3H]LTB_4$ were separated by rapid filtration of the incubation mixtures through Whatman GF/C (for intact PMNL) or GF/F (for PMNL membranes) glass fiber filters (Whatman Laboratory Products, Clifton, NJ), the filters were washed three times with 4 ml of PBS at 4°C, radioactivity in the filters was quantified, and specific binding was calculated by substracting nonspecific binding from total binding. Identical replicate aliquots of 1-2×10^6 PMNLs and of PMNL membranes consisting of 75-150 µg of protein in a total of 250 µl of buffer were incubated at 4°C for 90 min with 30 µg of a-Id IgG or nonimmune IgG, washed and incubated with 24.5 nCi of $[^{125}I]$ protein A for 60 min at 4°C. The PMNLs and isolated membranes then were washed three times, and bound radioactivity was quantified and corrected for binding in the absence of exogenous IgG to derive values for specific binding.

RESULTS

Loss of high-affinity receptors for LTB_4 from the surface of PMNLs chemotactically deactivated by incubation with 10 nM LTB_4 was significant after 1 min and reached a mean maximum after 20 min of 82% and 61%, respectively, as assessed by binding of $[^3H]LTB_4$ and a-Id (5). A combination of inhibitors of PMNL proteases did not prevent the LTB_4-induced decrease in surface receptors for LTB_4 (5). Incubation of membranes isolated from PMNL with 100 nM LTB_4 at 37°C resulted in loss of $[^3H]LTB_4$ binding activity with a time-course similar to that observed in intact PMNL, which attained a mean loss of 59% after 20 min (5). Disruption of deactivated PMNL by sonication failed to expose intracellular LTB_4 receptors, as indicated by similar mean recoveries of 20% and 7% of $[^3H]LTB_4$ binding activity from intact and sonicated PMNL after deactivation (5).

DISCUSSION

The rapid and reversible course of desensitization of receptor binding activity in chemotactic deactivation has been attributed to either alterations in combined site structure, shedding of the receptors from the cell surface, or translocation of receptors to other cellular compartments (Fig. 1). The translocation of receptors in deactivated PMNL might involve movement into the plasma membrane with or without binding to cytoskeletal proteins (Fig. 1-1) or internalization by one or more endocytic pathways (Fig. 1-3). Changes in receptor structure might include altered conformation, in part due to changes in association of LTB_4 receptors with G-proteins (Fig. 1-2), biochemical modification such as phosphorylation by protein kinases (Fig. 1-4), or surface proteolysis (Fig. 1-5). The consistent findings of LTB_4 receptor desensitization in isolated membranes, as well as in intact PMNL, favor translocation in the membrane (Fig. 1-1), but do not exclude changes in association of the receptors with G-proteins (Fig.1-2). The lack of effects of protease inhibitors, the failure to recover modified forms of the LTB_4 receptor protein, and the failure of sonification to release intracellular binding sites, are against covalent alterations and endocytosis (Fig. 1-3 to 5). Alterations in the display or disposition of LTB_4 receptors in PMNL plasma membranes thus remains the most likely cellular basis for LTB_4-induced chemotactic deactivation of PMNL. A precedent for this mechanism is found in the redistribution of PMNL receptors for peptide chemotactic factors by lateral segregation into actin- and fodrin-rich microdomains of the plasma membrane or into other membrane compartments (6,7).

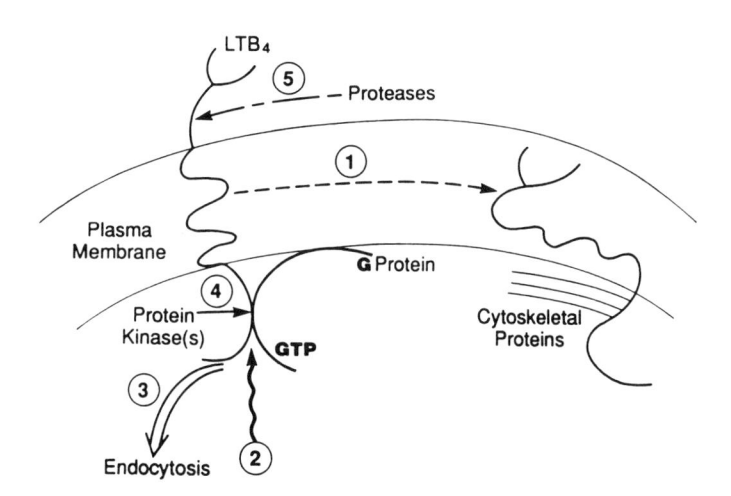

FIG. 1. Possible mechanisms of LTB_4-induced desensitization of PMNL receptors for LTB_4. G protein = guanine nucleotide-binding protein, GTP = guanosine triphosphate, 1 - 5 = sites of theoretical effects of LTB_4, which lead to receptor desensitization in chemotactic deactivation.

ACKNOWLEDGEMENT

This study was supported in part by grant HL 31809 (Edward J. Goetzl) from the National Institutes of Health.

REFERENCES

1. Goetzl, E.J., and Pickett, W.C. (1981):*J. Exp. Med.* 153:482.
2. Goldman, D.W., and Goetzl, E.J. (1984):*J. Exp. Med..* 159:1027.
3. Sherman, J., Goetzl, E.J., and Koo, C.H. (1988):*J. Immunol.* 140:3900.
4. Gifford, L., Chernov-Rogan, T., Harvey, J., Koo, C.H., Goldman, D., and Goetzl, E.J. (1987):*J. Immunol.* 138:1184.
5. Boggs, J.M., Koo, C.H., and Goetzl, E.J. (1990):*Clin. Res.* 38:359A.
6. Jesatis, A.J., Tolley, J.O., Bokoch, G.M., and Allen, R.A. (1989):*J. Cell Biol.* 109:2783.
7. Sarndahl, E., Lindroth, M., Bengtsson, T., Fallman, M., Gustavsson, S., Stendahl, O., and Andersson, T. (1989):*J. Cell Biol.* 109:2791.

DESENSITIZATION OF THE LEUKOTRIENE B_4 RECEPTOR BY PARTIAL AGONISTS

*D. Kiel, R.E. Zipkin, and *+S.J. Feinmark

Departments of *Pharmacology and +Medicine, Columbia University, New York, NY 10032 USA and Biomol Research Laboratories Inc., Plymouth Meeting, PA 19462 USA

Leukotriene (LT) B_4 activates human polymorphonuclear leukocytes (PMNL) causing aggregation, adherence to endothelium, superoxide production and release of granular enzymes (6). Prior exposure of PMNL to LTB_4 induces homologous desensitization in chemotaxis (3) and degranulation assays (5). A similar desensitization to LTB_4-induced degranulation (2) and superoxide generation (1) has also been shown after pretreatment of PMNL with 5(S),12(S)-DHETE, an LTB_4 isomer formed by transcellular metabolism requiring both platelets and PMNL. We have studied the effects of 5(S),12(S)-DHETE and a synthetic LTB_4 analog, LTB_4-aminopropylamide (LTB_4-APA) in order to elucidate the mechanism of LTB_4 receptor desensitization.

5(S),12(S)-DHETE and LTB_4-APA were found to be partial agonists at the human PMNL LTB_4 receptor. Both compounds weakly induced PMNL aggregation at concentrations exceeding 1 uM. Although LTB_4 activation of PMNL causes an increase in intracellular calcium (4), a dose-related increase in inositol trisphosphate (IP_3) accumulation has not been demonstrated directly in human PMNL. LTB_4 increased [^{3}H]IP_3 production in myo-[2-^{3}H]inositol labelled PMNL, in a dose-dependent manner (EC_{50}=1 nM) which paralleled the induction of PMNL aggregation (EC_{50}=5 nM). IP_3 generation by both 5(S),12(S)-DHETE and LTB_4-APA was shifted two to three orders of magnitude to the right and reached a plateau at a level lower than that induced by LTB_4. Thus, the ability of these compounds to increase IP_3 in neutrophils correlated with their biological activity.

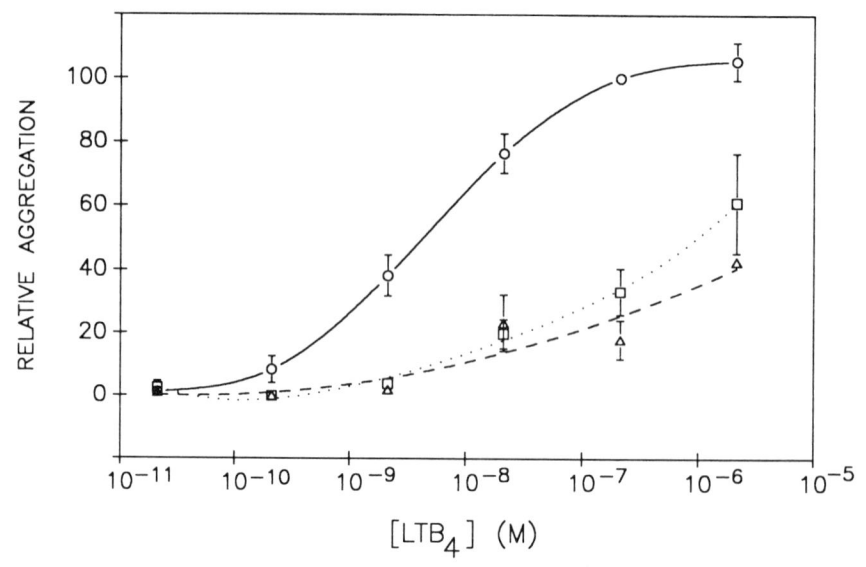

FIG. 1. LTB$_4$-induced aggregation of human PMNL. PMNL (4 x 10^6 in 0.3 ml) were pretreated at 37°C for one min with either vehicle (○), 5(S),12(S)-DHETE (2 uM; □) or LTB$_4$-APA (300 nM; △), and then cytochalasin B (5 ug/ml) for an additional 5 min. Aggregation was induced by the addition of LTB$_4$. (Kiel and Feinmark, submitted).

Pretreatment with either of these partial agonists antagonized LTB$_4$-induced aggregation of human PMNL (Figure 1). LTB$_4$-APA (300 nM) or 5(S),12(S)-DHETE (2 uM) reduced the PMNL response to LTB$_4$, and depressed the dose-response curves. These data suggest that the antagonism occurs in a non-competitive manner. This is also supported by the observation that the simultaneous addition of 5(S),12(S)-DHETE with LTB$_4$ failed to reduce the aggregatory response in contrast to the marked inhibition caused by pretreatment. The response of PMNL to fMLP was unaffected by pretreatment with either partial agonist which demonstrates that these compounds cause homologous desensitization.

To determine if LTB$_4$ stimulation of desensitized cells resulted in a decreased formation of IP$_3$, myo-[2-^{3}H]inositol-labelled human PMNL were pretreated with LTB$_4$-APA (300 nM) at 37°C for six minutes, washed twice and stimulated with LTB$_4$. The accumulation of IP$_3$ in LTB$_4$-APA pretreated PMNL was significantly reduced in comparison to control cells.

Since these partial agonists antagonize the biological responses of PMNL to LTB$_4$ in a non-competitive manner, we studied whether pretreatment with these compounds altered the number or affinity of PMNL LTB$_4$ receptors. Scatchard analysis of [^{3}H]LTB$_4$ binding to whole cells was carried out at 4°C and the data were fit by computer to a two-site model using

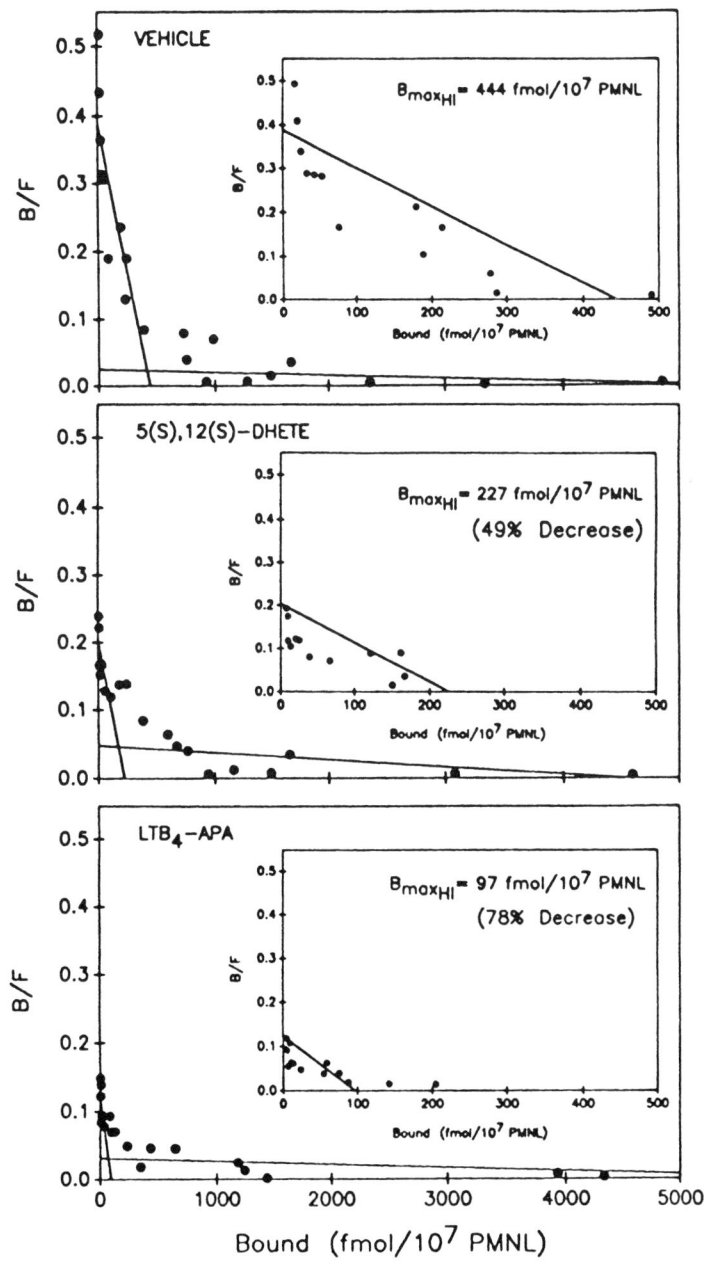

FIG. 2. Scatchard analysis of [^{3}H]LTB$_4$ binding to human PMNL. PMNL were pretreated at 37°C with vehicle (top), 5(S),12(S)-DHETE (2 uM; middle) or LTB$_4$-APA (330 nM; bottom). After washing, [^{3}H]LTB$_4$ binding was measured in the presence of increasing cold LTB$_4$. Bound ligand was separated from free by rapid filtration through a glass fiber filter and the radioactive material was quantified by liquid scintillation counting. The insets show the LIGAND generated line for high affinity binding on an expanded axis. The data points in the inset were recalculated to remove the low affinity component of binding. (Kiel and Feinmark, submitted).

LIGAND (Fig 2). PMNL exhibited both high (k_D=0.57 nM, B_{max}=444 fmol/10^7 PMNL) and low-affinity (k_D=111 nM, B_{max}=5436 fmol/10^7 PMNL) LTB_4 receptors. Cells pretreated at 37°C with either partial agonist had no change in the affinity or number of low-affinity sites, but we found striking differences in the number of high affinity receptors with no change in the k_D. PMNL pretreated with 5(S),12(S)-DHETE exhibited a 49% loss of high-affinity LTB_4 receptors, while cells pretreated with LTB_4-APA showed a 78% decrease in high-affinity receptor number (Fig 2, insets). This reduction in LTB_4 receptor number correlates with the ability of these partial agonists to antagonize LTB_4-induced aggregation.

In summary, these experiments indicate that 5(S),12(S)-DHETE and LTB_4-APA are partial agonists at the human PMNL LTB_4 receptor where they induce aggregation and IP_3 accumulation in parallel; these compounds antagonize LTB_4-induced PMNL aggregation and IP_3 formation in a non-competitive manner; and, pretreatment of human PMNL with these partial agonists causes a loss of high-affinity LTB_4 receptors from the cell surface which correlates with their antagonistic activity.

REFERENCES

1. Claesson, H.-E., and Feinmark, S.J. (1984): Biochim. Biophys. Acta, 804:52-57.
2. Feinmark, S.J., Lindgren, J.Å., Claesson, H.-E., Malmsten, C., and Samuelsson, B. (1981): FEBS Lett., 136:141-144.
3. Goetzl, E.J., Boeynaems, J.M., Oates, J.A., and Hubbard, W.C. (1981): Prostaglandins, 22:279-288.
4. Goldman, D.W., Gifford, L.A., Olson, D.M., and Goetzl, E.J. (1985): J. Immunol., 135:525-530.
5. O'Flaherty, J.T., Wykle, R.L., McCall, C.E., Shewmake, T.B., Lees, C.J., and Thomas, M. (1981): Biochem. Biophys. Res. Commun., 101:1290-1296.
6. Samuelsson, B. (1983): Science, 220:568-575.

S.J.F. is an American Heart Association-Boehringer Ingelheim established investigator. This work was supported by grant AI-26702 from the National Institutes of Health.

ONO-LB-457 : A NOVEL AND ORALLY ACTIVE LEUKOTRIENE B4 RECEPTOR ANTAGONIST

K. Kishikawa, N. Matsunaga, T. Maruyama, R. Seo, M. Toda, T. Miyamoto and A. Kawasaki

Minase Research Institute, Ono Pharmaceutical Co., Ltd., Shimamoto, Mishima, Osaka 618, Japan.

Leukotriene B4 (LTB4) has been reported to have various pharmacological actions such as neutrophil chemotaxis, aggregation, degranulation, adhesion to endothelial cell and lung parenchymal contraction. A high level of LTB4 was detected in lesions of human inflammatory diseases, for example, psoriasis, gout, rheumatoid, colitis and myocardiac ischemia (6). Theses results suggest that LTB4 might play an important role in development of inflammatory diseases, and the specific LTB4 antagonist might be useful for their treatment. Therefore we have developed ONO-LB-457 (5-[2-(2-Carboxyethel)-3-{ 6-(para-methoxyphenyl)-5E-hexenyl } oxyphenoxy] valeric acid) which is a potent and orally active. In the present study, we evaluated its pharmacological properties as an LTB4 antagonist *in vitro* and *in vivo*.

METHODS

^{3}H-LTB4 binding assay

Polymorphonuclear leukocytes (PMNLs) were prepared from the human venous blood, the peritoneal fluid of guinea pig or of casein-treated rat. PMNLs (10^7 cells/ml) were incubated with 1 nM of ^{3}H-LTB4 at 4 °C for 20 min in the presence of antagonists. PMNL-bound ^{3}H-LTB4 was separated from free ^{3}H-LTB4 by vacuum filtration. Specific binding was defined as the difference between total binding and binding in the presence of 3 µM LTB4 (nonspecific binding) (3).

Neutrophil aggregation

Human PMNL (10^7 cells/ml) in Hank's-0.5 % bovine serum albumin (BSA) medium (pH 7.4) were preincubated with ONO-LB-457 at 37 °C for 1 min prior to the addition of LTB4 (10 nM). Aggregation was monitored as change in light transmission using the multi channel aggregometer (2).

Neutrophil degranulation

Human PMNLs (10^7 cells/ml) in Hank's-0.5% BSA medium (pH 7.4) containing 5 µg/ml cytochalasin B were preincubated with ONO-LB-457, and then the reaction mixtures were incubated with LTB4 (0.3 µM) at 37 °C for 10 min. The results were expressed as % release of total myeloperoxidase in the cells.

Myotropic activity on guinea pig lung parenchymal strip

The measurement of myotropic activity was carried out previously described (4). Lung parenchymal strips were preincubated with ONO-LB-457 at 37 °C for 15 min, and then LTB4 (30 nM), LTC4 (10 nM) or LTD4 (10 nM) was added. Contractile responses of parenchymal strips were normalized relative to 10 µM histamine.

Transient neutropenia in guinea pig

ONO-LB-457 was injected i.v. in guinea pigs 1 min prior to administration of LTB4 (0.1 µg/kg i.v.). Blood samples were collected at 0.5, 1, and 2 min after LTB4 treatment to determine the leukocyte count using blood cell counter. The result was expressed as % of the pre-injection count (5).

Neutrophil accumulation in guinea pig skin

ONO-LB-457 was administered p.o. in guinea pigs 30 min before the intradermal injection of LTB4 (100 ng/site). Two hours after LTB4 injection, the animals were sacrificed and myeloperoxidase (MPO) activities, the neutrophil maker enzyme, in the skins were measured as neutrophil accumulation as previously described (1).

RESULTS AND DISCCUSION

In the binding assay, ONO-LB-457 inhibited specific ^{3}H-LTB4 (1 nM) binding for LTB4 receptor of human PMNL. From the comparison with the inhibitory constant (Ki) values of several

species, ONO-LB-457 had highest affinity for human PMNL-LTB4 receptor (TABLE 1).
TABLE 1. Binding affinity of ONO-LB-457 for PMNL LTB4 receptor of several species

Species	Ki (nM)
human	6
guinea pig	18
rat	86

In *in vitro* assay using isolated human PMNL, ONO-LB-457 inhibited LTB4-induced PMNL aggregation in a dose dependent manner. The concentrations causing 50 % inhibition (IC50) was 2.4 µM. ONO-LB-457 also inhibited LTB4-induced PMNL degranulation in a dose dependent manner. IC50 value was 3.0 µM. It has been reported that PMNL aggregation and degranulation are induced *via* the high and low affinity LTB4 receptors respectively. Therefore these results suggest that ONO-LB-457 antagonizes to LTB4 on the both high and low affinity LTB4 receptors of human neutrophil. ONO-LB-457 had no agonistic activity at all doses used in both assays (1 µM-10 µM). ONO-LB-457 specifically inhibited LTB4-induced contraction of lung parenchymal strips (IC50=0.7 µM), but failed to inhibit LTC4 and LTD4-induced contractions. In *in vivo* assay, intravenous administration of ONO-LB-457 prevented LTB4-induced transient neutropenia in guinea pig in a dose dependent manner (FIG. 1).

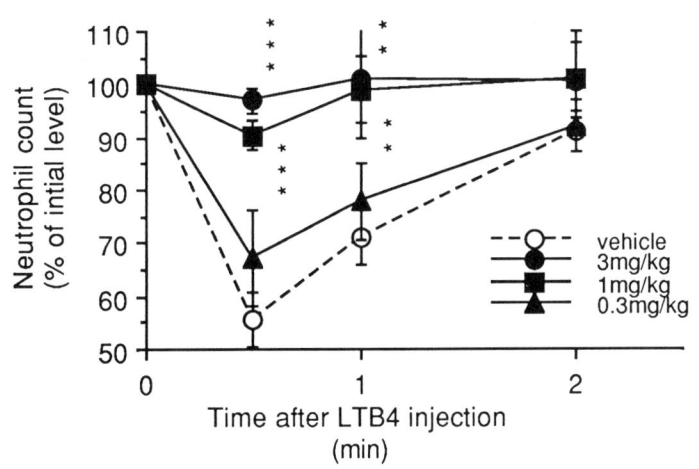

FIG. 1. Effect of ONO-LB-457 on LTB4-induced transient neutropenia in guinea pig

Each value represents mean ± SE (n=5-8).
**: p<0.01, ***: p<0.001 Significantly different from vehicle.

Oral administration of ONO-LB-457 suppressed LTB4-induced neutrophil accumulation in the skins in a dose dependent manner (FIG. 2), and its suppression (30 mg/kg) lasted for more than 6 hours. These results indicate that ONO-LB-457 is a potent, orally active and long acting LTB4 antagonist and this compound should allow the evaluation of the role of LTB4 in development of inflammatory diseases.

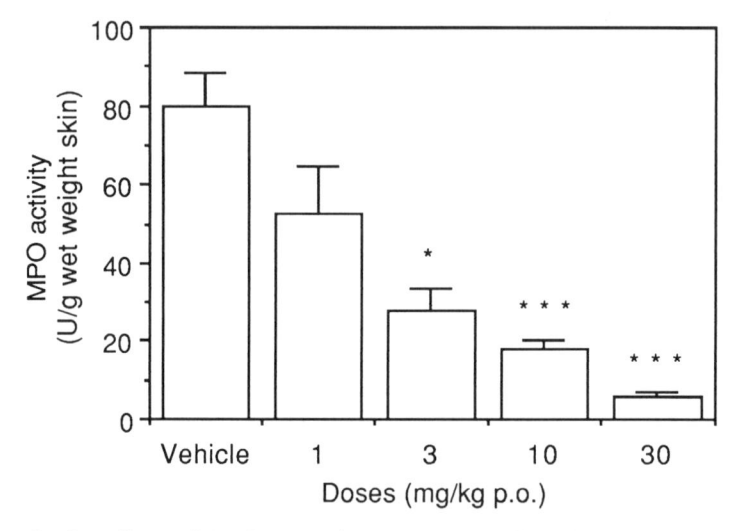

FIG. 2. Effect of ONO-LB-457 on LTB4-induced PMNL accumulation in guinea pig skin
Each value represents mean ± SE (n=10).
*: $p<0.05$, ***: $p<0.001$ Significantly different from vehicle.

REFERENCES

1. Bradley, P. P., Priebat, D., A. Christensen, R. D., and Rothstein, G. (1982): J. Invest. Dermatol. 78: 206-209.
2. Cunningham, F. M. (1980): J. Pharm. Pharmacol., 32: 377-380.
3. Kreisle, R. A., and Rarker, C. W. (1985): J. Immunology, 134: 3356-3363.
4. Lawson, C. F. (1988): J. Lipid Mediators, pre-issue: 3-12.
5. Sweatman, W. J. F., and Brandon, D. W. (1987): J. Pharmacological Methods, 18: 227-237.
6. Thomas, R. J., Gordon, L., Chi-Chung, C., Philip D. (1989): In: Leukotrienes and Lipoxygenases : Pharmacology and Pathophysiology of Leukotrienes, edited by J. Rokach, pp. 309-403. Elsevier, Amsterdam.

SYNTHESIS AND STRUCTURE-ACTIVITY RELATIONSHIPS OF A SERIES OF SUBSTITUTED-PHENYLPROPIONIC ACIDS AS A NOVEL CLASS OF LEUKOTRIENE B4 ANTAGONISTS

M. Konno, S. Sakuyama, T. Nakae, N. Hamanaka,
T. Miyamoto, and A. Kawasaki

*Minase Research Institute, Ono Pharmaceutical Co., Ltd.,
Shimamoto, Mishima, Osaka 618, Japan*

INTRODUCTION

Leukotriene B4 (LTB4) exerts a variety of pharmacologic actions including leukocyte chemotaxis and chemokinesis (2), neutrophil aggregation (6) and degranulation (10), enhanced vascular permeability (9), and a bronchoconstrictor activity via an indirect mechanism involving stimulation of the release of cyclooxygenase products (1). Furthermore, high level of LTB4 are detected in the inflammatory site in the lesions of human inflammatory diseases by lots of reseachers (3, 4, 5, 7, 8).

The synthesis of LTB4 antagonist is important to know the pathophysiological role of LTB4 itself and it may also provide the therapeutic value for inflammatory diseases mediated by LTB4. We describe here the synthesis and structure-activity relationship studies of β-phenylpropionic acids-containing compounds as high affinity and orally active LTB4 antagonists.

STRUCTURE ACTIVITY RELATIONSHIPS

The substitution of the triene unit of LTB4 at C7 to C9 with benzene ring resulted in the compound **1**. This compound showed a high binding affinity for rat neutrophil LTB4 receptors, but a poor affinity for human neutrophils.

Another modifications were carried out by the ring closure between C4 and C9 to give the potent compound **2**, whose IC50 value for human neutrophil LTB4 receptors was 0.18 μM. The introduction of the amide part of compound **1** into compound **2** resulted in the trisubstituted compound **3**. This compound had a high binding potency, however, it did not show antagonist activity but agonist activity. The replacement of the allylic alcohol group in the compound 3 with p-methoxystyrene unit afforded the potent compound 4. This one inhibited LTB4 (10^{-8}M)-induced human neutrophils aggregation with IC50 value of 3.6 µM, which had no agonist activity. We concluded that the propionic acid group was crucial for the receptor binding through the optimization of compound 4.

Possible conformers of LTB4

1 IC$_{50}$ 12 µM

2 IC$_{50}$ 0.18 µM

3 IC$_{50}$ 0.02 µM Agonist

4 IC$_{50}$ 0.045 µM Antagonist

IC$_{50}$ values: Binding Assay (human neutrophils)

We next examined the effect of different linkages between the terminal amide group and benzene ring. Compounds with ketone, methylene and ether functions as a connecting group are slightly less potent than compound 4 with the corresponding amide function.

4 IC$_{50}$ 0.045 µM

5 IC$_{50}$ 0.1 µM

6 IC$_{50}$ 0.2 µM

7 IC$_{50}$ 0.09 µM

8 IC$_{50}$ 0.03 µM

9 IC$_{50}$ 0.0036 µM ONO-LB-428

IC$_{50}$ values: Binding Assay (human neutrophils)

However, the shortening of chain length resulted in a 3-fold increase in binding potency, and a greater enhancement was observed with the reduction of ketone to hydroxy group. The IC50 value of ONO-LB-428 was 3.6 µM, which is approximately the same potency as that of native LTB4 (2.9 µM). This agent also showed potent antagonist activity, however, it was not suited for further development as a drug because of its poor pharmaceutical stability. So the pharmaceutically stable ether analog 7 was selected for further modifications. Also its chemical modifications were much easier than that of other analogs.

We investigated the effects of the substitution pattern of benzene ring in compound 7. The ortho isomer of compound 7 (ONO-LB-448) showed a 6-fold greater affinity than the meta-substituted compound 7, but it was short acting *in vivo* when given by an oral administration. The carboxylic acid analog 11 (ONO-LB-457) showed an equal binding potency to ONO-LB-448, but had a longer duration of action *in vivo*. Further experimentation is necessary to explain fully this interesting observation.

ONO-LB-457, which was the most promising compound, was easily prepared as a crystalline solid by 8 steps in good yield as follows.

CONCLUSION

Some potent and orally active antagonists of LTB4 were found out through the interphenylation approach. ONO-LB-457 was the most promising agent. Detailed biological evaluations will be reported separately.

REFERENCES

1. Bray, M. A., Cunningham, F. M., Ford-Hutchinson, A. W., and Smith, M. J. H., (1981): Br. J. Pharmacol., 72: 483.
2. Ford-Hutchinson, A. W., Bray, M. A., Doig, M. V., Shipley, M. E., and Smith, M. J. H. (1980): Nature, 286: 264.
3. Grabbe, J., Czarnetzki, B. M., Rosenbach, T., and Mardin, M., (1984): J. Invest. Dermatol., 82: 477.
4. Klickstein, L. B., Shapleigh, C., and Goetzl, E. J. (1980): J. Clin. Invest., 66: 1166.
5. O'Driscoll, B. R. C., Cromwell, O., and Kay, A. B., (1984): Clin. Exp. Immunol., 55: 397.
6. Palmblad, J., Malmsten, C. L., Udén, A. M., Rådmark, O., Engstedt, L., and Samuelsson, B., (1981): Blood, 58: 658.
7. Rae, S. A., Davidson, E. M., and Smith, M. J. H., (1982): Lancet, II: 1122.
8. Sharon, P., and Stenson, W. F., (1984): Gastroenterogy, 86: 453.
9. Sirois, P., Roy, S., Borgeat, P., Picard, S., and Vallerand, P. (1982): Prostaglandins, Leukotrienes and Medicines, 8: 157.
10. Smith, R. J., Iden, S. S., and Bowman, B. J. (1984): Inflammation, 8: 365.

SULPHIDOPEPTIDE LEUKOTRIENES IN ASTHMA

Tak H. Lee, Stephen P. O'Hickey, Crawford Jacques, Richard J. Hawksworth, Jonathan P. Arm, Pandora Christie, Bernd W. Spur, Attilio E.G. Crea.

Department of Allergy and Allied Respiratory Disorders, Guy's Hospital, London SE1 9RT. UK.

INTRODUCTION

Arachidonic acid (AA) released from membrane phospholipids during cell activation may be oxidatively metabolized by the enzymes of the cyclooxygenase or lipoxygenase pathways. AA is metabolized by the cyclooxygenase pathway to prostaglandins and thromboxane. The 5-lipoxygenase pathway generates 5 - hydroperoxy - eicosatetraenoic acid (5-HPETE) or is converted enzymatically to the unstable intermediate leukotriene (LT) A_4. LTA_4 is metabolized by an epoxide hydrolase to LTB_4, or by a LTC_4 synthase to LTC_4. LTC_4 is cleaved by gamma-glutamyl-transpeptidase to LTD_4, which is converted by a dipeptidase to LTE_4. LTB_4 is a potent chemoattractant for neutrophils, while the sulphidopeptide leukotrienes (LTC_4, LTD_4 and LTE_4) are potent spasmogens for non-vascular smooth muscle and comprise the activity previously recognized as slow reacting substance of anaphylaxis (SRS-A).

Identification in asthma:

Lam and colleagues analysed the bronchoalveolar lavage (BAL) fluid from 17 subjects with mild to severe asthma and from 9 healthy controls (7). Leukotrienes were resolved from the BAL samples by reverse phase - high performance liquid chromatography (RP-HPLC). LTE_4 was detected in the BAL fluid of 15 asthmatic subjects, LTD_4 was found in the BAL fluid of 2 asthmatic subjects and LTC_4 was not detected. The identity of LTE_4 was confirmed by its ultraviolet absorbance spectrum and by fast atom bombardment mass spectroscopy. Leukotrienes were not detected in the BAL fluid of healthy subjects.

The sulphidopeptide leukotrienes are potent bronchoconstrictor agents when inhaled. However, the airways of asthmatic subjects are not as hyperresponsive to those agonists as they are to histamine or methacholine. Griffin and colleagues reported that the concentration of LTD_4 required to elicit a 30%

fall in airflow at 30% vital capacity (V_{30}) in asthmatic subjects was on average only 1/3 that necessary to elicit a response in normal subjects (6). Barnes and colleagues demonstrated that the airways of a group of 6 asymptomatic asthmatic subjects were 11-fold more reactive to histamine than those of normal controls, but were 4- to 5-fold more responsive to LTC_4 and LTD_4.

Adelroth demonstrated a significant correlation between airways responses to methacholine to those of LTC_4 and LTD_4 in 12 asthmatic and six mon-asthmatic subjects. They also demonstrated a correlation between airways responsiveness to methacholine and relative responsiveness to LTC_4 and LTD_4 (i.e. the dose of methacholine required to elicit a given airway response ÷ the dose of LTC_4 or LTD_4 necessary to evoke the same response). Subjects with the most responsive airways demonstrated the lowest relative responsiveness to LTC_4 and LTD_4 as compared to methacholine (1).

When the airways responses to LTE_4 were compared with those to histamine and methacholine in 20 asthmatic subjects and 6 normal subjects (9) there was a correlation between the dose of LTE_4 causing a 35% fall in sGaw (PD_{35} sGaw) with both the histamine PD_{35} sGaw or the methacholine PD_{35} sGaw.

However, in contrast to the results reported for LTC_4 and LTD_4 the relative potency of LTE_4 compared to histamine and methacholine was greater in asthmatic than in normal subjects (4).

The differences between our findings for LTE_4 and those reported for LTC_4 and LTD_4 may have been due to patient selection, or to methodological differences between studies. We have therefore directly compared the potencies of histamine and methacholine to those of LTC_4, LTD_4 and LTE_4 in 6 asthmatic and 6 normal subjects (4). The airways of asthmatic subjects were 14-fold, 15-fold, 5-fold, 9-fold and 194-fold more responsive than the airways of normal subjects to histamine, methacholine, LTC_4, LTD_4 and LTE_4, respectively. Furthermore, while LTC_4 and LTD_4 were 100- to 150-fold more potent than LTE_4 in constricting the airways of normal subjects, they were only 4- to 5-fold more potent than LTE_4 in asthmatic subjects.

Thus, the airways of asthmatic subjects demonstrated a selective and marked hyperresponsiveness to LTE_4. These results may reflect the existence of leukotriene receptor subtype heterogeneity within the human airway.

The mechanism of aspirin sensitivity is unknown but probably depends upon inhibition of cyclooxygenase. The evidence that inhibition of cyclooxygenase leads to bronchoconstriction via an increased generation of spasmogenic leukotrienes is compelling. In subjects with aspirin-induced asthma (AIA) ingestion of aspirin was accompanied by the release of immunoreactive LTC_4 into nasal secretions (5). LTC_4 was not released following ingestion of aspirin in subjects without AIA or in subjects with

AIA following desensitisation. In addition, an asthmatic attack as a result of aspirin challenge in aspirin sensitive asthmatic subjects leads to an increase in LTE$_4$ levels in urine (Christie and Lee - unpublished).

An additional hypothesis for the mechanism of aspirin sensitivity suggests that there is an increased target organ sensitivity to leukotrienes. Airways responsiveness to histamine and LTE$_4$ was therefore evaluated in five subjects with AIA and in a control group of asthmatic subjects without AIA (3). LTE$_4$ was on average 145 times more potent than histamine in eliciting bronchoconstriction in subjects without AIA. In contrast LTE$_4$ was 1,870 times more potent than histamine in constricting the airways of subjects with AIA. Furthermore, following oral desensitisation to aspirin there was a mean 20-fold decrease in the sensitivity of the airways to LTE$_4$, but no change in airways responsiveness to histamine. These data suggest that a selective airways hyperresponsiveness to LTE$_4$ may contribute to the pathophysiology of AIA, and that the efficacy of desensitisation may be due in part to a specific down-regulation of receptors for LTE$_4$ within the airways.

The role of leukotrienes in airways hyperresponsiveness in asthma: Pretreatment of guinea pig tracheal spirals with LTE$_4$ enhanced the subsequent contractile response to histamine (8). In contrast concentrations of LTC$_4$ and LTD$_4$ which elicited the same contractile response as LTE$_4$ did not increase the contractile response of guinea pig tracheal spirals to histamine. Indomethacin (10μM), a cyclooxygenase inhibitor, blocked the LTE$_4$-induced phenomenon. Similarly, the selective TP receptor antagonist GR32191 (3μM), inhibited LTE$_4$-induced hyperresponsiveness. In the presence of indomethacin (10μM), a non-contractile dose (4nM) of U46619, a thromboxane A$_2$ mimetic, was able to mimic the hyperresponsiveness induced by LTE$_4$ of guinea pig tracheal strips. These results suggest that LTE$_4$ selectively augments histamine responsiveness in guinea pig tracheal tissues and that the mechanism for the effect may be mediated by a prostanoid, possibly via the TP receptor.

Since LTC$_4$ and LTD$_4$ are converted to LTE$_4$ and because LTE$_4$ may persist at the site of contraction for the longest period of time, we investigated the capacity of LTE$_4$ to enhance airways histamine responsiveness in both asthmatic and normal subjects (2). Inhalation of LTE$_4$ to produce a mean fall in sGaw of 41% led to a mean 3.5-fold decrease in the dose of histamine required to elicit a 35% fall in sGaw (PD$_{35}$ sGaw) ($p<10^{-5}$). Inhalation of methacholine to elicit a comparable fall in sGaw was not followed by any significant change in airways histamine responsiveness. Changes in airways histamine responsiveness were maximal at 4 to 7 hours after inhalation of LTE$_4$ and had returned to baseline values by one week. In addition a 50-fold higher dose of LTE_4 in normal subjects which produced a 38% fall in sGaw did not enhance airways responsiveness to histamine. Recent work suggests that airways responsiveness to histamine is also enhanced to a comparable degree in asthmatic subjects following inhalation of LTC_4 and LTD_4 (O'Hickey, Arm and Lee - unpublished). Six normal and 7 asthmatic subjects underwent histamine inhalation challenge at 1, 4 and 7 hours after saline control and bronchoconstriction induced by LTC_4, LTD_4 LTE_4 and methacholine. Airways responsiveness was determined as the dose of agonist required to induce a 35% fall in specific airways conductance. In asthmatic subjects prior inhalation of LTC_4 enhanced airways responsiveness to histamine, when compared to saline inhalation, by 2.8-, 3.9- and 2.9-fold at 1, 4 and 7 hours respectively after inhalation (p<0.001). LTD_4 enhanced histamine responsiveness by 2.1-, 2.9- and 2.1-fold after inhalation (p<0.001) and LTE_4 enhanced histamine responsiveness by 2.4-, 3.0- and 1.8-fold after inhalation (p<0.001). Methacholine inhalation did not alter significantly the histamine responsiveness throughout the time course. In normal subjects inhalation of LTC_4, LTD_4 and LTE_4 did not alter airways responsiveness to histamine.

SUMMARY

Bronchial asthma is characterized by airways inflammation and airways hyperresponsiveness. It is unlikely that the pathophysiology of asthma and bronchial hyperresponsiveness can be explained on the basis of a single cell or a single class of mediators. Nevertheless, the possibility that leukotrienes may contribute to the pathogenesis of the inflammatory, vasoactive and spasmogenic components of bronchial asthma is suggested by the properties of these lipid mediators, the preferential capacity of inflammatory cells to generate leukotrienes and the presence of leukotrienes in the airways of asthmatic subjects.

The sulphidopeptide leukotrienes are potent bronchoconstrictor agonists when inhaled. The airways of asthmatic subjects are hyperresponsive to leukotrienes as to other bronchoconstrictor agonists. Nevertheless, the airways responsiveness of asthmatic subjects to these agonists demonstrate several unusual properties. While the airways of asthmatic subjects are relatively less responsive to LTC_4 and LTD_4, compared to agents such as histamine or methacholine, they demonstrate a marked and selective hyperresponsiveness to LTE_4, suggesting a possibly unique role for this mediator in the pathogenesis of airways hyperresponsiveness. In addition an increased sensitivity of the airways to LTE_4 may contribute to the mechanism of aspirin-induced asthma. The capacity of the sulphidopeptide leukotrienes to increase the airways responsiveness of normal subjects to methacholine and of asthmatic subjects to histamine is further evidence for a role for these substances in the pathogenesis of bronchial asthma.

REFERENCES
(1) Adelroth, E., Morris, M.M., Hargreave, F.E., et al (1986): Airway responsiveness to leukotrienes C_4 and D_4 to methacholine in patients with asthma and normal controls. N. Engl. J. Med., 315:480-484.
(2) Arm, J.P., Spur, B.W., Lee, T.H. (1988): The effects of inhaled leukotriene E_4 on the airways responsiveness to histamine in asthmatic and normal subjects. J. Allergy Clin. Immunol., 82:654-660.
(3) Arm, J.P., O'Hickey, S.P., Spur, B.W. et al (1989): Airways responsiveness to histamine and leukotriene E_4 in subjects with aspirin-induced asthma. Am. Rev. Respir. Dis., 140:148-153.
(4) Arm, J.P., O'Hickey, S.P., Hawksworth, R.J., et al (In press): Asthmatic airways have a disproportionate hyperresponsiveness to LTE_4 as compared to normal airways, but not to LTC_4, methacholine and histamine. Am. Rev. Resp. Dis.
(5) Ferreri, N.R., Howland, W.C., Stevenson, D.D. et al (1988): Release of leukotrienes, prostaglandins and histamine into nasal secretions of aspirin-sensitive asthmatics during reaction to aspirin. Am. Rev. Respir. Dis., 137:847-854.
(6) Griffin, M., Weis, J.W., Leitch, A.G. et al (1983): Effects of leukotriene D_4 on the airways in asthma. N. Engl. J. Med., 308:436-439.
(7) Lam, S., Chan, H., Le Riche, J.C., et al (1988): Release of leukotrienes in patients with bronchial asthma. J. Allergy Clin. Immunol., 81:711-717.
(8) Lee, T.H., Austen, K.F., Corey, E.J. et al (1984): Leukotriene E_4-induced airway hyperresponsiveness of guinea pig tracheal smooth muscle to histamine and evidence for three separate sulphidopeptide leukotriene receptors. Proc. Natl. Acad. Sci. USA., 81:4922-4925.
(9) O'Hickey, S.P., Arm, J.P., Rees, P.J., Spur, B.W., Lee, T.H. (1988): The relative responsiveness to inhaled leukotriene E_4, methacholine and histamine in normal and asthmatic subjects. European Resp. J., 1:913-917.

ROLE OF ARACHIDONIC ACID METABOLITES IN THE PATHOGENESIS OF ACUTE LUNG INJURY

Andrew J. Lonigro, Alan H. Stephenson and Randy S. Sprague

Departments of Medicine and Pharmacology
St. Louis University School of Medicine
St. Louis, MO 63104 USA

Acute lung injury in humans, termed the adult respiratory distress syndrome (ARDS), is characterized clinically by nonhydrostatic pulmonary edema, systemic hypoxemia, pulmonary hypertension and decreased compliance of the lungs (3). Although products of arachidonic acid metabolism have been implicated as participants in each of the aforementioned pathophysiologic changes (5,6,11), it is to the question of nonhydrostatic pulmonary edema that the present work is directed. Implicit in the concept of nonhydrostatic pulmonary edema is a change in the permeability characteristics of the microvasculature. In view of reports that leukotriene synthesis occurred in several cells resident within the lung, as well as in the isolated perfused lung, and that the sulfidopeptide leukotrienes, LTC_4, LTD_4 and LTE_4, when administered, possessed the ability to enhance microvascular permeability (1,12,13), we postulated that, in acute lung injury, lipoxygenase products of arachidonic acid metabolism were the agents responsible for the enhanced microvascular permeability resulting, thereby, in the accumulation of extravascular lung water. This hypothesis was lent considerable credence when we found that leukotrienes C_4, D_4 and B_4 were elevated in the bronchoalveolar lavage fluid of patients with the adult respiratory distress syndrome when compared to normal volunteers (10).

To address this hypothesis, it was necessary, as a first step, to demonstrate that lipoxygenase products are produced by the lung in several models of acute lung injury, but not produced by edema resulting from increases in microvascular hydrostatic pressure. To this end, we decided to evaluate two models of acute lung injury in intact dogs, one that was neutrophil-independent and one that was neutrophil-dependent.

METHODS

Heartworm- and microfilaria-free, adult male mongrel dogs (20-30 kg), fasted overnight but allowed free access to water, were anesthetized with pentobarbital sodium (30 mg/kg, i.v.) followed by its continuous i.v. infusion (0.05 mg/kg/min), a dose sufficient to maintain anesthesia in the absence of neuromuscular blockade (9). Neuromuscular blockade was produced with pancuronium bromide (loading dose: 0.1 mg/kg, i.v.; maintenance dose: 40 µg/kg/h, i.v.). A 10 mm endotracheal tube was inserted through a tracheostomy and the animals were ventilated (Harvard Ventilator) with room air at 12-15 breaths/min with a tidal volume of 15 ml/kg. The frequency of ventilation was adjusted such that arterial pH and PCO_2 were within the range considered to be normal for unanesthetized dogs. Blood samples for pH, PCO_2 and PO_2 determinations were collected anaerobically and analyzed within 5 min (BNS3-Mk2, Radiometer). A Swan-Ganz catheter was advanced into the main pulmonary artery via a peripheral vein for continuous measurement of mean pulmonary arterial pressure (Ppa) and to obtain aliquots of mixed venous blood for blood gas determination and for assay of products of arachidonic acid metabolism. Catheters were also placed into the aorta for measurements of mean systemic arterial pressure (Psa) and to obtain arterial samples for blood gas measurements and for eicosanoid assays. Via thoracotomy, a catheter was placed into the left atrium through the atrial appendage for continuous measurement of mean left atrial pressure (Pla). In some experiments, the left main pulmonary artery was isolated and fit with an electromagnetic flow probe and, distal to the flow probe, an external vascular occluder (IBM, OC-8). A catheter was placed into the superior vena cava via the jugular vein for administration of ethchlorvynol (15 mg/kg) or phorbol myristate acetate (10 or 20 μg/kg). The jugular vein catheter was used for the rapid injection of a thermal-dye bolus for estimates of cardiac output (total pulmonary blood flow) and extravascular thermal volume of the lungs. For the production of hydrostatic pulmonary edema, a 16-Fr Foley catheter with a 20 ml inflatable balloon was placed into the left atrium via the left atrial appendage. The catheter was advanced to the level of the mitral annulus to insure that, when the balloon was inflated, the total pulmonary venous circulation was subjected to increased hydrostatic pressure.

Estimates of extravascular lung water (EVLW) were made by the measurement of extravascular thermal volume (EVTV) and by a gravimetric method (7,9). For measurement of EVTV, a 5-Fr thermistor-tipped catheter (Model 96020-5F Edwards Laboratories) was placed into a femoral artery. EVTV, reported as the mean of 2-3 determinations, was quantified by a microprocessor-based system (9310 Computer, Edwards Laboratories) which compares the mean transit-times of an indicator confined to the vascular space with one which distributes throughout the entire thermal mass of the lung. Thus, a bolus of iced 5% dextrose, containing 2 mg of indocyanine green dye, was injected rapidly into the superior vena cava. The dye concentration and thermal curves were measured simultaneously by withdrawing blood via the 5-Fr thermistor-tipped catheter through the cuvette of a dye-densitometer (Model D402-A Waters). The cardiac output was calculated as the integral of the area under the thermal curve divided by the duration of the curve. Immediately following the last EVTV measurement, an aliquot of systemic arterial blood was withdrawn for measurement of hemoglobin concentration. The pulmonary hila, pulmonary artery and aorta were then clamped, and the lungs removed for gravimetric determination of EVLW.

In an attempt to define more clearly the relationship between leukotriene generation and increases in EVLW, an isolated blood-perfused lung preparation was developed. In brief, after the animals had been anesthetized as described above, a left lateral thoracotomy was performed and the pulmonary artery supplying the left lower lobe was identified and isolated. Following heparin administration, 700 units/kg, i.v., 700 ml of blood were removed and used to perfuse the isolated left lower lobe. The left lower lobe was suspended from a force transducer (Grass FTO3C) and perfused under Zone III conditions at 38°C with blood containing papaverine (3×10^{-4}M) to prevent changes in perfusion pressure and, thereby, changes in the surface area available for fluid filtration.

The height of the venous reservoir was adjusted so that lobar venous pressure (Ppv) could be altered as desired. Lobar arterial (in-flow) pressure, lobar venous (outflow) pressure, perfusate flow rate and airway pressure were measured continuously. Pulmonary microvascular pressure (Pmv) was measured by the double occlusion method (2). This technique involves the simultaneous occlusion of the inflow and outflow tubing with valves that caused minimal fluid displacement. The occlusions were maintained for 3-5 seconds and the resulting equilibrium pressures in the lobar artery and vein were considered to be Pmv (2). For measurement of the pulmonary capillary filtration coefficient (Kfc), the weight gain of the isolated lobe over time in response to increased outflow pressure was recorded. To accomplish this, at a constant rate of perfusion, Ppv was increased rapidly from 8 to 15 cm H_2O by altering the height of the venous reservoir. The increase in Ppv was maintained for 7 min and lung weight was monitored continuously. In response to the abrupt increase in Ppv, the initial rapid increase in lung weight reflects an increase in lobar blood volume due to recruitment and distension of the pulmonary vasculature. The subsequent slower rate of gain in lobar weight reflects the accumulation of fluid in extravascular areas secondary to an increased rate of fluid filtration through the microvasculature. The slower component of the weight gain was used to calculate the Kfc. Since fluid movement across the microvasculature is related to both Kfc and Pmv, the determination of Kfc demands that Pmv be known. Microvascular pressure was determined immediately before and 7 min after the initiation of increased Ppv. The Kfc was determined by dividing the initial change in rate of weight gain, by the change in Pmv. All weight gain values were corrected to a lung weight of 100 g. Kfc is reported as ml/min/cm H_2O/100 g lung tissue.

Leukotriene, prostaglandin and thromboxane concentrations in blood, edema fluid and bronchoalveolar lavage fluid (BALF) were determined by immunoassay following extraction and purification as previously described (4,7,9,10).

RESULTS

As a first step in defining a role for lipoxygenase-mediated products of arachidonic acid metabolism as mediators of the increased pulmonary microvascular permeability and nonhydrostatic edema formation, we used ethchlorvynol (ECV), a sedative-hypnotic drug, to produce acute lung injury in anesthetized dogs (8). Ethchlorvynol had been reported to produce ARDS in drug abusers who administered it intravenously. Ethchlorvynol exhibited an interesting property in that it affected solely the first capillary bed encountered. Thus, if it were administered intravenously, only the lungs were affected. If given into a limb, edema developed in that limb and nowhere else. Because of this property we were able to produce not only bilateral acute lung injury, but also injury confined to one lung (8). Animals sustaining a bilateral acute lung injury developed progressive, systemic hypoxemia and bilateral nonhydrostatic pulmonary edema. Thus, 120 min after introduction of ECV, arterial PO_2 had decreased by 12±3% and EVLW had increased by 164±34%. The control LTC_4 concentration in systemic arterial plasma was 5.3±3.1 pg/ml which did not change in response to ECV administration. In contrast, the concentration of LTC_4 in pulmonary edema fluid, 120 min after ECV had been given, was 35.2±10.8 pg/ml, nearly sevenfold that of the arterial plasma ($P<0.01$). Since several cell types found in the lung are capable of synthesizing leukotrienes, the measurement of larger concentrations of LTC_4 in the pulmonary edema fluid than in the plasma, does not, in itself, define the relationship between increased concentrations of LTC_4, on the one hand, and the development of acute lung injury on the other. To relate LTC_4 generation to the development of acute lung injury, experiments were designed to confine the injury to one lung (Fig. 1). In the latter studies, bronchoalveolar lavage was used to obtain fluid from both the injured and uninjured lung prior to, as well as following the induction of unilateral acute lung injury with ECV. The concentration of LTC_4 in the lavage fluid obtained from the injured lung increased from a control value of 10.2±1.6 to 24.2±3.4 pg/ml

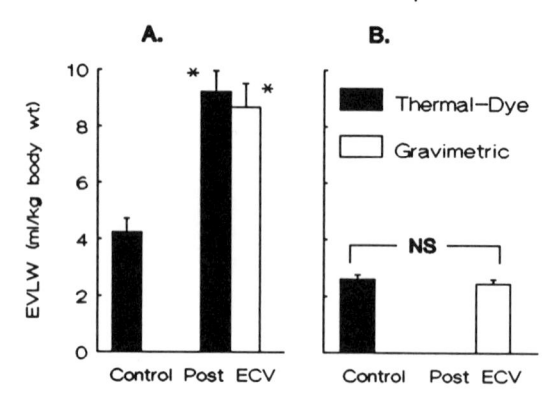

Figure 1. Effects of ethchlorvynol (ECV, 9 mg/kg) given into the right lung, on extravascular lung water (EVLW) in right (A) and left (B) lung. *P<0.05 from control.

(P<0.01) 120 min after ECV administration; whereas, the concentration of LTC_4 in BALF obtained from the uninjured lung did not change over the course of the experiment and did not differ from the concentrations of LTC_4 measured before ECV administration into the injured lung (Fig. 2) (8,9).

Although the studies described above demonstrated that a product of lipoxygenase-mediated arachidonic acid metabolism, capable of causing increased microvascular permeability, was found in the injured lung after ECV-induced acute lung injury, the results do not establish a causal relationship between leukotriene production and edema formation. In highly preliminary experiments designed to address this question directly, an inhibitor of lipoxygenase activity, nordihydroguaiaretic acid (NDGA), was administered (20 mg/kg, i.v. loading dose; 6 mg/kg/h maintenance dose) prior

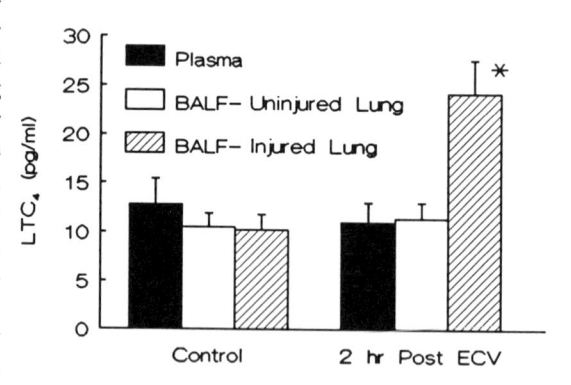

Figure 2. Effect of 9 mg/kg, ethchlorvynol (ECV) given into the right lung, on LTC_4 in plasma and bronchoalveolar lavage fluid (BALF) from the injured and the uninjured lung. Values are means ± SE. *P<0.01 from all other values.

to the induction of acute lung injury with ECV. This dose of NDGA resulted in no change in blood gases, EVLW or hemodynamic measurements. Unilateral ECV administration in the presence of NDGA resulted in an increase in the injured lung EVLW of 75±8% 120 min after the administration of the ECV which was considerably less than the 133±20% increase in EVLW observed in animals that were not pretreated with NDGA. Similarly, in the animals receiving NDGA prior to the induction of acute lung injury, LTC_4 in lavage fluid from the injured lung 120 min after administration of the ECV was 7.2±2.8 pg/ml in contrast to the value of 17.1±4.8 pg/ml measured in dogs receiving solely the NDGA vehicle. Thus, the administration of NDGA prior to the induction of acute lung injury with ECV resulted in a decrease in LTC_4, indicating at least partial inhibition of leukotriene synthesis and a concomitant reduction in extravascular lung water. Moreover, in the latter group of animals, there was a significant correlation between the amount of extravascular lung water measured at the end of the experiment and LTC_4 concentrations determined simultaneously. In a separate set of experiments, increases in EVLW were brought about by increasing hydrostatic pressure by inflation of a balloon in the left atrium. When increases in EVLW were brought about to equal those which had occurred in response to ECV, leukotrienes in BALF were not increased. All of the above described studies are consistent with the hypothesis that a product of lipoxygenase-mediated arachidonic acid metabolism participates in those microvascular changes which result in the increased permeability of acute lung injury.

Any comprehensive description of the role of lipoxygenase products as a final common pathway for the development of nonhydrostatic pulmonary edema demands that they be identified in dissimilar models of acute lung injury. To this end, we developed a model of acute lung injury induced by the intravenous administration of phorbol myristate acetate (PMA) which differs from the ECV model in that PMA-induced lung injury is dependent upon the presence of circulating neutrophils and is associated with sustained increases in pulmonary arterial pressure. In anesthetized dogs, the administration of PMA (20 µg/kg) produced increases in extravascular lung water and mean pulmonary arterial pressure, whereas cardiac output, left atrial pressure and arterial PO_2 decreased. Concentrations of immunoreactive LTD_4 and LTB_4 in BALF increased from control values of 75±24 and 406±282 pg/lavage to 177±52 ($P<0.05$) and 2446±980 pg/lavage ($P<0.05$), respectively, 60 min after PMA administration. Total leukocyte count decreased significantly by 30 min and remained depressed for the remainder of the experiment (7).

In the course of performing the experiments with PMA, it was noted that when PMA was administered at a lower dose, namely 10 µg/kg, there was no associated increase in extravascular lung water, nor were leukotrienes increased in bronchoalveolar lavage fluid; whereas, at the higher dose of 20 µg/kg, both extravascular lung water and leukotriene concentration in lavage fluid increased. Both doses produced increases in pulmonary arterial thromboxane concentrations and pulmonary artery pressures. In order to evaluate a possible relationship between increases in pulmonary arterial pressure and the generation of thromboxane, additional experiments were performed in which thromboxane synthesis was inhibited with the thromboxane synthetase inhibitor, OKY-046, or with the cyclooxygenase inhibitor, indomethacin, prior to the administration of a "low" dose of PMA (10 µg/kg). Thromboxane concentrations in arterial blood were significantly inhibited by the use of either OKY-046 or indomethacin. Surprisingly, however, only

OKY-046 eliminated the increase in pulmonary artery pressure in response to "low" dose PMA. In the case of those animals pretreated with indomethacin, the increase in pulmonary artery pressure as a result of PMA administration was actually enhanced. Moreover, the latter animals behaved as if they had been treated with a "high" dose of PMA in that leukotrienes were elevated in bronchoalveolar lavage fluid, extravascular lung water was significantly increased and arterial PO_2 was significantly reduced (Fig. 3). One interpretation of these results is that the blockade of cyclooxygenase activity with indomethacin was associated with diversion of arachidonic acid away from the cyclooxygenase pathway into the lipoxygenase pathway resulting in the generation of leukotrienes which, in turn, enhanced both microvascular permeability and pulmonary arterial pressure.

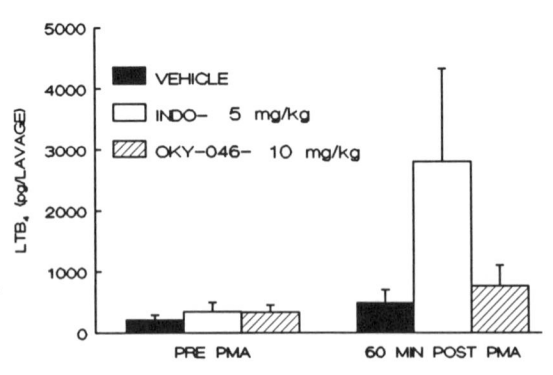

Figure 3. Effect of PMA (10 μg/kg, i.v.) on LTB_4 in bronchoalveolar lavage fluid after saline (Vehicle), indomethacin (INDO) or OKY-046 pretreatment. Values are means ± SE. *$P<0.05$ from PRE PMA.

In order to clarify further relationships between leukotriene production and microvascular permeability, attempts were made in anesthetized intact dogs to block leukotriene synthesis with either diethylcarbamazine (DEC) or BW755C, prior to the administration of PMA. Although the dogs remained hemodynamically stable after the administration of the leukotriene synthesis inhibitor alone, upon administration of PMA in the presence of the inhibitor, hemodynamic instability rapidly ensued, blood pressure was unable to be maintained and the animals succumbed to shock. To avoid the problems of hemodynamic stability in intact animals, an isolated perfused lung preparation was developed. Either DEC (5×10^{-3}M) or the vehicle for DEC (10 ml 0.9% NaCl) was added to the perfusate reservoir 15 min before the administration of PMA. Neither DEC nor its vehicle produced changes in

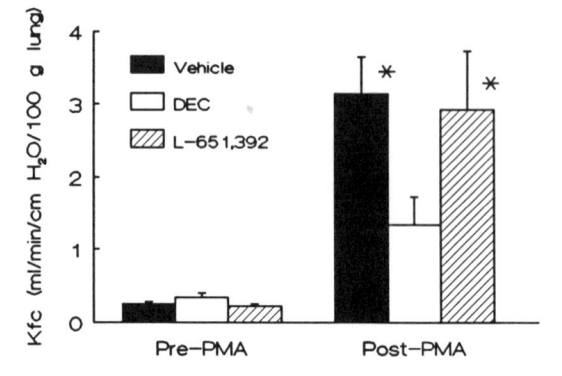

Figure 4. Effect of PMA (4.2×10^{-8} M) on capillary filtration coefficient (Kfc) after saline (Vehicle), diethylcarbamazine (DEC) or L-651,392 pretreatment. Values are means ± SE. *$P<0.05$.

Ppa, Ppv, Pmv or Kfc. PMA (18 μg) was added to the perfusate reservoir to achieve a final circulating concentration of 4.2×10^{-8}M. Administration of PMA to vehicle-pretreated lobes produced an increase in Kfc from a control value of 0.25 ± 0.04 to 2.96 ± 0.67 g/min/cm H_2O/100 g lung wt (P<0.01) (Fig. 4). There were no changes in Ppa, Ppv or Pmv. Administration of PMA to DEC pretreated lobes resulted in no change in Kfc or in any other of the perimeters measured. These results demonstrate that, in the isolated perfused lung, PMA produces an increase in pulmonary microvascular permeability which is prevented by the leukotriene synthesis inhibitor, DEC.

Caution regarding premature conclusions relating leukotriene generation and enhanced microvascular permeability in acute lung injury was introduced by two results obtained with the isolated blood-perfused lung preparation. First, we have been unable to obtain evidence that leukotrienes are increased either in the perfusate or in BALF of the isolated perfused lung in response to PMA administration. Moreover, in the same system, we have been unable to demonstrate that leukotrienes are suppressed by inhibitors of their synthesis. Second, an inhibitor of leukotriene synthesis, chemically dissimilar from DEC, namely, L-651,392, did not attenuate the increase in Kfc produced by PMA (Fig. 4).

DISCUSSION

Evidence is presented in support of the hypothesis which states that lipoxygenase products of arachidonic acid metabolism participate in the increased microvascular permeability which is responsible for the edema formation of acute lung injury. Thus, in two animal models of acute lung injury, one neutrophil-dependent (PMA) and the other neutrophil-independent (ECV), leukotrienes were identified either in the pulmonary edema fluid or in the bronchoalveolar lavage fluid following induction of injury with either agent. In the case of etchchlorvynol, which allows the induction of unilateral acute lung injury, extravascular lung water was increased solely in the injured lung, as were the leukotrienes. When leukotriene synthesis was attenuated with the lipoxygenase inhibitor, NDGA, both the accumulation of EVLW, as well as leukotriene concentrations were decreased. Similarly, in the case of PMA, only those doses which increased leukotriene concentrations were associated with increased EVLW. In the case of smaller doses of PMA, namely, 10 μg/kg, no injury was seen in the lungs unless the animals had been pretreated with indomethacin, a cyclooxygenase inhibitor. In the latter experiments, the released arachidonic acid appeared to have been diverted from the cyclooxygenase pathway to the lipoxygenase pathway leading to increased synthesis of leukotrienes and to the development of nonhydrostatic pulmonary edema. Hydrostatic pulmonary edema was not associated with leukotrienes in BALF. Finally, in an isolated perfused canine lung lobe preparation, in which estimates of microvascular permeability coefficients and microvascular pressures could be made, less clear results have been obtained. Thus, on the one hand, administration of diethylcarbamazine, a leukotriene synthesis inhibitor, attenuated increases in microvascular permeability coefficients in response to PMA administration. On the other hand, a chemically dissimilar inhibitor of leukotriene synthesis, L-651,392, had no effect on PMA-induced increases in Kfc. Moreover, we have been unable to demonstrate in the isolated perfused lung preparation either increased or decreased leukotrienes in response to PMA or leukotriene synthesis inhibitors, respectively. Whether these latter results will ultimately be explained by in vitro vs. in vivo considerations or by the lack of a causal relationship between leukotriene generation and altered microvascular permeability in acute lung injury awaits further definition.

REFERENCES

1. Albert, R., Greenberg, M., and Henderson, W. (1983): Chest, 83:855-865.
2. Hakim, T., Dawson, C., and Linehan, J. (1979): J. Appl. Physiol., 47:145-152.
3. Petty, T., and Ashbaugh, D. (1971): Chest, 60:233-239.
4. Lonigro, A., Sprague, R., Stephenson, A., and Dahms, T. (1988): J. Appl. Physiol, 64:2538-2543.
5. Sprague, R., Stephenson, A., Dahms, T., and Lonigro, A. (1986): J. Appl. Physiol., 61:1058-1064.
6. Sprague, R., Stephenson, A., Dahms, T., Asner, N., and Lonigro, A. (1987): Chest, 92:1088-1093.
7. Sprague, R., Stephenson, A., Dahms, T., and Lonigro, A. (1990): Prostaglandins, 39:439-450.
8. Stephenson, A., Sprague, R., Dahms, T., and Lonigro, A. (1984): J. Appl. Physiol., 56:1252-1259.
9. Stephenson, A., Sprague, R., Dahms, T., and Lonigro, A. (1987): J. Appl. Physiol. 62:732-738.
10. Stephenson, A., Lonigro, A., Hyers, T., Webster, R., and Fowler, A. (1988): Am. Rev. Respir. Dis., 138:714-719.
11. Stephenson, A., Sprague, R., and Lonigro, A. (1990): J. Appl. Physiol., In Press.
12. Voelkel, N., Stenmark, K., Reeves, J., Mathias, M., and Murphy, R. (1984): J. Appl. Physiol. 57:860-867.
13. Woodword, D., Weichman, B., Gill, C., and Wasserman, M. (1983): Prostaglandins, 25:131-142.

FURTHER EVIDENCE THAT LEUKOTRIENES ARE THE MAJOR MEDIATORS OF ALLERGIC CONSTRICTION IN HUMAN BRONCHI.

Thure Björck, Yoshiteru Harada[1], Barbro Dahlén*, Olle Zetterström*, Gunnar Johansson**, Louis Rodriguez***, Per Hedqvist and Sven-Erik Dahlén.

Departments of Physiology, Thoracic Medicine*, Clinical Immunology**, Thoracic Surgery*** and Institute of Environmental Medicine, Karolinska Institutet, S-104 01 Stockholm, Sweden.

INTRODUCTION.

Allergic bronchoconstriction can be studied in vitro by challenge of isolated human bronchi with stimuli that cause IgE-dependent release of mediators. In bronchi from non-atopic subjects, anti-human IgE may be used to cross-link and activate cells which carry IgE on the cell surface. This probe thus mimics the release process triggered by specific allergen in atopics. Using anti-IgE as a tool, we have previously reported in this series of publications that the cysteinyl-leukotrienes (LTC_4, LTD_4 and LTE_4) are strong candidates as mediators of IgE-dependent constriction of human bronchi (1). In this chapter, we present further evidence in support of this concept. First, we report on the influence of new and more selective drugs on the response to challenge of bronchi from non-asthmatics with anti-IgE. Secondly, we show that the mechanisms characterized in bronchi from non-asthmatics are present also in bronchi obtained from atopic asthmatics.

MATERIALS AND METHODS

Parts of macroscopically normal lung tissue were collected at surgery and immediately placed in ice-cooled phosphate buffer. The dissection of bronchi was performed in chilled buffer and commenced within 30 min after resection. Spirally cut strips of bronchi with an inner diameter of 3-7 mm were placed in organ baths filled with

---

[1]/present address: Department of Pharmacology, Kitasato University School of Medicine, Kanagawa, Japan.

Tyrode's solution kept at 37°C and gassed with 5% CO_2 in O_2. Mechanical responses were recorded isometrically on a Grass Model 7 Polygraph using Grass FT 03C force displacement transducers (resting tension 5 mN). Substances were added under non-flow conditions, and responses were expressed in percent of the maximal contraction produced at the end of the experiment by addition of histamine 100µM and acetylcholine 100µM.

On two occasions, bronchi were prepared from lung tissue of patients with asthma. Both patients were male (41 and 53 years of age), had asthma of 5-10 years duration, and required regular treatment with inhaled bronchodilators and corticosteroids (budesonide). Atopy was diagnosed on the basis of history, skin prick test and measurements of specific and total IgE. At the time of surgery, they demonstrated bronchial hyperresponsiveness to inhaled histamine.

Rabbit anti-human IgE was raised by injection of a human myeloma IgE, purified and checked for specificity. Allergens were from Pharmacia, Sweden. MK-886 and ICI-198,615 were gifts from Drs A. Ford-Hutchinson, Merck Frosst, Canada, and R.D. Krell, ICI Americas, respectively. Synthetic leukotrienes were provided by Merck Frosst Canada, Cascade Biochemicals UK and Biomol US. All other drugs and chemicals were from Sigma.

RESULTS.

By increasing the titer of anti-IgE (1/100 000 - 1/300) with half a log order of magnitude every 10 min, a dose-dependent contraction response was obtained in the isolated bronchi. The response to the highest dose of anti-IgE amounted to about 60% of maximal tissue contractility. The influence of pharmacological antagonists and inhibitors was compared for the highest dose of anti-IgE (1/300) and expressed in percent of the control contraction.

Pretreatment with a combination of H_1- and H_2- antihistamines (mepyramine and metiamide) did not affect the response to anti-IgE (Fig. 1A), suggesting that histamine did not mediate this contraction response. In contrast, the potent and selective leukotriene receptor antagonist ICI-198,615 (4) caused a significant and substantial inhibition of the contraction response to anti-IgE (Fig. 1A). We have documented that the dose of ICI-198,615 used in these experiments rendered the bronchi almost insensitive to exogenous leukotrienes without interfering with bronchial reactivity to histamine or acetylcholine. Furthermore, the specific leukotriene biosynthesis inhibitor MK-886 (3) inhibited the anti-IgE provoked contraction response to the same extent as ICI-198,615 (Fig. 1A). The dose of MK-886 used did not alter bronchial reactivity to exogenous leukotrienes or histamine.

There was however a distinct component of the anti-IgE response which appeared resistant to either ICI-198,615 or MK-886. Interestingly, when ICI-198,615 was combined with the antihistamines, the bronchi failed to respond to anti-IgE (Fig. 1A), although reactivity to acetylcholine was unaffected.

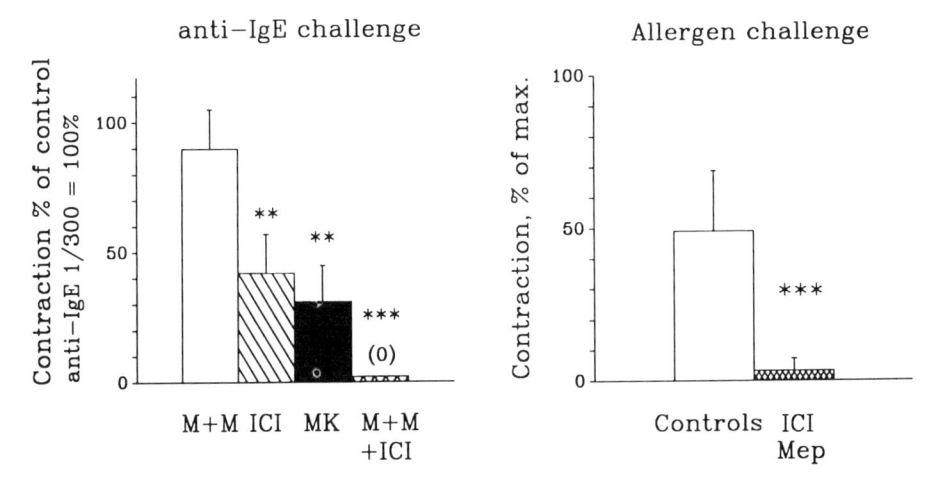

Fig. 1. **A.** *Contractions evoked by cumulative challenge with anti-IgE (1/300) in human bronchi. Responses in percent of parallel controls after pretreatment with: mepyramine 1μM and metiamide 1μM (M+M, n=8, open column), ICI 198,615 1μM (ICI n=4, hatched column), MK-886 30μM (MK n=5, filled column) or the combination of mepyramine, metiamide and ICI 198,615 (M+M+ICI, n=6, cross-hatched column).* **B.** *Influence of mepyramine (1μM) and ICI 198,615 1μM (n=5, cross-hatched column) on Schultz-Dale contractions evoked by challenge with specific allergen (Kiwi antigen, house dust mite or birch pollen in bronchial strips from two asthmatics (controls open column, n=10). Stars denote significant difference from control (Mann-Whitney U-test).*

Finally, it was tested if this synergism between the antihistamines and the leukotriene receptor antagonist existed also in bronchi from asthmatic patients. In the first patient, a Schultz-Dale contraction was elicited with an extract of Kiwi fruit. In the next case, sensitivity to two different antigens (house dust mite and birch pollen) made it possible to perform two antigen challenges in each strip. The results from provocations with these three antigens in bronchial strips from the two patients were pooled (Fig. 1B). As for the non-atopic bronchi challenged with anti-IgE, the combination of the receptor-antagonist ICI-198,615 with histamine-antagonism, resulted in almost complete inhibition of the response to specific allergen in bronchi from asthmatics.

DISCUSSION.

Leukotriene receptor antagonism or inhibition of leukotriene biosynthesis caused a striking and similar inhibition of the responses to anti-IgE, whereas this reaction was resistant to singular blockade of histamine receptors. However, the combination of these two classes of antagonists caused marked synergism and in fact prevented the reaction. There was no evidence of unspecific effects of the drugs used. Furthermore, the Schultz-Dale contractions elicited by challenge of bronchi from atopic asthmatics were also almost extinguished by the combined pretreatment with antihistamines and the leukotriene receptor antagonist ICI-198,615. It remains to investigate the relative role of histamine and leukotrienes in asthmatic bronchi but the strong correlation with the data from the anti-IgE experiments suggests that also in this case, leukotrienes are the major mediators whereas histamine accounts for the residual component.

It is concluded that histamine and the cysteinyl-leukotrienes are the exclusive mediators of IgE-dependent contractions of isolated human airways. The relative importance of this mechanism in the in vivo situation remains to define. The applicability of these in vitro findings appear to gain support from recent observations indicating that leukotriene antagonism provides significant protection against allergen induced asthma in man (2). The combined treatment with antihistamines and antileukotriene drugs may be of benefit in the treatment of asthma.

ACKNOWLEDGEMENTS

Supported by grants from the Swedish MRC (14X-9071,14X-4342), the Swedish Association Against Chest and Heart Diseases, the Swedish Association Against Asthma and Allergy (RmA), the Swedish National Board for Laboratory Animals (CFN), the Scientific Council of the Swedish Association Against Use of Experimental Animals in Research, the Institute of Environmental Medicine, the Swedish Environment Protection Board (5324060-2), and Karolinska Institutet.

REFERENCES

1. Dahlén, S.-E., Björck, T, Kumlin, M., Granström, E., and Hedqvist, P (1990): In: *Advances in Prostaglandin, Thromboxane and Leukotriene Research,* Vol. 20, edited by B. Samuelsson, S.-E. Dahlén, J. Fritsch and P. Hedqvist, pp. 193-200, Raven Press, New York.

2. Dahlén, S.-E., Dahlén, B., Eliasson, E., Johansson, H., Björck, T., Whitney, J., Binks, S., King, B., Stark, R., and Zetterström, O. In: *Advances in Prostaglandin, Thromboxane and Leukotriene Research*, Vol. 21, edited by B. Samuelsson, R. Paoletti, P. Ramwell, G.C. Folco and E. Granström, Raven Press, (this volume).

3. Rouzer, C.A., Ford-Hutchinson, A.W., Morton, H.E., Gillard J.W.(1990): *J Biol Chem.* **265**: 1436-1442.

4. Snyder, D.W, Giles, R.E., Keith, R.A., Yee, Y.K, Krell, R.D (1987): *J Pharm Exp Ther* **243**: 548-556.

FORMATION OF PGD$_2$ AFTER ALLERGEN INHALATION IN ATOPIC ASTHMATICS

K. Sladek[*], J.R. Sheller, G.A. FitzGerald, J.D. Morrow and L.J. Roberts, II.

Depts. of Medicine and Pharmacology, Vanderbilt University, Nashville TN 37232.
[*] N. Copernicus Academy of Medicine, Skawinska 8, 31-066 Krakow, Poland.

INTRODUCTION

Prostaglandin D$_2$ is the principal cyclooxygenase product released from activated mast cells (3), and is a potent bronchoconstrictor in man. Murray and coworkers (6) have shown that PGD$_2$ is released into the lower airway of sensitive asthmatics after instillation of allergen. Because PGD$_2$ may play a role in allergic bronchoconstriction, we measured the appearance of a urinary metabolite of PGD$_2$ in the urine of 8 atopic asthmatics challenged with inhaled allergen. In addition, we measured the appearance of LTE$_4$ and histamine in urine, and determined the effect of the cyclooxygenase inhibitor, indomethacin, on pulmonary function and mediator release after allergen inhalation.

METHODS

In a blinded randomized fashion, eight non smoking atopic asthmatics underwent allergen inhalation on two separate occasions after taking placebo or indomethacin (50mg) every 8 hrs for two days and on the morning and noon of the study day. Pulmonary function was measured, and urine obtained at baseline and at hourly intervals for 8 hrs after allergen inhalation. Subjects with a 20% or greater fall in FEV$_1$ from baseline values 3 or more hours after allergen inhalation were considered to have a late response.

A major urinary metabolite of PGD$_2$, 9α,11β-dihydroxy-15-oxo-2,3,18,19-tetranorprostane-1,20-dioic acid (PGD-M), was measured using gas chromatography/mass spectrometry in the negative ion mode (GC/MS/NICI) (4). Histamine production was assessed by measuring urinary excretion of N$^\tau$-methylhistamine by GC/MS/NICI (5), and LTE$_4$ was measured by HPLC followed by RIA using an antibody which cross-reacted 55% LTC_4, 100% LTD_4, 51% LTE_4, 67% LTF_4.

RESULTS

Allergen inhalation caused an early fall in FEV_1 in all subjects, and was associated with a late response in five subjects. Allergen inhalation caused a significant early rise in urinary excretion of PGD-M (Fig 1). The baseline levels of PGD-M were significantly reduced after indomethacin, and the rise in PGD-M after allergen was abolished. Despite significant blockade of cyclooxygenase products, indomethacin did not affect the pulmonary function response to inhaled allergen.

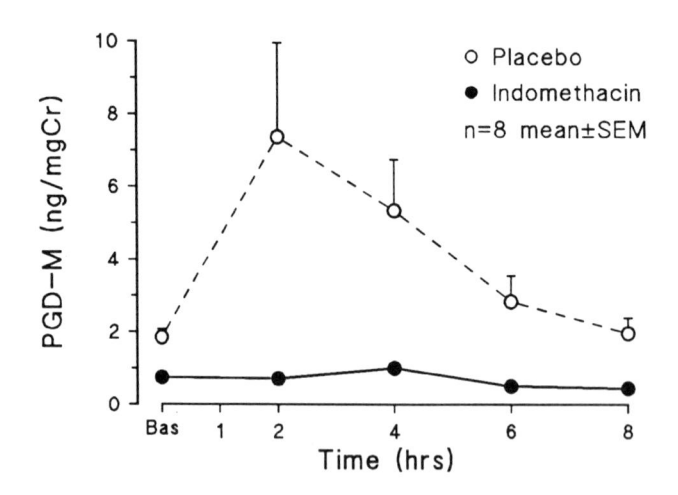

Figure 1. Effect of allergen inhalation on the urinary excretion of PGD-M in 8 subjects on placebo or indomethacin.

Urinary methyl histamine levels rose only slightly but not significantly early after allergen inhalation (Fig 2). The histamine levels were not affected by indomethacin.

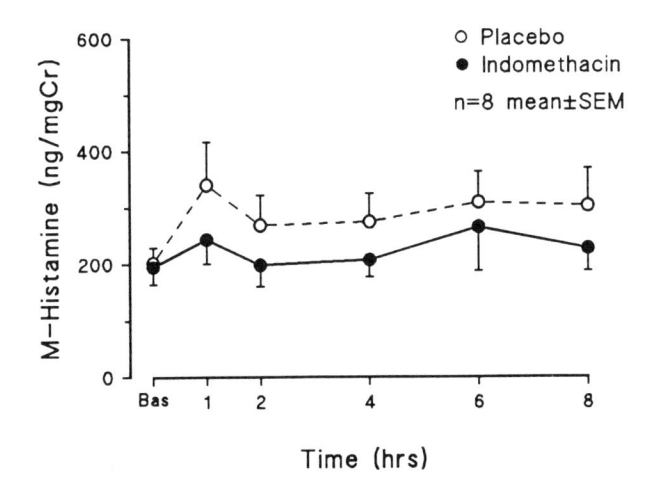

Figure 2. Effect of allergen inhalation on the urinary excretion of N^τ-methylhistamine in 8 atopic asthmatics on placebo or indomethacin.

As we have previously shown (7), LTE_4 levels in the urine increased early after allergen inhalation, and were also unaffected by indomethacin.

In the five subjects with a late response, there was no late rise in urinary PGD-M, histamine or LTE_4.

DISCUSSION

The increased urinary excretion of PGD-M acutely following allergen inhalation suggests that inflammatory cells, such as mast cells and/or macrophages, are activated acutely in man *in vivo* to synthesize cyclooxygenase products, specifically PGD_2. Although PGD_2 is a potent bronchoconstrictor, blocking its synthesis with indomethacin did not alter allergic bronchoconstriction, suggesting that PGD_2 is not crucial for the early pulmonary function response to inhaled allergen.

Cyclooxygenase inhibition may also prevent synthesis of "beneficial" prostaglandins, such as the bronchodilators PGI_2 and PGE_2, or cause an increase in the amount of constrictor 5-lipoxygenase products formed by activated cells (2). However, recent studies with potent thromboxane/prostaglandin receptor antagonists have shown only modest effects on allergic bronchoconstriction (1). Moreover, we found that indomethacin was not associated with an increase in the

5-lipoxygenase product, LTE_4, formed after allergen inhalation. Thus the role for constrictor prostaglandins in the pulmonary function response to allergen in man is limited.

There was no late rise in the urinary levels of the preformed mast cell mediator, histamine, nor the products of arachidonate metabolism, PGD_2 and LTE_4, in the five subjects with a late response to allergen, suggesting that these mediators are not directly responsible for the late bronchoconstriction, and that a second wave of mast cell activation does not occur during the late response.

REFERENCES

1. Beasley, R.C., Featherstone, R.L., Church, M.K., Rafferty, P., Varley, J.G., Harris, A., Robinson, C., Holgate, S.T. (1989) J. Appl. Physiol., 66:1685-93.

2. Dworski R., Sheller J.R., Wickersham N.E., Oates, J.A., Brigham, K.L., Roberts, L.J., FitzGerald, G.A. (1989) Am. Rev. Respir. Dis. 139:46-51.

3. Lewis, R.A., Soter, N.A., Diamond, P.T., Austen, K.F., Oates, J.A., Roberts, L.J. (1982) J. Immunol., 129:1627-1631.

4. Morrow, J.D., Duckworth, T.A., Zackert, W.E., Prakash, C., Blair, I.A., Oates, J.A., Roberts, L.J. (Manuscript in preparation).

5. Morrow, J.D., Parsons, W.G., and Roberts, L.J., II. (1989) Prostaglandins, 263-274.

6. Murray, J.J., Tonel, A.B., Brash, A.R., Roberts, L.J., Gasset, P., Workman, R., Capron, A., Oates, J.A. (1986) N. Engl. J. Med., 315:800-804.

7. Sladek, K., Dworski, R., FitzGerald, G.A., Sheller, J.R. (1990) Am. Rev. Respir. Dis. (in press).

METABOLISM OF ARACHIDONIC ACID BY FOÀ-KURLOFF CELLS
FROM GUINEA PIG LUNGS AND SPLEEN

P. Sirois, K. Maghni, C. Robidoux, A. Hallée
J. Laporte, S. Cloutier and *P. Borgeat

Department of Pharmacology, Faculty of Medicine,
University of Sherbrooke, Sherbrooke, P.Q. J1H 5N4
*Inflammation and Immunologie-Rhumatologie,
CHUL, Quebec, P.Q. G1V 4G2

INTRODUCTION

Foà-Kurloff cells commonly called Kurloff cells (for review, see 7) are mononuclear cells found only in guinea pigs. They have a large inclusion body identified as a mucoprotein-sulphated mucopolysaccharide complex associated with a glycoprotein. Kurloff cells have been found both in tissues and in peripheral blood and were shown to increase in numbers under physiological conditions in female guinea pigs and in males following estrogen treatment (3). These cells possess both lymphocyte and monocyte features but their role is not yet known. The aim of the present study was to purify pulmonary and splenic Kurloff cells and analyse their potential for releasing metabolites of arachidonic acid.

MATERIAL AND METHODS

Kurloff cells have been isolated from the spleen and lungs of Dunkin-Hartley female guinea pigs (200-300 g) treated with 17-β-estradiol. Lung cells were obtained after enzymatic digestion and elutriation as described by Pelé et al. (5). Further purification was done by Percoll gradient centrifugation. The spleen cells were obtained after mechanical dispersion and purification by continuous Percoll gradient centrifugation. Kurloff cells were stained by periodic acid-Schiff (PAS) for counting and ultrastructure study was done by electron microscopy.

Freshly isolated pulmonary and splenic Kurloff cells (1×10^6 cells/ml) have been incubated with arachidonic acid and/or calcium ionophore A23187. Prostaglandin E_2 (PGE_2) and thromboxane B_2 (TxB_2) have been measured in cell supernatant with enzyme immunoassays as described by Pradelles et al. (6). Arachidonic acid metabolism via the 5-lipoxygenase pathway was studied in supernatants using reverse phase high performance liquid chromatography (RP-HPLC) (1).

RESULTS

The enzymatic digestion and mechanical dispersion of lungs of estrogen-treated guinea pigs allowed to obtain approximately 700×10^6 cells. After the Percoll gradient, 50×10^6 Kurloff cells (density of 1.100 g/ml) were recovered with a purity and a viability close to 100 %. As shown in Figure 1, Kurloff cells have an ellipsoid nucleus and a single large homogenous electron-dense inclusion body, a Golgi apparatus with microvesicles of variable densities and an abundant endoplasmic

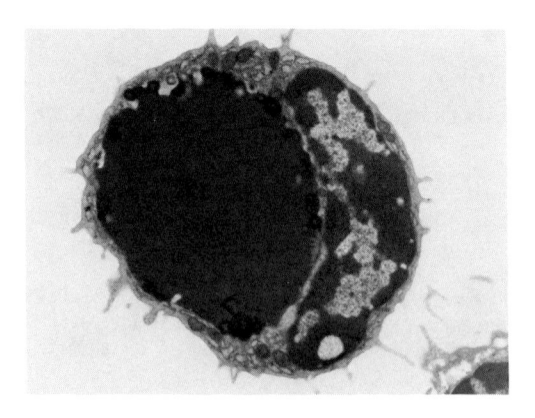

FIG. 1. Electron micrograph of a Kurloff cell purified from a guinea pig lung.

reticulum. Mechanical dispersion of splenic tissue has allowed to obtain 900 x 10^6 cells. After purification, approximately 150 x 10^6 cells were obtained with an almost total purity and viability. Their appearance was identical to those of the pulmonary Kurloff cells.

As shown in Table 1, control pulmonary and splenic Kurloff cells released very low amounts (low picogram range) of PGE_2 and TxB_2. In the presence of 2 µM ionophore A23187, the cells released a little more PGE_2 and TxB_2 but the increase was not significant. However, in the presence of 10, 30 and 100 µM arachidonic acid, PGE_2 and TxB_2 synthesis increased sharply. For instance, PGE_2 biosynthesis increased by 62-, 1 500- and 2 500-fold. In the supernatants of spleen cells incubated with 10, 30 and 100 µM arachidonic acid, the release of PGE_2 was also very marked although slightly less than with lung cells. Thromboxane release was stimulated by treatment of spleen cells with arachidonic acid but was by far less marked.

TABLE 1. Eicosanoid release by pulmonary and splenic Kurloff cells

	arachidonic acid (µM)			ionophore	control
	10	30	100	2 µM	
Lungs*					
PGE_2	0.125±0.013	2.930±0.260	4.950±0.930	0.005±0.002	0.002±0.0006
TxB_2	0.290±0.057	0.386±0.092	0.324±0.109	0.036±0.011	0.011±0.003
Spleen*					
PGE_2	0.120±0.020	0.860±0.120	2.200±0.290	0.008±0.004	0.002±0.0004
TxB_2	0.180±0.050	0.250±0.100	0.330±0.150	0.080±0.040	0.040±0.006

* ng/ml/10^6 cells   n = 3-8 experiments

Lipoxygenase products in cell supernatants were analysed by RP-HPLC. The chromatography profile obtained with supernatants of unstimulated cell suspensions did not show any absorption peak corresponding to lipoxygenase

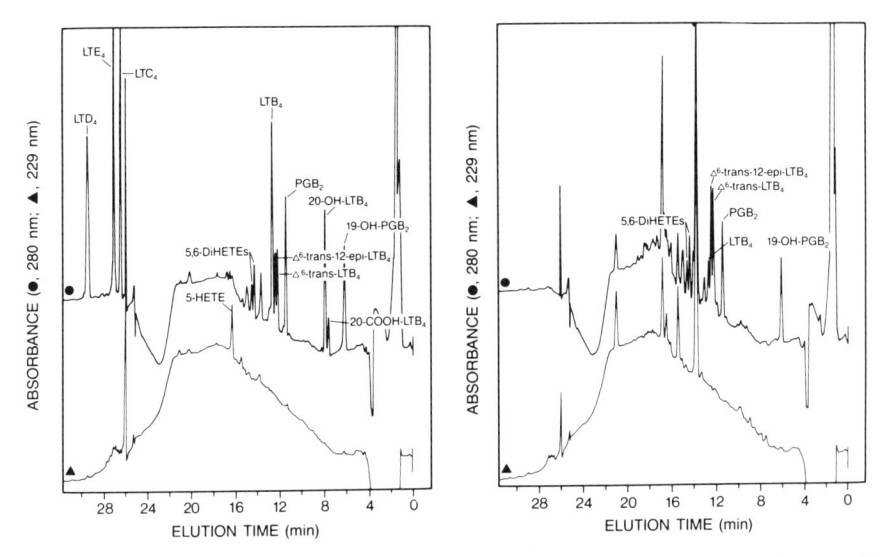

FIG. 2. The left panel shows a RP-HPLC chromatogram of a mixture of lipoxygenase products obtained from human neutrophils stimulated with the ionophore A23187, and supplemented with synthetic peptido-leukotrienes. The right panel shows the chromatograms of the denaturated supernatant of pulmonary Kurloff cells incubated with 2.5 µM LTA$_4$. PGB$_2$ (12.5 ng) and 19-OH-PGB$_2$ (12.5 ng) were used as internal standards.

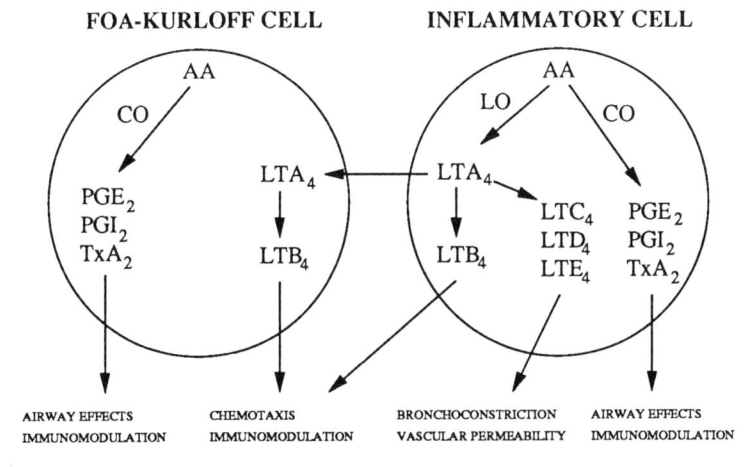

FIG. 3. Putative interactions between Kurloff cells and other inflammatory cells in the transcellular biosynthesis of leukotriene B$_4$.

products. Pulmonary or splenic Kurloff cells did not produce detectable amounts of LTB$_4$ or peptido-leukotrienes following stimulation with either ionophore A23187 or arachidonic acid. However, when Kurloff cells have been incubated with exogenous leukotriene A$_4$, they produce leukotriene B$_4$ as shown in the right panel of Figure 2. On the left hand side of Figure 2, a chromatogram of leukotriene standards is presented.

DISCUSSION

This study presents a technique for the isolation and full purification of pulmonary and splenic Kurloff cells. Electron microscopy confirms that the ultrastructure of the cells is well preserved with our technique. These cells were shown to have the potential to synthesize very significant amount of prostaglandins after incubation with arachidonic acid. The release of thromboxane by these cells was less marked. Our results also show that these cells do not have or express lipoxygenase activity since no lipoxygenase products were formed following incubation with arachidonic acid and/or ionophore A23187. However, they produced LTB_4 following incubation with LTA_4. No peptido-leukotrienes were formed.

The ability of Kurloff cells to generate large amounts of PGE_2 could have important physiological significance. Kurloff cells are located in very specific organs and the amounts of eicosanoids that are produced could modulate the activity of a number of systems. For instance, pulmonary Kurloff cells are located very close to type II pneumocytes that can produce surfactant following PGE_2 stimulation. Furthermore, Kurloff cells were shown to possess some of the characteristic features of human cytotoxic cells (2). It is possible that Kurloff cells could modulate the activity of the immune system. Although Kurloff cells were not shown to produce leukotrienes following stimulation with arachidonic acid and/or ionophore A23187, it is possible that due to their close proximity to a number of inflammatory cells, they could be fed the substate LTA_4 and by transcellular metabolism release LTB_4 (Figure 3). A similar mechanism has been described between platelets and neutrophils (4).

In conclusion, Kurloff cells have demonstrated peculiar metabolic activities. They possess the characteristic features of both lymphocytes and monocytes. They express cyclooxygenase activity like the monocytes and do not express 5-lipoxygenase activity like the lymphocytes. Furthermore, the biologic features of these cells also belong to both lymphocytes and monocytes. The strategic localization of Kurloff cells and their metabolic activities support their involvement in the physiopathology of many systems.

REFERENCES

1. Borgeat, P. and Picard, S. (1988): *Anal. Biochem.* 171: 283-289.
2. Debout, C., Quillec, M. and Izard, J. (1984): *Cell. Immunol.* 87: 674-677.
3. Ledingham, J.C.G. (1940): *J. Pathol. Bacteriol.* 50: 201-219.
4. McGee, J.E. and Fitzpatrick, F.A. (1986): *Proc. Nat. Acad. Sc. USA* 83: 1349-1353.
5. Pelé, J.P., Robidoux, C. and Sirois, P. (1989): *Inflammation* 13: 103-123.
6. Pradelles, P., Grassi, J. and Maclouf, J. (1985): Anal. Chem. 57: 1170-1173.
7. Revell, P.A. (1977): *Intern. Rev. Cytol.* 51: 275-314.

15(S)-HYDROXYEICOSATETRAENOIC ACID (15-HETE) IS THE MAJOR ARACHIDONIC ACID METABOLITE IN HUMAN BRONCHI

M. Kumlin, E. Ohlson, *T. Björck, M. Hamberg, **E. Granström, †B. Dahlén, †O. Zetterström, and *S.-E. Dahlén.

Departments of Physiological Chemistry, *Physiology, **Reproductive Endocrinology and †Thoracic Medicine, Karolinska Institutet, S-104 01 Stockholm, Sweden.

The conversion of arachidonic acid via the 15-lipoxygenase pathway has been reported to be an important route of transformation in several cells and tissues (cf. Ref. 4). 15-HETE was identified as the major metabolite of arachidonic acid in lung tissue from an asthmatic patient (2) and also shown to be the major monohydroxy acid formed in lung tissue from two atopic asthmatics (1). In the present investigation, we have studied the in vitro conversion of arachidonic acid into monohydroxy acids in the human lung. The formation of 15-HETE in human bronchi was characterized and the amounts of 15-HETE formed in tissue specimens from three asthmatic patients were compared to those found in tissue from non-asthmatic individuals.

EXPERIMENTAL PROCEDURE

Human lung tissue, obtained immediately after resection from patients undergoing surgery, was processed and incubated as described (6). Briefly, incubations were performed in PBS (pH 7.4, 37°C, 10-90 min) in the presence of different stimuli and terminated with 3 vols. of ice-cold ethanol supplemented with the internal standard 16-hydroxyheneicosatrienoic acid (16-HHnTrE) (cf. Ref. 6). Products were identified and quantitated on RP-HPLC with the use of authentic standards. On three occasions it was possible to obtain lung tissue from asthmatic individuals, one woman with endogenous asthma and two atopic asthmatic men.

RESULTS AND DISCUSSION

Incubation of chopped human bronchi, in buffer alone, for 10 min at 37 °C resulted in the production of large quantities of a compound which coeluted with authentic 15-HETE in three different RP-HPLC systems. The compound showed a single uv-absorption maximum at 235 nm, and gas chromatographic-mass spectrometric analysis of the methyl ester trimethylsilyl ether of the compound produced findings consistent with previously published data for 15-HETE (2). Furthermore, stereochemical analysis of the compound revealed an (S) configuration of the C-15 hydroxyl. Based on these analytical data the compound was identified as 15(S)-hydroxy-5,8,11,13-eicosatetraenoic acid.

Addition of exogenous [^{14}C]arachidonic acid (75 μM) caused a substantial increase in the yield of 15-HETE, and the major part of the converted radioactivity (mean ± SE: 53 ± 3 %, n=11) was recovered at the retention time of 15-HETE on RP-HPLC. The remainder of the radioactivity was distributed among several smaller fractions: prostaglandins and thromboxanes accounted for 33 ± 2 %, n=11 and dihydroxy-eicosatetraenoic acids (di-HETEs) contained together 9 ± 1 %, n=11 of the radioactivity.

Exogenous arachidonic acid dose-dependently stimulated the formation of 15-HETE in the bronchi with maximal levels reached at about 75-100 µM of substrate. However, stimulation with calcium ionophore A23187 alone, or in combination with exogenous arachidonic acid (75 µM), did not alter the levels of 15-HETE obtained in the absence of A23187 (Fig. 1). Neither did an immunological challenge of the bronchi with anti-IgE influence the production of 15-HETE as compared to unstimulated controls (Fig. 1).

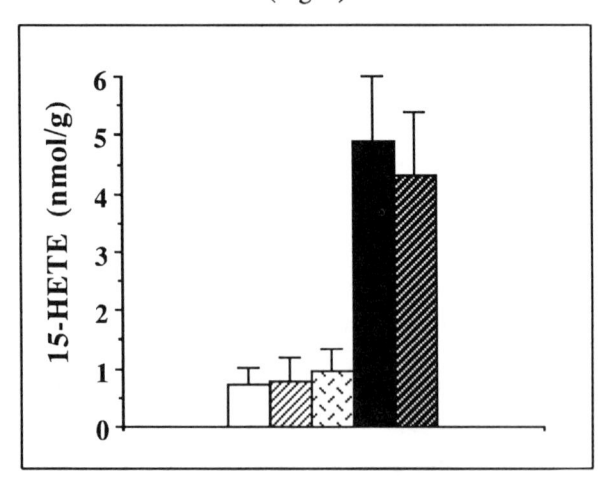

FIG. 1. *Stimulus dependent formation of 15-HETE in human bronchi in vitro.* Specimens of chopped human bronchi were incubated for 10 min at 37°C in buffer alone (☐), or in the presence of ionophore A23187 (2.5 µM,▨), anti-Ige (10 µg/ml.▨), arachidonic acid (75 µM,■), or the combination of arachidonic acid and A23187 (▨). Amounts of 15-HETE formed were quantitated from peak areas on RP-HPLC with 16-HHnTrE as internal standard. Results are means ± SE, n=5 for each stimuli.

Pretreatment with the lipoxygenase inhibitor NDGA (30 µM) reduced the production of 15-HETE in the bronchi, whereas indomethacin (10 µM) had no significant effect. This supports that the formation of 15-HETE in the human bronchi was catalyzed by a 15-lipoxygenase.

Time-course studies of the response to 75 µM of arachidonic acid showed peak formation of 15-HETE after about 10 min of incubation, but approximately the same levels were retained throughout the 90 min course of the experiments. When exogenous 15-HETE was added to bronchial fragments, small amounts of products eluting at the retention times of isomers of 8,15-diHETEs were observed, as well as 15-keto-eicosatetraenoic acid. However,the major part (> 80%) of the added 15-HETE remained intact after 45 min of incubation. The corresponding hydroperoxy acid (15-HPETE) was rapidly converted into 15-HETE and about the same metabolic profile as described for 15-HETE was seen after addition of this compound. No lipoxins were detected under any of these conditions, i.e. incubations with arachidonic acid or 15-H(P)ETE with or without ionophore challenge. These results indicate that the 15-HETE formed in the bronchi was not to any considerable extent catabolized within this tissue. However, when human bronchi were incubated in the presence of LTA$_4$ or co-incubated with human granulocytes small amounts of lipoxins could be detected, as reported elsewhere in this volume (7).

In order to elucidate the cellular origin of the 15-lipoxygenase activity, the epithelial layer was removed from bronchial fragments. The epithelium denuded bronchi where incubated in the presence of exogenous arachidonic acid with or without ionophore A23187. The amounts of 15-HETE obtained in incubations of the epithelium denuded fragments were substantially diminished to about 30 % of the amounts formed in the native bronchi, indicating an epithelial location of the 15-lipoxygenase. In line with these observations human tracheal epithelial cells obtained post mortem has been reported to produce 15-HETE (5). Furthermore, formation of 15-HETE has also been described in epithelial cells isolated from surgical specimens of human nasal turbinates (3) and in cultured human bronchial epithelial cells in response to exogenous arachidonic acid (9). Recently, human eosinophils and tracheal epithelial cells were described as the richest cell sources for 15-lipoxygenase activity (4).

When specimens of bronchi and lung parenchyma from the same donors were incubated in parallel in the presence of arachidonic acid and ionophore A23187, the amounts of 15-HETE obtained in the bronchi were about ten times higher (per gram of tissue) than those found in the peripheral parenchyma. Another dissimilarity between the two compartments was the observed effect of ionophore A23187 on the yield of monohydroxy acids. In the bronchi, ionophore stimulation did not modify the formation of either 15-HETE or 5-HETE, whereas in the parenchyma the ionophore stimulation significantly increased the production of 5-HETE.

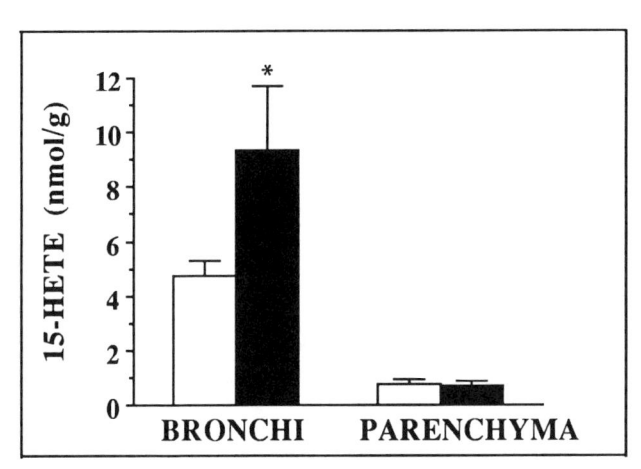

FIG. 2. *Arachidonic acid induced formation of 15-HETE in bronchi and lung parenchyma from asthmatic and non-asthmatic donors.* Tissues were incubated for 10 min at 37°C in the presence of arachidonic acid (70-75 µM) with or without ionophore A23187 (2.5µM). Results are presented as nmol 15-HETE formed per gram of tissue from non-asthmatics (open bars, n=5-8) and asthmatics (filled bars, n=3). Means ± SE.
* $P<0.05$, versus amounts formed in tissue from non-asthmatic individuals.

In this series of experiments, it was possible to include lung tissue from three asthmatic patients. Interestingly, the amounts of 15-HETE formed in the bronchi of the asthmatic patients were under all conditions higher than in the non-asthmatic donors (Fig.2). The levels of 15-HETE in the parenchyma of the asthmatic patients were, however, not different from the amounts normally detected (Fig. 2). Neither did the formation of 5-HETE vary significantly between tissue specimens from asthmatics and non-asthmatics. If 15-HETE predominantly was derived from eosinophils, ionophore stimulation would have been expected to result in increased production of 5-HETE as well. Since this was not the case, we suggest that epithelial cells in the airways mainly were responsible for the increased formation of 15-HETE in the bronchi of the asthmatics.

Taken together, 15-HETE was the major metabolite in human bronchi and the proposed 15-lipoxygenase activity appeared to be located in the airway epithelium. Although a number of biological activities has been reported for 15-HETE and/or 15-HPETE, the importance of the remarkable production of 15-HETE in human bronchi remains to be evaluated. However, the present findings with elevated amounts of 15-HETE in bronchial specimens from three asthmatic patients, and previously published data by us (1,2) and others (8), raise the possibility that 15-HETE may somehow be involved in the airway inflammation characteristic of asthma.

ACKNOWLEDGMENTS

This work was supported by the Swedish Medical Research Council (Project 03X-5915, 14X-09071), the Swedish Association Against Chest and Heart Diseases, the foundation in Memory of Bengt Lundqvist, the Swedish Society for Medical Research, the Swedish Association Against Asthma and Allergy (RmA), the Swedish National Board for Laboratory Animals (CFN), the Scientific Counsil of the Swedish Association Against Use of Experimental Animals in Research, the Institute of Environmental Medicine, the Swedish Environment Protection Board (5324069-3), and Karolinska Institutet.

REFERENCES

1. Dahlén, S. -E., Hansson, G., Hedqvist, P., Björck, T., Granström, E., and Dahlén, B. (1983): *Proc. Natl. Acad. Sci. USA*, 80: 1712-1716.
2. Hamberg, M., Hedqvist, P., and Rådegran, K. (1980): *Acta Physiol. Scand*, 110: 219-221.
3. Henke, D., Danilowicz, R. M., Curtis, J. F., Boucher, R. C., and Eling, T. E. (1988): *Archs. Biochem. Biophys.*, 267: 426-436.
4. Holtzman, M. J., Pentland, A., Baenzinger, N. L., and Hansbrough, J. R. (1989): *Biochim. Biophys. Acta*, 1003: 204-208.
5. Hunter, J. A., Finkbeiner, W. E., Nadel, J. A., Goetzl, E. J., and Holtzman, M. J. (1985): *Proc. Natl. Acad. Sci. USA*, 82: 4633-4637.
6. Kumlin, M., Hamberg, M., Granström, E., Björck, T., Dahlén, B., Matsuda, H., Zetterström, O., and Dahlén, S.-E. (1990): *Archs. Biochem. Biophys.*, (in press).
7. Lindgren, J. Å., Edenius, C., Kumlin, M., Dahlén, B., and Änggård, A. *Adv. Prostaglandin, Thromboxane, Leukotriene Res.*, this volume.
8. Murray, J. J., Tonnel, A. B., Brash, A. R., Roberts, L. J. II, Gosset, P. G., Workman, R., Capron, A., and Oates, J. A. (1986): *N. Engl. J. Med.*, 315: 800-804.
9. Salari, H., and Chan-Yeung, M. (1989): *Am. J. Respir. Cell Mol. Biol.*, 1: 245-250.

METABOLISM OF ARACHIDONIC ACID IN HUMAN ALVEOLAR MACROPHAGES FROM PATIENTS WITH SARCOIDOSIS

V. De Rose*, M.T. Crivellari**, T. Viganò**, G.C. Folco**, L. Trentin^, M Masciarelli^, G. Semenzato^, E. Pozzi* and G. Gialdroni Grassi§

* Clin. of Respiratory Diseases, University of Turin, Osp. S. Luigi Gonzaga Regione Gonzale 10, 10043 Orbassano (TO) - ** Inst. of Pharmacol. Sciences, University of Milan, Via Balzaretti 9, 20133 Milano - ^ Inst. of Clinical Medicine, University of Padua, Via Giustiniani 2, 35128 Padua - § Inst. of Respiratory Disease, University of Pavia, Via Taramelli 5, 27100 Pavia.

INTRODUCTION

Sarcoidosis is a multisystem chronic granulomatous disorder of unknown etiology characterized by hightened immune processes at the site of disease activity (4). In particular an enhanced recruitment and activation of immunocompetent cells, i.e. alveolar macrophages and T cells, takes place within the alveolar structures.

Once activated, these cells have a wide spectrum of effector functions including secretion of a variety of mediators that play an important role in the evolution and modulation of local immune processes in sarcoidosis (10). Among the products released from alveolar macrophages (AM), arachidonic acid (AA) metabolites are known to modulate inflammatory and immune reactions.

Prostaglandin E_2 (PGE_2) has been shown to suppress various lymphocyte functions such as T lymphocyte proliferation (2) and lymphokine secretion (3) as well as to inhibit Ia antigen expression on macrophages (9). In addition, AM isolated from experimentally induced immune granuloma are capable of metabolizing AA to 5-lipoxygenase (5-LO) products that may sustain the tissue reactions (5). Therefore the relative amounts of AA metabolites released by AM could be important, in modulating the granulomatous inflammatory response. The present study was designed to investigate the capacity of AM, from patients with sarcoidosis in different states of disease activity, to release PGE_2 and leukotriene B_4 (LTB_4) in vitro at resting conditions and following a phagocytic stimulus.

MATERIALS AND METHODS

Study population

26 patients with biopsy-proven sarcoidosis (mean age: 42 ± 10 years) were studied. Disease activity was evaluated according to the following criteria: a) percentage and absolute number of T cells recovered from the bronchoalveolar lavage (BAL) and b) positivity of the ^{67}Ga scan. Using these criteria 14 patients had active sarcoidosis (AS, T cells > 30%, ^{67}Ga positivity), while 12 patients showed inactive disease (NAS, T cells < 30%, ^{67}Ga negativity).

None of them had received steroids or antiinflammatory nonsteroidal drugs in the last three months. 5 normal subjects (mean age: 39 ± 8 years) were evaluated as controls (C). All subjects were non smokers.

Cell purification and culture

AM were obtained by BAL. Lavage fluid was filtered, centrifuged and total and differential cell counts were obtained. The cell pellet was resuspended in RPMI 1640 containing 10% foetal calf serum, 100 U/ml penicillin and 100 mcg/ml streptomycin. Following a 2 hours incubation at 37°C in 5% CO2 air, the non-adherent cells were removed by washing. Opsonized zymosan (500 mcg/ml) was then added to some culture tissue dish, in order to evaluate mediator's release by stimulated and unstimulated AM. Supernatants were collected at 30', 60', 120', 24 h.

PGE_2 and LTB_4 assay

PGE_2 and LTB_4 levels were determined by enzyme immunoassay according to Pradelles et al. (6).

Statistical analysis was performed using Dunn test (1) for the comparison among the three groups and a one-way analysis of variance for the evaluation of responses to zymosan stimulation.

RESULTS

The time course of PGE_2 release in basal conditions showed detectable levels only at 24 h; a similar profile was observed in stimulated AM. No significant differences among groups were observed (data not shown).

As far as LTB_4 is concerned, basal release was higher during the first 30'-60' of culture and showed a tendency to lower at 24 h; this behaviour was observed in both normal and sarcoid cells.

Only minute amounts of the hydroxyacid were released at resting conditions both by normal and sarcoid AM. Opsonized zymosan was unable to increase LTB_4 production at 30' in AM from control subjects, while triggered a significant increase ($p < 0.001$) in cells from sarcoid patients with active disease. After 24 h of culture AM from all groups exhibited a significant response to zymosan stimulation, that was

FIG. 1.   Release of LTB$_4$ by human alveolar macrophages after 30' in culture

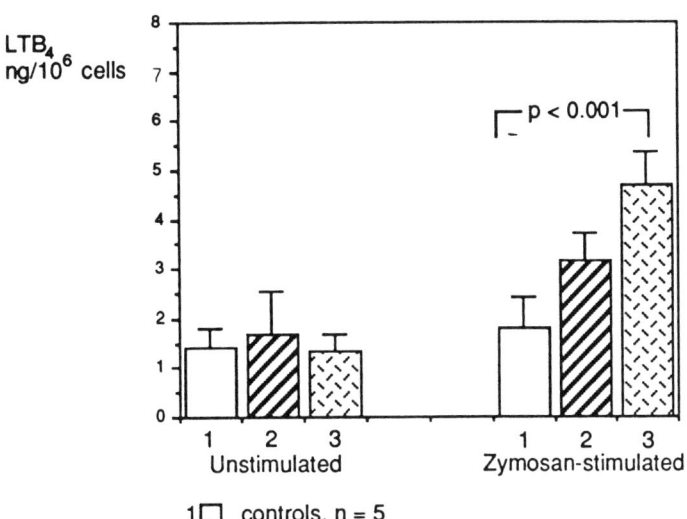

$p < 0.001$

LTB$_4$ ng/10^6 cells

Unstimulated
Zymosan-stimulated

1 □ controls, n = 5
2 ▨ patients with non active sarcoidosis, n = 12
3 ▨ patients with active sarcoidosis, n = 14

FIG. 2   Release of LTB$_4$ by human alveolar macrophages after 24 h in culture

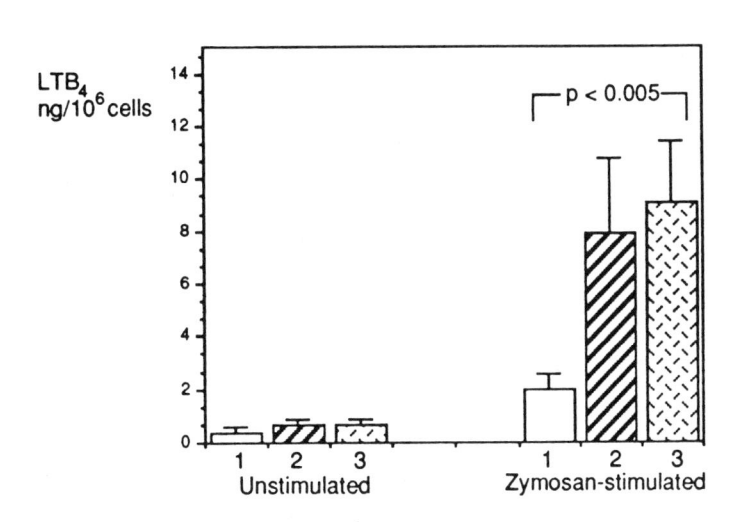

$p < 0.005$

LTB$_4$ ng/10^6 cells

Unstimulated
Zymosan-stimulated

1 □ controls, n = 5
2 ▨ patients with non active sarcoidosis, n = 12
3 ▨ patients with active sarcoidosis, n = 14

higher in sarcoid AM, particularly from patients with active disease (C: $p < 0.05$, NAS: $p < 0.02$, AS: $p < 0.005$ of stimulated vs unstimulated).

Comparing LTB_4 levels released by stimulated AM from the three groups, a statistically significant difference was observed between patients with AS and C, both at 30' and 24 h of culture (Fig. 1, 2).

Pretreatment with indomethacin (3×10^{-6} M) blocked PGE_2 production at 24 h in zymosan-stimulated cells from all sarcoid patients withouth any change in LTB_4 values (data not shown).

DISCUSSION

AM have been implicated as being central to the evolution of granulomatorus inflammatory responses in the lung; activation of these cells results in the production of a variety of biologically active molecules which may suppress or potentiate the immune response. In the present study we have investigated the capacity of sarcoid AM to release PGE_2 and LTB_4 in comparison with nor mal AM. No difference in PGE_2 production was found between sarcoid and normal AM; AM from sarcoid patients, however, respond to a phagocytic stimulus with a marked production of LTB_4 that is highest in patients with AS. The use of cycloxygenase inhibitors does not confirm the existence of a feed-back mechanism between products of the oxidative pathways of AA in sarcoid AM.

LTB_4 is a 5-LO product of AA metabolism that has potent chemotactic activity for polymorphonuclear and mononuclear leucocytes (7); its release by sarcoid AM may play a role in the amplification of the granulomatous response by recruiting mononuclear phagocytes from the blood into the lung.

REFERENCES

1) Dunn, G. (1964): Technometrics, 6: 241-250
2) Goodwin, J.S., Ceuppens, J. (1983): J. Clin. Immunol. 3: 295-300
3) Gordon, D., Bray, A.M., and Morley, J. (1976): Nature, 262: 401-404
4) Hunninghake, G.W., and Crystal, R.G. (1981): N. Engl. J. Med., 305: 429-432
5) Kunkel, S.L., Chensue, S.W., Mouton, C., and Higashi, G.I. (1984): J. Clin. Invest., 74: 514-520
6) Pradelles, P., Grassi, J., and Maclouf, J. (1985): Anal. Biochem., 57: 1170-1173
7) Rola-Pleszczynski, M., Chavaillaz, P.A., and Lemaire, I. (1985): Prostaglandins leukotrienes Med., 23: 207-210
8) Smith, M.J.H. (1981): Gen. Pharmacol., 12: 211-216
9) Snydec, D.S., Beller, D.I., and Unanue, E.R. (1982): Nature, 299: 163-165
10) Thomas, P.D., and Hunninghake, G.W. (1987): Am. Rev. Respir. Dis., 135:747-760

THE COMPARATIVE NASAL EFFECTS OF PROSTAGLANDIN D_2 IN NORMAL AND RHINITIC SUBJECTS

P Howarth, S Walsh and C Robinson*

Medicine I and *Clinical Pharmacology, Southampton General Hospital, Southampton S09 4XY, UK.

Introduction

Allergic rhinitis is a common condition affecting 10 - 15% of the westernised world, giving rise to the symptoms of pruritis, sneezing, rhinorrhoea and nasal blockage. These symptoms are considered to be secondary to the release of vasoactive and inflammatory mediators from sensitized cells within the nasal mucosa (3). Two possible contributing cells are mast cells and eosinophils. Nasal biopsies or smears in both seasonal and perennial allergic rhinitis identify an increase in mast cells and eosinophils within the nasal mucosa as compared to normal subjects. Both these cell types possess IgE Fc receptors and can directly interact with allergen to release locally active mediators. Measurement of mediators within the nasal cavity by lavage identifies the release of histamine, tryptase and prostaglandin D_2 following local nasal airways allergen challenge (7), indicative of mast cell degranulation. Nasal biopsy also identifies ultrastructural evidence of mast cell degranulation.

Histamine is the major preformed mast cell mediator and local nasal challenge with histamine induces the symptoms of rhinitis, producing itching, sneezing, rhinorrhoea and nasal blockage. These effects are predominantly H_1-receptor mediated. Treatment with H_1-receptor antagonists in clinical disease, however, while alleviating itching, sneezing and rhinorrhoeea is without effect on nasal blockage (4). Mediators other than histamine are thus likely to be of greater relevance to the pathogenesis of nasal blockage. As prostaglandin D_2 (PGD_2) is the major prostanoid produced on immunologic challenge of mast cells we have investigated the nasal effects of PGD_2 in atopic rhinitic and non-atopic non-rhinitic subjects.

Subjects and methods

Eight non-atopic non-rhinitic and 8 atopic rhinitic subjects participated. Each subject underwent a dose-response study to PGD_2 (Salford Ultrafine Chemicals and Research Limited) and to the diluent vehicle (0.9% saline and methanol) while 10 of the subjects (6 normal and 4 rhinitics) also underwent single dose challenge with PGD_2 and vehicle to investigate the time course of action of PGD_2. All nasal challenges were undertaken bilaterally with a metered dose pump spray delivering 3.8 - 60.9nmol PGD_2 per nostril in incremental doses for the dose response study, and 60.9nmol PGD_2 per nostril for the time course of action study. The nasal response was monitored in all instances by measurement of nasal airways resistance (NAR) by active posterior rhinomanometry using a Mercury NR6 rhinomanometer. In addition, on the time course of action study days record was made of nasal pruritis, number of sneezes and quantity of nasal secretions.

Subsequent to these studies the effect of the alpha agonist, oxymetazoline hydrochloride (Kirby Warwick Pharmaceuticals Limited, Suffolk, UK) on the nasal response to PGD_2 (60.9nmol per nostril) was investigated in 4 subjects by comparing the nasal response to PGD_2 before and after topical oxymetazoline (0.4gms) pretreatment or saline pretreatment. The nasal effects of PGD_2 were monitored in this study by measurement of NAR.

Statistical analysis

Baseline NAR in the two groups on the dose-response days were compared within groups for the PGD_2 and vehicle challenge days by the Wilcoxon's signed rank test and between groups using the Mann-Whitney U test for non-paired data. Page's test for trends was used to investigate the dose-response relationship between PGD_2 and increments in NAR. The dose response curves were analysed, with respect to the differential effect of PGD_2 over that of vehicle challenge alone, both as maximal increase in NAR for each PGD_2 dose and as area under the dose-response curve for each 30 minute period as calculated by trapezoid integration. Between group comparisons were undertaken using the Mann-Whitney U test. On the time course of action study absolute values of NAR at each time point post challenge were compared with the pre-challenge baseline values using the Wilcoxon's signed rank test.

Results

There was no significant difference between the mean ($\pm$ sem) NAR values (Pasec ccs^{-1}) in the rhinitics (0.27 $\pm$ 0.03) or non-rhinitics (0.22 $\pm$ 0.01) prior to challenge. Prostaglandin D_2 nasal insufflation produced a significant dose-dependant increase in nasal airways resistance in both atopic rhinitic and non-atopic non-rhinitic subjects ($p<0.001$), while vehicle was without significant effect. Within group comparisons of the increase in NAR due to PGD_2 identified no significant difference between the rhinitics and non-rhinitics whether the data was analysed as maximal increase in NAR or as area under the NAR-dose curve. The mean percentage increase in NAR area under the curve (Auc) in the two groups for the incremental doses of PGD_2 is identified in table I.

TABLE I Mean percentage increase in NAR Auc following PGD_2 nasal challenge

Group	PGD_2 (nmol/nostril)				
	3.8	7.6	15.2	30.4	60.9
Non-rhinitic	15.5	41.6	90.3	174.2	523.4
Rhinitic	23.7	66.1	91.5	145.2	137.0*

*2 rhinitics unable to complete because of severe nasal blockage

Single dose PGD_2 (60.9nmol/nostril), in the time course study, caused a rapid increase in NAR, significant by 2 minutes ($p<0.01$), which peaked at 10 minutes (171% increase above baseline) and was significantly greater than baseline up to the 50 minute measurement ($p<0.05$). There was no significant difference between the rhinitics and non-rhinitics in the duration or magnitude of response ($p<0.05$). PGD_2 did not induce sneezing or rhinorrhoea. Nasal irritation was reported by all 4 rhinitic subjects and 3 of the 6 non-rhinitic subjects.

Oxymetazoline pre-treatment abolished the nasal response (NAR) to PGD_2 nasal insufflation while saline pre-treatment had no effect.

Discussion

These results identify that topically administered prostaglandin D_2 induces an highly significant dose-dependent increase in nasal airways resistance in both rhinitic and non-rhinitic subjects. The time course of action study revealed a rapid onset of action which was sustained following single dose administration (60.9nmol/nostril) for up to 50 minutes. The increase in NAR was associated with some nasal irritation but no sneezing or rhinorrhoea. Although some rhinitic subjects exhibited nasal hyperresponsiveness to the effects of PGD_2, with increases in NAR above that experienced by the non- rhinitics, overall there was no significant difference between the rhinitic and non-rhinitic groups in their nasal response to PGD_2, as assessed either by the magnitude or duration of response.

These results would suggest that prostaglandin D_2 is likely to play a prominent role in the genesis of nasal blockage in allergic rhinitis. Nasal biopsies after nasal allergen exposure identify mast cell degranulation and nasal lavage reveals increased recovery of PGD$_2$ consistent with mediator secretion. Pre-treatment with aspirin protects against pollen-induced increases in NAR with challenge in some rhinitic subjects (5) and the combination of terfenadine and flurbiprofen has been shown to be significantly superior to terfenadine plus placebo in the treatment of seasonal allergic rhinitis, especially with respect to nasal blockage (1). The lack of complete protection with the combination of terfenadine and flurbiprofen could be related to the involvement of other mediators, such as leukotriene C4 or kinins (3), in the nasal response to seasonal allergen exposure in sensitized individuals, or related to the lack of complete obliteration of PGD$_2$ production by flurbiprofen. While flurbiprofen is a potent cyclooxygenase inhibitor it has recently been identified that prostanoids can be generated *in vivo* by a non-cyclooxygenase pathway involving free radical formation (6). In this instance PGD$_2$ production would be uninfluenced by flurbiprofen.

The vasoconstrictor, oxymetazoline, prevented the increase in NAR with PGD$_2$ in this study. This suggests that the effects of PGD$_2$ on NAR are vascular, which is consistent with the concept that changes in NAR are largely determined by volume changes within the nasal venous sinisoids. The identification that the PGD$_2$ metabolite, $9\alpha\ 11\beta$ PGF$_2$, which is equipotent to PGD$_2$ on the muscular TP receptor is ineffective in inducing nasal blockage (7) would suggest that the vascular effects of PGD$_2$ within the nose are mediated directly through the vascular DP receptor. To fully elucidate the contribution of of PGD$_2$ to nasal blockage in allergic rhinitis it would be necessary to investigate the effects of specific antagonism of PGD$_2$ at the DP receptor. Such antagonists are not available for clinical use. These studies would, however, suggest that PGD$_2$ is likely to be an important mediator of nasal blockage in allergic rhinitis.

1. Brooks C D and Karl K J. (1988): J Allergy Clin Immunol. 81: 1110 - 1117.
2. Harrison K, Robinson C, Brewster H and Howarth P H. (1990) in 7th International Conference on Prostaglandins and related compounds. P 323 FondazioneGiovanniLorenzini Italy.
3. Howarth P H. (1989): In Rhinitis Mechanisms and Management edited by I Mackay pp 33 - 53.
4. Howarth P H and Holgate S T. (1984): Thorax. 39: 668 - 672.
5. Mclean J A, Bacon J R, Mathews K P and Banas J. (1983): J Allergy Clin Immunol 72: 187.
6. Morrow J D, Hill K E, Burk R F, Nammour T M, Badr K F and Roberts L J. (1990) in 7th International conference on Prostaglandins and related compounds. p12. Fondazione-GiovanniLorenzini Italy.
7. Naclerio R M, Proud D, Peters S P, Silber G, Kagey-Sobotka A, Adkinson N F and Lichtenstein L M. (1986): Clin Allergy 16: 101 - 110.

INHIBITION OF ENDOTHELIN-INDUCED BRONCHOCONSTRICTION BY OKY-046, A SELECTIVE THROMBOXANE A2 SYNTHETASE INHIBITOR, IN GUINEA PIGS

F. Nambu, N. Yube, N. Omawari, M. Sawada, T. Okegawa, A. Kawasaki, and S. Ikeda*

Minase Research Institute, Ono Pharmaceutical Co., Ltd., Shimamoto, Mishima, Osaka 618 and * Central Research Laboratories, Kissei Pharmaceutical Co., Ltd., Matsumoto 399, Japan

INTRODUCTION

Endothelin (ET)-1 is a newly described peptide isolated from culture supernatant of porcine aortic endothelial cells (8). ET-1 induces vascular (8) and airway smooth muscle contractions in both *in vivo* (7) and *in vitro* (3). Although a role of ET-1 in the pathogenesis of asthma is unknown, its production in the vicinity of bronchial smooth muscle (1) and increased level of ET-1 in bronchoalveolar lavage (BAL) fluid during asthmatic attack (5) may suggest that this peptide could affect adjacent bronchial tone. Accordingly, we examined pharmacological activities of ET-1 on guinea pig airways and possible contributions of arachidonic acid metabolites, histamine and parasympathetic nervous system to ET-1-induced bronchoconstriction.

MATERIALS AND METHODS

Male Hartley guinea pigs (210-470g) were anesthetized with pentobarbital sodium (75 mg/kg, i.p.) and artificially ventilated with a constant volume of 5 ml at 70 strokes/min. Bronchoconstriction was measured as previously described (4). ET-1 was intravenously administered at a dose of 1 μg/kg except for the dose-finding study.

In an experiment where thromboxane (Tx) B2 and 6-keto-PGF1α were measured, blood and BAL fluid samples were obtained just before and 1 min after ET-1 injection. Both samples were centrifuged (1700 x g, 10 min, 4 °C) and the resultant supernatant was extracted with acetic acid and purified with SEP-PAK® C18 column, Bond Elut®DEA column and thin layer chromatography for radioimmunoassay for TxB2 and 6-keto-PGF1α were performed subsequently.

OKY-046 [a TxA2 synthetase inhibitor (2)] was administered i.v. 2 min or i.d. 30 min prior to ET-1 injection. ONO-8809 (a TxA2/PG endoperoxide receptor antagonist) and ONO-1078 [a peptide leukotrienes (LTs) receptor antagonist(6)] were administered i.d. 1 hr and i.v. 1 min prior to ET-1 injection, respectively.

Statistical analyses were based on two-way ANOVA or Student's t-test for unpaired design with probability value $p<0.05$ regarded as significant.

RESULTS

ET-1, when administered i.v., caused dose-related increase in insufflation pressure at doses ranging from 0.1 to 3 µg/kg. Higher doses of ET-1 exhibited biphasic bronchoconstriction and one out of three animals used died within 10 min following injection of a maximal dose (3 µg/kg) of ET-1.

Pretreatment with indomethacin (2 mg/kg, i.v.) almost abolished ET-1 (1 µg/kg, i.v.)-induced bronchoconstriction although neither mepyramine (1 mg/kg, i.v.) nor atropine (1 mg/kg, i.v.) inhibited airway responses to ET-1 injection.

OKY-046 elicited dose-related inhibitory effects on ET-1-induced bronchoconstriction at doses ranging from 0.1 to 1 mg/kg, i.v. (FIG. 1) and 3 to 30 mg/kg, i.d. ONO-8809 attenuated ET-1-induced bronchoconstriction in a

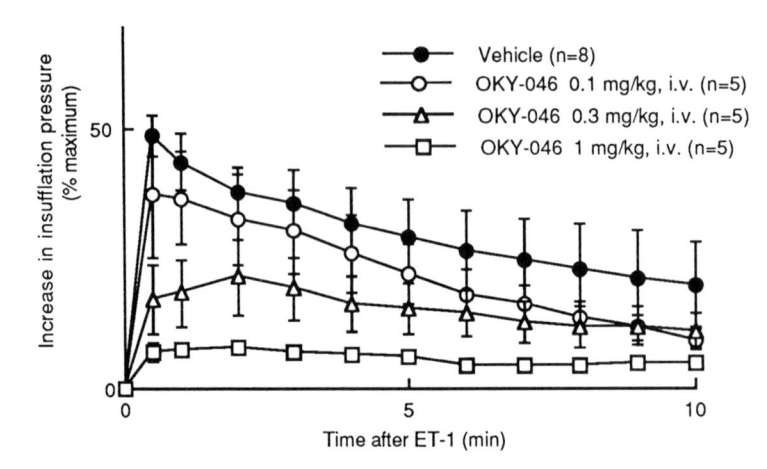

FIG. 1. Effect of OKY-046 on ET-1-induced bronchoconstriction in guinea pigs. OKY-046 was intravenously administered 2 min prior to ET-1 (1 µg/kg, i.v.) injection. Each value represents the mean±S.E.

dose-dependent manner at doses ranging from 10 to 30 µg/kg, i.d. On the other hand, ONO-1078, a peptide LTs receptor antagonist, did not show any inhibitory effects on ET-1-induced bronchoconstriction at 1 mg/kg, a dose which prevents peptide LTs-induced bronchoconstriction.

Both plasma and BAL fluid levels of TxB2 significantly elevated following i.v. injection of ET-1, and OKY-046 inhibited these increases in TxB2 levels in a dose-dependent manner (Table 1).

Table 1. Effects of OKY-046 and indomethacin (Indo) on TxB2 levels following ET-1 injection

Group	Doses mg/kg,i.v.	Plasma (pg/ml) Before[a]	Plasma (pg/ml) After[b]	BAL fluid (pg/ml) Before[a]	BAL fluid (pg/ml) After[b]
Control	-	447.2±56.4**	1046.4±111.0	52.8±11.9*	245.7±57.8
OKY-046	0.1	ND[c]	794.8±292.2	ND[c]	176.3±66.2
	1	ND[c]	403.4±73.7**	ND[c]	89.6±21.1*
Indo	2	ND[c]	127.0±18.3***	ND[c]	47.0±11.2*

Each value represents the mean±S.E. *, ** and *** indicate significant differences compared to control value (After) where $p<0.05$, $p<0.01$ and $p<0.001$, respectively.
[a] Before: just before ET-1 injection, [b] After: 1 min after ET-1 injection [c] ND: not determined

Although 6-keto-PGF1α levels in both plasma and BAL fluid did not change following ET-1 injection, OKY-046 dose-dependently elevated both plasma and BAL fluid levels of 6-keto-PGF1α. Indomethacin decreased both TxB2 and 6-keto-PGF1α levels.

DISCUSSION

In the present study, we investigated possible contributions of arachidonic acid metabolites, histamine and parasympathetic nervous system to ET-1-induced bronchoconstrictions *in vivo*. ET-1-induced bronchoconstriction was abolished by the pretreatment of indomethacin but not by mepyramine and atropine, suggesting that contractile cyclooxygenase products may be involved in mediating ET-1-induced bronchoconstriction. Since TxA2 has an extremely potent contractile activity on airway smooth muscle, we examined the effect of OKY-046 on ET-1-induced bronchoconstriction. The results showed that OKY-046 dose-dependently attenuated airway response to ET-1. To ascertain whether inhibitory effect of OKY-046 could be due to the inhibition of TxA2 synthesis, effect of a TxA2/PG endoperoxide receptor antagonist, ONO-8809, was examined. ONO-8809 inhibited bronchoconstriction induced by ET-1 in a dose-dependent manner, indicating that bronchoconstrictor activity of ET-1 is predominantly mediated by TxA2 generated by stimulation of ET-1. On the other hand, it is well known that TxA2 is also produced by peptide LTs. Accordingly, we examined the effect of ONO-1078, a peptide LTs receptor antagonist, on ET-1-induced bronchoconstriction because there is a possibility that ET-1 could stimulate the production of TxA2 through LTs production. However, ONO-1078 did not show any inhibitory effects on ET-1-induced bronchoconstriction. To further support the hypothesis that TxA2 is involved in ET-1-induced bronchoconstriction, plasma and BAL fluid levels of TxB2 and 6-keto-PGF1α were measured. The results clearly showed that both plasma and BAL fluid levels of TxB2 elevated following i.v. injection of ET-1 and that OKY-046 and indomethacin significantly inhibited these increases in TxB2 levels.

The data described here suggest that TxA2 is a promising and potent candidate for mediating ET-1-induced bronchoconstriction and involvement of peptide LTs, histamine and parasympathetic nervous system can not be counted.

REFERENCES

1. Black, P.N., Ghatei, M.A., Bretherton-Watt, D., Takahashi, K., Krausz, T., and Bloom, S.R. (1989) : *Am. Rev. Respir. Dis.*, 139 : A52.
2. Hiraku, S., Taniguchi, K., Wakitani, K., Omawari, N., Kira, H., Miyamoto, T., Okegawa, T., Kawasaki, A., and Ujiie, A. (1986) : *Japan. J. Pharmacol.*, 41 : 393-401.
3. Lagente, V., Chabrier, P.E., Mencia-Huerta, J.-M., and Braquet, P. (1989) : *Biochem. Biophysic. Res. Commun.*, 158 : 625-632.
4. Nambu, F., Motoishi, M., Omawari, N., Okegawa, T., Kawasaki, A., and Ikeda, S. (1990) : *Japan. J. Pharmacol.*, 52 : 307-317.
5. Nomura, A., Uchida, Y., Kameyama, M., Saotome, M., Oki, K., and Hasegawa, S. (1989) : *Lancet, II* : 747-748.
6. Obata, T., Katsube, N., Miyamoto, T., Toda, M., Okegawa, T., Nakai, H., Kosuge, S., Konno, M., Arai, Y., and Kawasaki, A. (1985) : *Advance in Prostaglandin, Thromboxane and Leukotriene Research*, edited by O. Hayaishi and S. Yamamoto, pp229-231. Raven Press, New York.
7. Uchida, Y., Ninomiya, H., Saotome, M., Nomura, A., Ohtsuka, M., Yanagisawa, M., Goto, K., Masaki, T., and Hasegawa, S. (1988) : *Eur. J. Pharmacol.*, 154 : 227-228.
8. Yanagisawa, M., Kurihara, H., Kimura, S., Tomobe, Y., Kobayashi, M., Mitsui, Y., Yazaki, Y., Goto, K., and Masaki, T. (1988) : *Nature*, 232 : 411-415.

THE EFFECTS OF A 5-LIPOXYGENASE INHIBITOR ON ANTIGEN-INDUCED MEDIATOR RELEASE, LATE-PHASE BRONCHOCONSTRICTION AND CELLULAR INFILTRATES IN PRIMATES

ROBERT H. GUNDEL, CAROL A. TORCELLINI, COSMOS C. CLARKE, SUDHA DESAI, EDWARD S. LAZER AND CRAIG D. WEGNER

Boehringer Ingelheim Pharmaceuticals Inc., Ridgefield, CT 06877

Recent studies suggest that the pathological abnormalities seen in bronchial asthma are the consequence of pro-inflammatory cell infiltrates and the release of preformed and newly generated bronchoactive and vasoactive mediators (2). The leukotrienes are metabolites of arachidonic acid formed via the lipoxygenase pathway (8). The peptido-leukotrienes (LTC_4, LTD_4, LTE_4) are extremely potent bronchoconstrictors being approximately 1000 fold more potent than histamine or methacholine (3). Furthermore, LTB_4 has been shown to be one of the most potent chemotactic agents for neutrophils (5). Thus, the leukotrienes represent a class of biologically active compounds that may mediate altered lung function and the development of airway inflammation in response to allergen exposure.

BI-L-239, (2,6-dimethyl-4-[-2-(4-fluorophenyl)ethenyl]phenol), a novel leukotriene synthesis inhibitor, has been recently synthesized and characterized (7). This compound has impressive in vitro activity inhibiting 5-lipoxygenase in human neutrophils (IC_{50} = 0.12uM).

The purpose of this study was to examine the effects of BI-L-239 in a primate model of antigen-induced mediator release, early and late-phase bronchoconstriction and pro-inflammatory cell influx into the lungs.

METHODS

Adult male cynomolgus monkeys (Macaca fascicularis) were anesthetized with an intramuscular injection of ketamine hydrochloride (4 mg/kg) and xylazine (1 mg/kg), intubated with a cuffed endotracheal tube and seated in an upright position in a specially designed support chair. Ketamine (4 mg/kg) was used to supplement anesthesia when needed. Baseline respiratory system resistance (Rrs), measured by discrete frequency forced oscillations superimposed on tidal breathing as previously described (9), was recorded over a 15 minute time period followed by either vehicle or drug aerosol treatment. Rrs was monitored for an additional 10 minutes post inhalation treatment. Antigen inhalation challenge was administered by intermittent positive pressure breathing with a Bird Mark 7A respirator and micronebulizer (model #8158) at 15 breaths per minute for 2 minutes. Following antigen challenge Rrs was monitored for 10 minutes (early response) after which the animals were removed from the chair, placed in the supine position and bronchoalveolar lavage (BAL) was performed with a pediatric bronchoscope (Olympus, model 3C10). Following BAL each animal was allowed to recover from anesthesia and returned to their cage. To monitor the late-phase response, each animal was re-anesthetized with the ketamine/xylazine mixture, intubated, seated in the support chair and Rrs was monitored over a 15 minute time period. Rrs measurements were recorded at 4, 6, 8 and 24 hours post antigen inhalation. In order to examine antigen-induced changes in airway cellular composition, BAL was performed during the peak late-phase response on the opposite lung that was lavaged during the early response. Airway cellular composition was analyzed with Wright stained cytocentrifuge preparations. The BAL levels of immunoreactive LTC_4 (i-LTC_4) and immunoreactive PGD_2 (i-PGD_2) were measured by radioimmunoassay. Inhibition of mediator generation and bronchoconstriction were determined by comparing drug treated studies to bracketing control studies in each animal. The data were evaluated statistically using Fischer's t-test where a P value of administered dexamethasone. In contrast, inhaled beclomethasone, administered 10 minutes prior to antigen challenge, did not alter LTC_4 less than or equal to 0.05 was considered statistically significant.

RESULTS

Antigen inhalation resulted in a dramatic increase in i-LTC_4 and i-PGD_2 recovered in BAL 20 minutes post challenge (Table 1). Inhaled BI-L-239, administered 10 minutes prior to antigen challenge, provided a dose-dependent inhibition of LTC_4 generation (Table 2). The efficacy

TABLE 1: *Mediators Recovered in Monkey BAL Fluid* (mean ± SEM)

Challenge	i-LTC4 (ng)	i-PGD2 (ng)
Baseline	1 ± 0.7	2 ± 0.9
PBS	2 ± 0.5	2 ± 1.2
Ascaris	45 ± 9	32 ± 7

TABLE 2: *Inhibition of Antigen-Induced Mediator Release*

Compound	Dose	n	% Inhibition i-LTC	i-PGD2
BI-L-239	1 mg/ml, aerosol	6	35 ± 74	0 ± 76
	3 mg/ml, aerosol	5	61 ± 17	30 ± 12
	10 mg/ml, aerosol	6	73 ± 12*	52 ± 14
Dexamethasone	1 mg/kg, i.m.	7	71 ± 6*	51 ± 8*
Beclomethasone	2 mg/ml, aerosol	5	0 ± 19	0 ± 18

Aerosolized compounds were administered 10 minutes prior to antigen challenge. Dexamethasone was administered -24, -4 and -1 hour prior to antigen challenge. Values represent mean ± SEM. *($P<0.05$).

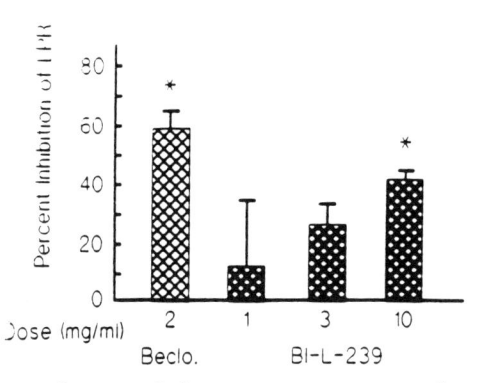

FIG. 1. The effects of aerosol drug treatment on antigen-induced late-phase response. % inhibition calculated by comparing drug studies to bracketing control studies. Values represent the mean ± SEM (n=5).

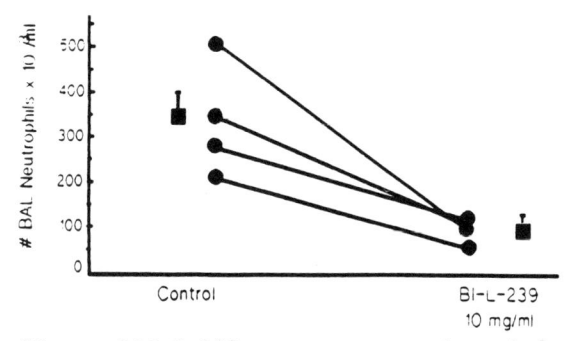

FIG. 2. The effects of BI-L-239 treatment on antigen-induced neutrophil influx into the airways.

of aerosolized BI-L-239 (10 mg/ml) was similar to that of chronically generation. A single aerosol administration of BI-L-239, 10 minutes prior to antigen inhalation, provided dose-related inhibition of the peak late-phase bronchoconstriction response (Figure 1). Inhaled beclomethasone also significantly inhibited the late-phase response. Neither BI-L-239 nor beclomethasone significantly inhibited the early (immediate) peak bronchoconstriction (data not shown). The antigen-induced neutrophil influx into the airways, associated with the late-phase response, was also inhibited (63% mean) with BI-L-239 treatment (Figure 2).

DISCUSSION

The leukotrienes are products of arachidonic acid metabolism with potent pro-inflammatory and bronchoconstricting effects which may be relevant to pathogenesis of asthma. We have previously demonstrated that antigen inhalation in sensitive monkeys results in the generation and release of leukotrienes and prostaglandins into the airways which are recoverable and quantifiable in BAL fluid (6). Our present study demonstrates that acute treatment with a lipoxygenase synthesis inhibitor or chronic treatment with dexamethasone will block the generation and release of leukotrienes. Interestingly, while the peptidoleukotrienes are known to be very potent bronchoconstrictors, significant inhibition of leukotriene production did not alter the peak increase in Rrs immediately following antigen inhalation. However, it should be emphasized that in these studies only the peak increase in Rrs was monitored (usually occurring 5 minutes post antigen inhalation) and not the duration of the early response. It may be that inhibition of leukotriene synthesis would decrease the duration of this response, a subject that will be examined in future studies.

Inhibition of leukotriene generation did, however, significantly block the development of the late-phase response. This observation is in agreement with reports by Delehunt and co-workers in which a leukotriene receptor antagonist inhibited late-phase bronchoconstriction in a sheep model of asthma (4). Furthermore, Abraham and associates have reported that LTD_4 inhalation caused immediate and late-phase bronchoconstriction in dual responder sheep (1). These data suggest that the production and release of leukotrienes following antigen inhalation may initiate events relating to the late-phase response. One such event may be the influx of pro-inflammatory cells into the lungs. In the present study neutrophil influx was significantly reduced in all animals treated with BI-L-239 suggesting that a 5-lipoxygenase product may be mediating this response to antigen inhalation.

SUMMARY

Inhaled BI-L-239 significantly inhibited i-LTC_4 generation, late-phase bronchoconstriction and the influx of neutrophils into the lungs. We conclude that leukotriene generation and release within the lungs, following allergen exposure, in part mediate altered lung function and contribute to the development of airway inflammation. As such, treatment with a selective 5-lipoxygenase inhibitor may aid in the treatment of bronchial asthma and other allergic diseases.

REFERENCES

1. Abraham, W.M., Russi, E., Wanner, A., Delehunt, J.C., Yerger, L.D., Chapman, G.A. (1985): *Prostaglandins*, 29:715-726.
2. Barnes, P.J., Chung, K.J., Page, C.P. (1988): *Pharm. Rev.*, 40:49-84.
3. Dahlen, J.E., Hedquist, P., Hammerstrom, B., Samuelsson, B. (1980): *Nature*, 288:484-486.
4. Delehunt, J.C., Perruchoud, A., Yerger, L., Marchette, B., Stevenson, J.S., Abraham, W.M. (1984): *Am. Rev. Respir. Dis.*, 130:748-754.
5. Ford-Hutchinson, A.W., Bray, M.A., Doig, M.U., Shipley, M.E., Smith, M.J.H. (1981): *Nature*, 286:264-265.
6. Gundel, R., Torcellini, C., Clarke, C., Watrous, J., Homon, C., Kinkade, P., Farina, P., Wegner, C. (1988): *Physiologist*, 31:A91. (abstract).
7. Lazer, E.S., Wong, H.C., Wegner, C.D., Graham, A.E., Farina, P.R. (1990): *J. Med. Chem.*, 33 (in press).
8. Piper, P.J. (1984): *Physiol. Rev.*, 64:744-761.
9. Wegner, C.D., Jackson, A.C., Berry, J.D., Gillespie, J.R. (1984): *Annu. Rev. Physiol.*, 55:47-61.

INHIBITION OF ALLERGIC BRONCHOCONSTRICTION IN ASTHMATICS BY THE LEUKOTRIENE-ANTAGONIST ICI-204,219

Sven-Erik Dahlén[1], Barbro Dahlén[2], Eva Eliasson[2], Heléne Johansson[2], Thure Björck[1], Maria Kumlin[3], Karin Boo[4], Jeff Whitney[5], Sue Binks[5], Barbara King[5], Ron Stark[5] and Olle Zetterström[2].

Departments of Physiology[1], Thoracic Medicine[2], Physiological Chemistry[3] and Institute of Environmental Medicine[1], Karolinska Institutet, S-104 01 Stockholm, Sweden, and ICI Pharmaceuticals, Clinical Research Departments, S-411 21 Göteborg[4], Sweden and Mereside[5], SK10 4TG Cheshire, England.

INTRODUCTION.

Several lines of evidence indicate that the cysteinyl-containing leukotrienes (LT) C_4, D_4 and E_4 are potential mediators of airways obstruction in asthma. Nevertheless, it has been difficult to prove involvement of leukotrienes in asthmatic reactions, probably because the drugs initially used to test this hypothesis were lacking in potency and/or bioavailability. Recently, however, a more suitable generation of selective leukotriene antagonists has appeared. The most potent receptor antagonist so far described, ICI-198,615, blocks the action of the cysteinyl-leukotrienes on human bronchi in the nanomolar dose range (3). A closely related compound, ICI-204,219 (4-[5-cyclopentyloxycarbonylamino-1-methylindol-3-ylmethyl]-3-methoxy-N-O-tolylsulfonylbenzamide) has the same pharmacodynamic profile as ICI-198,615, but superior oral bioavailability (1). It was recently documented that ICI-204,219 indeed is an effective antagonist of inhaled LTD_4 in man (2). Here we report that ICI-204,219 also produces significant inhibition of the bronchoconstrictor response to allergen in atopic asthmatics.

SUBJECTS AND EXPERIMENTAL PROCEDURES.

Ten atopic asthmatic men (23-56 years of age; mean forced expiratory volume in 1.0 second ($FEV_{1.0}$) 94% of predicted, range 77-109) with documented airways hyperresponsiveness to inhaled histamine gave their informed consent to participate in the study which was approved by the ethical committee (Dnr 89:120). Two of the patients inhaled bronchodilators and corticosteroids daily, one patient was on cromoglycate whereas the remaining subjects used bronchodilators only when required. Before the provocations, anti-asthmatic drugs were withdrawn according to standard guidelines.

Bronchial provocation with specific allergen (cat dander, dog dander or birch pollen) was performed by tidal breathing from a dosimeter controlled jet nebulizer (Spira Electro 2, Respiratory Care Center, Finland and KEBO Care Sweden). Pulmonary function was measured on a Vitalograph MDI Compact (KEBO Care Sweden). The dose of allergen was increased by half a log order of magnitude every 20 min until $FEV_{1.0}$ was decreased by 20%. This dose of allergen was defined as the provocative dose. The subjects were challenged at three different occasions being at least three weeks apart. At the first session (open control), the sensitivity for allergen was determined. At the two succeeding sessions, cumulative challenge with allergen was repeated 2h after ingestion of either placebo or

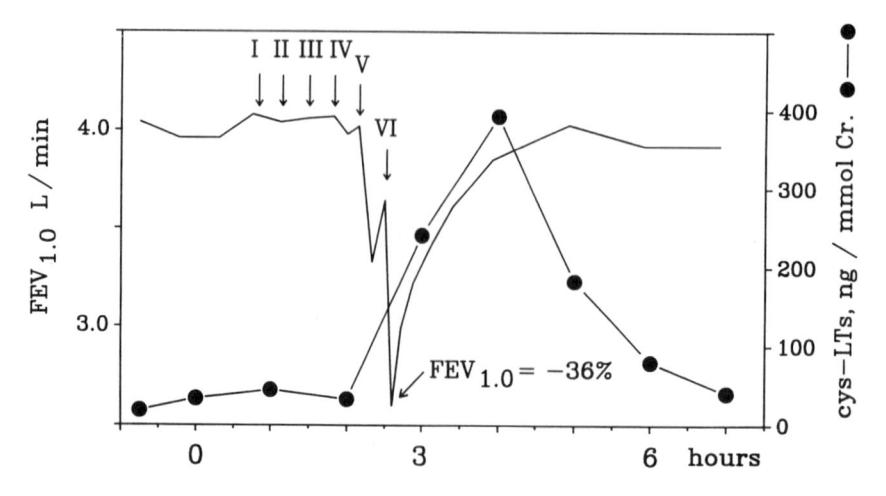

FIG. 1. Bronchial provocation with cat dander in an atopic asthmatic subject. The dose of allergen was increased by half a log order every 20 min (I-VI). Airways response followed by measurements of forced expiratory volume in 1.0 second ($FEV_{1.0}$, solid line, left ordinate). Concentration of immunoreactive cysteinyl-leukotrienes (cys-LTs) in urine indicated by filled circles and expressed as ng per mmol of excreted creatinine (Cr; right ordinate).

20 mg of ICI-204,219 under double-blind conditions. During sessions II and III, urine was collected every hour and the concentration of cysteinyl-leukotrienes was determined by radioimmunoassay.

RESULTS

As exemplified in Figure 1, inhalation of specific allergen caused a fall in $FEV_{1.0}$ which was paralleled by increased excretion of cysteinyl-leukotrienes into the urine (Fig. 1). The allergen-challenge was very reproducible, as evidenced by almost identical sensitivity to allergen at the control and placebo sessions (Fig. 2). In contrast, after pretreatment with the leukotriene-antagonist ICI-204,219, there was generally a conspicuous increase in the dose of allergen tolerated by the subjects (Fig. 2). For the group as a whole, the response to the provocative dose of allergen was in fact inhibited by almost 60% (Fig. 2).

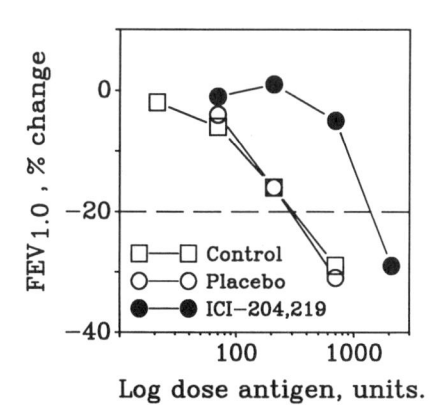

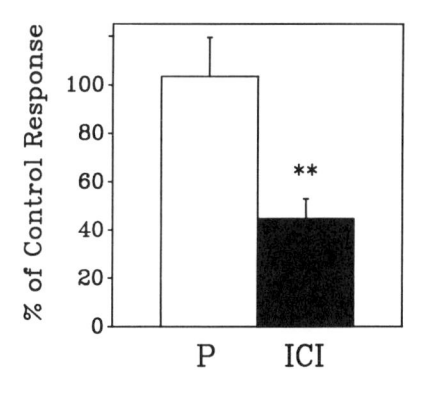

FIG. 2. *Left panel*: Changes in forced expiratory volume in 1.0 second ($FEV_{1.0}$) in response to cumululative challenge with antigen at the three test sessions in one of the subjects. Note reproducibility of provocation response from control session after intake of placebo, but displacement of the dose-response relation to the right after treatment with the leukotriene-antagonist ICI-204,219.
Right panel: Response to the provocative dose of allergen 2 h after ingestion of either placebo (P) or 20 mg of ICI-204,219 (ICI). The provocative dose was determined at the first session. The fall in $FEV_{1.0}$ caused by this particular dose of allergen at the two succeeding provocations was expressed in percent of the response at the first session. Means ± S.D. for all ten patients. Stars denote p<0.01 (Mann-Whitney U-test).

DISCUSSION

It is well established that the cysteinyl-leukotrienes are potent bronchoconstrictors. In line with observations by others (4), we found that bronchial provocation of atopic asthmatics with allergen increased the concentration of cysteinyl-leukotrienes in the urine, indicating allergen-induced release of leukotrienes Moreover, the leukotriene antagonist ICI-204,219 unambiguously inhibited the bronchoconstriction induced by provocation with specific allergen in the asthmatics. Therefore, it can be concluded that as far as allergen-induced bronchoconstriction in man is concerned, the cysteinyl-leukotrienes fulfil all three classical criteria (stimulus-evoked release, appropriate biological activity, and inhibition of the response by a selective antagonist) required to prove a mediator function. This particular dose of the leukotriene antagonist inhibited about 60% of the acute response to allergen. Future studies will determine whether or not this is the maximal influence of leukotriene-antagonists on this type of response. In any event, the demonstration that a significant component of the response to allergen-challenge in man can be ascribed to leukotrienes prompts for the evaluation of leukotriene-antagonism in the clinical treatment of asthma.

ACKNOWLEDGEMENTS

Supported by grants from the Swedish Medical Research Council (project 14X-09071, 03X-5915), the Swedish Association Against Chest and Heart Diseases, the Swedish Association Against Asthma and Allergy (RmA), the Swedish National Board for Laboratory Animals (CFN), the Scientific Council of the Swedish Association Against Use of Experimental Animals in Research, the Institute of Environmental Medicine, the Swedish Environment Protection Board (5324060-2), and Karolinska Institutet.

REFERENCES

1. Krell, R.D., Aharony, D., Buckner, C.K., Keith, R.A., Kusner, E.J., Snyder, D.W., Bernstein, P.R., Matassa, V.G., Yee, Y.K., Brown, F.J., Hesp, B., and Giles, R.E. (1990): *Amer Rev Respir Dis* **141**: 978-987.

2. Smith, L.J., Geller, S., Ebright L., Glass, M., and Thyrum, P.T. (1990): *Amer Rev Respir Dis* **141**: 988-992.

3. Snyder, D.W., Giles, R.E., Keith, R.A., Yee, Y.K., Krell, R.D. (1987): *J Pharm Exp Ther* **243**: 548-556.

4. Taylor, G.W., Taylor, I., Black, P., Maltby, N.H., Turner, N., Fuller, R.W., and Dollery, C.T. (1989): *Lancet* **1**, 584-588.

EFFECT OF A LEUKOTRIENE ANTAGONIST ON EXPERIMENTAL AND CLINICAL BRONCHIAL ASTHMA

T. Nakagawa[1], Y. Mizushima[1], A. Ishii[2], F. Nambu[3], M. Motoishi[3], Y. Yui[4], T. Shida[4], T. Miyamoto[4]

Department of Internal Medicine, St. Marianna University, School of Medicine, 2-16-1 Sugao, Miyamae-ku, Kawasaki 213[1]; Department of Medicine and Physical Therapy, University of Tokyo, School of Medicine, 7-3-1 Hongo, Bunkyo-ku, Tokyo 113[2]; Research Institute, Ono Pharmaceutial Co.,LTD., 3-1-1 Sakurai, Shimamoto-cho, Osaka 618[3]; Department of Internal Medicine, National Sagamihara Hospital, 18-1 Sakuradai, Sagamihara 228[4], Japan.

Leukotriene(LT)C_4, D_4, and E_4, which constitute the biological activities of slow-reacting substance of anaphylaxis (SRS-A), have been shown to play the crucial role in the pathophysiology of bronchial asthma. Since the specific LT receptor antagonist seems to possess beneficial effect on this allergic disorder, the present investigations were designed and performed employing the drug designated as ONO-1078, i.e. 4-oxo 8-[p-(4-phenylbuthyloxy)benzol] amino -2-(tetrazol-5'-yl)-4H-1-benzopyran hemihydrate. ONO-1078 was proved previously to antagonize the actions of LT C_4, D_4 and E_4 in various experimental models(2,3).

This chapter describes our recent findings regarding the inhibitory effects of this novel LT receptor antagonist on experimental and clinical bronchial asthma.

EFFECT ON LUNG ANAPHYLAXIS IN GUINEA PIGS

To evaluate whether this compound could exhibit inhibitory effects on experimental asthma, guinea pig lung anaphylaxis experiments in vitro and in vivo were performed(1).

in vitro study

As the in vitro model, Schultz-Dale reactions were performd. Male Hartley guinea pigs were passively sensitized by rabbit anti-ovalbumin(OA) serum 2 days before use. The animals were killed, and the tracheal strips were prepared and suspended in organ bathes. The tissues were then incubated with mepyramine as the H_1-receptor antagonist, with ONO-1078 or FPL 55712 as the LT receptor antagonist before OA antigen challenge.

The challenge with OA resulted in a rapidly developing and sustained contraction. The initial phase of contraction was significantly inhibited by the addition of mepyramine(10μ g/ml), while the late phase was significantly inhibited by the addition of ONO-1078 (1-10 μ g/ml). The combined use of mepyramine and ONO-1078 significantly inhibited both initial and late phases of the contraction. FPL 55712 (10μ g/ml) also elicited significant inhibitory effect on the late phase of the contraction.

in vivo study

Endogenous LT_s-mediated lung anaphylaxis experiments were subsequently performed. Male Hartley guinea pigs were passively sensitized by guinea pig anti-OA serum containing IgE antibodies 8 days before use. The animals were injected i.p. with ONO-1078, followed by i.v. injections of mepyramine and indomethacin. Inhalation challenge with OA was performed, and the respiratory resistance and flow-patterns were measured by the modified Mead's methods.

The inhalation challenge of OA antigen to sensitized guinea pigs pretreated with mepyramine and indomethacin resulted in developing late phase bronchoconstriction. Concomitant pretreatment with ONO-1078 inhibited this antigen-induced bronchoconstriction in vivo in a dose-dependent manner(3,10,30 mg/kg).

CLINICAL APPLICATION FOR HUMAN BRONCHIAL ASTHMA

Based upon these immunopharmacological findings, the clinical application of ONO-1078 to asthmatic subjects was subsequently performed.

At first, 7 normal volunteers were challenged bronchially with LTD_4 and histamine, before and after 7 day-medication of 75 mg or 150 mg/day of ONO-1078. ONO-1078 could inhibit this LTD_4-induced bronchoconstriction in a dose-dependent fashion (FIG.1), while showed no effect on histamine-induced bronchoconstriction.

Then, 7 asthmatic patients sensitive to house dust (HD) were challenged bronchially with HD, before and after 7 day-medication of 150 mg/day ONO-1078. The results demonstrated that this compound could also exert inhibition in the antigen-induced bronchoconstriction in sensitive asthmatic patients.

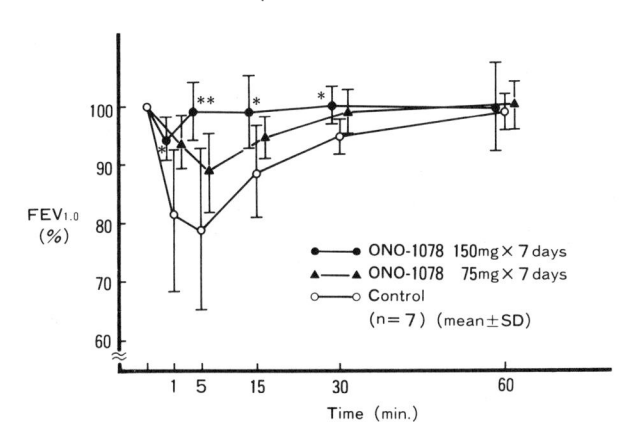

FIG.1 Bronchial provocation tests induced by LTD_4 in 7 normal volunteers. *$p<0.05$, **$p<0.01$ as compared to the control values.

Clinical trials are currently under way in adult patients with bronchial asthma, mild-moderate degree. Symptom scores and concomitant usage of bronchodilators/steroids have been evaluated for the judgement of clinical usefulness. The data accumulated up to now revealed that the overall efficacy reached more than 80% in these asthmatic patients.

THE CONCLUDING REMARKS

The results obtained so far clearly indicate that ONO-1078 is a specific LT receptor antagonist as evident by the guinea pig experiments and human bronchial provocation tests and show that this compound can significantly reduce hazardous symptoms such as wheezing and dyspneal attacks in asthmatic patients.

REFERENCES

1. Ishii, A., Nakagawa, T., Nambu, F., Motoishi, M., and Miyamoto, T. (1990) : Int. Archs Allergy appl. Immun., in press.
2. Obata, T., Nambu, F., Kitagawa, T., Terashima, H., Toda, M., Okegawa, T., and Kawasaki, A. (1987) : In Advances in Prostaglandin, Thromboxane, and Leukotriene Research, Vol. 17, edited by B. Samuelsson, R. Paoletti and P. W. Ramwell, pp. 540-543 Raven Press, New York.
3. Toda, M., Nakai, H., Kosuge, H., Konno, M., Arai, Y., Miyamoto, T., Obata, T., Katsube, N., and Kawasaki, A. (1985) : In Advances in Prostaglandin, Thromboxane, and Leukotriene Research, Vol. 15, edited by O. Hayaishi and S. Yamamoto, pp. 307-308, Raven Press, New York.

THE PHARMACOLOGICAL PROFILE OF SK&F 104353-Z_2, A POTENT, SELECTIVE INHALED ANTAGONIST OF CYSTEINYL LEUKOTRIENES, IN NORMAL MAN.

JM EVANS, [*]PJ PIPER and JF COSTELLO

Department of Thoracic Medicine, King's College School of Medicine and Dentistry, London SE5 9PJ, UK. and [*]Department of Pharmacology, Royal College of Surgeons of England, London WC2A, UK.

The cysteinyl leukotrienes(LT) C_4, D_4 and E_4 are potent bronchoconstrictors when inhaled by both normal and asthmatic human subjects, with a potency 1,000 times greater than histamine (1). To establish the role of LTs in asthma requires the use of potent, selective LT receptor antagonists in various models of asthma and in clinical asthma. For these to be successful it is necessary to first establish the potency and duration of activity of any potential LT antagonists in man. One method of examining the activity of such an antagonist is to study the effect of the compound on LTD_4-induced bronchoconstriction since inhalation challenge testing with LTD_4 in normal human subjects has been found to be highly reproducible and safe (2).

SK&F 104353-Z_2 [the disodium salt of 2(S)-hydroxy-3(R)-[2-carboxyethyl)thio]-3-[2-(8-phenyloctyl)phenyl]-propanoic acid] is a novel LT-antagonist (pA_2 = 8.6 in guinea pig trachea) which is structurally related to LTD_4 (3). In animal models, in vivo, SK&F 104353 is an active LT antagonist by the inhaled route with predicted activity in man at doses between 100ug and 800ug (4).

As SK&F 104353 is delivered by the inhaled route and has a similar chemical structure as that of the naturally occurring agonist LTD_4 it is conceivable that this compound might have a short duration of action due to either rapid clearance from the bronchial tree or because of rapid metabolism by the same enzymes available for the natural agonist. In addition, such a LT antagonist might be expected to possess partial agonist activity. Since the duration of activity was initially unknown, our previous studies with inhaled SK&F 104353 therefore examined the effect of this antagonist, at a nebulised dose of 800µg, at 15 minutes and 4 hours after inhalation. A single concentration of LTD_4 was used for each subject which was known to reduce baseline measurements of specific airways conductance (sGaw) by at least 50%. SK&F 104353 protected against LTD_4-induced bronchoconstriction at both time points to a similar degree with the 800µg dose (mean maximum percentage fall in sGaw with LTD_4: at 15 min: 55.5% placebo vs 14.3% SK&F 104353, n = 8, p<0.001; at 4 hours: 53.3% placebo vs 24.2% SK&F 104353, n = 6, p <0.001). At an inhaled dose of 100µg after 4 hours, SK&F 104353 was also active against LTD_4-induced broncho-constriction (mean maximum percentage fall in sGaw: 53.5% placebo vs 24.3% SK&F 104353, n = 6, p<0.001). We have now studied the potency and selectivity of inhaled SK&F 104353 at a nebulised dose of 100µg on LTD_4 and histamine dose-response curves in a double-blind, placebo controlled randomised crossover trial.

METHODS

Six normal, healthy male volunteers, mean age 32 years (range 28-37 years) were studied. All were non-smokers with normal pulmonary function and with no history of allergic or respiratory disease. Informed consent was obtained from each subject and the study was approved by the ethics committee of King's College Hospital.

The study took place on four days and each was separated by at least a week. On each study day, the subject attended the laboratory and baseline measurements of pulmonary function were made using forced expiratory volume in one second (FEV_1), sGaw and maximum flow at 30% of vital capacity above residual volume ($\dot{V}max_{30}$) from a partial expiratory flow-volume curve. SK&F 104353 (100µg) or matching placebo was then inhaled as a bufferred nebulised solution from an ultrasonic nebuliser (Pulmosonic, DeVilbis) by tidal breathing from a mouthpiece for ten minutes. The volume of the solution left in the nebuliser reservoir was measured after this to provide an estimate of the dose of drug inhaled. On completion of the nebulised treatment the pulmonary function tests were repeated. Fifteen minutes after inhaling the drug or placebo the appropriate agonist challenge was commenced with the inhalation of normal saline from a Wright nebuliser by tidal breathing from a face mask for two minutes and sGaw and $\dot{V}max_{30}$ were measured. Following this, either histamine starting at a concentration of 10^{-4} mol/litre or LTD_4 starting at 2.0×10^{-7} mol/litre was inhaled in the same way. Increasing concentrations of agonist were given at 3.2 (1/2 log_{10})-fold increments until at least a 35% fall in sGaw from the post-saline values occurred or the maximum concentration of 10^{-1} mol/litre histamine or 2.0×10^{-4} mol/litre LTD_4 had been reached. Dose-response curves were constructed with the response recorded as a percentage of the post-saline values. The provocation concentration (PC) of agonist which produced a 35% fall in sGaw ($PC_{35}sGaw$) from the post-saline values and a 30% fall in $\dot{V}max30$ ($PC_{30}\dot{V}max_{30}$) were determined by linear interpolation of the curves. Following the active drug a provocation concentration was not achieved with LTD_4 and the PC value was obtained by overlying of the placebo dose-response curve for that subject.

RESULTS

The mean nebulised dose of SK&F 104353 was 100µg in the LTD_4 challenges and 97µg in the histamine challenges (Table 1). Baseline measurements of pulmonary function were similar for both placebo and drug at pre-dosing and there was no significant change in these measurements following either placebo or SK&F 104353.

TABLE 1. Nebulised volumes of solutions of placebo and SK&F 104353

	Placebo	SK&F 104353	DOSE [µg]
LTD_4	[a]1.7 (0.1)	2.0 (0.2)	100.0 (11)
Histamine	2.1 (0.4)	1.9 (0.3)	97.0 (13)

[a] Mean (SD)

The LTD_4 and histamine challenges were all completed within two hours of inhaling the treatment solution. The dose-response curves for LTD_4 were shifted to the right after SK&F 104353 when compared with placebo in all subjects. The geometric mean shift was 10.4-fold for sGaw and 10.8-fold for $\dot{V}max_{30}$ (Table 2). There was no significant shift in the histamine dose-response curves for any subject (Table 2). No serious side effects were found with inhaled SK&F 104353 and the inhaled drug was well tolerated.

TABLE 2. Geometric mean provocation concentrations of LTD_4 and histamine after placebo and SK&F 104353 (100μg)

	Placebo	SK&F 104353
LTD_4 ($\times 10^{-5}$ mol l^{-1})		
$PC_{35}sGaw$	2.40	24.9
$PC_{30}\dot{V}max_{30}$	1.92	20.5
Histamine ($\times 10^{-2}$ mol l^{-1})		
$PC_{35}sGaw$	4.92	4.59
$PC_{30}\dot{V}max_{30}$	6.50	5.73

DISCUSSION

SK&F 104353 has been shown to be a potent LTD_4 antagonist in normal human airways at a nebulised dose of 100ug within two hours of inhaling the drug. The antagonism would seem to be selective since there was no effect on histamine-induced bronchoconstriction. There was no evidence of partial agonist activity and inhaled SK&F 104353 was well tolerated. Since the duration of activity of this compound has been found to be at least four hours in our previous studies, SK&F 104353 has considerable potential as a pharmacological tool for use in clinical studies to investigate the role of LTs in the asthmatic response.

REFERENCES

1. Barnes N.C., Piper P.J. and Costello J.F. (1984): Thorax, 39:500-504.
2. Barnes N.C., Zakrzewski J.T., Piper P.J. and Costello J.F. (1985): Br. J. Clin. Pharmacol., 20:554P.
3. Hay D.W.P., Muccitelli R.M., Tucker S.S., Vickery-Clark L.M., Wilson K.A., Gleason J.G., Hall R.F., Wasserman M. A. and Torphy T.J. (1987): J. Pharmacol. and Exp. Ther., 243:474-481.
4. Torphy T.J., Newton J.F., Wasserman M.A., Vickery-Clark L., Osborn R., Bailey L.S., Yodis L.A.P., Underwood D.C. and Hay D.W.P. (1989): J. Pharmacol. and Exp. Ther., 249:430-437.

PROSTANOID CONTRACTIONS IN HUMAN ISOLATED PULMONARY MUSCLE PREPARATIONS: INHIBITION BY BAY u3405.

X. Norel, C. Labat, *P. Gardiner and C. Brink

CNRS URA 1159, Centre Chirurgical Marie Lannelongue, 133 av. de la Résistance, 92350 Le Plessis Robinson, France and *Bayer UK LtD, Research Department Stoke Court, Stoke Poges, SL2 4LY, England.

INTRODUCTION

The aim of the present study was to examine the effects of several prostanoids on human isolated bronchial and pulmonary arterial muscle preparations in the presence and absence of a potent TxA_2 antagonist, BAY u3405.

MATERIALS AND METHODS

Parts of the human bronchus and pulmonary artery were dissected free of surrounding lung tissues and set up as rings (initial loads of 2-3 g) in 10 ml organ baths containing Tyrode's solution (mM): NaCl, 139.2; KCl, 2.7; $CaCl_2$, 1.8; $MgCl_2$, 0.49; $NaHCO_3$, 11.9; NaH_2PO_4, 0.4 and glucose, 5.5; pH 7.4; gassed with 5% CO_2 in 95% O_2 at 37°C. Following the equilibration period (90 min) and after two histamine (50μM) contractions, two different protocols were performed. First, bronchial and pulmonary arterial muscle ring preparations were incubated for 30 min with an antagonist (BAY u3405 or AH23848; 0.1 μM) and subsequently a cumulative concentration-effect curve was produced using a contractile agonist (U46619, PGD_2, $PGF_{2\alpha}$, histamine or endothelin). Secondly, pulmonary isolated arterial muscles were incubated (BAY u3405; 30 min), contracted with histamine (50 μM) and relaxed with prostacyclin (PGI_2), iloprost or butaprost. Changes in force were measured from isometric recordings and expressed in grams (g). The EC_{50} value (concentration of agonist which produced 50% of the maximal response) was interpolated from the individual concentration-effect curves and transformed into pD_2 values (negative logarithms of EC_{50} values). All results are presented as means $\pm$ SEM and statistical analysis was performed using the Student's t test for paired variates.

The drugs and their sources were: histamine dihydrochloride, $PGF_{2\alpha}$, PGI_2, PGD_2 and U46619 (Sigma Chemical Co., St. Louis, MO., USA). Endothelin was obtained from (Novabiochem, Cléry-en Vexin, France). Butaprost, AH23848 and BAY u3405 were a gift (BAYER UK LtD, England) and iloprost from Schering (RFA).

RESULTS

The data presented in Figure 1 demonstrate that U46619 was more potent than PGD$_2$ in both types of preparations.

FIGURE 1. Prostanoid contractions in human isolated bronchial and pulmonary arterial muscle preparations.

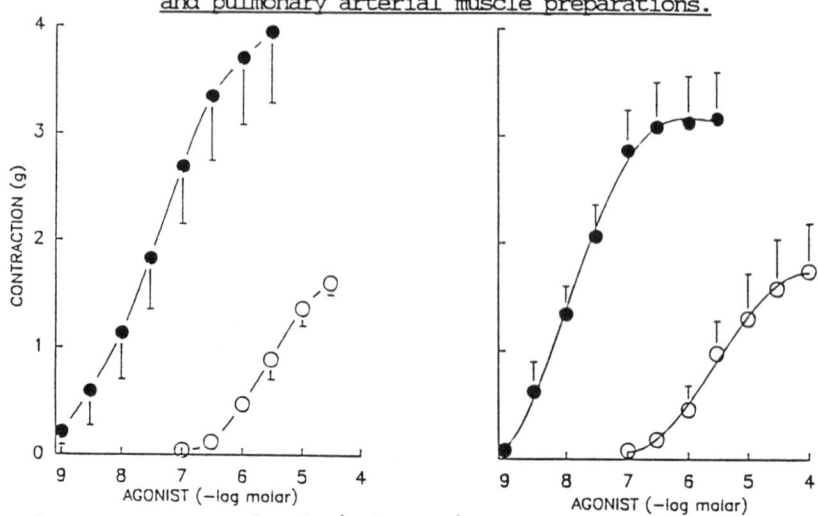

Curves were produced in bronchial (left panel) or arterial tissues (right panel) to U46619 (●) or PGD$_2$ (O). Values are means ± SEM of 4 lungs.

TABLE 1. Inhibitory action of BAY u3405 on U46619 contractions in human isolated pulmonary muscle preparations.

Preparations	(N)	Antagonist (0.1 µM)	U46619 (pD$_2$ value)
Bronchus	(4)	control	7.54 ± 0.21
	(4)	u3405	5.54 ± 0.24
	(5)	AH23848	7.34 ± 0.28
Artery	(4)	control	7.44 ± 0.19
	(4)	u3405	5.19 ± 0.14
	(4)	AH23848	7.62 ± 0.19

Values are means ± SEM and N indicates the number of lungs.

The results shown in Table 1 indicate that at an equimolar concentration BAY u3405 caused a significant dextral shift (300-fold) of the U46619 curves whereas AH23848 was without effect. AH23848 (1 µM) caused a 10-fold shift in the U46619 curves in bronchial preparations. In bronchial tissues the inhibitory activity of BAY u3405 was also observed against PGF$_{2\alpha}$-induced contractions (Figure 2). The histamine and endothelin concentration-effect curves (Figure 3) were not modified by the BAY u3405 antagonist.

FIGURE 2. Inhibitory activity of BAY u3405 on PGF$_{2\alpha}$ contractions in human isolated bronchial and pulmonary arterial muscle preparations.

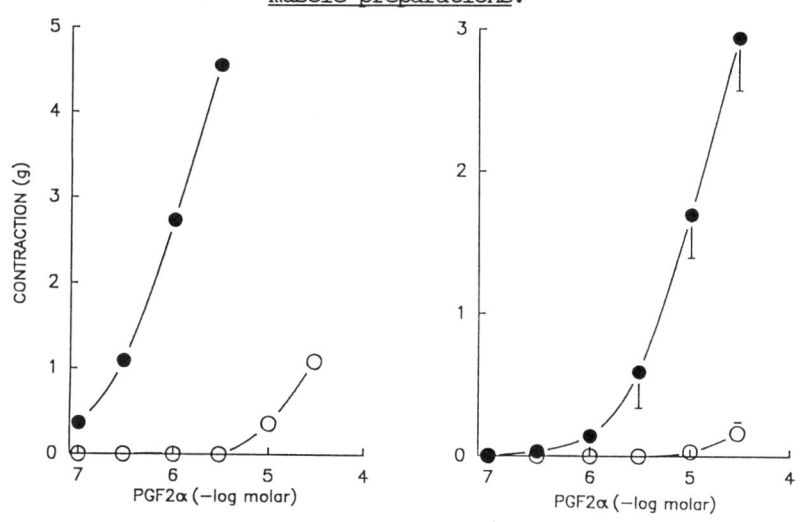

Curves were produced in bronchial (left panel; N=1) or arterial tissues (right panel; N=4) after Tyrode's solution (●) or BAY u3405 (0.1 μM; O) incubations.

FIGURE 3. Effect of BAY u3405 on human isolated bronchial and pulmonary arterial muscle preparations contracted with histamine or endothelin.

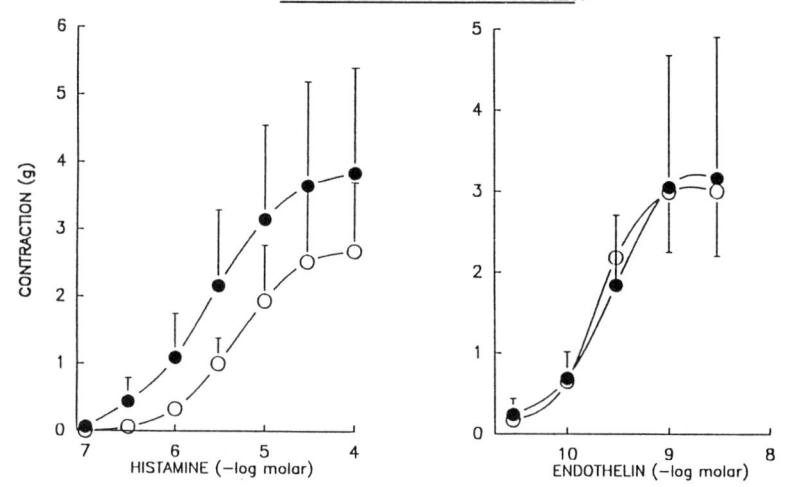

Curves were produced in bronchial (left panel; N=4) or arterial tissues (right panel; N=4) after Tyrode's solution (●) or BAY u3405 (0.1 μM; O) incubations. Values are means ± SEM.

The relaxant effect of PGI_2 on histamine-induced contracted arterial preparations was not altered subsequent to a 30 min incubation with BAY u3405 (0.1 μM; control pD_2 value, 6.68 $\pm$ 0.11 and BAY u3405, 6.52 $\pm$ 0.14; n=4). Results obtained with iloprost or butaprost were also not modified by BAY u3405.

DISCUSSION

The U46619 pD_2 values reported by Armour et al., (1) were similar to those observed in bronchial ring preparations (Table 1) and these data confirm the results reported by Lumley et al., (6) on human isolated pulmonary arterial muscle preparations. McKenniff et al., (7) showed similar results for the potency of U46619 in bronchial muscle preparations which had been pretreated with a number of receptor antagonists and enzyme inhibitors. These data suggest that the local endogenous release of mediators does not alter the sensitivity of the preparations to the TxA_2-mimetic. BAY u3405 is considerably more potent than AH23848 on human isolated pulmonary muscle preparations. The effects of specific TxA_2 antagonists (4,2,6) support the notion of a single site, TP receptor (5,3), through which prostanoids may be acting (7). This report also provides evidence for this concept. These data suggest that contractile prostanoids may be acting via the same site in human airway and pulmonary vascular muscle preparations.

REFERENCE

1. Armour, C.L., Johnson, P.R.A., Alfredson, M.L., and Black, J.L. (1989): Eur. J. Pharmacol., 165:215-222.

2. Brittain,R.T., Boutal, L., Carter, M.C., Coleman, R.A., Collington, E.W., Geisow, H.P., Hallet, P;, Hornby, E.J., Humphrey, P.P.A., Jack, D., Kennedy, I., Lumley, P., McCabe, P.J., Skidmore, I.F., Thomas, M., and Wallis, C.J. (1985): Circ., 72: 1208-1218.

3. Coleman, R.A., and Sheldrick, R.L.G. (1989): Br. J. Pharmacol., 96: 688-692.

4. Jones, R.L., Peesapati, V., and Wilson, N.H. (1982): Br. J. Pharmacol., 76:423-438.

5. Kennedy, I.R., Coleman, R.A., Humphrey, P.P.A., Levy, G.P., and Lumley, P. (1982): Prostaglandins, 24: 667-689.

6. Lumley, P., White, B.P., and Humphrey, P.P.A. (1989): Br. J. Pharmacol., 97: 783-794.

7. McKenniff, M., Rodger, I.W., Norman, P., and Gardiner, P.J. (1988): Eur. J. Pharmacol., 153:149-159.

Advances in Prostaglandin, Thromboxane, and Leukotriene Research, Vol. 21,
edited by B. Sameulsson et al.
Raven Press, Ltd., New York © 1990.

WY-50,295 TROMETHAMINE: A NOVEL INHIBITOR OF LEUKOTRIENE-MEDIATED REACTIONS

Barry M. Weichman, Joseph W. Berkenkopf, David Grimes, Richard J. Heaslip, Robert J. Sturm, and Joseph Y. Chang

Immunopharmacology Division, Wyeth-Ayerst Research, Princeton, NJ 08543-8000 USA

The leukotrienes (LT), a family of 5-lipoxygenase (5-LO) metabolites of arachidonic acid (AA), have been postulated to play key roles in the etiology of several allergic and inflammatory diseases, such as asthma, rhinitis, and inflammatory bowel disease (3). Inasmuch as both the peptidoleukotrienes (pLT), LTC_4, LTD_4 and LTE_4, and the dihydroxyleukotriene, LTB_4, possess biological actions relevant to these diseases, the identification of drugs capable of inhibiting the biosynthesis of both LT classes represents an attractive therapeutic target. Whereas initial compounds identified as 5-LO inhibitors were, in general, not orally active or functioned as nonselective antioxidants, newer generations of specific 5-LO inhibitors have been identified which are poised to help define the role of LTs in pathophysiology. In our laboratories, WY-50,295 tromethamine [S-α-methyl-6-(2-quinolinylmethoxy)-2-napthalene acetic acid, tromethamine salt; Fig. 1] has been pharmacologically characterized as a potent, orally active, and long-acting 5-LO inhibitor, that has the advantage of also functioning as a pLT receptor antagonist.

5-LIPOXYGENASE INHIBITION

WY-50,295 tromethamine inhibited LT biosynthesis in isolated rat peritoneal exudate cells, mouse resident peritoneal macrophages, human peripheral blood neutrophils, and fragmented sensitized guinea pig lung in a concentration-dependent manner with IC_{50} values ranging from 0.055 to 1.79 μM (Table 1). In these studies, WY-50,295 tromethamine inhibited the production of members of both LT classes, and was effective when the cells were challenged with three different cellular stimuli (A23187, zymosan, or antigen). Selectivity for the 5-LO pathway was suggested in that WY-50,295 tromethamine did not alter prostaglandin synthesis. For example, in rat peritoneal exudate cells, WY-50,295

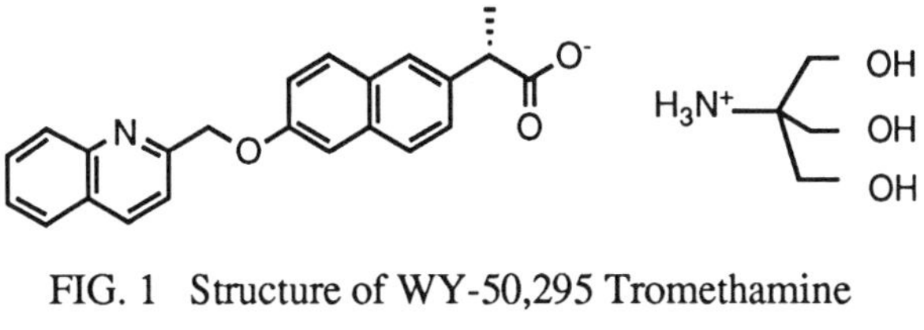

FIG. 1 Structure of WY-50,295 Tromethamine

TABLE 1. In Vitro Inhibition of Leukotriene Biosynthesis by WY-50,295 Tromethamine

Preparation	Stimulus	5-LO Product	IC$_{50}$ [95%CL]: µM
Rat Peritoneal Exudate Cells	A23187	LTB$_4$	0.055 [0.012, 0.26][a]
Mouse Peritoneal Macrophages	Zymosan	LTC$_4$	0.16 [0.11, 0.23][c]
Human Peripheral Blood Neutrophils	A23187	LTB$_4$	1.79 [0.31, 10.3][a]
			0.92 [0.05, 15.9][b]
Guinea Pig Fragmented Lung	Antigen (Ovalbumin)	pLT	0.63 [0.18, 2.21][c]

[a]At 1 µM exogenous AA; [b]At 0.01 µM exogenous AA; [c]Endogenous AA

tromethamine at 10 µM did not affect PGE$_2$ or TxB$_2$ biosynthesis. The 5-LO inhibitory effects of WY-50,295 tromethamine appeared reversible inasmuch as washing drug-treated human blood neutrophils twice with buffer restored LTB$_4$ production to control levels.

Using the 5-LO present in a 100,000 x g supernatant of glycogen-elicited guinea pig peritoneal exudate cells, WY-50,295 tromethamine inhibited the conversion of [^{3}H]-AA into LTB$_4$ and 5-HETE in concentration- and substrate-dependent manners. At 50 nM AA, the IC$_{50}$ values for inhibiting LTB$_4$ and 5-HETE were 5.7 µM and 21 µM. Inasmuch as the 5-LO inhibitory activity decreased as the substrate concentration was increased from 5 nM to 500 nM, the results imply that WY-50,295 tromethamine may inhibit the 5-LO enzyme via competitive substrate inhibition, and therefore differs mechanistically from two other 5-LO inhibitors, A-64077 and L-663,536. A-64077, which is believed to inhibit the 5-LO by chelation of an iron molecule integral to the enzyme's activity (1), equally inhibited LTB$_4$ and 5-HETE and was independent of substrate concentration. In contrast, L-663,536, which inhibits 5-LO translocation (2), was inactive in this cell-free 5-LO preparation.

WY-50,295 tromethamine appeared selective for the 5-LO in that the drug did not inhibit rabbit platelet 12-LO or soybean 15-LO. In the 12-LO studies, 100 µM WY-50,295 tromethamine increased the conversion of [^{3}H]-AA into 12-HETE by 55-65% at substrate concentrations of 0.5 nM-10 µM. Additionally, WY-50,295 tromethamine did not affect ram seminal vesicle PGH synthetase at 100 µM or human platelet or synovial fluid PLA$_2$ at 50 µM.

The 5-LO inhibitory activity of WY-50,295 tromethamine was biochemically quantitated in vivo as inhibition of LTB$_4$ production in the rat pleural cavity following induction of a reverse passive Arthus reaction (RPAR; 4). When administered orally 1, 3, or 18 h prior to induction of the RPAR, WY-50,295 tromethamine inhibited LTB$_4$ in a dose-dependent manner with ED$_{50}$ values of 2.0, 1.7, and 6.3 mg/kg, respectively (Table 2); the slopes of the dose-response curves were parallel. Whereas the potencies of A-64077, L-663,536, and ICI-207,968 were similar to that of WY-50,295 tromethamine at the 1 h pretreatment

TABLE 2. Inhibition of LTB$_4$ Biosynthesis in the Rat Pleural Cavity Following Induction of a Reverse Passive Arthus Reaction

Pretreatment Time:	1 Hour	3 Hours	18 Hours
Drug		ED$_{50}$ (95% C.L.) mg/kg p.o.	
WY-50,295 Tromethamine	2.0 (1.0-4.1)	1.7 (0.6-4.9)	6.3 (2.6-15.4)
L-663,536	2.9 (0.7-12.4)	5.8 (1.0-34)	36% Inh (30mg/kg)
A-64077	2.3 (0.7-7.9)	7.8 (2.8-21)	6% Inh (50mg/kg)
ICI-207,968	2.2 (0.5-10.0)	25% Inh (10mg/kg)	Not tested

time, the other 5-LO inhibitors appeared less potent at 3 and 18 h, suggesting that WY-50,295 tromethamine was longer acting in the rat. Further, WY-50,295 tromethamine (225 mg/kg p.o. - 1 h pretreatment) did not inhibit TxB$_2$ production in the pleural cavity.

LEUKOTRIENE RECEPTOR ANTAGONISM

WY-50,295 tromethamine exhibited LTD$_4$ antagonist activity both in vitro and in vivo at concentrations/doses similar to that at which 5-LO inhibition occurred. The drug competed specifically for the [^{3}H]-LTD$_4$ binding site in guinea pig lung membranes with a K$_i$ of 2.8 µM, similar to that of LY-171,883. In isolated guinea pig trachea, WY-50,295 tromethamine competitively antagonized LTD$_4$-induced contractions with a pA$_2$ of 6.06 and a Schild plot slope of 1.06. A-64077 and L-663,536 did not antagonize the LTD$_4$-induced contractions. On isolated human bronchial muscle rings that were highly sensitive to LTD$_4$, WY-50,295 tromethamine (10 µM) shifted the LTD$_4$ concentration-response curve to the right by approximately 30-fold (C. Brink, personal communication). The drug did not antagonize LTD$_4$ on bronchi that were weakly responsive to LTD$_4$.

In anesthetized, ventilated guinea pigs, WY-50,295 tromethamine antagonized the i.v. LTD$_4$-induced bronchoconstriction with ED$_{50}$ values of 1.3 mg/kg i.v. (5 min pretreatment) and 6.6 mg/kg p.o. (4 h pretreatment). Neither A-64077 (30 mg/kg i.v.) nor L-663,536 (10 mg/kg i.v.) antagonized the LTD$_4$-induced bronchoconstriction. WY-50,295 tromethamine (10 mg/kg i.v.) appeared selective for LTD$_4$, since it did not antagonize histamine- or PAF- induced bronchoconstriction.

ANTIASTHMATIC ACTIVITY

On isolated trachea from sensitized guinea pigs, the initial histamine-dependent phase of antigen (ovalbumin)-induced contraction was not significantly affected by WY-50,295 tromethamine, whereas the drug inhibited the second, sustained LT-dependent phase in a concentration-dependent manner over the range of 0.1-10 µM. At 40 min after antigen, the IC$_{50}$ was 0.43 µM. When evaluated in the presence of mepyramine and indomethacin, the antigen concentration (0.001-10 µg/ml ovalbumin)-response curve was almost completely inhibited by 3 and 10 µM WY-50,295 tromethamine. In both protocols, WY-50,295 tromethamine was more potent and efficacious than either A-64077 or L-663,536.

TABLE 3. Inhibition of Leukotriene-mediated Bronchoconstriction in Guinea Pigs

Compound	LTD$_4$	Ovalbumin	Ratio[a]
	ED$_{50}$ (mg/kg i.v.)		
WY-50,295 Tromethamine	1.3	2.5	1.9
A-64077	Inactive (30)	17	-
L-663,536	Inactive (10)	10	-
WY-48,252	0.07	1	14.3
LY-171,883	0.4	4.2	10.5
FPL-55,712	0.12	4.8	40

[a]Ratio of Ovalbumin ED$_{50}$/LTD$_4$ ED$_{50}$

In sensitized guinea pigs pretreated with mepyramine, indomethacin, and propranolol, the i.v. ovalbumin-induced bronchoconstriction was inhibited by WY-50,295 tromethamine with ED$_{50}$ values of 2.5 mg/kg i.v. (5 min pretreatment) and 7.3 mg/kg p.o. (4 h pretreatment). Peak oral antiasthmatic activity was noted at 4-6 h with significant activity maintained through 18 h (ED$_{50}$ = 11 mg/kg p.o.). Four hours after dosing, WY-50,295 tromethamine was 6-fold more potent than A-64077, whereas L-663,536 at doses up to 10 mg/kg p.o. exhibited little activity. The activity of WY-50,295 tromethamine against antigen-induced bronchoconstriction presumably resulted from both the 5-LO inhibition/ LTD$_4$ receptor antagonism mechanisms inasmuch as reference LTD$_4$ antagonists (e.g. WY-48,252, LY-171,883, FPL-55712) required 10-40-fold higher i.v. doses to inhibit the antigen vis a vis the LTD$_4$-induced response (Table 3). In contrast, WY-50,295 inhibited antigen- and LTD$_4$- induced effects at similar doses, whereas the other 5-LO inhibitors only inhibited the antigen response.

In summary, WY-50,295 tromethamine is a novel inhibitor of LT-mediated events, since it can both prevent LT biosynthesis by virtue of its ability to inhibit the 5-LO, and block the effects of the peptidoleukotrienes by virtue of its ability to antagonize pLT receptors. Its potency, oral bioavailability, and duration of action make it an attractive drug for treating LT-mediated diseases.

Acknowledgements. The authors thank Ms. L. Marinari, Ms. D. Holloway, Ms. B. Hardysh, Mr. T. Lock, and Mr. B. Sickels for their expert technical assistance and Ms. M. Tulanowski for her patience in the preparation of this manuscript.

REFERENCES

1. Carter, G.W., Young, P.R., Albert, D.H., Bouska, J.B., Dyer, R.D., Bell, R.L., Summers, J.B., Brooks, D.W., Gunn, B.P., Rubin, P., and Kesterson, J. (1989): In: Leukotrienes and Prostanoids in Health and Disease, edited by U. Zor, Z. Naor, and A. Danon. pp 50-55. Karger, Basel.
2. Rouzer, C.A., Ford-Hutchinson, A.W., Morton, H.E., and Gillard, J.W. (1990): J. Biol. Chem. 265: 1436-1442.
3. Samuelsson, B. (1981): Int. Archs. Allergy appl. Immunol. 66 (Suppl 1): 98-106.
4. Weichman, B.M., Berkenkopf, J.W., Cullinan, C.A., and Sturm, R.J. (1987): Agents Actions 21: 351-354.

LEUKOTRIENES IN CEREBROSPINAL FLUID OF THE CONSCIOUS CAT: EFFECT OF PLATELET-ACTIVATING FACTOR AND PYROGENS[*]

F. Coceani, I. Bishai, J. Lees, and N. Hynes

Research Institute,
The Hospital for Sick Children,
Toronto, Ontario, Canada M5G 1X8

It has been recognized for some time that brain is endowed with an enzyme system for the formation of leukotrienes(LT) (7). According to current knowledge, LTB_4 synthesis is distributed diffusely, while the synthesis of peptidoleukotrienes prevails in certain regions such as the hypothalamus. Limited information, however, is available on the activity of the synthetic enzymes *in vivo* and its modification by stimuli.

In addressing this issue, our objective has been to ascertain whether leukotrienes are normally present in cerebrospinal fluid (CSF) and, if so, whether their levels are amenable to pharmacologic manipulation. Platelet-activating factor (PAF) was chosen among the potential stimulators in light of data, in the brain and elsewhere, linking this etherophospholipid with the leukotrienes in certain pathophysiological conditions. Pyrogens were also studied with the intent of verifying that leukotrienes, unlike prostaglandin E_2 (PGE_2) (3), have no role in the development of fever and associated manifestations forming the host defense reaction.

BASAL CONTENT OF LEUKOTRIENES

Experiments were carried out in conscious cats and CSF was withdrawn from the third ventricle via an indwelling cannula (see 4). As shown in Table 1, peptidoleukotrienes could be measured in nearly all samples when they were assayed as the total product (SP-LT) after enzymatic conversion to LTE_4. Conversely, native LTE_4 was detected in only about 30% of the samples, implying that LTC_4 and/or LTD_4 account for most of the SP-LT activity. Indeed, separate experiments employing a highly specific radio-immunoassay procedure confirmed the presence of LTC_4 in CSF. LTB_4 levels, on the other hand, were exceedingly low and, in many cases, were below detection. SP-LT content

---
[*]added at press time

TABLE 1. *Ventricular concentration of leukotrienes under basal conditions*

	CSF content	
Leukotriene	Above detection (pg/ml)	Below detection (no. of samples)
SP-LT [a]	325 ± 14 (103)	6
LTC_4	244 ± 41 (4)	0
LTE_4	317 ± 45 (10)	21
LTB_4	30 ± 2 (23)	18

Values are means ± S.E. for number of samples given in parentheses. All compounds were measured by radioimmunoassay. Note that the antibody against LTC_4 crossreacted minimally with LTD_4 (1%) and LTE_4 (<0.1%).
[a] CSF was treated with a crude preparation of γ-glutamyl-transpeptidase and the resulting product was expressed as LTE_4 (6).

was fairly consistent among experiments and, in a given experiment, remained constant through repeated sampling over a period of several hours.

EFFECT OF INTRACEREBROVENTRICULAR PAF

PAF caused a sustained rise in body temperature (mean ΔT, 1.7°C) when given intraventricularly (icv) as a 1-μg bolus. CSF levels of SP-LT also increased about 5-fold in treated animals; however, the elevation was confined to the latent period and the uprise phase of the hyperthermia. Among the individual leukotrienes, LTC_4 was elevated after treatment (3-fold increase), while LTB_4 levels remained unchanged. PAF action was not selective for the peptido-leukotrienes, but was also directed on the cyclooxygenase pathway. Significantly, there was a sustained increase in PGE_2 (from about 30 to 450 pg/ml CSF), and this event has conceivably a bearing on the development of the hyper-thermia.

PAF-induced stimulation of SP-LT synthesis was prevented by treatment with the PAF antagonist, BN52021 (1 μg icv) (2). Likewise, 5-lipoxygenase inhibitors, differing in structure and mode of administration (U-60,257, 75 μg icv; L-651,392 10 mg/kg p.o.) (1,5), reversed the PAF activation. In contrast, pretreatment with indomethacin (500 μg icv) caused a greater response, and SP-LT levels exceeded basal values about 9-fold. Of note is the fact that PAF hyperthermia was enhanced by 5-lipoxygenase inhibitors, while indomethacin had an opposite effect.

In brief, our findings demonstrate a stimulatory effect of PAF on the synthesis of peptidoleukotrienes *in vivo*. Surprisingly, LTB$_4$ was not affected by the treatment, and the reason for this negative finding remains unclear. The identity of the cell, or cells, producing peptidoleukotrienes in response to PAF remains to be ascertained; however, the absence of significant pleocytosis (data not shown) argues against the involvement of infiltrating leucocytes.

EFFECT OF PYROGENS

Endotoxin and recombinant IL-1 had no effect on CSF levels of the peptidoleukotrienes and LTB$_4$ when given intravenously, respectively, as a bolus or by continued infusion. Likewise, both pyrogens (given as a bolus) were ineffective by the intraventricular route. The negative result occurred despite the sustained fever, and it was in sharp contrast with a consistent elevation in PGE$_2$ (see 4). Indeed, no change was noted even when subjecting the animal to the combined treatment of intraventricular endotoxin and indomethacin, a situation in which any stimulation of leukotriene synthesis would expectedly have been magnified.

Collectively, the above findings and the general lack of correlation between leukotriene synthesis and activation of heat-conserving mechanisms argue against the involvement of the leukotrienes in any stage of the fever process and reaffirm the prime role of PGE$_2$ as a pyrogenic agent.

CONCLUSION

Our studies indicate that the peptidoleukotrienes are a normal constituent of the CSF and tentatively identify the active species with LTC$_4$. The conclusion accords with the demonstration of specific receptors for this leukotriene in brain tissue. Synthesis of the peptidoleukotrienes is stimulated by PAF and this finding supports a pathogenetic role for the compounds in inflammatory processes and the reactive changes to injury. No evidence was obtained for the involvement of leukotrienes in the initiation of fever and fever-associated events proper of the host response to bacterial infection.

ACKNOWLEDGEMENTS

This work was supported by the Medical Research Council of Canada. Compounds BN52021, U-60,257 and L-651,392 were provided by, respectively, Drs. P. Borgeat, M. Bach (Upjohn), and A. Ford-Hutchinson (Merck Frosst).

REFERENCES

1. Bach, M. K., and Brashler, J. R. (1989): In: *Advances in Prostaglandin, Thromboxane, and Leukotriene Research, vol. 19*, edited by B. Samuelsson, P. Y.-K. Wong, and F. F. Sun, pp. 511-514. Raven Press, New York.

2. Braquet, P., Touqui L., Shen, T. Y., and Vargaftig, B. B. (1987): *Pharmacol. Rev.*, 39:97-145.

3. Coceani, F., Bishai, I., Hynes, N., Lees, J., and Sirko, S. (1989): In: *Leukotrienes and Prostanoids in Health and Disease. New Trends Lipid Mediators Research, vol. 3*, edited by U. Zor, Z. Naor, and A. Danon, pp. 183-186. Karger, Basel.

4. Coceani, F., Lees, J., and Bishai, I. (1988): *Am. J. Physiol.*, 254:R463-R469.

5. Guindon, Y., Girard, Y., Maycock, A., Ford-Hutchinson, A. W. et al. (1987): In: *Advances in Prostaglandin, Thromboxane, and Leukotriene Research, vol. 17*, edited by B. Samuelsson, R. Paoletti, and P. W. Ramwell, pp. 554-557. Raven Press, New York.

6. Hoppe, U., Hoppe, E. M., Peskar, B. M., and Peskar, B. A. (1986): *FEBS Lett.*, 208:26-30.

7. Miyamoto, T., Lindgren, J. Å., Hokfelt, T., and Samuelsson, B. (1987): *FEBS Lett.*, 216:123-127.

Subject Index

Acetohydroxamic acids, pharmacokinetics of, 110–111
Acetylcholinesterase, as label in radioimmunoassays, 319–322
Acute inflammatory reactions, PGE$_1$ and, 948
Acute lung injury, arachidonic acid metabolites and, 421–428
Adhesion, of lipids, 553–555
Aggregation, and chronic granulomatous disease (CGD), 561–564
Allergies,
  leukotrienes and, 429–432, 461–464
  PGD$_2$ formation and, 433–436
  rhinitis and, 449–452
  see also Respiratory illness
Alveolar macrophages, metabolism in human cells, 445–448
Anaphylactoid purpura, thromboxane (TxA$_2$) and, 645–648
Angiogenesis, eicosanoid action in, 623–626
Antagonists, dual, 929–937
Antigen-induced mediator release, lipoxygenase and, 457–460
Antimetastatic actions, of prostacyclin analogs in mice, 913–916
Antiproliferative agents,
  activity modulation, 887–890
  inhibitory effects of, 922–923
Aplysia, neuromodulator production in, 715–721
Arachidonate 5-lipoxygenase, immunohistochemical study, 21–24
Arachidonate 12-lipoxygenase cDNA, cloning and expression from porcine leukocytes, 29–32
Arachidonic acid, 173–176
  acute lung injury and, 421–428
  asthma and, 415–418
  astroglial cell pathways, 743–747
  calcium ions and, 257–260
  cell signalling process and, 220
  cytochrome P450-dependent metabolites, 185–196, 675–682
  and erythropoietin, 831–834
  15-HETE, 441–444
  glomerular microcirculation and, 683–688
  human neutrophils and, 553–555
  ion transport inhibition and, 209–212
  Lewis lung carcinoma cells and, 895–900
  lipoxins (LX), 701–706
  metabolism by Foa-Kurloff cells, 437–440
  and PAF receptor mediated production in LPS primed P338D1 cells, 249–255
  PGD$_2$ cardio- and hemodynamic profile, 591–593
  phospholipase A$_2$, 573–576, 831–834
  Raji cells and, 133–136
  sarcoidosis and, 445–448
  in seminal fluids, 197–200
  steroidal regulation, 815–818
  see also Leukotrienes
Arthritis, PGE$_1$ and, 950
Aspirin,
  coronary artery thrombosis and, 603–606
  lupus patients and, 611–614
  PGG/H synthase and heme binding, 77–80
  PGI$_2$ synthesis and, 153–155
  reverse phase HPLC profiling and, 312–314
  Rosaprostol effects on gastrointestinal bleeding, 789–792
  TxA$_2$ synthesis and, 153–154
  withdrawal effects, 157–159
Asthma,
  antigen-induced mediator release and, 457–459
  leukotriene antagonist effects on bronchial asthma, 465–468
  MK-571 effects, 11–12
  PGD$_2$ formation and allergen inhalation, 433–436
  sulphidopeptide leukotrienes and, 415–418
Astrocytes, eicosanoid synthesis and, 739–742
Astroglial cell pathways, 743–747
Atherosclerosis, EPA and, 241–243
Attachment, eicosanoid synthesis by, 261–264
Autocrine function, in porcine cells, 671–674

B lymphocytes,
  biosynthesis of leukotriene B$_4$, 1005–1011
  and leukotriene A$_4$ hydrolase, 133–136
BAY U 3405; Thromboxane antagonist, 355
Binding sites, photoaffinity labeling of leukotrienes, 395–398
Biosynthesis, of leukotriene B$_4$, 1005–1011
Blood cells,
  metabolizing enzymes and, 33–36
  platelet activating factor (PAF), 221–236, 383–386, 617–620
  polymerase cloning from, 33–36
  see also Platelets
Blood pressure, cytochrome P450-dependent metabolites and, 675–682
Blot analysis,
  of arachidonate 5-lipoxygenase of porcine leukocytes, 21–24
  for LCTs, 291–294
BN 50726, as dual antagonist, 932–933
BN 50727, as dual antagonist, 933–935
BN 50739, as dual antagonist, 935
Bone marrow transplant, 525–528
Bronchoconstriction,
  ET-1 induced in guinea pigs, 453–456
  15-HETE and, 441–444
  leukotriene-antagonist ICI-204,219 and, 461–464
  leukotrienes and, 429–432
  PGD$_2$ formation and, 433–436

Calcium ions,
  and arachidonic acid release, 257–260
  GC action in suppression of PLA$_2$ and, 265–271
Cancer,
  antimetastatic action of stable prostacyclin analogs in mice, 913–916
  host immunocompetence and, 917–920
  lipoxygenase inhibition and human leukemia, 921–924

osteoblastic cell calcification, 847–850
prostacyclin analogues and in vivo tumor model, 901–908
13-HODE synthesis and tumor cell adhesion, 909–911
tumor cell proliferation by TxA$_2$ and, 925–928
Capillary leak syndrome and, 525–528
Carcinoma,
 antimetastatic action of stable prostacyclin analogs in mice, 913–916
 13-HODE synthesis and tumor cell adhesion, 909–911
 Lewis lung carcinoma cells, 895–900
Cardiac transplant patients, 649–653
Cardiovascular disease,
 cytochrome P450-dependent metabolites and, 193–196
 non-steroidal drug effects, 153–155
 thromboembolism, 355–358
 see also Coronary arterial thrombosis
Cardiovascular surgery, 13-HODE synthesis and, 667–670
Catecholamine-stimulated PGI$_2$ production, 659–662
CD23,
 IgE regulation and, 983–988
 signalling pathway in human B cells, 997–1003
Cell signalling, modification of eicosanoid system and, 217–224
Cellular Cyclooxygenase (COX) activity, biochemical and pharmacological manipulation, 45–51
Central nervous system,
 hepoxilins and, 731–734
 P-450 activity and, 201–204
 PGE$_2$ synthesis in chick spinal cord, 735–738
 phosphatidic acid and, 287–290
 sleep-wake regulation, 723–730
Chemoattractants, neutrophil activation and protein 1 of *N. Gonorrhoeae*, 545–550
Chemotactic deactivation,
 of human leukocytes, 399–401
 ONO-LB-B457 and, 407–410
Chick spinal cord, PGE$_2$ synthesis, 735–738
Child Syndrome, fibroblasts failure to proliferate in response to interleukin 1A, 835–838
Chronic granulomatous disease (CGD), leukotriene B$_4$ and, 561–564
Chronic myeloid leukemia, lipoxygenase and, 883–886
Cornea, metabolic pathway of arachidonic acid, 185–194
Coronary artery thrombosis,
 aspirin and, 603–606
 GR32191 and, 599–602
 13-HODE synthesis and, 667–670
 ONO-8809, 599–602
 thromboxane-dependent platelet activation and, 617–621
 see also Cardiovascular disease
Critical limb ischemia (CLI), iloprost and, 583–589
Crohn's disease, and smoking, 777
Cyclooxygenase,
 bone resorption and, 839–840
 and eicosanoid synthesis, 169–172
 EPA and DHA ethylesters and, 233–235

induction in osteoblasts and bone metabolism, 839–842
 inhibitory effects on bone formation, 841
 in mouse osteoblastic cells, 53–58
 PGE$_2$ production and, 840
Cyclopentenone prostaglandins, glutathione biosynthesis and, 859–861
Cytochrome P450,
 brain synthesis and cerebrovascular action, 201–204
 ion transport inhibition and, 209–212
 monooxygenase metabolites of arachidonic acid, 201–204
Cytochrome P450-dependent metabolites, 185–191, 675–682
 brain activity and, 201–204
 cardiovascular disease and, 193–196
 renal activity and, 689–692
 see also Arachidonic acid
Cytokines,
 antitumor cytostatic activity and, 879–882
 cartilage destruction and repair, 955–966
 parasitic diabetes and, 975–982

Defibrotide, rabbit renal activity and, 711–714
Dexamethasone (DEX),
 lipocortins (LCT) effects, 291–294
 PLA$_2$ suppression and, 266–267
DI-M-PGE$_2$, T cell formation and, 851–854
Diglyceride kinase (DGK), 281–286
Docosahexaenoic acid (DHA), 233–238
Dual antagonists, 929–937

EDRF (Endothelium Derived Relaxing Factor), 223, 637–643
Eicosanoids,
 after fatty acid modification, 237–240
 in angiogenesis, 623–626
 cell signalling and, 217–224
 critical approach to assays, 295–302
 cyclooxygenase-derived by parasitic nematode, 509–512
 global ischemia and, 749–752
 mechanisms of, 161–163, 577–580
 as mediators and modulators of inflammation, 537–543
 metabolizing enzymes and blood cells, 33–36
 in murine macrophages, 169–172
 PGE$_2$ production and, 249–255
 phospholipase D (PLD), 281–285
 synthesis by attachment, 261–264
 synthesis of and murine macrophages, 169–172
 synthesis by spinal cord astrocytes, 739–742
 tumor cell proliferation and by TxA$_2$ and, 925–928
 see also Arachidonic acid; Leukotrienes
Eicosapentaenoic acid (EPA),
 effects on fatty acids, 233–235
 ingestion effects, 241–244
ELISA, and immunoquantification of thromboxane synthase in human tissues, 307–310
Endometrial cells, progesterone and prostaglandin release, 823–826
Endometrial prostaglandins, 820

SUBJECT INDEX

Endometrial stromal cells, steroidal regulation of arachidonic acid uptake and, 815-818
Endothelial cells,
  fatty acid modification and eicosanoid production, 237-240
  13-HODE synthesis and, 667-670, 909-911
  nitric oxide in porcine cells, 671-674
  PGD_2-induced P31 in, 891-894
  PGH synthase and, 141-144
  tumor cell adhesion, 909-911
Endothelial Derived Relaxation Factor (EDRF), 223, 637-643
Endothelial mediators, 627-635
  Guanidino compounds and, 637-643
  leukotrienes and, 663-666
  in peripheral resistance, 595-597
  see also Leukotrienes
Endothelium-induced bronchoconstriction, 453-456
Enzyme immunoassay,
  critical approach to, 295-301
  lupus patients and aspirin activity, 611-614
Eosinophil activation, parasitic diabetes and, 975-982
Epidermal growth factor, linoleic acid metabolism and, 843-846
Epinephrine, myometrial adenylate cyclase activation and, 812-814
Epithelial Lipoxygenases,
  biochemical characterization of, 37-39
  evidence of selective expression, 37-40
Epoxyeicosatrienoic acids (EET), biosynthesis of, 193-196
Epoxygenase metabolites, role in intracellular signal transduction, 827-830
Epstein Barr virus (EBV), CD23 molecules and, 997-1003
Erythropoietin, phospholipase A_2 activation and, 831-834
Essential thrombocytosis (ET), 883-886
Ethylesters, cyclooxygenase and EPA/DHA, 233-235

Fatty acids,
  bone resorption and, 839-840
  cell signalling process and, 217-224
  EPA and DHA ethylesters and, 233-235
  fish oil and, 229-232
  modification of and eicosanoid production, 237-240
  n-3 supplementation effects, 245-248
  in osteoblasts, 53-58, 639-642
  see also Cyclooxygenase
FCE 22178, glomerular thromboxane synthase regulation and, 707-710
Fetal rat brain, ischemia and eicosanoid metabolism, 749-752
15-HETE,
  description of, 441-444
  storage in human neutrophils, 105-108
Fish oil,
  and prostanoid formation in man, 225-228
  vascular disease and, 229-232
Foa-Kurloff cells, metabolism and, 437-440

Gastric mucosal eicosanoids, effects of protective and damaging substances, 785-788

Gastrointestinal bleeding,
  rosaprostol and, 789-792
  and ulcer healing activity, 793-797
Gastrointestinal system,
  lipoxygenase products in gastric damage and protection, 753-760
Gastrointestinal tract, effects of smoking, 777-779
Ginkgolides, as dual antagonists, 930-932
Global ischemia, eicosanoid metabolism in fetal rat brain, 749-752
Glomerular microcirculation, effects on, 683-688
Glucocorticosteroid (GC) action, 265-271
Glutathione biosynthesis,
  antiproliferative activity modulation and, 887-890
  and cyclopentenone prostaglandins, 859-861
GR32191,
  aspirin and, 603-606
  coronary artery thrombosis and, 599-602
GR63799X, selectivity research, 379-382
Guanidino compounds, and endothelial mediators, 637-643

Heparin, 299-301
Hepatocytes, photoaffinity labeling of leukotrienes, 395-398
Hepoxilin A_3, actions in rat brain, 731-734
Human alveolar macrophages, metabolism in, 445-448
Human cyclooxygenase gene, cloning and characterization of, 61-64
Human endothelial cells, and prostaglandin H synthase, 141-144
Human keratinocytes, LTB_4 formation and, 863-866
Human leukocytes, see Leukocytes
Human myometrial adenylate cyclase activation, 811-814
Human platelet, see Platelet
Human umbilical vein endothelial cells (HUVEC), 149-151
Hydroperoxides, PGH synthase and, 137-140
Hypertension, and pregnancy, 807-810

Iloprost, clinical studies of, 583-589
Immunoassays, see Radioimmunoassays
Immunochemistry, of leukotriene B_4, 387-392
Immunocompetence, stable prostacyclin analogues and, 917-920
Immunoquantification, of thromboxane synthase in human tissues, 307-310
In vivo production,
  of prostaglandins, 125-128
  selective thromboxane synthase inhibition and, 165-168
Indomethacin,
  PGH synthase and, 137-140
  TxA_2 synthesis and, 154
Inflammatory disorders,
  15-HETE storage in human neutrophils and, 105-108
  lupus, 611-614
  PGE_1 and, 948
Interleukin-1, tumor necrosis factor and, 222-223
Internal mammary arteries, 13-HODE synthesis and, 667-670

SUBJECT INDEX

Ion transport inhibition, 209-212
Ionophore A23187, 311-314
  GC action in suppression of PLA_2 and, 265-271
Ischemia,
  acute myocardial ischemia in perfused rabbit heart, 939-942
  CLI (Critical limb ischemia) and iliprost, 583-589
  eicosanoid metabolism after global ischemia, 749-752
  eicosanoid metabolism in fetal rat brain, 749-752
Islet cells, neonatal, 287-290
Isoproterenol (ISO), myometrial adenylate cyclase activation, 812-814
Isotope dilution mass spectrometry, 315-318

6-KetoPGFia, rebound elevation after aspirin withdrawal, 157-160
Kurloff cells, metabolism and, 437-440

Late-phase bronchoconstriction, leukotrienes and, 457-459
Leukemia,
  lipoxygenase and, 883-886
  lipoxygenase inhibition and, 921-924
Leukocytes, purification of 15-Lipoxygenase as evidence of presence of isozymes, 101-104
Leukotoxins,
  bronchoconstriction and, 433-436
  in human respiratory illness, 569-571
Leukotriene A_4, in human endothelial cells, 663-666
Leukotriene A_4 hydrolase,
  B-Lymphocytic cell line *Raji* and, 133-136
  in human cell lines, 41-44
Leukotriene B_4
  biological effects in B lymphocytes, 1005-1011
  biosynthesis of, 387-392, 1005-1011
  and chronic granulomatous disease (CGD), 561-564
  densitization of, 403-405
  in human endothelial cells, 663-666
  ONO-LB-B457, 407-410
  substituted phenylpropionic acids as antagonists, 411-413
Leukotriene C_4,
  cardiac responses in rat isolated hearts, 115
  inhibition of output from rat, 113-116
  inhibition and radioimmunoassay (RIA) of eicosanoids, 114
  microcirculation in ethanol-induced gastric injury, 771-776
  preparation of isolated tissues for study of inhibition, 113-114
  treatment with Ph CL28A and, 115
Leukotriene production, *see* Lipoxin
Leukotriene synthesis, and smoking, 777-779
Leukotriene-antagonist ICI-204, 219, 461-464
Leukotrienes, 173-176, 181-187
  actions and biochemistry, 221
  allergic bronchoconstriction and, 429-432, 461-464
  antagonist effects on bronchial asthma, 465-468
  in B-lymphocytic cell line *Raji*, 133-136
  bone marrow transplant and, 525-528
  bronchoconstriction and, 429-432
  burn toxins and, 569-571
  in cardiac transplant patients, 649-653
  chemotactic deactivity of human leukocytes, 399-401
  inhibitory effects on cell proliferation, 922-923
  late-phase bronchoconstriction and, 457-459
  leukotriene-antagonist ICI-204,219 and, 461-464
LTA_4,
  biosynthesis of LTB_4 and, 1005-1011
  immunochemistry and, 387-392
  Raji cells and, 133-136
LTB_4,
  biosynthesis and biological effects in B lymphocytes, 1005-1011
  chemotactic deactivation, 399-401
  human keratinocytes and, 863-866
  as inflammatory mediator, 565-568
  rat polymorphonuclear leukocytes and, 181-184
LTC_4, 177-179
  eicosanoid output from rat isolated lungs, 114
LTE_4,
  capillary leak syndrome and, 525-528
  metabolism of radioisotopic variants, 177-180
  measurement by immunoassays using acetylcholinesterase as label, 319-322
  murine macrophages and eicosanoid synthesis, 169-172
  peripheral vascular disease (PAD) patients and, 655-657
  photoaffinity labeling, 395-398
  quantification of, 1006
  regulation of production and action by MK-571 and MK-886, 9-20
  skin reactions and, 565-568
Lewis lung carcinoma cells, 895-900
Ligands, structure of, 339-340
Limb of Henle's loop, ion transport inhibition and by P450 metabolites, 209-212
Linoleic acid,
  epidermal growth factor, 843-846
  transformation in leaves of corn, 117-124
Lipid remodeling, 553-555
Lipocortins (LCT), dexamethasone (DEX) and, 291-294
Lipoperidoxidation, in rat pancreas transplantation, 573-576
Lipopolysaccharides (LPS), priming of P3888D1 cells, 250-252
Lipoxins,
  coincubation of GM-CSFrh-primed PMN and platelets, 94
  conversion of leukotriene A_4, 89-92
  formation in human platelets, 97-100
  generation and biological activities of rainbow trout, 557-560
  GM-CSF-primed PMN, 94
  human respiratory epithelium and, 89
  leukotriene production, 96
  platelet-dependent metabolism of LTA_4, 97
  receptor-activated interactions between human platelets and cytokine-primed neutrophils, 93-96
  regulation in rat mesangial cells (MC), 701-706
  release of arachidonic acid in human neutrophils and, 553-555

SUBJECT INDEX

Lipoxygenase activation, interleukin-1 transduction signal and, 517-520
Lipoxygenase inhibition, antiproliferative effects of, 921-924
Lipoxygenase metabolites,
 glomerular microcirculation and, 683-688
 renal activity and, 689-692
Lipoxygenase products, in gastric damage and protection, 753-760
Lipoxygenases,
 in astroglial cell pathways, 743-747
 characterization of promoter of human gene, 1-8
 cloned in eukaryotic and prokaryotic systems, 25-27
 evaluation of inhibitors, 109
 from human leukocytes, 101-104
 immunohistory of epithelial tissue, 39-40
 inhibition and development of hydroxamic acids and hydroxyureas, 109-112
 as inhibitor on antigen-induced mediator release, 457-460
 12-lipoxygenase enzyme and neuromodulator production, 715-721
 in myeloproliferative disorders, 883-886
 pharmacokinetics of, 111-112
 mRNA expressed in rat pancreatic islets, 17-20
LPS priming, 250-254
 inhibitor effects, 252-254
LTA_4,
 biosynthesis of leukotriene B_4, 1005-1011
 immunochemistry and, 387-392
 Raji cells and, 133-136
LTB_4,
 chemotactic deactivation, 399-401
 human keratinocytes and, 863-866
 as inflammatory mediator, 565-568
 rat polymorphonuclear leukocytes and, 181-184
 see also Leukotrienes
LTC_4, 177-179
 eicosanoid output from rat isolated lungs, 114
 see also Leukotrienes
LTE_4,
 capillary leak syndrome and, 525-528
 metabolism of radioisotopic variants, 177-179
 see also Leukotrienes
Lung disease, cancer, 895-900
Lupus, thromboxane (TxA_2) and, 611-614

Manoalide, and PAF receptor mediated production in LPS primed P338D1 macrophage-like cells, 249-255
Marine invertebrates, prostaglandins and, 129-132
Mass spectrometry,
 assay for PGD-M, 315-318
 PAF analysis, 323-326
Mast cells, eicosanoid synthesis by attachment, 261-264
Menopause, treatment of, 799-806
Mesangial cells (MC), lipoxin regulation in rat, 701-706
Metabolism, 181-193
 of alveolar macrophages in human cells, 445-448
 15-HETE and, 441-444
 by Foa-Kurloff cells, 437-440
 glomerular microcirculation and lipoxygenase metabolites, 683-688
 guanidino compounds and endothelial mediators, 637-643
 Lewis lung carcinoma cells and, 895-900
 linoleic acid metabolism and epidermal growth factor, 843-846
 phospholipase A_2 in rat pancreas transplantation, 573-576
 problems of in eicosanoid assay, 295-297
 radioisotopic variants of LTE_4 and, 177-179
 sarcoidosis and arachidonic acid, 445-448
Metastasis,
 lung cancer, 895-900
 prostacyclin analogues and, 902-908
 and stable prostacyclin analogs in mice, 913-916
 stable prostacyclin analogues and modulation of host immunocompetence, 917-920
 tumor cell proliferation by TxA_2 and, 925-928
 see also Cancer; Carcinoma cells; Tumors
MK-571, and asthmatic patients, 11-12
MK-886, as inhibitor in production of leukotrienes, 12-15
Molsidomine, reaction with prostacyclin, 655-657
Murine macrophages, eicosanoid action, 169-172
Murine tumors, Lewis lung carcinoma cells, 895-900
Myeloproliferative disorders, lipoxygenase and, 883-886

N. Gonorrhoeae, Protein 1 studies, 545-550
Naproxen, TxA_2 synthesis and, 154
Neonatal islet cells, phosphatidic acid and, 287-290
Nephrotoxicity, cytochrome P450-dependent metabolites and, 689-692
Neutrophil functions,
 chemoattractants and neutrophil activation and protein 1 of *N. Gonorrhoeae*, 545-550
 and chronic granulomatous disease (CGD), 561-564
 15-HETE storage in human neutrophils, 105-108
 lipoxins in human neutrophils, 553-555
 receptor-activated interactions between human platelets and cytokine-primed neutrophils, 93-96
 and vascular disease, 229-232
Nitric oxide (NO),
 autocrine function in porcine cells, 671-674
 endothelial mediators and, 627-635
Nociception, eicosanoid synthesis and, 739-742
Nocloprost, gastroprotective and ulcer healing activity, 793-797
Norepinephrine (NE), myometrial adenylate cyclase activation and, 812-814
Northern blot analysis, of lipocortin (LCT), 291-294
NSAIDs,
 cartilage destruction and repair, 955-966
 renal function and, 968-972

Ocular tissues, P450 system in, 185-194
ONO-8809, anti-thrombotic effect of, 599-602
ONO-LB-B457, research on, 407-410
Osteoblastic cells,
 calcification, 847-850

cyclooxygenase induction in, 839-842
cyclooxygenase in mouse osteoblastic cells, 53-58
prostaglandins and, 848-849
Ovarian hormones, uterine contractility and, 799-806
Oxygen free radicals, infection and, 222
Oxygenation, of arachidonic acid, 553-555

PAF,
 acute myocardial ischemia in perfused rabbit heart, 939-942
 analysis by mass spectrometry, 323-326
 see also Platelet activating factor
PAF antagonists, development of TCV-309, 943-946
Pain, eicosanoid synthesis and, 739-742
Pancreas,
 PLD in, 287-290
 transplantation and phospholipase A_2, 573-576
Paracetamol, TxA_2 synthesis and, 154-155
Parasitic diabetes, 975-982
Parasitic nematodes, eicosanoids derived from, 509-512
Peripheral resistance, prostaglandins role in, 595-597
Peripheral vascular disease (PAD), 655-657
 fish oil and, 229-232
 see also Vascular disease
Peritoneal cells, dexamethasone (DEX) and, 291-294
PGB_1, reverse phase HPLC profiling and, 311-314
PGD_2,
 cardio- and hemodynamic profile, 591-593
 CLI and iloprost, 583-589
 formation of, 433-436
 intracellular glutathione and, 887-890
 P31 induction, 891-894
 rhinitis and nasal effects of, 449-452
 seminal fluids and, 197-199
 sleep-wake regulation, 723-730
PGD-M, mass spectrometric assay, 315-318
PGE_1,
 adjuvant arthritis and, 950
 analogues and potential therapeutic effects, 972
 antiinflammatory effects, 947-953
 immune complex induced tissue injury, 949
 immune responses, 947-953
 marine lupus and, 950-951
 myometrial adenylate cyclase activation and, 812-814
 regulation of acute inflammatory reactions, 948
PGE_2,
 gastroprotective and ulcer healing activity, 793-797
 PAF receptor mediated production in LPS primed P338D1 macrophage-like cells, 249-255
 role in bone metabolism, 840-841
 synthesis in chick spinal cord, 735-738
 T cell formation and, 851-854
PGF_2 compounds, formation in vivo by non-cyclooxygenase free radical catalyzed mechanism, 125-128
PGF Synthase, see Prostaglandin F Synthase
PGG/H synthase,
 aspirin and heme binding, 77-80
 serum induction and superinduction, 65-68
PGH synthase,
 enzyme evidence, 141-144

hydroperoxides and indomethacin interaction, 137-140
 indomethacin and, 137-140
 properties of trypsin-cleaved, 81-84
 salicylates and, 149-151
PGI_2,
 acute myocardial ischemia in perfused rabbit heart, 939-942
 secrection of, 145-147
 in vivo synthesis and non-steroidal anti-inflammatory drugs, 153-156
PGI_2 synthesis, 153-155
Phosphatidic acid, in signal transduction, 287-290
Phosphatidylinositol, 105-108
Phospholipase A_2,
 activation, 831-834
 purification of, 273-275
 in rat pancreas transplantation, 573-576
 in rat vascular smooth muscle cells, 277-280
 suppression of and GC action, 265-271
Phospholipase D (PLD), 281-288
 in pancreatic islet, 287-290
Photoaffinity labeling, of leukotriene binding, 395-398
Piperidinothieno diazepines, as dual antagonists, 932-935
Piriprost, inhibitory effects of, 921-924
Piroxicam, TxA_2 synthesis and, 154
Plasma, molsidomine reaction with prostacyclin, 655-657
Platelet,
 properties of the purified receptor, 343-344
 purification and characterization of, 339-346
 receptor isolation, 342
 TxA_2 receptor in erythroleukemia cells, 344-345
 see also Ligands
Platelet activating factor (PAF), 221-222
 determination by high resolution mass spectrometry, 327-330
 EPA effects, 233-236
 modulation of activity, 383-386
 during pregnancy, 807-809
 TxA_2 and, 617-620
Platelet-derived growth factor (PDGF),
 eicosapentaenoic acid ingestion and, 241-244
 linoleic acid metabolism and, 843-846
Platelet-derived histamine releasing factor (PDHRF), modulation of platelet aggression, 532-536
Platelets, aggregation chronic granulomatous disease (CGD), 561-564
Polymerase cloning, from blood cells, 33-36
Polymorphonuclear leukocytes (PMNL), 554-556, 1005-1011
 activation of densitization of, 403-405
 chemotactic deactivation, 399-401
 in human endothelial cells, 663-666
 molsidomine reaction with prostacyclin, 655-657
Polyunsaturated fatty acids (PUFA), DHA and, 233-238
Porcine cells,
 autocrine function in, 671-674
 western blot analysis, 21-24
Pregnancy,
 antihormone effects, 802-804
 hypertension and, 807-810

myometrial adenylate cyclase activation during, 811–814
Progesterone, prostaglandin release and, 823–826
Propanolol, effects of, 283–285
Prostacyclin,
  activation and biosynthesis in humans, 607–609
  anaphylactoid purpura and, 645–648
  anti-atherogenic actions, 221
  molsidomine reaction, 655–657
  nitric oxide (NO) and, 627–635
  non-steroidal drug effects, 153–155
  PGI_2 production, 659–662
  secretion of and protein phosphorylation, 145–148
  selective thromboxane synthase inhibition and, 165–168
  tobacco consumption and, 615–618
Prostacyclin analogues,
  antimetastatic action of stable prostacyclin analogs in mice, 913–916
  modulation of host immunocompetence, 917–920
  in vivo tumor model effects, 901–908
Prostaglandin E_2,
  effects on cell-associated interleukin one, 513–515
  modulation of platelet activity by, 383–386
  regulation of tumor expression, 521–524
Prostaglandin E, as a regulator of inflammation, 947
Prostaglandin F Synthase, 85–89
Prostaglandin H_2, characterization through radiodination, 331–337
Prostaglandin H synthase, human endothelial cells and, 141–144
Prostaglandin H synthase gene, elevated in RAS transformed cells, 73–76
Prostaglandin release, progesterone and, 823–826
Prostaglandin synthesis, regulation by differential expression of gene encoding, 69–72
Prostaglandins,
  anti-inflammatory effects, 947–953
  antineoplastic and antiviral activity through heat shock, 867–874
  antitumor cytostatic activity and, 879–882
  bone metabolism and, 840–841
  calcium ions in suppression of PLA_2, 265–271
  cancer patient survival and, 875–878
  cartilage destruction and repair, 955–956
  in chick spinal cord, 735–738
  Critical limb ischemia (CLI), 583–589
  endometrial, 820
  excessive prostaglandin E_2 synthesis, 835–838
  formation of PGD_2, 433–436
  human uterine contractility and, 799–806
  immune responses, 947–953
  in vivo production, 125–128
  induction of heat shock protein synthesis and, 867–874
  inflammatory regulation, 948
  intracellular glutathione and, 887–890
  in LPS primed P338D1 macrophage-like cells, 249–255
  lupus and, 950–951
  marine invertebrates and, 129–132
  myometrial adenylate cyclase activation and, 811–814
  and non-steroidal anti-inflammatory drugs, 153–156
  nsaid-induced renal dysfunction and, 967–974
  osteoblastic cell calcification and, 847–850
  P31 induction in PGD_2-treated endothelial cells, 891–894
  PGD-M mass spectrometric assay, 315–318
  PGG/H synthase, 65–68, 77–84, 137–151
  PGH synthase and indomethacin, 137–140
  PGI_2, secretion, 145–147
  regulation of acute inflammatory reactions, 949–950
  reverse phase HPLC profiling and, 311–314
  rhinitis and, 449–452
  role in kidney, 967–968
  scintillation proximity assays, 303–306
  seminal fluids and, 197–199
  sleep-wake regulation, 723–730
  steroidal regulation of arachidonic acid uptake and, 815–818
  T cell formation and, 851–854
  therapeutic effects of PGE_1 analogues, 972
  tissue injury and, 949
  see also specific prostaglandins by name
Prostanoids,
  endogenous, 761–765
  formation of and dietary fish, 225–228
  GR63799X selectivity research, 379–382
Protein kinase C (PKC), 265–268, 545–547
Protein phosphorylation,
  N. Gonorrhoeae, 545–550
  prostacyclin secretion and, 145–148
Protein synthesis, dexamethasone (DEX) and, 291–294

Rabbit renal cortex, purification of PLA_2 and, 273–275
Radioimmunoassays,
  critical approach to, 295–301
  of leukotrienes using acetylcholinesterase as label, 319–322
  metabolism of radioisotopic variants, 177–180
  scintillation proximity assays, 303–306
Raji cells, leukotrienes in, 133–136
Rat brain,
  eicosanoid metabolism after global ischemia, 749–752
  hepoxilins and, 731–734
  P-450 activity and, 201–204
  see also Central nervous system
Rat mesangial cells, lipoxins in, 701–706
Rat peritoneal macrophages, calcium ion effects, 257–260
Rat vascular smooth muscle cells, PLA_2 activation, 277–280
Renal activity, 177–179
  aspirin withdrawal effects, 157–159
  cytochrome P450-dependent metabolites and, 689–692
  defibrotide and, 711–714
  FCE 22178 and glomerular thromboxane synthase regulation, 707–710
  high urinary TxB_2, 525–528
  vasoconstriction with thromboxane mimetic, 693–699
  see also Urinary metabolites

SUBJECT INDEX

Respiratory illness,
  acute lung injury and arachidonic acid metabolites, 421-428
  asthma, 11-12, 415-418, 433-436, 457-459, 465-468
  endothelin-induced, 453-456
  leukotoxins and, 569-571
  leukotriene antagonist effects on bronchial asthma, 465-468
  Lewis lung carcinoma cells, 895-900
  lipoxygenase inhibitors and, 457-460
  lung cancer, 895-900
  PGD$_2$ formation and bronchoconstriction, 433-436
  rhinitis, 449-452
  see also Asthma; Bronchoconstriction
Rhinitis, PGD$_2$ effects, 449-452
Rosaprostol, effects on aspirin-induced gastrointestinal bleeding, 789-792
RPMI 1640 culture, LCTs and, 291-295

Salicylates, inhibition of de novo synthesis by, 149-151
Sarcoidosis, and arachidonic acid, 445-448
Scintillation proximity assays, 303-306
Seminal fluids, arachidonic acid and, 197-200
Signal transduction,
  in P338D1 cells, 254
  phosphatidic acid and, 287-290
Skin,
  leukotrienes and burn toxins, 569-571
  LTB$_4$ as inflammatory mediator, 565-568
Sleep-wake regulation, PGD$_2$ and, 723-730
Spinal cord astrocytes, eicosanoid synthesis and, 739-742
Steroidal regulation, of arachidonic acid uptake, 815-818
Steroids, uterine contractility and, 799-806
Substituted phenylpropionic acids, as antagonists, 411-413
Sulphidopeptide leukotrienes, in asthma, 415-418
Superoxide dismutase (SOD), 301
Superoxide formation, and chronic granulomatous disease (CGD), 561-564

TCV-309, as potent PAF antagonist, 943-946
13-HODE synthesis,
  cardiovascular surgery and, 667-670
  and tumor cell adhesion, 909-911
Thromboembolism, arachidonic acid induced, 355-358
Thromboxane, cell signalling process and, 221
Thromboxane B$_2$, rebound elevation after aspirin withdrawal, 157-160
Thromboxane receptor antagonists (TxRa's),
  pathological states and, 353-354
  platelet activation, 353
  prolonged action in man, 351-354
  prolonged inhibitions of responses to platelets and, 353-354
  renal vasoconstriction effects, 157-159, 693-699
Thromboxane synthesis,
  and aspirin, 153-154
  immunoquantification of in human tissues, 307-310
  and indomethacin, 154
  and naproxen, 154

  and paracetamol, 154-155
  and piroxicam, 154
  and smoking, 777-779
Thromboxane synthesis inhibitors (TSi's),
  FCE 22178 and, 707-710
  mechanism-based inactivation of, 161-163
  renal vasoconstriction effects, 693-699
  selective inhibition studies, 165-168
  see also Thromboxane (TxA$_2$)
Thromboxane (TxA$_2$), 599-602
  activation and biosynthesis in humans, 607-609
  anaphylactoid purpura and, 645-648
  aspirin and, 157-159, 603-606
  in cardiac transplant patients, 649-652
  characterization through radiodination, 331-337
  FCE 22178 and glomerular thromboxane synthase regulation, 707-710
  increased formation and antiphospholipid syndrome, 529-532
  ligands for TxA$_2$ receptor, 339
  lupus patients and, 611-614
  non-steroidal drug effects, 153-155
  platelet activation and, 617-620
  role in platelet aggregation, 339
  tobacco consumption and, 615-618
  tumor cell proliferation and, 925-928
  use in treatment of ischemia, thromboembolic and respiratory diseases, 355
  in vivo synthesis and non-steroidal anti-inflammatory drugs, 153-156
Thromboxane (TxB$_2$), capillary leak syndrome and, 525-528
Tissue content, of thromboxane synthase, 309
Tobacco consumption, TxA$_2$ secretion and, 615-618
Tumors,
  antimetastatic action of stable prostacyclin analogs in mice, 913-916
  cell proliferation by TXA$_2$ and, 925-928
  host immunocompetence and, 917-920
  interleukin-1 and, 222-223
  Lewis lung carcinoma cells, 895-900
  prostacyclin analogues and, 901-908
  13-HODE synthesis and tumor cell adhesion, 909-911

U-937 cells, LCTs and, 291-295
Ulcer, Nocloprost and healing activity, 793-797
Urinary metabolites, LTE$_4$ radioisotopic variants and, 177-179
Uterine contractility, and prostaglandins, 799-806

Vascular disease, fish oils' effects on, 229-232
Vascular smooth muscle cells, PLA$_2$ activation, 277-280
Vasoactive peptide mediators, gastric damage and, 761-765
Vasoconstriction, with thromboxane mimetic, 693-699

Western blot analysis,
  of arachidonate 5-lipoxygenase of porcine leukocytes, 21-24
  of lipocortin (LCT), 291-294

Zymosan, 311-314

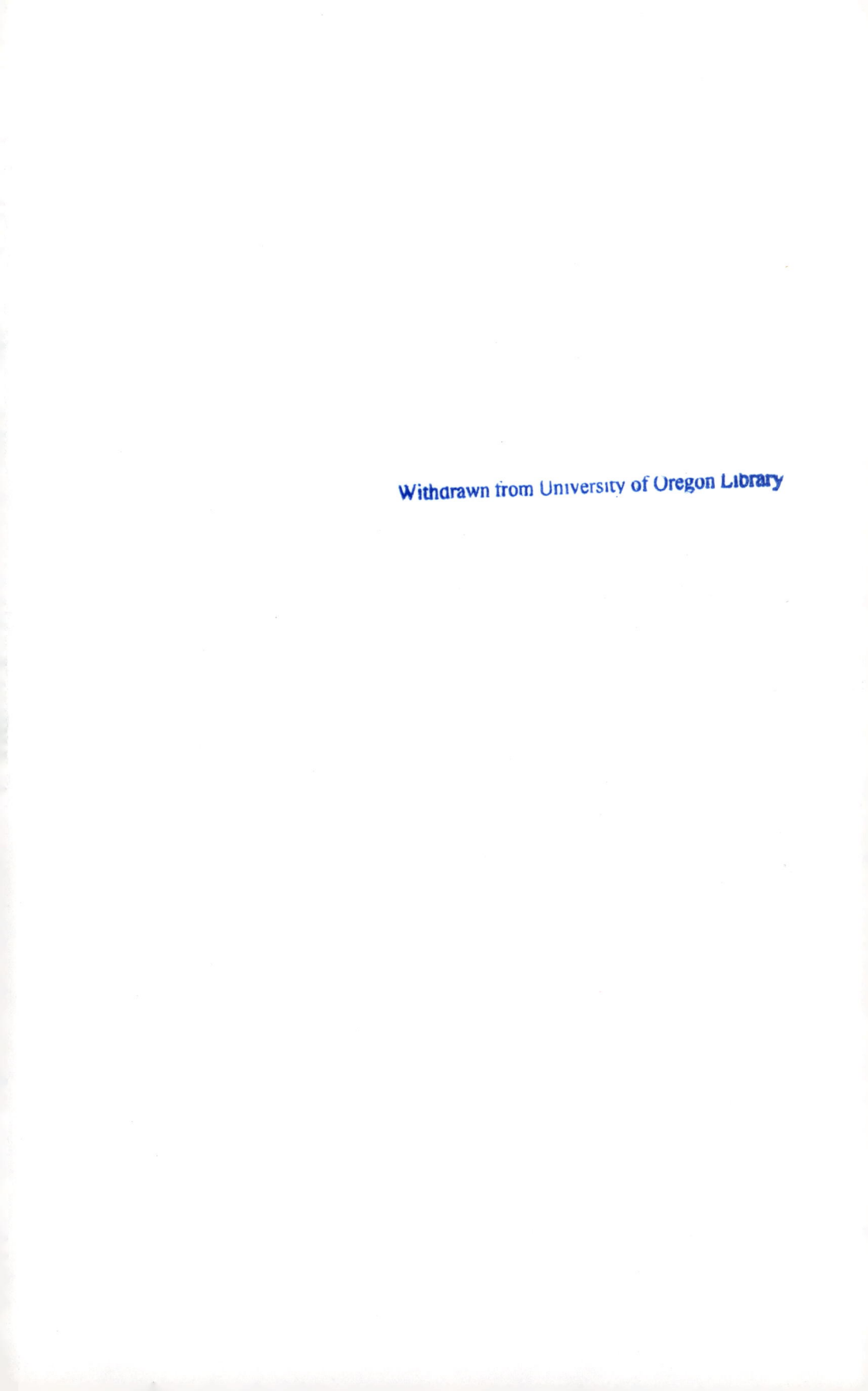